OTHER TITLES OF INTEREST FROM GR/ST. LUCIE PRESS

Ecological Validity of Neuropsychological Testing

Detecting Malingering and Deception: Forensic Distortion Analysis (FDA)

Disorders of Executive Functions: Civil and Criminal Law Applications

Neuropsychology for the Attorney

Diagnosing and Treating Aphasia: Alexander Luria's System Approach to Brain-Behavior Relationships (Video)

The Neuropsychological Analysis of Problem Solving

Principles and Practices of Disability Management in Industry

Neurobehavioral Assessment Format (NAF): A Manual for the Clinical Assessment of Patients with Neurologically Related Disorders

Head Injury and the Family: A Life and Living Perspective

The Disability Evaluation: Practical Guide for Physicians

Traumatic Brain Injury Rehabilitation Training Consortium Monograph Series

Traumatic Brain Injury Rehabilitation Training Consortium Video

For more information about these titles call, fax or write:

GR/St. Lucie Press
100 E. Linton Blvd., Suite 403B
Delray Beach, FL 33483

TEL (561) 274-9906 • FAX (561) 274-9927
E-MAIL information@slpress.com
WEB SITE http://www.slpress.com

D1480276

Neuropsychological Rehabilitation

Fundamentals, Innovations and Directions

Neuropsychological Rehabilitation

Fundamentals, Innovations and Directions

Edited by José León-Carrión

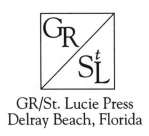

GR/St. Lucie Press
Delray Beach, Florida

Printed and bound in the U.S.A. Printed on acid-free paper.
10 9 8 7 6 5 4 3 2 1

ISBN 1-57444-039-X

Phone: (561) 274-9906
Fax: (561) 274-9927
E-mail: information@slpress.com
Web Site: http://www.slpress.com

Published by
GR/St. Lucie Press
100 E. Linton Blvd., Suite 403B
Delray Beach, FL 33483

Dedicated to
my wife, María del Rosario,
and to my sons,
Umberto and Román,
with love.

José León-Carrión

Irreversibility is an illusion, a subjective impression, the product of exceptional initial conditions.

—Albert Einstein

Each solution of a problem creates new unresolved problems. The more difficult the original problem and more daring the attempt to resolve it is, the more interesting will be these new problems.

—Karl Popper

TABLE OF CONTENTS

PART III: REHABILITATION OF NEUROCOGNITIVE PROCESSES

FOREWORD

As President and Chief Executive Officer of the Brain Injury Association, and as President of the International Brain Injury Association, I frequently get asked to write a foreword or introduction for a book about brain injury. I generally decline because the book is not up to speed nor does it fill a need.

When I was asked to write the foreword for *Neuropsychological Rehabilitation: Fundamentals, Innovations and Directions* being edited by Professor José León-Carrión, I gave a reluctant "yes" depending upon the content and authors.

After reviewing the content and reading the chapters, I can now give an enthusiastic "two thumbs up." Professor León-Carrión has assembled a world class group of authors. He has organized the material to flow from the historical review of neuropsychological rehabilitation to cutting edge information on innovative treatment and emerging issues in neurorehabilitation of persons with brain injury. This is a very comprehensive book that covers every possible concern about brain injury. For the physician, there are chapters on neuroimaging, gene therapy, sleep disorders, post-traumatic epilepsy, and neuropharmacological treatment. For the therapist, case manager, or interested family member, there are chapters that explain self-awareness, children's issues, behavior problems following brain injury, education, the design of neuropsychological rehabilitation programs, evaluation of programs, and models for rehabilitation of persons with brain injury.

Overall, this is a serious attempt to organize a comprehensive review of neurorehabilitation of persons with brain injury. The authors come from different cultural backgrounds, giving the book an international perspective not always found in books about brain injury, which is very needed as the brain injury movement spreads around the globe. The International Brain Injury Association will be able to utilize this book worldwide.

Neuropsychological Rehabilitation: Fundamentals, Innovations and Directions is a very useful book and a welcome contribution to the field.

George A. Zitnay, Ph.D.
Brain Injury Association
Washington, DC

PREFACE

Neuropsychological Rehabilitation: Fundamentals, Innovations and Directions has been conceived as an instrument for all professionals concerned with the treatment and return to community of those citizens who have had a traumatic brain injury. Two central ideas form the foundation of this book. The first is that scientific intervention (treatment) can be successful. The second is that neuropsychologists must be open to theoretical and technological advances and not necessarily fixated from the start on the idea of reversibility.

As part of the first principle, neuropsychologists must have confidence and assurance, knowing the process that they are going to use will be successful. In the same way, neuropsychologists must be satisfied that the instruments and techniques they are using will be helpful. If they have doubts about their capacity and their rehabilitation techniques, they may fail. Neuropsychologists must be imaginative and must be boldly prudent in the use of all their knowledge and techniques in order to serve rehabilitation successfully. There are, undoubtedly, many possible ways of achieving neuropsychological rehabilitation.

This success is, in my opinion, closely related to the objectives pursued when planning the neuropsychological rehabilitative course for a patient. As Einstein said, "Irreversibility is an illusion, a subjective impression, the product of the initial exceptional conditions." All is possible; it is only a question of relativity. Likewise, we have to consider that in neuropsychological rehabilitation, the pursuit of neuropsychological functioning reversibility can be an illusion. Therefore, we have to adapt rehabilitation procedures and goals to the new cerebral conditions that are exceptional, too. The neuropsychologist is searching for the new neuropsychological coherence of the patient according to his/her new brain condition. In others words, when the neuropsychologist and the family are trying to restore the patient to who he/she was before the injury, their objective can be no more than an illusion. The cerebral conditions, emotional and affective aspects, and the experience and social skills of the patient before the brain injury were exceptional and unique; the new conditions of the patient after the brain injury are also exceptional and unique but different, with a high level of plasticity. Thus, neuropsychological rehabilitation must pursue the construction of a new personal reality and new neurocognitive functioning, starting with the patient's new conditions. In fact, there is no limit to how far a patient may go. No one is the same after a traumatic accident, even when there is no brain injury; therefore, it is less likely someone will be the same after a severe and direct accident to the brain.

Nothing in brain injury rehabilitation is reversible or irreversible; it all depends on the goals of the rehabilitation. Through neuropsychological rehabilitation, the outcome can be a new combination of traits that make up the person, possibly with some better adaptability and social functioning than before and probably with the same basic characteristics as before. We cannot forget that, in nature, some amount of change is predictable. Because rehabilitation tries to achieve a new neuropsychological understanding (coherence) of the patient, the person's initial psychological condition should not become an objective. Instead, a new direction, where neurocognitive entropy after a brain injury takes precedence, should become the goal of rehabilitation.

This book deals with these principles as a whole to offer the professional a framework of realistic information necessary in order to begin the successful treatment of patients with brain injury.

In planing neuropsychological rehabilitation, the neuropsychologist must know comprehensively the fundamentals of this discipline. In order to set a plan of action, neuropsychologists must know the context in which they are going to develop the neuropsychological program of treatment. The history and the culture of each nation or state, in terms of healthcare, will considerably affect the type of treatment that can be offered. For example, a treatment plan in a European country with a national healthcare system will differ from the plan in a country where healthcare is privatized. In the first case, treatment is usually paid for by the government, and, therefore, techniques, procedures, and professionals available are limited by funding and budgets. In the second case, resources will depend on the income level of the patient.

In addition, neuropsychological rehabilitation can be planned using different models. Neuropsychologists must be clear about which model they are using. There are models centered on the patient and models centered on the illness; each one suggests different strategies, methods, procedures, and needs. Likewise, the role played by neuropsychological and neuroimaging assessment is fundamental in order to choose the rehabilitation model. Neuropsychologists and the directors of the centers where they work must, in a like manner, know the efficiency of the treatments that they apply and have the appropriate techniques to evaluate the rehabilitation program. All these elements are reviewed in the first part of this book.

The second part of the book offers chapters focused on different types of treatments that can be applied simultaneous with or in the absence of neuropsychological rehabilitation. These chapters cover the role of the neuropsychologist in intensive care, during coma or persistent vegetative state, in gene therapy, in neural transplants, etc. Neuropharmacological treatment following brain injury, the problems that arise in treating post-traumatic epilepsy, and the rehabilitation of sleeping disorders are also considered. Good and effective neuropsychological rehabilitation cannot be developed if it is not started before or developed simultaneously with a physical rehabilitation program. It is important to realize that neuropsychologists have and can develop a role throughout the treatment continuum.

The third part of this book focuses on rehabilitation of the different cognitive processes that can be affected by a brain injury. All are of special interest because, for so long, it was believed that the only way to manage these limitations was through compensation, especially in organic memory deficit and post-traumatic aphasia.

The fourth part of this book discusses frequently overlooked topics having to do with the *treatment* of patients with brain injury. Personality disorders, affective disorders, suicide attempts, and violent behavior are aspects that neuropsychologists have to treat with their best tools, knowledge, and touch. Because the ultimate goal of rehabilitation is a return to society, a number of chapters are dedicated to training for social skills and rehabilitation for employment, leisure activities, and community inclusion.

Finally, the book considers special topics such as brain injury in children and the problems of returning to school. In the United States, TBI is the largest killer and disabler of children, thus impacting one's lifelong experience. Teachers, parents, and neuropsychologists have to understand specific models and strategies to respond to these students' educational, family, and social needs. The book also considers patients with special needs, for example, the growing Hispanic population in the United States. Of great interest to a variety of medical practitioners will be the concluding chapter on the economic and legal aspects of neuropsychological rehabilitation.

ACKNOWLEDGMENTS

My thanks and appreciation to:

- The Brain Injury Association, especially to Dr. George Zitnay, for its support and efforts in helping the cause of people with brain injury.
- The International Brain Injury Association (IBIA), of which I am proud to be a member. We share the visions of a better quality of life and a higher human dignity for all people who have sustained a brain injury, wherever they are.
- Professor Helio Carpintero and Professor M. Victoria del Barrio, for their support and friendship through the years.
- Daniel Garcia Contreras, Director of the Instituto Universitario de Sevilla (for American students), for his help in English translation.
- All my colleagues and friends from the Traumatological Hospital, "Virgen del Rocio," for the cooperation and collaboration we have maintained over the years.
- My patients, from whom I learn a great deal.
- My students and collaborators. They suffer with me and encourage me with their questions and interests. Without them, this work would be more difficult.

José León-Carrión
Facultad de Psicología
Universidad de Seville

ABOUT THE EDITOR

José León-Carrión, Ph.D., is head of the Human Cognitive Neuropsychology Laboratory and professor of neuropsychology at the University of Seville in Spain. He is also director of the Postgraduate Program in Neuropsychology at the University of Seville. Dr. León-Carrión is vice president of the Brain Injury Association of Spain and vice president of the International Brain Injury Association. He has published numerous articles in international journals and is the author of *Manual of Human Neuropsychology*. He holds membership in the International Neuropsychological Society, European Brain Injury Society, and European Association of Psychological Assessment.

PART I:

FUNDAMENTALS

A Historical View of Neuropsychological Rehabilitation: The Search for Human Dignity

José León-Carrión

Facultad de Psicología
Universidad de Seville, Seville, Spain

INTRODUCTION

The history of neuropsychological rehabilitation is closely linked to the advances made in the study of the brain and to the concerns with human dignity. In the following pages, we will see how these two factors have played a central role in the creation of the centers where the neuropsychological consequences of brain damage could be treated. Not having the scientific and technical means to tackle the sequela of brain lesions has been linked to the scientific and pseudo-scientific beliefs on the subject. The story is exciting because the brain has not always been considered an organ having the same functions. Nor have, of course, social life and health aspects always been approached in the same manner. Naturally, the treatment of what we now call neuropsychological sequela was a luxury during times when basic survival was difficult and feeding oneself was complicated. Too many factors influenced treatment, and too many events have taken place until the present time. Now in the developed nations, fortunately, technical knowledge and social, economic, and administrative sensitivity coincide so that any citizen may make use of the results of a discipline such as neuropsychological rehabilitation, which, although in its early stages of development, shows promise and progress in its body of knowledge and in its implementation approaches. Extremely important socially dynamic and structural changes and scientifically abundant events have taken place that have led to the current conception of the brain. These transformations did not take place suddenly but rather over time—day by day, period by period—going beyond individuals and concrete facts to shape the body of knowledge about the brain that we now have.

Nevertheless, there are social developments and individual achievements that have marked the milestones leading us to an overview of the conception of the brain throughout the evolution of humanity (León-Carrión, 1995).

In shaping the story of the treatment of brain lesions, one can generally say that there is a ladder with many steps, which has been leading to different rooms. Many concepts have remained in these rooms for centuries; some have remained for long stays while others have had short stays. The first steps and rooms in the shaping of neuropsychology were related to the polemic about two organs that competed as the seat of the soul: the heart and the brain. The next polemic, once it was established that it the brain that was the organ that interprets conscience, places itself in two opposing positions: localizationism vs. antilocalizationism. On one side were those who maintained that the brain was a heterogenous mass in which parts with different functions could be indicated, and on the other were those who maintained that the brain was a homogenous mass, all of it equivalent, and that it was not possible to identify any parts with any functional assignment.

From the earliest times of human history, the treatment given to people who had suffered some type of accident with physical lesions, especially with brain lesions, has been varied. All cultures have not treated these persons in the same manner, nor have they done so consistently or even consistently within the same geographical zones. Among primitive peoples, those children who exhibited some sort of deformity were either allowed to die or were put to death; the adults with lesions who developed physical or psychic deficits were separated from the group and were considered persons of no consequence either socially or in a family context. Of course, at that time this did not constitute a social problem; separating someone from the group was considered normal. However, the majority of them, because of their precarious state of health and the harsh living conditions that they had to face, died at a very early age.

THE EARLY STAGES: PRE-RATIONAL ANTECEDENTS AND THE WORLD OF MAGIC

The oldest known data about the treatment of problems related to brain damage date back to over 12,000 years ago during the Mesolithic Age. Skulls with oval 16–18 mm diameter trephinations on their left side have been found by the Dnieper River. Surprisingly, these patients seem to have survived "surgical" interventions, since the holes that had been made in the bone appear healed with the presence of new bone tissue. Similarly, it was the norm and not the exception in the skulls found that these trephinations performed in the skulls healed (Haeger, 1988, p. 12).

If we move on to ancient Egypt, papyrus documents have been found in which reference is made to persons with disabilities and deformities and about the type of treatment given to skull fractures and to the relation of the brain and/or spinal lesions and their paralysis. In the bas-reliefs found in some pharaohs' tombs, figures with physical injuries appear. Some mummies have been found with splints and other devices used for the treatment of physical trauma. For instance, there is a bas-relief of the Eighteenth Dynasty in which a prince appears with his lower right extremity atrophied, exhibiting a talipes equinus probably due to poliomyelitis. The prince carries a type of crutch that indicates he experienced motor difficulties. The most famous case of a head injury is that of Seqenere Tao, a king of the Seventeenth Dynasty (Figure 1.1), who took part in the war to rid his country of its foreign rulers, the Hyksos (Filer, 1995).

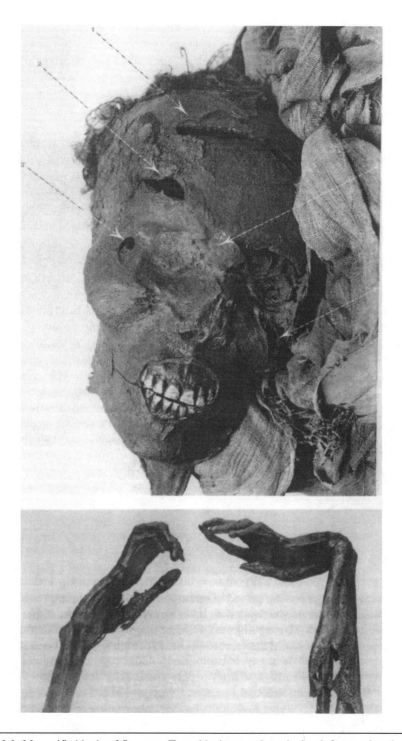

Figure 1.1: Mummified body of Sequenre Tao with six wounds to the head, face, and neck, made by weapons used by the Hyksos and inflicted on the battlefield, which resulted in his dealth. X-ray analysis shows that the bone around one of these wounds to the forehead had partially re-grown, indicating that this injury was sustained months ago and probably caused paralysis in one of his arms (see Filer, 1995). (From G.E. Smith. *The Royal Mummies* [Catalogue Géneral du Musée dú Caire], Cairo 1912, plates I and II.)

However, although the Egyptians earned well deserved fame as embalmers, they did not have good knowledge about the human body nor about its functioning. For a long time the Egyptians believed that any internal disorder of the human body was due to the effects of some supernatural agent—the gods, the dead—that entered the body of the individual and took possession of it. Therefore, the rehabilitation "techniques" and "treatment" also had to be supernatural. Those that knew most about these problems were the magicians and sorcerers who worked with enchantment formulas, ointments, and potions. Because the ointments gradually took on a greater importance than the enchantments, physicians were born. But the latter were hesitant to treat those disorders for which they did not have remedies and referred the more difficult patients to the sorcerers. The physicians and the magicians lived in harmony together. Nevertheless, Egyptian medicine developed a great reputation throughout the entire Orient.

The Egyptians knew relatively little about the internal functioning of the human body, and their notions of the brain were limited, although they did have quite a bit of knowledge about the face, skull, hair, etc. It has been described that when some of the pharaohs with skull deformities (Figure 1.2) from difficulties at birth suffered more or less severe epileptic attacks, these attacks were interpreted as a special form of communication with the gods. With others, skull trephinations were performed to draw out the bad humors and the demons that might be lodged in the body. The procedure was likely to have been used either to treat head injuries (relieving pressure) or for magical practice.

In the Smith papyrus of the Eighteenth Dynasty exists one of the first, if not the first, descriptions of the treatment of brain trauma. In this papyrus there is a description of ten cases. The surgeon makes a distinction between superficial injuries (i.e., those that did not fracture the bone) and those that perforated it. In the first case, the surgeon feels very secure and confident that he will be able to treat the injury and heal the wound. He would use only a bandage of fresh meat, a compress soaked in fat and honey, which he would

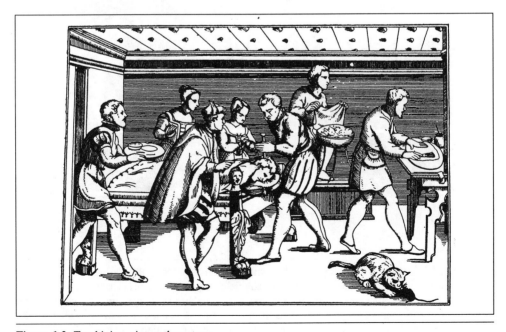

Figure 1.2: Trephining, sixteenth century.

place over the injury, whose edges he would have previously joined with two ribbons. When the injury was deep, the surgeon had doubts about his success but went ahead with the treatment, focusing his efforts especially on preventing movement of the skull. To achieve this, he would place the patient in a seated position, secured by two brick supports that prevented him from moving. Those patients who survived were treated with oil unctions on the head, neck, and back. With this type of treatment, the majority of patients probably died, and with those who did manage to survive, we have no idea of what sequelae they suffered.

It is interesting to analyze part of the contents of this papyrus found by Edwin Smith that describes 48 cases of surgery, with information on the different types of brain lesions.[1]

> *If you visit a man with a deep head wound, you must touch it, even if the injured person trembles terribly. Ask him to raise his head and notice if it hurts to open his mouth and if his heart beats weakly.*

> *Notice also if he has saliva around his mouth and if it drips or not, and if he bleeds through the nose and ears, and if his neck is rigid and he cannot move his head and cannot look at his shoulders and chest.*

> *You must look at him and say: "He who has a deep wound in the head, with injury up to the bone of the skull, clenches his teeth and bleeds through the nose and ears, and suffers neck rigidity, I will free of his torment."*

> *As soon as you see him clench his jaws spasmodically, apply heat to him so that he will feel better and can open his mouth. Keep it open with the help of the threads, fat and honey, until the crisis reaches a climax.*

> *If later on you notice that the patient has fever as a result of the skull injury, place your hands on him. If then you notice that his forehead is damp with sweat, that the neck tendons are tense, his face is red, that his breath smells like sheep urine, that his mouth is closed, his eyebrows are distended and he looks like he has cried, you must look at him and tell him: "He who suffers from a deep wound to his head which reaches his skull, cannot open his mouth and has a rigid neck, will be incurable."*

> *But you notice that this man has become pale and shows signs of exhaustion.*

> *You must keep his mouth open with a piece of wood wrapped in cloth and give him fruit juice. He must sit upright between the brick supports, until the symptoms subside.*

It seems that it was with Greek medicine that we have, for the first time in antiquity, a concern for the well-being of the citizens. This becomes manifest through the "Hippocratic collection."[2] In it, dietetic, hygienic, and gymnastic advice and method is valued over speculation. The Hippocrats had a fundamentally enlightened religious ethic, and therefore, their therapeutic resources were based on the divine condition of the *physis*. The economic relation between the Greek *asclepius* (physician) and his patient followed certain rules. The first one was that the physician had to think about his art above all and about how to heal the patient; therefore, he must not think about the wages he was going to receive for his work. His goal was to heal and learn from what nature could teach him. The second rule was that at the moment of setting his fee, he had to take into consideration the economic situation of the patient and set his fees accordingly, but without abuse or inhumanity. Finally, sometimes the physician could render his services without charging a fee because he wanted fame (especially with foreign patients), or because he was paying back favors received previously, or because he had a love for his profession and patients (Laín-Entralgo, 1969).

For the Hippocratic school, the brain is an important organ because it governs intelligence and regulates the majority of body functions. But it is in the work *The Sacred Disease*[3] where one can read the best discussion in antiquity on brain functions, noting that epileptic patients have been studied in depth. Hippocrates did not consider epilepsy a sacred illness but believed it had natural causes. He believed that men considered it sacred out of ignorance about its symptoms and its causes, even though a very exhaustive description of the epileptic syndrome existed. The Hippocratic physicians define the epileptic symptomatology as the patient feeling an aura and a feeling of premonition, followed by the attack which, when sensed by the patient, causes him to go to a removed location in order to lie down. The attack would start with a cry or another sound made by the patient. Afterwards, he would gnash his teeth, foam at the mouth, and kick his legs. His intelligence would darken, and he would suffer convulsions in one part of his body; he might expel excrements and after a while, he should recover. The psychological causes of epilepsy, according to the Hippocratic school, were the patients' fears, but its physiological causes could be found in the brain. It will be the inferior vena cava and the one coming from the spleen of the aorta, when the air passages were obstructed, that were cited as causes of epilepsy.

For the Hippocratic physicians, the brain was the organ from which we felt joy and fear, from where we think, see, and hear, and from where we are capable of distinguishing beauty from ugliness, good from bad, and that which is pleasant from that which is not. The Hippocratic physicians also recommended the use of trephination for the treatment of mild brain injuries.

This was the scientific climate that existed in Greece. In Athens during the age of Pericles (499–429 B.C.), there was a great splendor in the Helenistic civilization. It was then that patients with physical lesions began to be treated. Several types of hospitals were founded, as well as convalescence homes, in places that were beneficial because of their climate and their waters. In the face of this, individuals with congenital deformities in Greece, especially in Sparta, were considered unnatural and were excluded from society. Children born with deformities were displayed in public places. For a period of time it was decreed that children with any type of deformity be thrown off of Mount Taigeto. Mental diseases were not excluded from these religious rites, much less those ailments that came about during the course of life, especially those caused by wars. Those suffering from the latter had a right to receive compensation since they were different from other ailments that were considered of divine origin (Bellet, 1990; Ruano, 1993).

We must stress that from the point of view of therapy, in Athens the assistance was not the same for slaves as it was for freemen. According to Plato,[4] there were three aspects that made the difference. First, slaves were not seen by Asclepiads or by physicians well versed in the medical arts of the medical schools but instead by physicians' helpers who had no better association than that of having been close to their master, normally as a slave, to serve him and help him. From this proximity they had learned some external routines about healing. Second, medicine for slaves was something akin to "veterinary science for men." With this approach to the treatment of illnesses, communications between physician and patient were kept down to the indispensable. Finally, treatment was not individualized; instead, general healing criteria were applied. The only discrimination was quantitative (i.e., it was directed either toward a child or toward an adult, toward a large person or toward a small one).

However, when the patient was a freeman and wealthy, the type of therapy changed considerably, and the treatment and diagnosis of the patient was individualized. The Asclepiads used the following therapeutic resources. First, the physician would instruct the patient and those close to him about the illness without giving them a lecture because his mission was not to make a physician out of his patient. Second, he used verbal persuasion, and he would not prescribe anything to the patient until he had convinced him about the efficacy of the treatment to cure the illness. Finally, the Greek physicians made use of the biographical adequacy of the treatment (i.e., the treatment had to adjust itself to the biography of the patient and to the temporal course of the ailment while observing the suitability of the medical intervention) (Laín-Entralgo, 1969, pp. 30–31).

In imperial Rome, citizens had the right to take the life of those children who were born with any type of physical lesion if, once shown to five neighbors, the latter gave their consent. This right to life and death was later broadened even more to the point that a father could deprive of life his child with lesions after its birth without the consent of anyone. Nevertheless, the practice of infanticide was not common in Rome except during times of corruption and decadence, although in these times deformed or invalid children were abandoned or thrown into the Tiber River in flower baskets. It was also common practice in Rome to use injured children as beggars for profit. Similarly, there was widespread sale of children with these problems, which naturally worsened their physical conditions (Ruano, 1993).

It was not until Galen in the second century B.C., one of the first authors of antiquity, that we find the first writings about brain damage and brain functions. His great surgical experience was obtained while he was the official physician of the school of gladiators of Pergamum and from his experiments of anatomical dissection with monkeys. These activities placed him in an outstanding position, such was his knowledge of the anatomy of the nervous system and of brain trauma. His writings on the spinal cord and on the brain and spinal nerves, in which he associated certain types of lesions to the paralysis of certain parts of the body, are famous. For him, an injury in the anterior parts of the brain interfered with the sensory perception registry, posterior injuries caused disorders in the memory, and those of the "ventriculus medius" caused problems in reasoning. For Galen, it was necessary and unavoidable to perform a detailed clinical examination of all patients, noting and detailing all symptoms and setting up a hierarchy of them so that later a diagnostic judgement could be issued and the necessary technique could be proposed (Figure 1.3).

Galen's concepts on the nervous system, which come from his research, are important. He located and distributed seven cranial pairs (he lacked the olfactory and pathetic nerves), and he failed in the anatomy of the "nervus trigeminus." He located the recurrent, rachidian, and cervical nerves; the nervous ganglions; and part of the sympathetic system. In his biological theory, psychic life (psychic pneuma) has its seat in the brain and runs through the nervous system, with the cerebral ventricles responsible for the psychological processes. According to him, the blood that is carried through the arteries to the brain is transformed into the psychic pneuma, which later will be distributed through the nerves.

Consequently, before the Middle Ages and with these concepts, the "centers" of rehabilitation, treatment, and clinical learning are heterogenous, although there were different theoretical schools and schools of learning both in the Greek and in the Roman world. However, hospitals appeared only with the advent of Christianity during the reign of the Emperor Constantine, and they multiplied during the Middle Ages. In reality these

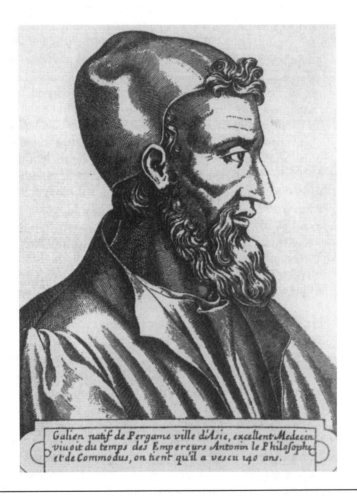

Galien natif de Pergame ville d'Asie, excellent Medecin viuoit du temps des Empereurs Antonin le Philosophe et de Commodus, on tient qu'il a vescu 140 ans.

Figure 1.3: Figure of Galen from the sixteenth entury.

hospitals, rather than being hospitals in a modern sense, resembled a type of dispensary in the best of cases and more often were asylums or places to seek shelter (Figure 1.4).

THE MIDDLE AGES: THE PRE-TECHNOLOGICAL AGE— THE SINNERS, THE POSSESSED, THE BEGGARS, AND THE CRIPPLED

From the scientific point of view and for our purposes, the Middle Ages was marked by two developments—the academic doctrine of the ventricles as the seat of mental power and the controversy between the heart and the brain as the seat of the soul and mental activity. Additionally, the Church attempted to keep control of the most important writings of Greek and Roman medicine. Thus, Nemesins in the fourth century established that the functions of the soul were located in the cerebral ventricles. The cerebral "ventriculus medius" was responsible for thought and reason, the anterior cerebral ventricle for emotions, and the superior ventricle for memory. Although he makes clear that while the soul cannot be located, the functions of the mind can, Saint Augustine (fourth

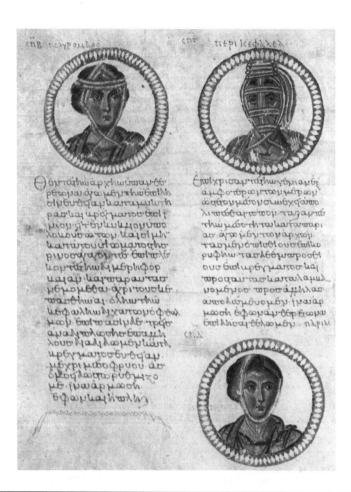

Figure 1.4: A text from the book of Sorano of Efeso (S.II A.D.) explaining different manners of bandaging the head.

or fifth century A.D.) differs with Nemesins and defines the first parts of the brain as the location for imagination and fantasy, the middle part as the place for reason, and the posterior part as the place of memory. Since the Aristotelian doctrine took some time to reach the "West" and did so only in the middle of the thirteenth century, medieval researchers followed the Platonic doctrine of locating the soul in the brain. When the Scholastics were at their peak of influence during that century, the Aristotelian doctrine that the heart was the seat of the soul began to be considered and taken into account (Figure 1.5).

The Middle Ages also meant, in some manner, a change in the way social life and public health were perceived. One must not forget that the majority of the medical writings of the Greeks and Romans were meant for the wealthy and leisure classes. Galen's patients were people close to the court circles and not slaves, peasants, or merchants. Thus, as Sigerist indicates (1956, pp. 35–36),

> *Galen's hygiene, although not unknown, did not have an important influence during the Middle Ages, since the social class for which it was meant no longer*

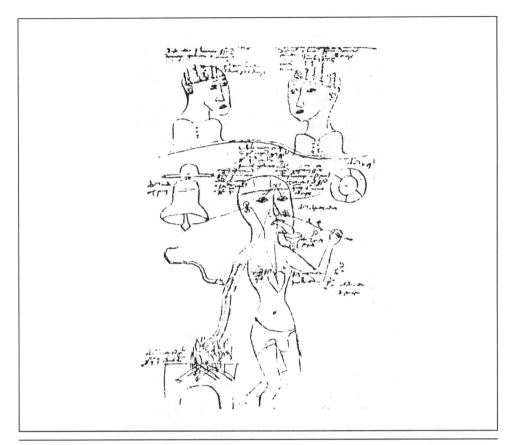

Figure 1.5: A medieval design about the Aristotelian sensory system. (From a catalogue of Incunabula in the Wellcome Historical Medical Library by F.N.L. Poynter. Oxford University Press, 1954, plate 8.)

existed. Christianity had revolutionized the western world. It arrived as the religion that promised redemption and cure, and addressed itself not only to the immaculate and the pure, but to everyone: the slaves, the prostitutes, the sinners. It stated that all men were equal before God, thus denying the class structure.... Things went so far as to have consulting a physician in the event of illness, become an obligation; physicians and medicine were seen as a source of secondary help for the preservation of life—the primary source of help coming naturally from heaven.

Laín-Entralgo (1969) indicates that as a matter of fact, between Hippocratic Greece and the Middle Ages, important developments emerged in the relationship between the physician and the patient:

1. The egalitarian condition of treatment;
2. The moral and therapeutical appraisal of pain;
3. The methodical incorporation of consolation into the work of the physician and in the care of dying or terminally ill patients;
4. The free assistance, as charity, of the needy patient; and
5. The incorporation of Christian religious practices in the care of the ill.

The Middle Ages in Europe was marked by invasions and by the Crusades, as well as by epidemics and plagues that struck the continent. This led to a large number of people suffering from important physical lesions. These people ordinarily had to survive by begging. During that time the roads of Europe were filled with beggars who were feared by all because of the existing superstitions and because of the spells they could cast.

The teaching and learning of medicine was fundamentally based on the review and study of the ancient texts, basically Greek and Roman. We know, for example, that in Salerno (Italy), Emperor Frederick II developed a formal curriculum for physicians. The latter had to study at least three years of logic and five years of medicine, practice anatomy through the dissection of pigs, perform one year of practice under the supervision of a tutor, and finally pass a skills exam. They were then extended a license that allowed them to work throughout the country. In any event, our modern university is a Middle Ages creation stemming from three bases: the professional schools, such as the school of medicine of Salerno and the law school of Bologna; the cathedral schools; and the monastic schools. During the Middle Ages, receiving a diploma from a university automatically gave one the right to practice medicine in any country in Europe (Figure 1.6).

It was not until the Gidenange of Rogerio of Sicily in 1140, and more effectively, the one of Frederic II of Barbarossa in 1231, that it was established that an official title was required in order to practice medicine. This prompted the appearance of the schools of medicine in the first universities: Montpellier, Salamanca, Oxford, Bologna, and Paris. According to Laín-Entralgo (ibid.), with these developments the figure of the physician/priest slowly disappears.[5]

Despite some positive developments, we could say that the Middle Ages, in the historical review we are doing, was a dark period in the treatment of physical injuries. People with some degree of injury or disability lived or survived confined or wandering and chased on the roads of Europe. They were considered beings who bore a curse as a punishment from God. It seems that only the Church's places of assistance provided them with some type of shelter. The majority of hospitals had a monastic or episcopal origin and were located next to cathedrals and bishops' or church palaces. In these hospitals, both pilgrims and sick persons were attended to, although the stay for the former was limited while that of the latter could be for an indefinite period of time. In Figure 1.7, one can see the Hôtel Dieu de Paris across from the cathedral of Notre Dame.

The connection of hospitals to ecclesiastical institutions made them places of assistance and shelter that were supervised by Church authorities and shaped by their Christian view of the world at a time when religion strongly shaped life in society. Therefore, these hospices were seen socially as part of the established religious concept of helping the needy in that society. However, during the Low Middle Ages, cities began to grow, and a budding city middle class began to appear. That is when the hospital centers changed both in their functions as well as in their organization. Some of them began to depend on the municipal governments, with lay direction and management. This fact added to the hospital a social spirit in addition to the religious one (Riera, 1985). Those people dedicated to the care of patients did not do so with an interest in making money but did it, instead, altruistically with the idea of service and sacrifice and of dedicating themselves to their fellow man.

During this period, madness or mental illness was contemplated from different perspectives. In the category of "mad" were those considered "victims" of the devil, the sinners, the nonbelievers, desperate lovers, dangerous individuals, and in a manner—buffoons. The "psychopathologic" characteristics or the "diagnostic criteria" that were

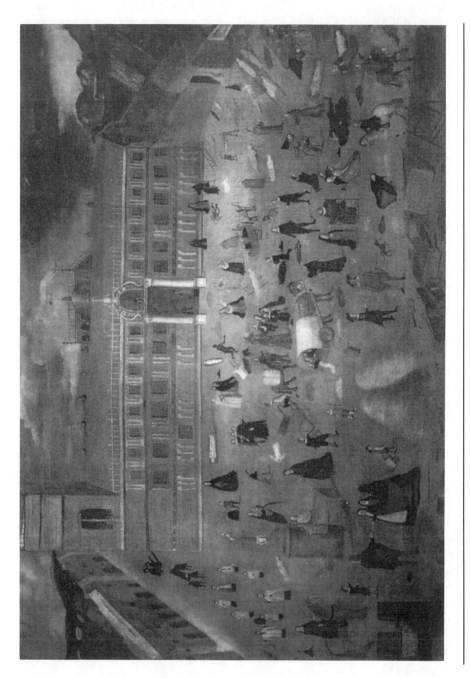

Figure 1.6: Anonymous painting of the explanade of the *Hospital de la Sangre* in Seville (Spain) during the 1649 plague. In this time the municipality was responsible for sanitary assistance. (From Hospital of Pozo Santo.)

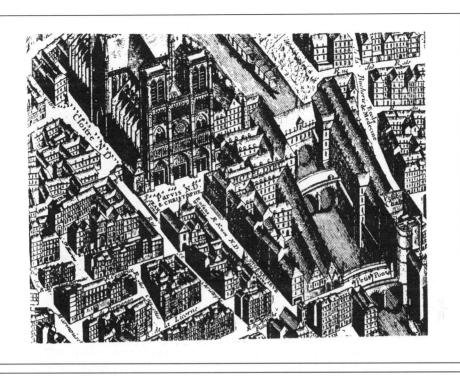

Figure 1.7: Representation of Hôtel Dieu in Paris in front of Notre Dame. This fact reflects the connection of the hospital to ecclesiastical institutions.

used to define a "mad" person during the medieval period were muteness, unreasoned laughter, melancholy vs. logorrheic behavior, instability, incoherence, limited capabilities, and wandering behavior. Additionally, also defined as such were those who exhibited vacillating speech, echolalia, the repetition of words or phrases, tautologic thought, the preference of monologue to dialogue, senseless gesticulation, changing tone of voice, frequent changes of identity, metaphoric expressions, and auto-referential discourse (Fritz, 1992).

As Gonzalez-Duro (1994, p. 12) indicates,

> ...crazy individuals survived immersed in the poverty which affected a good portion of the citizenry. Although they were relatively tolerated, they provoked contradictory feelings and were considered by the Church as possessed by the devil or under a spell. This remained so until the growing number of poor persons endangered the social order, and the rising middle class put into effect specific responses of social control, such as insane asylums, in which the demented wandering the streets were gathered. The first insane asylums were founded in the fifteenth century in the Hispanic kingdoms. Their appearance cast a modern view on the problem: in them, insanity was seen as a disease capable of being medically treated. But this progress was stopped. Spanish medicine was not able to give an adequate answer to the problem of insanity, because the Inquisition and the spirit of the Counter-Reformation prevented the development of psychiatric science. The insane asylums became horrendous jails, with hardly any functionality, and it was not possible for the insane, for the most part, to be socially excluded. That is why insanity was ever more present in society and impregnated the culture.

The insane were prohibited from marrying, receiving the Holy Sacraments, being ordained, testifying, and making a will. This was the approach that feudal society had toward those who, for some reason, were outside of what was considered "normal." The treatment of the mentally ill did not exist. As such, they remained or were "kept" hidden at home, and the members of the family community took over their custody rather than took care of them. Only a few were able to reach the religious "assistance" network of the convents, monasteries, etc. or were able to be taken to "hospital" institutions that were nothing more than places to gather these people and watch over them. In those cases when the patients were violent, there was no problem with having them sent to a prison. The pharmacopoeia of the time used sedatives with these patients, especially those derived from opium, antispasmodics, and emetics. Salvia was considered a brain nerve fortifier, and salvia wine was considered a good remedy against epilepsy. Diet, rest, isolation, advice, music, etc. were used less frequently therapeutically (Laharie, 1991).

The medical diagnosis and treatment are described by Laín-Entralgo (p. 70):

> *The physician approached the patient, asked him about his ailments, checked his pulse and his urine and labeled symptomatically the disease. The physician could proceed to prescribe treatment. Three main habits inspired—with a changing prevalence of one over the other—the assistance to the patient in Middle Ages monasteries: therapeutic empiricism, Christian charity, and the superstition of miracles. More or less basing himself on the few remains of therapeutical knowledge from antiquity which remained, the physician priest prescribed medicinal herbs, usually from the "hortus medicinalis" of the monastery itself, and dietetic rules, bleedings or baths. Charity, without a doubt, was the main moving force behind monastic medicine and probably very frequently shaped, under the form of spiritual and psychotherapeutic consolation, the behavior of the therapist. But the mentality of the time added many times practices that were more or less superstition—the use of relics, diverse rites—to the purely sacramental or merciful exercise* (Figure 1.8).

Given the influence existing concepts had at that time on the understanding of the brain, a thirteenth century encyclopedia titled *Proprietationes Rerum* ("on the properties of things") by Bartholomei[6] gives a summary of the existing views of the functioning of the brain during the Middle Ages. In it one can read that the brain is white in color because it has little blood, although it is rich in air, spirit, and much marrow substance. Therefore, it is like a "tabula rasa" ready to receive as many impressions and images as could be given to it. The brain is round so that it is better able to receive the spirits and better protect them; the more spirits it receives, the better the impulses will be changed into movement. The function of the ventricles is to promote the main functions of the brain (sensitivity, reasoning, memory, and imagination). Sensory impressions cause imagination in the third ventricle; they then pass to the middle ventricle so that they can be used as reasoning material, and the results of this whole process are stored as memory in the posterior ventricle.

But the doctrine that the heart is the seat of the soul is also present. Thus, Alfred of Sareshel,[7] around the year 1210, states that the brain received life from the psychic impulses from the heart through the soul. Conscience was not indispensable for the soul. Emotional disorders were transferred from the heart to the brain as the second organ. The brain received the radiations from the heart and reflected them as a perfect image, thus creating a perfect sensory perception (Pagel, 1958).

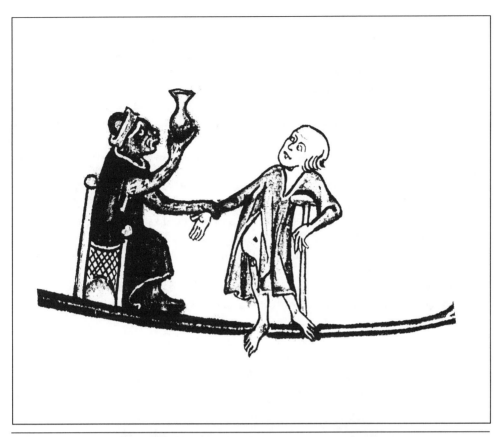

Figure 1.8: Satirical drawing with a monkey checking the pulse and the urine of the patient. (From Laín-Entralgo, pp. 80, 84.)

THE RENAISSANCE: CREATING THE CLIMATE FOR SCIENCE AND TECHNOLOGY—THE PATERNALISM

It is during the Renaissance (fifteenth to seventeenth centuries) that society began to take its first steps in recognizing its role and its responsibilities to its more needy members—the ill, the poor, and people with lesions. During this period, interest in medical problems increased, and texts were written resulting from this interest. From the point of view of the study of the brain, a change takes place. Speculation is no longer accepted regarding the seat of the soul unless it is through observation and mechanistic interpretations. From this period on, it was also legitimate and acceptable to try to prolong life as much as possible. Thus, Paracelso (1493–1541) wrote the *Liber de Longa Vita* in which he proposes the possibility of extending life for two fundamental reasons—because there is not a limit for the time of a life and because medicine was created by man precisely for the purpose of extending life, keeping the body healthy, and keeping it away from illness. Nevertheless, Paracelso is convinced that the heart is the seat of the soul and the center of life at the same time that he believes that the brain is the center of reason and the seat of some mental illnesses. The brain and the heart are related to one another through a constant flow of the spirits from the second to the first. Paracelso was a passionate student of alchemy and the occult sciences, and for this reason, he was a strong advocate of iatrochemistry and of metallotherapy. For him, gold, magnet, and the philosopher's stone were excellent therapeutic agents because they miraculously prolonged life. From the standpoint of treatment, he tried to use good and well-defined formulas with chemical principles extracted from little known drugs. His therapeutic goal was to establish a chemical balance in the human body (Figure 1.9). In any event, one must not forget that during the Renaissance, astrology also gained great importance and, combined with the theories of Galen, was very influential in the development of scientific understanding during this period.

During this period, medicine was located in the universities and convent cloisters. In France, for example, the master's degree or license to work was granted by the ecclesiastical authorities; in Paris, specifically, this was granted by the Canon of Notre Dame. If these physicians also taught, the Church took charge of their sustenance and support. But this dependence on the Church had its advantages and disadvantages. If a physician held any type of position, he had to forsake matrimony—even students of medicine had to remain celibate. On the other hand, rural medicine was left in the hands of barber-surgeons, since, for a long time, there was a repugnance on the part of the Church toward surgical acts (Figure 1.10). However, celibacy was modified by a cardinal decree in 1452, thus leading toward more progressive secularization of the profession.

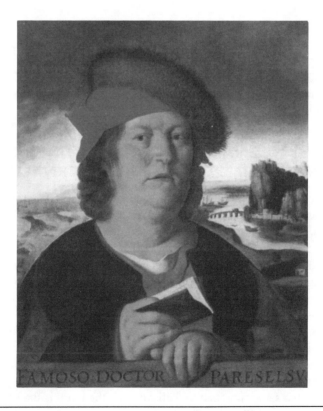

Figure 1.9: A portrait of Paracelso made in his time. The belief that man can try to prolong life as much as possible began with him.

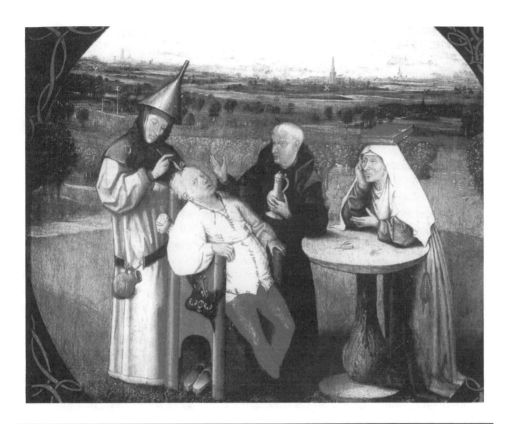

Figure 1.10: Caricature from the sixteenth century representing the barber-surgeons in their double job—cutting the hair and surgery.

In any event, the problems of persons with physical lesions were never attended to in a special manner and/or specifically. These people were grouped in the category of the poor or ill, even though it might have appeared that there could have been an improvement in terms of how they were treated. In this sense, their going to institutions and places of assistance, so that they could improve in some manner their conditions of living, was made easier. However, as Bellet (1990) indicates, these social actions may have another type of interpretation. Pity, the laws for the poor, the asylum for the deranged, etc. could also be interpreted as attempts on the part of the dominant classes to establish a closed order and a control over the poor, the insane, and, later on, over the disabled and persons with deformities and corporal physical lesions. This repressive, segregationist, internment attitude was followed by an attitude of assistance centered fundamentally on a public or private paternalism with a greater burden of humanist, moral and social objectives (Ruano, 1993).

It is also fair to indicate that the Inquisition[8] also aligned itself against physicians and surgeons fundamentally due to accusations of crimes of superstition (i.e., enchantments, spell casting, bewitchings). The inquisitors were firmly convinced that the physicians, especially the Morisco physicians, invoked demons and, therefore, committed acts of heresy. Through the written testimony of the trials by the Inquisition, we can learn how some physicians treated some illnesses. Below we translate the answer given by a

Morisco physician when asked by the inquisitor about the illnesses he cured (from Garcia-Ballester, 1976):

> *...hemiplegia, which is when someone has an extremity, an arm or a leg or an entire side of the body over which he has no control and is cold or frozen...the cold humor, having penetrated in some part of the body...stanch the blood coming out through the mouth or nose.... It also has cured and cures disorders of the female, such as those of the spleen and of the uterus, which prevents their normal purge and their not being able to become pregnant...for women who cannot give birth...in the event that their menstrual period does not come...and in the event that they have a low uterus, that she does not retain the seed of the man because she is filled with cold...if the reason for not becoming pregnant is because she has an abundant flow of blood...in the case when the woman becomes ill of the heart and has fainting spells...it has cured urinary illnesses. And if it is because of stone...and if the mentioned urinary illness is caused by fleshy excrescence, which is when thick humors lodge themselves in the neck which are called strangury...this defendant has cured and cures some eye illnesses, such as clouds lasting two years, that do not go beyond that, and when they are bloodshot and water a lot...another cure of great importance, which this defendant is accustomed of performing for those who suffer from the discharge of the head to the chest and from there to the lungs and creates a sore in it, which is a very dangerous illness, and that the cure, at the beginning of the illness, is to take, when they are going to go to sleep a dozen juniper berries, which are the fruit of the tall juniper trees, red or black...and that the mentioned juniper berries are also good to avoid the creation of stone, and it dissolves the existing stones and it also cures if they have blood in the urine....*

Figure 1.11 shows a document from a trial of the Inquisition against a Morisco physician in Spain.

The father of Spanish psychologists also suffered the devastating effects of the Inquisition. Juan Huarte de San Juan published in 1575 *Examen de Ingenio para la Ciencia*, which has been considered as the beginning of "Differential Psychology." Some passages of the book were prohibited by the ecclesiastical tribunal and were not republished in Spain between 1594 and 1846. Carpintero states (1994, pp. 40–41) that

> *the episode with the Inquisition should be known. A theology professor of the University of Baeza, Alonso Pretel, denounced the book to the Inquisition in Cordoba in 1579. As Granjel notes, that measure was justified "by the doctrine of Huarte regarding the organic relation between the brain and understanding and for accepting that it was possible that there be influences of temperament over free will; and during the Trial the entire chapter which made reference to the immortality of the soul was also censured. Huarte was rebuked for having dared to contradict at times the teachings of Aristotle and for not always bowing to the authority of Galen; it also caused suspicion that he conducted studies on the conditions or 'human inventiveness'" (Granjel 1980, 34–35). The book proposes the following doctrine: if men's rational souls are perfectly equal, in their metaphysical makeup, then the differences found in men must come from another level, that is to say, from the empirical constitution in which the connection of the soul is made with his body.*

An example of such repression can be found in the 1594 edition, where the inquisitors had suppressed the following paragraph:[9]

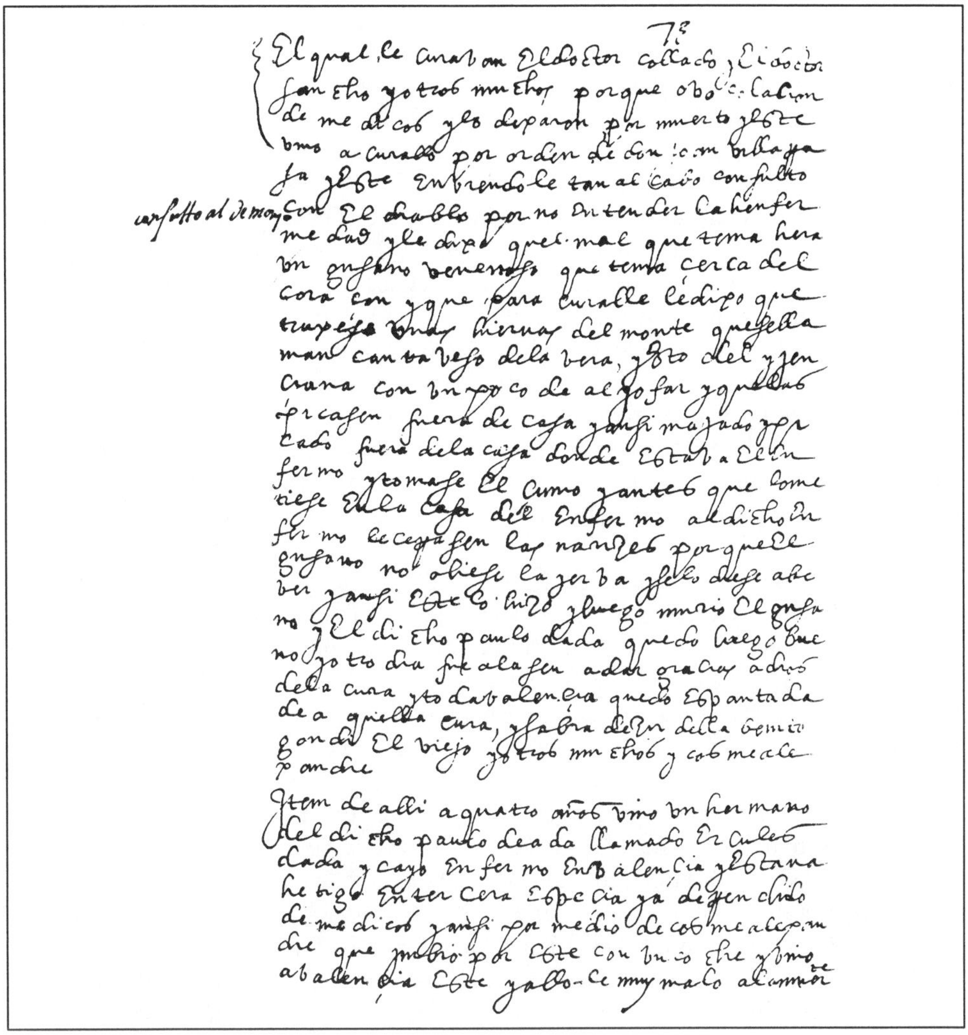

Figure 1.11: Reproduction of a document from a trial of the Inquisition against the Moorish physician, Jeronimo Pachet, in Spain.

Necessarily inside the brain there must be an organ for understanding and an organ for imagination and still another for memory. Because if all the brain were organized in the same manner, it would all be memory, all understanding, or all imagination. And we can see that there are other very different ones. So consequently, there must be a variety of instruments.

It was replaced by this paragraph:

Necessarily, in the brain there must be an organ for memory and an organ for the imagination. For understanding, nature did not create an instrument, as we stated before, although ghosts need it, as we will prove below.

This type of prohibition and censorship, which lasted in Spain for over five centuries, prevented the natural progress of ideas, concepts, and experimentation about the brain.

There is no doubt that the ideas of Huarte de San Juan are clearly those of a localizationist, despite the fact that when the brain is opened up, all of it appears the same, without differences; they preceded, for almost three centuries, the ideas of Franz Joseph Gall and his phrenology. Since the concepts of the Spanish author are supported more so upon modern cognitivism, the delay caused had an impact not just in Spain, but all over the known world, since Spain at that time was a kingdom "where the sun never set."

Huarte de San Juan's characteristics of memory are interesting historical notations of cognitive neuroscience. According to him, memory is an indispensable rational power, since without it, training and imagination are worthless. The role of memory is to store the registers without intervals for when they are needed by understanding. Thus, when memory is lost, the remaining "cognitive functions" will not be able to operate. There are, therefore, three types of memory: the first one is that which registers events easily but which forgets them just as easily; the second one is that which has difficulty retaining but which once it has retained, is capable of retaining for a long time; and finally, there is that which memorizes easily and takes a long time to forget. Obviously, this is an applied concept of memory and with the same spirit tries to offer an explanation for the problems of senility.

According to Huarte de San Juan (Figure 1.12), man learns the most in infancy, since he has more memory than in all the other stages of his life because his brain is very humid.[10] However, the aged have much more understanding because they have much dryness and are lacking in memory because they have little humidity. It is for this reason that the brain substance hardens and thus cannot receive the understanding of figures, just as hard wax cannot accept easily the figure of the seal, and soft wax does so easily. The reverse happens with the young, who, because of the great amount of humidity that they have in the brain, are lacking in understanding and are very nervous because of the great softness of the brain. It is easier to have memory in the afternoon than in the morning. This cannot be denied, but this does not happen for the reason that Aristotle states, but rather because the serum of the previous night has dampened and fortified the brain, and the sleeplessness of the entire day has dried it up and hardened it.

From the neurocognitive point of view, Huarte de San Juan indicates that the brain ventricles contain the seat of understanding, memory, and imagination where they collaborate jointly, which appears to be a rudimentary advance of the concept of the functional system proposed by Luria or of the neuronal assemblies proposed by D.O. Hebb.

Despite the modern "cognitive neuroscience" of Huarte de San Juan, the social changes that the discovery of the New World implied, and the fact that in other parts of Europe the ground work was being prepared for modern times, the Inquisition was an important influence on life in Spain. During the sixteenth century, Spaniards were entirely dedicated to the tasks of conquest and "westernizing" the newly discovered New World, which was translated into an enormous social effort. Nevertheless, the Inquisition still weighed heavily. While in Europe a new political context was being developed—the Reformation and the Counter Reformation—the Spanish Empire experienced a spiritual closing down as a reaction to the Protestant Reformation. In 1559, Emperor Philip II issued an order in which he forbid all his vassals from studying in European universities, except those of Bolonia, Rome, Naples, and Coimbra. This prohibition prolonged entrance into the modern age (Carpintero, 1994, p. 54).

During this period not everyone could nor wanted to go to the physician; the majority went to the healers, a practice so widespread that clerics, nobles, and even the Crown went

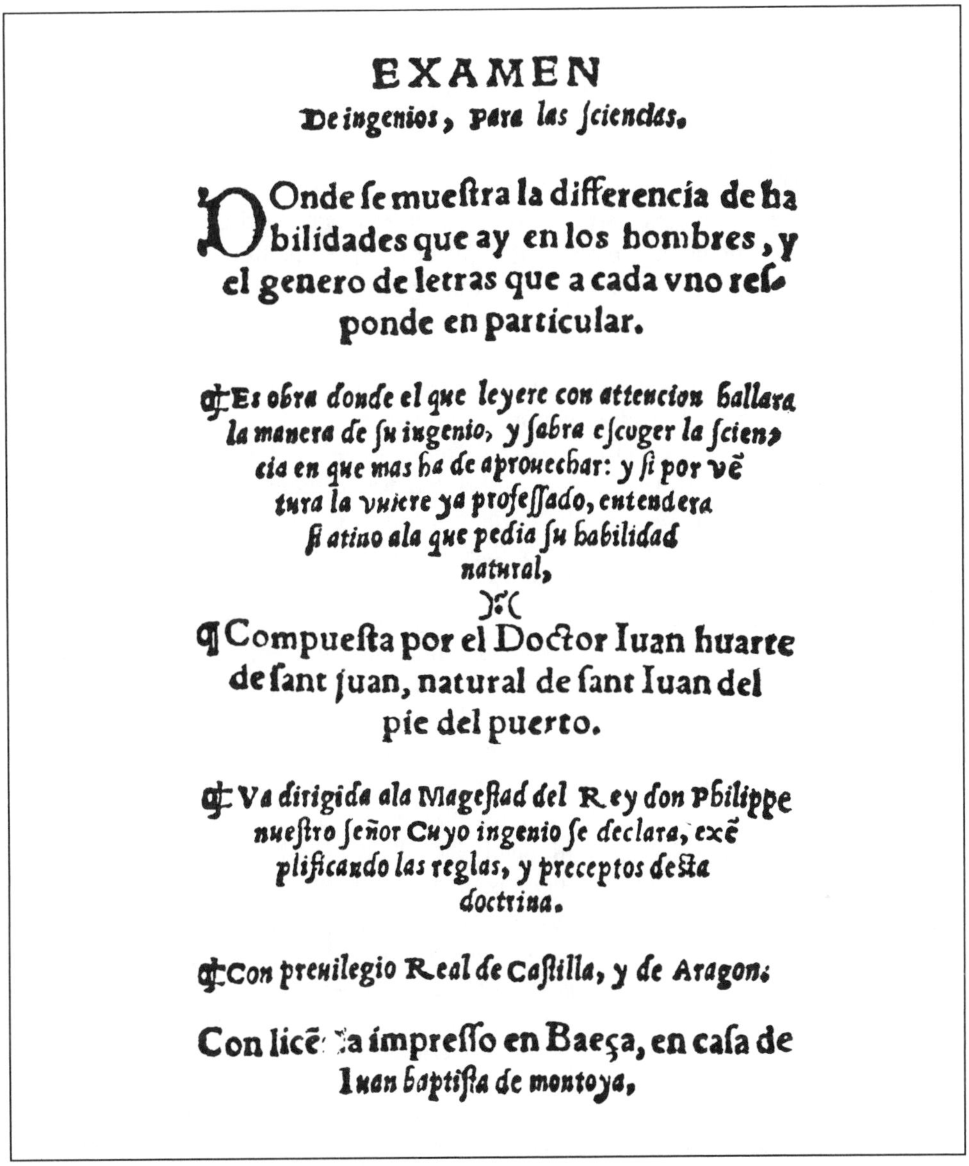

EXAMEN
De ingenios, para las sciendas.

Onde se muestra la differencia de ha bilidades que ay en los hombres, y el genero de letras que a cada vno res ponde en particular.

Es obra donde el que leyere con attencion hallara la manera de su ingenio, y sabra escoger la scien-cia en que mas ha de aprouechar: y si por vē tura la vuiere ya professado, entendera si atino ala que pedia su habilidad natural,

)(

Compuesta por el Doctor Iuan huarte de sant juan, natural de sant Iuan del pie del puerto.

Va dirigida ala Magestad del Rey don Philippe nuestro señor Cuyo ingenio se declara, exē plificando las reglas, y preceptos desta doctrina.

Con preuilegio Real de Castilla, y de Aragon.

Con licē za impresso en Baeça, en casa de Iuan baptista de montoya,

Figure 1.12: Reproduction of the cover of Huarte de San Juan's book *Examen De ingenios para las ciencias.*

to them. The physician was a person who was called on as a last resort or when there was no other option, because they had the reputation of charging much and healing little. Many of the physicians were also astrologers since the chairs of astrology were linked to the schools of medicine. Many physicians were more often sought out as astrologers than as physicians.

Later on, important advances gradually begin to appear in all social and cultural orders. In the area that interests us, the better educated and trained social classes began to accept, in some manner, the new philosophical concepts and scientific principles that had been struggling to be recognized for several centuries. Following Ruano (1993), we can point to an event that represents an important landmark in the attitude that society developed toward persons with physical deficits or physical lesions—the approval in England in 1601 of what was called the "law of the poor." With this law, local authorities were going to assume the responsibility of giving assistance to the ill, to the needy, and to all those who lacked the necessary means of survival. This law represents an important advance for the treatment of the problems of this type of people and achieves the first statute that made possible their care. In France, a law was passed regarding the teaching of medicine, and only and exclusively those persons who achieved master's degrees had the right to practice medicine. To obtain this degree, they would have to study for at least three years, with periods of review every four months and with final exams at the end. In addition, in their curriculum, practices in anatomy, in chemical and galenic pharmacy, and in the knowledge of the effects of plants also had to be present.

In France, it was Vicente de Paul (1591–1660) who founded an institution for the fundamental purpose of protecting children with some sort of handicap and who were victims of exploitation by being forced to beg. This charitable sisterhood, founded by Paul in 1617, was the first institution in the world that was established exclusively for the purpose of taking care of injured and disadvantaged children. These daughters of charity had as their doctrine Paul's norm (Figure 1.13): "...and they shall have as monastery the home of the sick...and as cloister the streets of the city or the rooms of the hospitals...." (Ruano, 1993).

In summary, charitable efforts were for a long time the only possibility of attention that people who were physically or mentally injured could enjoy. It is important to remember that the treatment of injured persons has been, throughout history, a matter of charity rather than a right or a real possibility. Nevertheless, scientific and social advances gradually contributed to create a new climate, especially in the physician/patient relationship. Illness and mental and physical lesions began to be better understood, and they eventually stopped being considered as a divine punishment. Since the lesions became accepted as illnesses, the physician ultimately had as his main role that of taking care of these people, being by their side, and helping them. According to Hildreth (1995, p. 251),

> in the institutions all sorts of patients mixed together—orphans, nursing infants, pregnant women, the insane, the feverish, victims of massive accidents and massive infections of general squalor and overcrowding: four to six patients per bed was the norm at the Hôtel-Dieu, last the individual patients situation varied according to his/her place in the social hierarchy of the hospital out-culture. Single beds, the best food, and eating halls were generally reserved for the hospital staff (who often were themselves convalescent patients). The hospitals had laberinthine support system of bakeries and farm, and other various auxiliary institutions which created an unwieldy and convoluted bureaucracy.

In France, other initiatives appear such as the "National Institution for Invalids" (Hôtel des Invalides), a great hotel whose purpose was to receive the war wounded or those wounded in battle situations. There is also the work done by Johann Peter Frank, a public health director in the Austrian Lombardy toward the end of the eighteenth century, in favor of socialized medicine. For him, the real social physician was one who was beside man from birth until death and who took care of keeping him away from the evil that might come upon him either from his physical or social surroundings.[11]

Regarding the concepts that existed about the brain at the time, there are some facts that should be mentioned. Descartes' mechanism appears, opening the mind/body debate and giving rise to the psychological concepts—the purely mentalist one and the materialist one—evolving from the mind and body as two different entities. According to Riese (1958, p. 123),

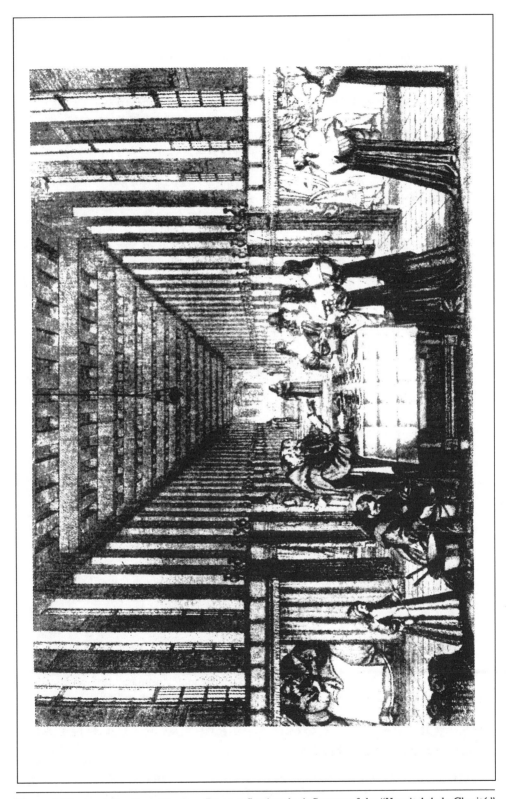

Figure 1.13: A painting from Abraham Bosse reflecting the infirmary of the "Hospital de la Charité."

That the soul perceives only in so far it is in the brain, seemed clearly established to Descartes for three reasons. In the first place, there are various maladies, which, though they affect the alone, yet bring disorder upon, or deprive altogether of the use of our senses. The second proof is, that though there be no disease in the brain (or in the members in which the organ of the external senses are), it is nevertheless sufficient to take away sensation from the part of the body where the nerves terminate, if only the movement of one of the nerves that extend from the brain to these members be obstructed in any part of the distance that is between the two. The last proof is that we sometimes feel pain as if in certain of our members, the cause of which, however is not in these members where is felt, but somewhere nearer the brain, through which the nerves pass that give to the mind the sensation of it.... For the first time in medical history, Descartes thus described the phantom limb, for which he offered the following explanation: "...the nerves before stretched downwards from the brain to the hand and then terminated in the arm close to the elbow, were there moved in the same way as they require to be moved before in the hand for the purpose of impressing on the mind in the brain the sensation of pain in this or that finger." This clearly shows, he concluded, that the pain of the hand is not felt by the mind in so far as it is in the hand but in so fair as it is in the brain.

In this context appears the work by Haller in which he establishes that the white matter in the brain and the cerebellum are the real base of sensations and movement. In 1664, *Cerebri anatomi* by Thomas Willis was published, which brought forth an entire model of anatomical procedures through which the cranial nerves were discovered (although incorrectly). A short time later, a supplementary text appeared on the pathology of the brain and the nerves, which dealt with epilepsy, hysteria, hypochondria, convulsions, and movement disorders. They were based on the books and the clinical experience of Willis. However, the interpretations made were still inspired by Galen's theories of animal spirits. Thus, he maintained that if blood did not reach the brain or was blocked, the nervous functions disappeared because the vital spirits could not reach the ventricles and become animal spirits. In such a manner, certain parts of the body become paralyzed by the nerves to which they are connected when the flow of animal spirits is interrupted. In 1671, he wrote,

we shall conclude after this manner, with a sufficiently probable conjecture, that the animal Spirit being brought from the Heas by the passage of the Nerves to every Muscle (and as it is very likely) received from the membranaceus fibrils, are carried by their passage into the tendinous fibres, there they are plentifully laid up as in fit Storehaus which Spirits, as they are naturally nimble and elastick, where ever they may, and are permitted, expanding themselves, leap into the fleshy fibres; then the force being finished, presently sinking down, they slide back into tendons, and so vicissively....

During this period, it was accepted that the nerves may stimulate the muscles; optics was developed, and the microscope was invented (León-Carrión, 1995).

THE MODERN AND CONTEMPORARY AGE: TECHNICAL AND SOCIAL ADVANCES

The eighteenth century begins the predominance of the medical systems. The *iatromechanical* of the Dutchman, Hermann Boerhaare, maintained that the body works through the solids submerged in the humors; thus, the human machine works through chemistry, heat, and the vital spirits through the foods that are mixed up with the digestive juices and the animal heat that allows them to be cooked and passed on to the blood so that they may later reach the brain where they become vital spirits. Thus, illness was a result of an imbalance between the solids due to changes with the air and the humors; it is for this reason that cold air ailments, hot air ailments, and damp air ailments existed. The other medical system of this century was the *iatrochemical* presented by the German, Friedrich Hoffmann, for whom the human body was a hydraulic machine for the circulatory movement of the humors. Illnesses occurred through the digestive system.

The eighteenth century marks the modern age. It begins with a climate of optimism, renovation and progress that can be seen everywhere. The scientific advances of the previous century contributed to the creation of this climate of expectation. There was great intellectual curiosity perhaps due to Newton's successes and the progress in experimental physics, all of which, no doubt, made the century start with the best expectations of progress in cities that were already lighted by electricity and in which science was the partner of progress. This climate set the ground work for the French Revolution of 1789, which caused a social change in all spheres of human life. However, the philosophy of the Enlightenment translated itself in a totally different tendency in matters of public health. Some philosophers and physicians did not defend the protection of the State, but, instead, they addressed themselves to the individual. The State is corrupt, they said, and an instrument of tyranny and oppression. Nothing good can come from the State. Man, on the other hand, is a reasonable being by nature; he is unhappy because he has not been enlightened; he becomes sick because he is ignorant; civilization has corrupted him by removing him from Nature. Man's natural state is to enjoy good health and happiness, and education is the means by which to achieve it (Sigerist, 1956, p. 81).

With the French Revolution, people begin to see a democratic society in which all the sick could be treated with equality, with dignity, and with the most scientific means. As Weiner indicates (1993, p. 127), "All contemporary doctors assumed that in exchange for the best care charity patients should sure clinical teaching. As citizen this was their duty. And unless their families objected, their cadavers would undergo dissection."

This, in fact, meant leaving the patient fundamentally at the mercy of physicians and medical students, with certain advantages and disadvantages; however, according to Weiner (op. cit.), in many ways the institutionalized patients were much better off after the revolution than before.

During this century, some hurdles were overcome, and the philosophy of humanitarianism and a form of understanding life and its problems from a perspective more centered on the human experience and on reason appeared. The prevailing attitude which, until that moment, had been fundamentally based on religious ideas and concepts experienced a serious crisis. From that period on, people began to proclaim that they were free and equal and that no social class had any right to exercise power over the rest. From the ideas of discipline, hierarchy, authority, and dogma, society moved on to those of independence and equality and also to a natural religion cloaked in concrete anti-Christianity feelings. It was the change from the mentality of Bossnet to that of Voltaire, to the criticism of all traditional convictions—from that of the Christian faith to even that of absolute monarchy, including the vision of history and social norms (Marias, 1986). It was an effective revolution of the mental assumptions of France, the leading nation in Europe at that time. Eighteenth century Europeans were faced with one of the greatest changes that western civilization has ever had to face. Just before the revolution, life expectancy was around 29 years of age. The birth rate was around 40% (see Table 1.1) with a tendency toward a decrease, and the mortality rate fluctuated from year to year—in 1778, it was 33% (Ruano, 1993).

Table 1.1: Population of Major European Cities in the Eighteenth Century (from Ruano, 1993, p. 20)

	Population
London	850,000
Paris	650,000
Amsterdam	200,000
Vienna	200,000
Madrid	150,000
Venice	130,000
Milano	130,000

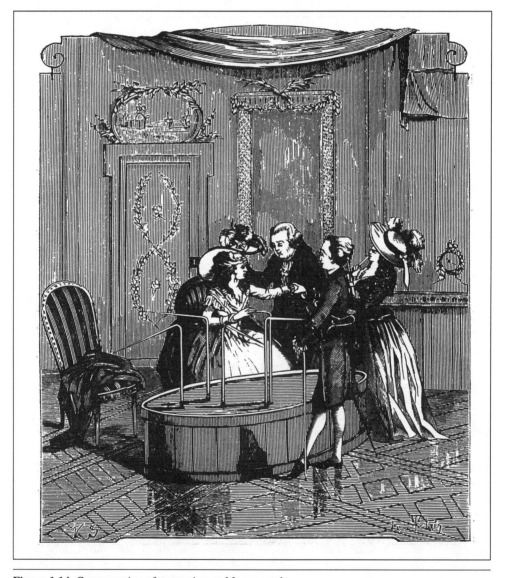

Figure 1.14: Group session of magnetism at Mesmer style.

From that moment on, the medical treatment given to people with injuries was also affected by the new and prevailing ideas. Therefore, during the eighteenth century, the attitudes regarding the injured that had been held up to then, which had considered the injured as different from the rest of society, begin to change. Along with the technical advances, new therapy techniques also appeared, such as the use of electricity. The first attempt to use electricity for therapeutic purposes was carried out by Jean Jallabert in 1740. This attempt, it seems, made it possible for a victim of paralysis to recover his health. From that moment on, the attempt was made to use it for the treatment of hemiplegias. The use of magnetism for healing purposes was followed by the use of magnetism with Mesmer's laying on of hands. His group sessions were carried out in a room where he would place a container full of acid water and metallic bars in which the patients, who were seated in a circle, had to hold in their hands (Figure 1.14). Then he would create the proper atmosphere by means of lighting, music, etc., and the effects were guaranteed. In 1784, a commission appointed by the Academy of the Sciences declared this method as incorrect. It is in this period that, primarily in France, formal medicine appears with the creation of chairs of legal medicine. At the same time surgery was no longer excluded from the environment of medical prestige and was dignified when the Gace College of Surgery was established in Paris in 1724; its studies were made equal to those of medicine.

With the discovery of electricity, the Galenic theory of the animal spirits also enters into crisis. Toward the end of the eighteenth century, the idea of connecting animal electricity with the nerves was something that excited the scientists. Note the discussion that Luigi Galvani and Alessandro Volta had. The former used electricity to stimulate the muscles of a frog and found that they contracted together with the intermittent production of electricity. Galvani published his findings in 1791 in his study *De Viribus Electricitatis In Motu Musculari Commentarius*, in which he drew the revolutionary conclusions that there was an inherent electricity in frogs and possibly in all living things. At the same time he seemed to indicate that the brain was the source of this inherent animal electricity and that it distributed it through the "Nervous System." It is the fiber extremities of the nerves that stored and condensed the electricity in the muscle fibers. Volta was opposed to the entire idea; although he accepted that metals may generate electricity and cause sensory effects on individuals, he did not admit that electricity was in the individuals but rather that it was in the metals. In the year 1800, using discs of different metallic makeup dampened in acid and separated by plugs (poles), he invented the voltaic battery (Figure 1.15).

At this time, the theories of Gall (1822–1825) and his phrenology also became famous. According to Pribam and Robinson (1985), Gall was the first person to present his hypothesis with data brought forth from clinical pathology, anatomy and neurology. For him, the brain was not a homogenous mass, but rather one in which mental functions and abilities could be located (Figure 1.16). Gall not only established that the cortex was something more that just a vascular tissue, but that it was also the seat of the principal organs of the brain. It is with him that the dignification of the brain began, despite the difficulties he had to go through in his personal and professional life (León-Carrión, 1991). But Gall was also an excellent anatomist from whose contributions we draw at least eight relevant points for neuropsychology:

1. His work showed that extraordinary development of the brain, especially the frontal lobe, is a fundamental characteristic of man.
2. His work showed that the cerebral cortex is not just a vascular tissue.

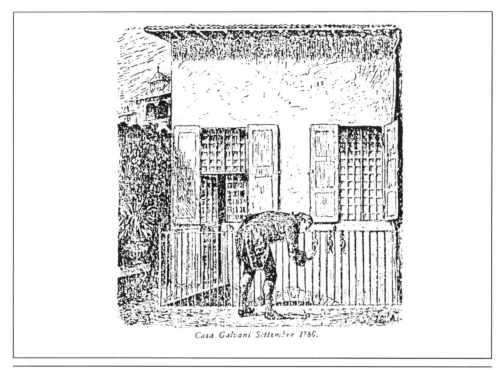

Casa Galvani Settembre 1786.

Figure 1.15: Galvani at his home in Bologne hanging up frog's legs. (From Reden von Emil Du Boys-Reimond, Vol. 2, Leipzig, 1798, p. 589.)

3. He established the current understanding of a basic division between white matter and grey matter.
4. He established the current knowledge of the paths of the central nervous system.
5. He established the difference between converging fibers (of association) and diverging fibers (projection).
6. He established a clear description of the cerebral commissures, understanding that each system is double with its parts symmetrically connected.
7. He established that the brain nerves do not have their origin in the brain but in the medulla.
8. He gave an explanation for the brain folds as fulfilling the need to gain space in the skull.

It is from this century that people begin to accept that people with physical lesions as no different from all the rest, that they are capable of leading a normal life if they are prepared and are given adequate means to be able to put into practice their capabilities and overcome their limitations. However, we must not forget that the French Revolution, which represents the change that the eighteenth century has brought about and which proclaimed the rights of man and of the citizens, was a middle class revolution. It was the middle class that arrived and placed itself in the positions of power. It was this revolution that led to liberal capitalism, which in turn was followed by the appearance in Europe of social inequality. These inequalities affected the poorer and less fortunate social classes. In reality the revolution turned against the poorest in society and created the progressive

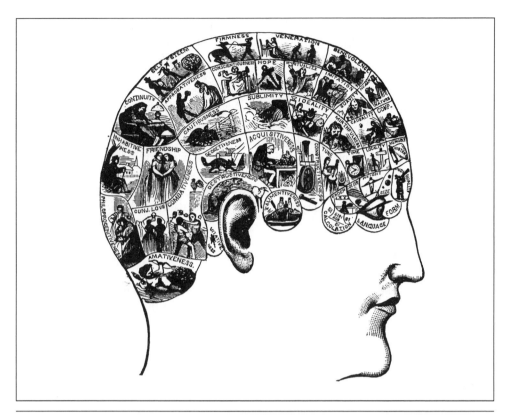

Figure 1.16: Representation from Gall Phrenological ideas. Each cerebral zone represented a mental function.

middle class. The revolution offered an excellent opportunity to carry out reforms in health and medicine, to the extent that the National Assembly gave medical reform a high priority. The reforms were carried out in spite of the conservative resistance of the hospitals. The internal organization of the hospitals was changed by centralizing services and also fighting corruption. Finally, patients were provided with individual beds, different wings of the hospitals were set aside for different types of illnesses, and patients were also hospitalized by age and by sex. The institutional control again fell into the hands of the physicians, and the nursing sisters lost their previous powerful role. Even the physical and architectural appearance of the hospitals underwent change, as well as the questions of health and hygiene (Weiner, 1993).

It was Napoleon (1769–1821), with his injured soldiers, who made one of the first attempts to offer professional rehabilitation to all. According to his criteria, those injured should receive, in addition to the necessary medical care due to them as a result of their physical condition, a special preparation with the goal of getting them to live in accordance with their nature as human beings. His idea was that their injuries should not become obstacles for the positive continuation of their lives, and, therefore, it was necessary to promote the responsibility of the State to provide the injured soldiers with the necessary resources. This fact was so important that when Napoleon died in 1893, he was buried with all solemnity in the pantheon of the invalids (Berges, 1989).

This existential initiative of Napoleon had had its precedents. King Luis of France had already created hospitals for injured military men. Some of these hospitals were designated for blind soldiers. Henry III of France created the Order of Christian Charity, which was concerned with injured soldiers and officers *"pour avoir bien servi."* In Spain, on June 21, 1573, an order was put into effect recognizing the payment of a special pension to several soldiers of the Spanish guard who had suffered injuries. Cristobal de Herrera asked Felipe II for the creation of an organization which would be at the service of the war disabled that the King had not authorized. In 1627, a Royal Order reached the Council of State complaining of the little attention that was being given to the injured soldiers "who received, in payment and reward for their services, hunger and nakedness." Latter in 1814, the depot for disabled soldiers was created, and training in arts and crafts was provided for these people—a type of center for occupational therapy. Those people who had been injured during military service were given preferential treatment in obtaining jobs in the government. These measures somehow tried to make up for the neglect in which soldiers had found themselves in comparison with other injured persons (Perez Leñero, 1961; Ruano, 1993).

During the second part of the nineteenth century, a social concern for the problems of injured persons surfaced, a movement which gave rise to the appearance of private initiatives and to the creation of numerous institutions with this goal. Fundamentally, they tried to study and solve the problems of these people. Gradually, hospitals dedicated to the treatment of the injured were founded. The professionals capable of helping the physically injured and the professional publications favored and provided a relevant and important alternative for the treatment and attention of the problems of these persons. In a survey of worldwide medical literature on, for example, paraplegia and medulla injury between 1800 and 1930, one can find 48 books and 518 articles (Ruano, 1993).

On the other hand, in the nineteenth century, important transformations appeared on the theories of the "Nervous System." There was a switch from the electrical nerve vibrations theory of Galvani to the theory of impulses and waves. Although practically no one dared argue that the nerves were electrical, no one dared affirm either how they functioned. Johannes Peter Miller describes in an 1826 textbook that the sensory nerves which appear to all function in the same manner were actually different and depended on the senses to which they were connected. Thus, while the mechanical irritation of a nerve may produce a luminous effect, that of another nerve produced pain and still that of another one, sounds. According to him, each of the sense nerves was not a mere passive conduit, but rather each one of them had special powers and qualities caused by stimulation. Two of his disciples achieved a spectacular advance in the study of the nervous system: Emil du Bois Reymond and Herman Von Helmhotz.

Du Bois-Reymond revealed nervous electricity and established that it is conducted in the nerves at a high speed comparable to that of telegraph messages. However, Helmholtz proved that the nerve messages move at a slower speed than telegraph messages. He reached this conclusion after experimenting with patients who were subjected to a simple apparatus that measured muscle relaxation and contraction; he discovered that nerve impulses moved at a speed of 35 m/sec. His experiments were easy to duplicate and always produced the same results.

The year 1800 brought forth those researchers who studied brain functions and the changes caused by chemical substances lesions. Thus, in 1809, the main active ingredient of the drug morphine was isolated. Toward the middle of the century, there was a strong development of chemical medicine, which was inaugurated with the discovery of surgical

Table 1.2: Tabulation of Part of Kingzett's 1878 Data on the Growth of Chemical Knowledge of the Brain (from McIlwain, 1958, p. 168)

Date	Investigator	Brief note of findings
1717	Hensing	Occurrence of phosphorus
1766	Spielmann	Study of ash
1790	Mönch	Oxalic acid by action of HNO_3
1790	Thouret	Soap-like material
1793	Fourcroy	PO_4, NH_3, Na, Ca; protein; (cholesterol)
1811	Vauquelin	Separations with EtOH and PB salts; P in organic combination; occurrence of S
1814	John	Vauquelin's compounds in man, calf, deer, chicken and crayfish
1826	Gmelin	Identification of cholesterol
1830	Lassaigne	Similar fractions from brain, retina and optic nerve
1834	Couerbe	Analysis of fractions of organic material. Reported changes in mental disorder
1841	Frémy	Degradation of phospholipid to olein and phosphoric acid
1847	Gobley	Phospholipids of the brain and of eggs; glycerophosphoric acid from lipids; lactic acid in the brain
1854	Bibra	Distribution of solids, fats and inorganic matter in the brain of mammals, birds and reptiles
1857	Müller	Creatine and some purines; inositol
1865–1882	Thudichum	Detailed chemical work including characterization of kephalin, sphingomyelin, phrenosine, sphingosine and cerebronic acid

For other collected historical data see Schlossberger (1856) and Thudichum (1874).

anesthesia. Studies on the effects and manner of acting of the substances appear, which, in turn, facilitated the understanding of the brain. The drugs were designed in structure on the basis of known central actions of radicals which they contained (McIlwain, 1958). Different authors also contributed to the knowledge of the inorganic constituents of the brain, as shown in Table 1.2.

The studies conducted by Paul Broca (1824–1880) achieved an important advance in the study and treatment of problems derived from brain damage. Broca's interest in the brain came from his relationship with professor Leuret at the Bicêtre Asylum and from his reading of the book *Anatomie comparée du systeme nerveux consideré dous res rapport avec Inteligence.*[12] In this book, we find the first description of the cerebral convolutions, and it states that their "number, shape, arrangement, and relationship are not haphazard."

For Leuret to not accept this implied a great lack of knowledge of the brains of animals. Each species has its brain structured in convolutions with characteristics exclusive to each species. Broca, in 1861, by using postmortem contrast methods, suggested the predominance of the left hemisphere for language, establishing that an injury in the posterior third of the frontal convolution of the left hemisphere caused aphemia, or what Trousseau called "aphasia." A few years later, Wernicke (1874) identified in the posterior third of the temporal convolution of the left hemisphere sensory aphasia, a disorder characterized by the loss of the ability to understand speech (Figure 1.17).

Toward the end of 1800, doubts surface regarding neuronal transmissions being totally electrical. An Austrian, Loewi, and an Englishman, Henry Hallet Dale, were pioneers in finding how electrical activity is transmitted from one nerve cell to another or from a cell to a muscular fiber. Their work obtained for them the Nobel Prize for Physiology in Medicine in 1936. They established that neuron transmission was chemical and that the impulses were transmitted chemically.

From 1800 on, a series of landmarks took place that lead to the birth and growth of neuropsychological and neuroscientific developments, which made it possible, in turn, to

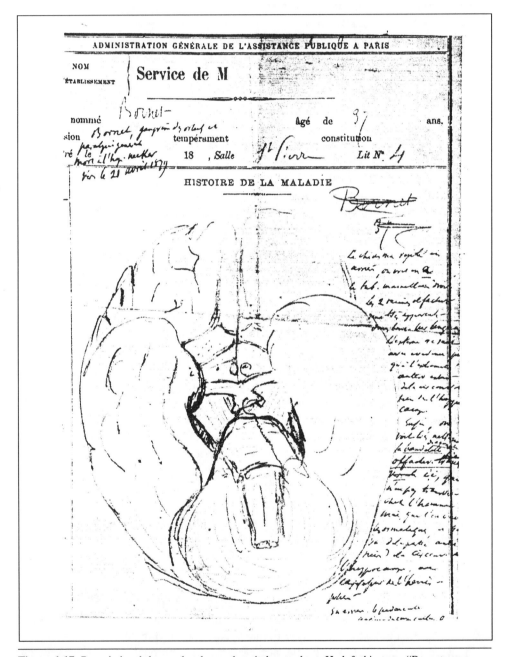

Figure 1.17: Broca's hand-drawn sketch on a hospital note sheet. He left this note: "Bornet, gangrene of toes and general paresis. Died at Hosp. Necker about 21 April 1879." (From Schiller, 1979. *Paul Broca*. Berkeley, CA: University of California Press.)

reach the design of neuropsychological rehabilitation programs. It began with the detection of subjects with brain damage through the present when a greater emphasis was placed on the treatment of these injuries (León-Carrión, 1995, pp. 25–27).

Doctors in the United States also had their vicissitudes, and their status had not been too high during the eighteenth and nineteenth centuries. Of the estimated 3,800 physicians existing during the period of the Revolutionary War, only 400 had medical degrees. At the beginning of the last century, the duration of study was 13 weeks, and it was not until 1847 that the American Medical Association recommended that there be at least 6 months of required study.[13] At this time, physicians were not a powerful group, nor were they well organized, and their organizations were not strong lobbies. On the other hand, the competition to try to get patients was normal and frequently occurred among these professionals. The reality of the type of assistance given at that time was that it was marked by the existence of a great variety of sects which promoted the excellence of their respective therapeutic methods. The end result was that as a group, they did not have a great amount of power to be able to have an impact on society so that they could influence public health policy. The first hospital in the United States was the Pennsylvania Hospital founded in 1751 by laymen, not physicians. Congress authorized the building of the first federal mental hospital in Washington, DC, in 1855 (the U.S. Government Hospital for the Insane).

Generally speaking, in the United States, the care of the ill was carried out in homes, and patients were sent to the few hospitals that existed only as a last resort. As Luchins indicates (1993, p. 35),

> The small number and size of the hospitals suggested that they were not in great demand. Associated with death and dying, with pest houses and paupers, as late as 1920 the hospital was widely regarded as a gateway to death. Hospitals exposed one to the dangers of "hospitalism" or sepsis; to contagious, infectious diseases; and to contact with low-class, unsavory people. Because of the sigma attached to it, self respecting people avoided treatment in hospitals. Even the poor viewed with horror the prospect of being hospitalized. Therefore, the hospital served mainly the very needy poor, such as domestic and impoverished workmen who could not pay for medical care, and boarders and lodgers who did not have an adequate place of residence in which to be nursed.

In 1870, there were fewer than 200 hospitals in the United States (Figure 1.18); none of them had more than 200 beds (Toner, 1873) for a population of 40 million inhabitants. For Cassedy (1991),

> the reality of American medicine has been marked by the country's free enterprise and money-making tradition, which has favored in a very special way private medicine and some very special institutions. This fact has its advantages and disadvantages. It has been the cause of a notable and clear delay in the appearance of a state-sponsored healthcare system in the manner of any advanced European nation, which in turn has had a direct effect in the disparities in the quality of care to the citizens based on their socioeconomic status.

Despite the number of years that have lapsed, the European healthcare system at this time is quite consolidated. All citizens have a right to healthcare simply by being citizens of the country. In the United States, there is no national healthcare system, and the citizens have to have their own healthcare insurance system. For the needier in society, there were

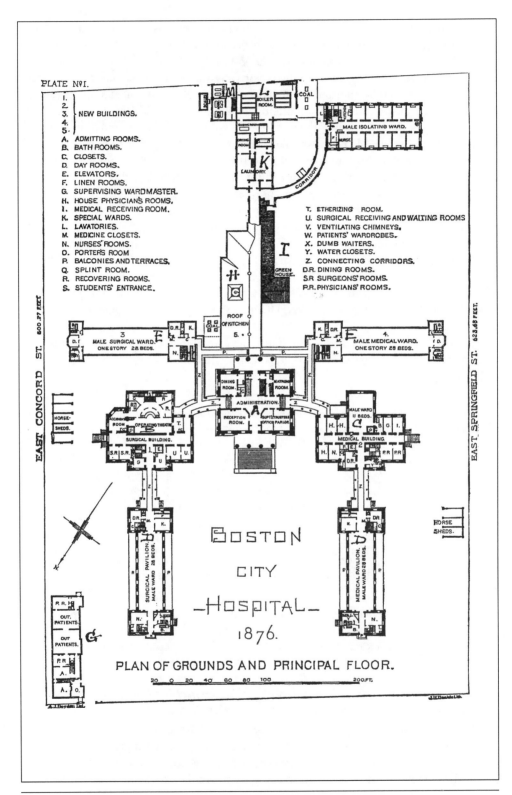

Figure 1.18: Plan of the grounds and principal floor of Boston City Hospital as it was in 1876.

welfare healthcare plans. Likewise in Europe, there is a social protection system for all those that suffer work injuries.

The care of persons who have suffered some type of injury moves enormous amounts of money and has an important social impact. As Pope and Parler (1991) indicate, in the United States alone, there are around 57 million people who suffer injuries every year, of which 1.3 million suffer cranial trauma; between 70,000 and 90,000 suffer moderate or sever traumatic brain injury, and between 10,000 and 20,000 suffer permanent spinal cord injury each year. Diller indicates (1994) that every 15 seconds, there is a case of cerebral injury—every 5 minutes, one of these persons dies, and another is left permanently disabled. For all of this, there are 152 independent rehabilitation hospitals with 700 specialized brain injury programs. According to Bistany (1994, p. 45),

> *As we move through the 1990s toward the 21st century, we are embarking on an economic revolution, particularly in healthcare. However, rehabilitation, which is an aspect of this health-care reform, is often forgotten and remains a "stepchild" of the medical profession. Although medicine has been a vital part of history for many thousand of years, rehabilitation medicine is barely 50 years old. Specialization in head injury rehabilitation is even younger, resulting in limited understanding and skepticism for many.*

In any event, the care of persons having suffered brain injury is seen today in the United States with increasing interest. According to Diller (1994, p. 279),

> *Rehabilitation of TBI has received a great deal of support from managed care systems that are profit seeking; this has led a number to abuses that have resulted in Congressional hearings and unfavorable publicity. As a result, Congress recently passed laws to correct this: (a) the Brain Injury Rehabilitation Quality Act of 1992, which protects the rights of each brain-injured patient in rehabilitation with a national set of standards and oversight; and (b) a bill to develop a national definition for TBI. This bill, "the TBI Act," mandates all states to add TBI to their data-reporting structures. It identifies the need for federal, state, and local resources to develop services for a defined condition.*

Consequently, all these vicissitudes have helped in the appearance of specific centers both in the United States and in Europe dedicated to the treatment of brain injuries. Numerous specialized publications have also appeared on the rehabilitation of brain injuries. Similarly, national and international associations have been formed with the purpose of studying and promoting the treatment of these types of injury. All of this has led to new approaches and better care of the sequelae of these types of injuries. We could say that the current situation approaches, as never before in human history, human dignity both in health as well as in sickness.

ENDNOTES

1. Quoted from Haeger (1988), p. 23.
2. Some consider the Hippocratic collection as the sum of the works of Hippocrates, while others consider it a collection of the medical writings of different tendencies.
3. Hippocrates. *Selected Work: The Sacred Disease*. London: Hilnemann, Loeb Classical Library, pp. 139–83.
4. See Laín-Entralgo (1969).
5. We must not forget that monastic medicine is very deeply rooted in medieval society. For the physician/priest, medical treatment was, above all, an act of love and the application of Christian principles.

6. Bartholomei Anglici Liber de Propietatibus Rerum. Argent, 1491. Lib V. Capt. 3.
7. Alfredus Anglicus van Sareshel. *De Motu Cordis.* Beitr. Z. Gesch. D. Philos. D.M.A. Vol. 23, 1–2. Muenster, 1923.
8. The Inquisition was an ecclesiastical tribunal established for the purpose of looking into and punishing crimes against the Faith. It was founded by Pope Innocent IV in 1248. The tribunal of the Inquisition, or Holy Office as it was commonly known, acted in secret, and its sentences were carried out as an "Auto de Fe" by the civil authorities. It was established in Spain by the Catholic Kings on a permanent basis in the fifteenth century. Napoleon banned it in 1808, and it was abolished in 1813 and revived several times later until it finally disappeared in 1835, although it was ineffective from the end of the eighteenth century. While it lasted, its effects were devastating for social life and for scientific progress.
9. Huarte de San Juan (1575, p. 117). Complete edition prepared by E. Torre for Editorial Nacional. Madrid, 1976.
10. Huarte de San Juan bases his differentiating theories on the four humors (p. 127).
11. Although Frank was a social physician, we must not forget that he was totally given to the ideas of the Enlightenment, "all for the people but without the people." The physicians of this period, as was the case with the monarchs, had a paternalistic attitude toward their patients. Since they were responsible for the health of the people, they were also responsible for dictating any and all measures which were, according to them, necessary to preserve it.
12. F. Leuret and P. Gratiolet. 2 vols. Paris. Didot, 1839–1857. This book is, in a manner of speaking, a homage to Luigi Rolando, the first to describe regular cerebral folds and the main vertical fissure that distinguishes the anterior half of a hemisphere from the posterior half.
13. One could say that in the United States, there were no institutions worthy of being called universities until 1847, when the Harvard scientific schools were created with the purpose of training engineers. Despite trying to attract, in those early years, important figures of American science, the cultural level and the scientific climate had no relation to the climate that existed in the European universities. This was finally achieved with the foundation of Johns Hopkins University, which was the first center of higher learning and research in the European model.

REFERENCES

Alfredus, A.S. (1923). De Motu Cordis. *Beitr. Gesch. D. Philos. d.M.A., 23,* 1–2. Muenster.

Bartholomei, A.L. (1491). *Propietatibus Rerum.* Argent. Lib V. Capt. 3.

Bellet, E. (1990). Analyse des processus d'exclusions et d'integration vis-à-vis des handicapés depuis 25 siècles. In *La formation professionnelle élément d'une politique d'integration des persones adultes handicapées* (p. 19). C.R.I.C.

Berges, G. (1980). Prólogo. In Aguilar (Ed.), *Stendhal.* Napoleón.

Bistany, D.V. (1994). Overview of the economics of rehabilitation in the United States. In A.-L. Christensen and B.P. Uzzell (Eds.), *Brain injury and neuropsychological rehabilitation: International perspectives* (pp. 245–256). Hillsdale, NJ: Laurence Erlbaum Associates.

Carpintero, H. (1994). *Historia de la psicología en España.* Madrid: Eudema Universidad.

Cassedy J.M. (1991). *Medicine in America: A short history.* Baltimore, MD: The Johns Hopkins University Press.

de San Juan, H. (1575). *Examen de ingenio para la ciencia.* Complete ed. prepared by E. Torre for Editorial Nacional, Madrid, 1976.

Diller, I. (1994). Federal planning with regard to traumatic brain injury in the United States. In A.-L. Christensen and B.P. Uzzell (Eds.), *Brain injury and neuropsychological rehabilitation: International perspectives* (pp. 269–280). Hillsdale, NJ: Laurence Erlbaum Associates.

Filer, J. (1995). *Disease.* London: British Museum Press.

Fritz, J.M. (1992). *Le discours du fou au Moyen Age. XIIe-XIIIe siècles.* Paris: Presses Universitaires de France.

Garcia-Ballester, L. (1976). *Historia social de la medicina en la España de los siglos XIII al XVI.* Madrid: Akal.

Gonzalez-Duro, E. (1994). *Historia de la locura en España.* Madrid: Temas de hoy (Temas I & II).

Granjel, L.S. (1980). *La medicina española renacentista*. Salamanca: Universidad de Salamanca.

Haeger, K. (1988). *The illustrated history of surgery*. Gothenburg: A.B. Wordbok.

Hildreth, M.H. (1995). Reform and innovation in hospital care and public health in revolutionary and early nineteenth century France. *Journal of the History of Behavioral Sciences, 31,* 250–254.

Hippocrates. *Selected work: The sacred disease*. London: Hilnemann, Loeb Classical Library.

Laharie, M. (1991). *La folie au Moyen Age. XIe-XIIIe siècles*. Paris: Le Léopard d'Or.

Laín-Entralgo, P.L. (1969). *El médico y el enfermo*. Madrid. Ediciones guadarrama.

León-Carrión, J. (1992). Indulgencia para Gall: La dignificación del cerebro. *Revista historia de la psicología 12,*(3,4), 429–432.

———. (1995). *Manual de neuropsicología humana*. Madrid: Siglo XXI.

Leuret, F., &Gratiolet, P. (1839–1857). *Anatomic comparèe du systeme nerveux consideré dous res rapport avec Inteligence* (2 vols.). Paris: Didot.

Lopez-Piñero, J.M. (1984). Introducción. Los estudios histórico-sociales sobre la medicina. In E. Lesky (Comp.), *Medicina social. Estudios y testimonios históricos. Colección Textos Clásicos Españoles de la salud Pública* (pp. 9–30). Ministerio de la salud y consumo. Secretaría General Técnica.

Luchins A.S. (1993). Social control doctrines of mental illness and the medical profession in nineteenth-century America. *Journal of the History of the Behavioral Science, 29,* 29–47.

Marias, J. (1986). In J.A. Garmendia & J. Rastrilla (Eds.), *Historia del arte y de civilizaciones*. Editorial S.M.

McIlwain, H. (1958). Chemical contributions, especially from the nineteenth century, to knowledge of the brain and its functioning. In *Acts of Anglo-American symposium: The brain and its functions* (pp. 167–190). Amsterdam: B.M. Israel.

Pagel, W. (1958). Medieval and Renaissance contributions to knowledge of the brain and its functions. In *Acts of Anglo-American symposium: The brain and its functions* (pp. 95114). Amsterdam: B.M. Israel.

Perez, Leñero J. (1961). *Ideario de la rehabilitación profesional de los Invalidos*. Ministerio de trabajo, Secretaría general Técnica.

Pope A.M., & Parler, A.R. (1991). *Disability in America: Toward a national agenda for prevention*. Washington, DC: National Academy Press.

Pribam, K.H., & Robinson, D.N. (1985). Biological contribution to the development of psychology. In C.E. Buxton (Comp.), *Points of view In the modern history of psychology* (pp. 345–381). New York: Academic Press.

Riera, J. (1985). *Historia, medicina y sociedad*. Madrid: Piramide.

Riese, W. (1958). Descartes' ideas of brain functions. In *Acts of Anglo-American symposium: The brain and its functions* (pp. 115–134). Amsterdam: B.M. Israel.

Ruano, A. (1993). *Invalidez, desamparo e indefensión en seres humanos*. Madrid: Fundación Mafre Medicina.

Sigerist, H. (1956). *Hitos en la historia de la salud pública*. Madrid: Siglo XXI. (*Landmarks in the history of hygiene*. London: Oxford University Press, Amen House).

Toner, J.R. (1873). Statistic of regular medical association and hospitals in the United States, 1872-73. *American Medical Association Transactions, 24,* 288–330. Cited in Luchins.

Weiner, D.B. (1993). *The citizen-patient in revolutionary and imperial Paris*. Baltimore, MD: The Johns Hopkins University Press.

Wernicke, C. (1874). *Der aphasische symptomen complex. Eine psychologische studie auf antomischer basis*. Breslau: M. Cohn and Weigart.

2

Neuropsychological Rehabilitation Models

Barbara P. Uzzell

Memorial Neurological Association
Houston, TX

INTRODUCTION

Neuropsychological rehabilitation has many definitions. Some say it is rehabilitation of cognitive losses only, but it is much broader; it is a method of restructuring lives in a social context. It includes integrated knowledge from neurophysiology, neurosurgery, neuropharmacology, neuroimaging, neuropsychology and psychology, and techniques adapted from occupational therapy, aphasiology, and special education. Often, it is elusive to the brain-damaged patient and their families who participate in it, to other professionals, and to administrators in health management. Many people in the field of neuropsychological rehabilitation like to think it began in the 1980s, but its origins in Europe and the United States are earlier (Boake, 1991). Other terms add to the confusion, especially "cognitive therapy," "cognitive remediation," and "cognitive retraining," and have dissimilar meanings denoting certain neuropharmacological, psychotherapeutic, or behavioral management programs. Neuropsychological rehabilitation is broader than any of these terms due to its restructuring of lives in a social context and does not represent retraining of cognitive abilities only.

Models for neuropsychological rehabilitation are not abundant. The paucity of models may be due to the failure of professionals in the field to agree on a theoretical framework for recovery from brain damage, the variety of behavioral manifestations after brain damage associated with particular brain structures, the elusiveness of accurate measurements of cognitive and behavioral functions, and the interactive effects of cognitive, social, and behavioral functioning in any given brain-damaged individual. Such reasoning not only prevails currently, but has in the past as well.

MAJOR MODEL OF NEUROPSYCHOLOGICAL REHABILITATION

Many say only one theory of neuropsychological rehabilitation is sound and all-inclusive. It is based on the theoretical principles of Alexander R. Luria (1963, 1980). The theory is derived from observable behaviors that comprise many basic processes coming from contributions of different levels and sites within the brain. The functional cortical system accounts for the organization of higher level thought processes. The theory distinguishes three hierarchical functional units of the brain: (1) the arousal unit responsible for regulating cortical tone; (2) the sensory-input unit responsible for receiving, analyzing, and storing information; and (3) the organizational and planning unit responsible for programming, regulation, and verification of activity. Each of these units is hierarchically organized into: (1) primary areas, which receive and send impulses to and from the periphery; (2) secondary areas, which perform information processing; and (3) tertiary areas, which receive input from two or more of the secondary areas and serve to integrate information. The three hierarchical functional units are essential to the execution of any cognitive task.

Disinhibition is present after brain damage. Recovery of functioning, according to Luria's theory, occurs when newly learned connections are established through mental retraining exercises specifically targeted at the basic processes that have been disrupted. Direct intervention is essential to the recovery and reorganization of the brain. The theory provides a conceptual framework for current neuropsychological rehabilitation programs (Christensen, Caetano, & Rasmussen, 1996).

OTHER MODELS

Another model has been the Process-Specific Approach (Sohlberg & Mateer, 1989), which uses techniques consistent with established scientific principles. Under this theory, a group of tasks targeting the same component of a particular cognitive process is systematically and repetitively administered according to the need for treatment. Tasks are arranged in a hierarchy, so as soon as a level of mastery is reached, higher level treatment targeting the same cognitive component is introduced. The neurological system for a specific function (e.g., visuomotor ability), is used to facilitate reorganization of this ability. Treatment is data-based and direct with a measure of treatment success made through generalization probes. The ultimate success is determined by improvements in level of vocational ability and independent living. The model is based in part on Luria's theory that direct retraining of cognitive processes results in reorganization of higher level thought processes.

Goals of neuropsychological rehabilitation have been clear—to improve cognitive and emotional functioning and quality of life. Many attempts to reach these goals are empirically driven, without hypothesizing improvement in underlying brain functioning. Two empirically driven models are worth mentioning since they are often seen. The first of these is generally know as the *Stimulation Model.* It assumes that any stimulation of cognitive functioning will improve mental abilities. The notion that stimulation is better than no stimulation at all is supported by this model. Tasks are not directed towards specific functioning based on concepts about functional brain organizations.

The second theory is the *No-Transfer-of-Training Model.* This model assumes that learning in one situation is not transferable to other situations. Patients are trained to perform specific tasks in naturalistic settings. Training is required for each task. Brain functioning is not considered in this model.

TESTING THE MODELS

Substantiating goal achievement has been difficult, regardless of the model used. There are enthusiastic, ardent supporters of neuropsychological rehabilitation and skeptical, harsh critics. While supporters may learn from the critics and vice-versa, the prognosis for fulfilling the goals of neuropsychological rehabilitation without participation in it is not favorable for most individuals with brain damage.

Neuropsychological rehabilitation models are tested in an area of clinical research that is always difficult, regardless of the field. Clinical research requires withholding a treatment under some conditions. This means that some subjects or participants will receive treatment and others will not, or the treatment will be delayed. If there is a critical period or "window of opportunity" for the brain to receive treatment, those not receiving treatment at that time may be in jeopardy. Indications from the plasticity of the nervous system suggest the earlier the treatment, the better (Stein, Glasier, & Hoffman, 1994; Kolb, 1996). Hampering the development of a theoretical model based on treatment timing is our limited knowledge about critical periods. It is also difficult for clinicians who are trained to treat to withhold treatment, even if the treatment is done under double-blind conditions.

Testing a model is difficult without quantification of treatment measures. Use of some models, such as the Process-Specific, are more easily quantifiable (Sohlberg & Mateer, 1989). Outcome measures, such as return to work and the duration of a work return, have also been chosen (Ponsford, Olver, & Curran, 1996) as evidence of the efficacy of treatments.

All models have to address spontaneous recovery, which can occur anytime, but which occurs more frequently during the early stages of brain insults. Individual behavior is examined over time with case studies, as group studies tend to mask individual differences is response to treatments. One case study design is to withdraw and reinstate treatment over time, examining the level and change in the data over the baseline with treatment. During multiple-baseline studies, measurements are often made of one behavior in multiple settings or one behavior across multiple subjects. Simultaneous treatments can also be measured by alternating treatments on a split-session schedule. These measures and other variations require careful, special statistical analysis (Kazdin, 1976).

PRINCIPLES UNDERLYING NEUROPSYCHOLOGICAL REHABILITATION

The first principle of recovery recognized by John Hughlings Jackson (1879) over 100 years ago, which is often forgotten today, is that symptoms of brain damage do not necessarily reveal the functions of damaged tissue, but, instead, more accurately reflect what the remaining areas of the brain can do after injury to a part. This concept is recognized in Luria's investigative system. Others, such as Henry Head (1926), conceptualized the remaining nervous system as "the new whole." Goldstein (1939) went further, stating that behaviors after brain damage represented the adaptive capacity to survive in an altered world.

During neuropsychological rehabilitation, the following question becomes important: are there dynamic changes in the central nervous system, such as regenerative or collateral sprouting, that are a direct result of treatments? The answer to this question remains speculative, although inroads are being made in this area (Risberg & Jensen, 1994). Most neuropsychological rehabilitation specialists believe the nervous system does change as a result of treatment, although they may disagree on what changes are occurring. Some favor static concepts of sparing, redundancy, and substitution rather than dynamic ones. Others believe that nervous system regrowth may be maladaptive at times. More definitive evidence may be available in the future about central nervous system implications for neuropsychological rehabilitation.

Neuropsychological assessments are often performed before and after treatment in an attempt to support the success or failure of the treatment model under investigation and to speculate about underlying neuronal changes. During assessment, the remaining brain of the whole organism is performing, not just, for instance, its hippocampus or visual cortex. Neuropsychological assessments have been quick to localize and describe brain lesions and rather reluctant to recommend treatment or to note treatment effects. Often overlooked is the high degree of variability encountered following brain lesions that may be attributed to variations in brains (or genetic factors) and distal effects of lesions.

Assessment for neuropsychological rehabilitation takes on new meaning for old techniques. Assessment measures must be carefully chosen to be sensitive to the targeted treatment behaviors and to minimize practice effects. Knowledge of preexisting patient conditions, such as learning disability, superior abilities, or culture differences, are required. Other variables, such as emotional state at the time of measurements, must be considered during assessment as well as during treatments.

TECHNIQUES USED TO ACHIEVE THE GOAL

Various procedures have been used to achieve the goal of neuropsychological rehabilitation. The one initially used was the *drill*. Most of us are familiar with this procedure from our participation in the educational system. There has been some evidence that this most often used technique can produce successful recall of basic orientation and safety information in densely amnesic patients (Goldstein & Malec, 1989). *Visual imagery* is another popular treatment technique (Moffat, 1984; Goldstein et al., 1988) that has been successfully used. *Computer programs* for retraining attention maintenance, visual processing, and reasoning/problem solving began to appear in the 1980s (Gianutsos & Klitzner, 1981). Many of these software programs remain useful, although placement of a patient in front of a computer screen with any available operational program does not guarantee effective treatment. Computer usage, as with any of these techniques, requires selectivity based on the model under investigation. Other commonly used treatment methods include *external aids, motor coding*, and various *verbal memory strategies* (Moffat, 1984).

Training methods may be similar across some models, but they may vary with the model. It was recognized early on that training must be theoretically based (Diller, 1976) to be effective. Training of cognitive conditions is seldom done in isolation, but rather in social situations artificially created with a therapist or in naturalistic settings. Training needs to be relevant to the individual's life (Hart & Hayden, 1986). The brain-damaged individuals bring not only their damaged cognitive abilities to treatment, but also bring their unique personality structure. Neuropsychological rehabilitation must address the impact of brain damage on the personality of the individual (Prigatano, 1986; Gordon & Hibbard, 1991), creating an environment for awareness of changes and necessary modifications required.

CONCLUSIONS

Luria's model for neuropsychological rehabilitation seems to dominate the field, although some chose the process-specific approach or no theoretical model at all. It is in the latter situation that trouble arises, since there is no theory to guide the treatment. Evaluation methodologies have been limited or nonexistent. Showing a relationship between treatment and changes in aspects of a brain-damaged individual's behavior is not easy. Reliability and validity of outcome measures to support a theory are difficult to obtain in groups, as well as in case studies (Robertson, 1994). What is needed is not more theories but scientific proof that theoretically based treatments work. Improved evaluation methodology and replication of findings in the future will, no doubt, provide answers to justify the underlying process of neuropsychological rehabilitation.

REFERENCES

Boake, C. (1991). History of cognitive rehabilitation following head injury. In J.S. Kreutzer & P.H. Wehman, (Eds.), *Cognitive rehabilitation for persons with traumatic brain injury* (pp. 3–12). Baltimore: Paul H. Brookes Publishing Company.

Christensen, A.-L., Caetano, C., & Rasmussen, G. (1996). Psychosocial outcome after an intensive neuropsychologically oriented day program: Contributing program variables. In B.P. Uzzell & H.H. Stonnington (Eds.), *Recovery after traumatic brain injury*. Mahwah, NJ: Lawrence Erlbaum Associates.

Diller, L. (1976). A model for cognitive retraining in rehabilitation. *Clinical Psychologist, 29*, 13–16.

Gianutsos, R., & Klitzner. (1981). *Computer programs for cognitive rehabilitation*. Bayport, NY: Life Science Associates.

Goldstein, G., & Malec, E.A. (1989). Memory training for severely amnesic patients. *Neuropsychology, 3*, 9–16.

Goldstein, G., McCue, M., Turner, S.M., Spanier, C., Malec, E.A., & Shelly, C. (1988). The efficacy study of memory training for patients with closed head injury. *The Clinical Neuropsychologist, 2*, 251–259.

Goldstein, K. (1939). *The organism*. New York: American Book Company.

Gordon, W.A., & Hibbard, M.R. (1991). The theory and practice of cognitive remediation. In J.S. Kreutzer & P.H. Wehman (Eds.), *Cognitive rehabilitation for persons with traumatic brain injury* (pp. 13–22). Baltimore: Paul H. Brookes Publishing Company.

Hart, T., & Hayden, M.E. (1986). The ecological validity of neuropsychological assessment and remediation. In B.P. Uzzell & Y. Gross (Eds.), *Clinical neuropsychology of intervention* (pp. 21–71). Boston: Martinus Nijhoff.

Head, H. (1926). *Aphasia and kindred disorders of speech*. Cambridge, MA: Cambridge University Press.

Jackson, J.H. (1879). On affections of speech from disease of the brain. *Brain, 2*, 323–356.

Kazdin, A.E. (1976). Statistical analyses for single-case experimental designs. In M. Hensen & D.N. Barlow (Eds.), *Single-case experimental designs: Strategies for studying behavior change* (pp. 265–316). New York: Pergamon.

Kolb, B. (in press). Brain plasticity and behavior during development. In B.P. Uzzell & H.H. Stonnington (Eds.), *Recovery after traumatic brain injury*. Mahwah, NJ: Lawrence Erlbaum Associates.

Luria, A.R. (1963). *The working brain*. New York: Basic Books.

———. (1980). *Higher cortical functions in man* (2nd ed.). New York: Basic Books.

Moffat, N. (1984). Strategies of memory therapy. In B.A. Wilson & N. Moffat (Eds.), *Clinical management of memory problems* (pp. 63–88). Rockville, MD: Aspen Publishers.

Ponsford, J.L., Olver, J.H., & Curran, C. (1996). Outcome following traumatic brain injury: An Australian study. In B.P. Uzzell & H.H. Stonnington (Eds.), *Recovery after traumatic brain injury*. Mahwah, NJ: Lawrence Erlbaum Associates.

Prigatano, G. (1986). *Neuropsychological rehabilitation after brain injury*. Baltimore: The Johns Hopkins University Press.

Risberg, J., & Jensen, L.R. The value of regional cerebral blood flow measurements in neuropsychological rehabilitation. In A.-L. Christensen & B.P. Uzzell (Eds.), *Brain injury and neuropsychological rehabilitation* (pp. 71–83). Hillsdale, NJ: Lawrence Erlbaum Associates.

Robertson, I.H. (1994). Methodology in neuropsychological rehabilitation research. *Neuropsychological Rehabilitation, 4,* 1–6.

Sohlberg, McM., & Mateer, C.A. (1989). *Introduction to cognitive rehabilitation, theory and practice*. New York: Guilford Press.

Stein, D.G., Glasier, M.M., & Hoffman, S.W. (1994). Pharmacological treatments for brain-injury repair: Progress and prognosis. In A.-L. Christensen & B.P. Uzzell (Eds.), *Brain injury and neuropsychological rehabilitation* (pp. 17–39). Hillsdale, NJ: Lawrence Erlbaum Associates.

3

Rehabilitation and Assessment: Old Tasks Revisited for Computerized Neuropsychological Assessment

José León-Carrión

Facultad de Psicología
Universidad de Seville, Seville, Spain

INTRODUCTION

All neuropsychological rehabilitation processes must begin with an adequate neuropsychological assessment capable of determining what psychological functions are impaired, what zone groups or neural networks are implicated, and what contribution each one makes to the injured functional system. The type of neuropsychological assessment will be fundamental in the design of the chosen therapeutic approach.

The neuropsychologist will perform the assessment to detect the neurocognitive, behavioral, or social deficits that the patient suffers. After the assessment, the neuropsychologist must establish the structural basis that provokes those deficits and the type of organizational deficit of the functional system that produces it. The last point is essential to design the techniques for the restructuring of the damaged functional system and to identify the rehabilitation methods chosen for the rehabilitation process.

However, it should be noted at this time that the neuropsychological assessment is not innocent (i.e., it may have repercussions). There are different assessment models that, in turn, lead to different neuropsychological rehabilitation models. There are two primary models: quantitative and qualitative. Neuropsychologists using a quantitative approach will create a rehabilitation design different from one created by those who focus on the qualitative aspects during the assessment process.

The *quantitative approach* in neuropsychological assessment is perfectly represented in the use of standardized tests and neuropsychological batteries. This is a psychometric model of assessment, and it is based on the results brain injury patients obtain in the tests they have performed. According to Smith (1975), the term "psychometric" literally means "measurements or the measurement of the speed and precision of the mental processes," in contrast to the traditional clinical assessment that assesses the patient's ability to respond to simple medical questions.

Therefore, the quantitative or psychometric approach has its strongest tradition in traditional psychological assessment based on the use of psychological tests and is associated with the traditional medical model and its methodology, procedures, and conception of the disease. Based on such results, the relationship between the injured brain and behavior can be inferred. The clearest representative of this quantitative approach in neuropsychological assessment is Ralph Reitan, whose neuropsychological battery has been considered preeminent in the neuropsychological testing field, in addition to being an objective assessment tool comparable to the WAIS in the measurement of intelligence or of the MMPI for personality. However, it is presently being surpassed by new techniques and procedures (León-Carrión, 1995a).

The *qualitative approach* to neuropsychological assessment is perfectly represented by the European neurological clinical tradition associated with the work of Alexander R. Luria. According to Luria and Majovski (1977), this approach assumes that the main aim of the neuropsychological assessment is to analyze the disorders of the specific higher cortical processes of a person. To this end, it bases itself on the neuropsychological principles of understanding neuropsychology as a discipline concerned fundamentally with the study of the role that the brain systems play in human psychological activity.

The qualitative neuropsychological assessment (Figure 3.1) has its own theoretical framework in a whole-human neuropsychological model. The qualitative assessment tries to ascertain the organic condition that has caused the behavioral disorder in order to analyze its influence in the complete psychological activity of the subject. Thus, once a focal lesion has been localized, its influence must be studied in one or several neurocognitive functional systems.

This type of analysis allows the establishment of those processes that are internally linked to the functional system of the injured person, and, above all, it establishes which other psychological processes of the patient are not functionally altered by the lesion. Therefore, the complete syndrome and its possibilities of recovery can be discovered. Thus, with this methodology, one can discover which modifications take place when there is an alteration in any function, as well as the possible mutual dependence (or relationship) between the different psychological processes. It facilitates the establishment of the specific steps of the neuropsychological treatment for a patient.

The neuropsychological assessment from the qualitative model (Figure 3.1) is a process that has as its objective the discovery of the final structure of the psychological changes that have happened after brain injury. This model stresses the fundamental neurocognitive, behavioral, affective, and/or social effects, as well as the secondary alterations. The neuropsychological data thus obtained from the patient will lead to a neuropsychological rehabilitation design of his/her primary and secondary deficits. This approach follows an experimental methodology: first, formulation, election, and assessment of the problem; second, formulation of a hypothesis; third, confirmation of the hypothesis; and fourth, formulation of a conclusion (León-Carrión, 1995a).

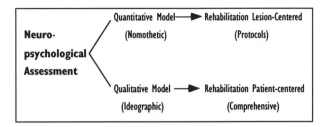

Figure 3.1: The two models of neuropsychological assessment lead to two different models of neuropsychological rehabilitation: one is centered in the lesion and the neurocognitive deficits the patients show using standard tools of rehabilitation. The other is centered in what functions are intact in a particular patient; it has a human neuropsychological frame and uses patient-adapted tools of rehabilitation.

ASSESSMENT AND REHABILITATION

The neuropsychological rehabilitation will depend, therefore, on the assessment model to which the psychologist is committed. Table 3.1 shows the main characteristics of the two principal models of neuropsychological rehabilitation.

Table 3.1: Characteristics of the Main Models of Neuropsychological Rehabilitation

Quantitative Model	Qualitative Model
• Substancialist	• Theoretical frame
• Normative	• Processual
• Magnitude	• Based on injured brain sites
• Based on injured brain sites	and intact brain sites
	• Looks for neuropsychological coherence

The neuropsychological rehabilitation *model* based on actuarial, psychometric, and quantitative data is based on the substancialist, normative, and magnitude assumptions. It focuses mainly on the disorder or deficits that the patient shows. The *substancialist* assumption refers to the deficits observed as the direct result of a lesion in the brain tissue. The *normative* assumption focuses on returning the patient to normalcy. The *magnitude* assumption requires that the progress achieved during rehabilitation be quantifiable in numbers and percentages.

The *qualitative* or *experimental* neuropsychological rehabilitation *model* stems from a fundamental point—the existence of a theoretical framework on human neuropsychological functioning. It is centered in processes more than in results and takes into account the deficits the patient exhibits, as well as the undamaged brain functions. The qualitative evaluators and rehabilitators always have a theoretical framework of human neuropsychological functioning that permits, from the initial interview, coherent focus on the diagnostic process. Therefore, the rehabilitation will make coherent the neuropsychological functioning of the patient after the brain damage.

The neuropsychological coherence is not only obtained by directly rehabilitating the deficits observed in the patient. Some deficits must be considered in relation to the *intact zones* of the brain that play a central role in the rehabilitation process. The neuropsychological rehabilitation must begin taking into account the undamaged functional zones. The neuropsychological rebuilding must initiate with what remains intact and not from what has been damaged. Thus, this qualitative model is *not* centered on returning the patient to his/her earlier normalcy (i.e., rehabilitation process is not centered on patients' return to being as they were before the brain damage) (León-Carrión, 1986). The main objective is to achieve, through the rehabilitation, neuropsychological coherence in patients.

Therefore, in planning the rehabilitation, neuropsychologists are not concerned solely with the quantitative data of the functional impairment or with the final results of the assessment. What neuropsychologists need to know from the assessment is which processes have contributed to the functional disorganization or to the loss of the neuropsychological coherence of the patient.

SEVILLA NEUROPSYCHOLOGICAL TEST BATTERY (BNS)

The following pages show efforts to computerize old tasks and tests of neuropsychological assessments, with the aim that they are useful in the planning of some of the neuropsychological rehabilitation aspects of patients with brain damage. They are tests with a strong psychometric and quantitative component but which can be used by the expert and trained neuropsychologist within the qualitative model (i.e., this battery is designed for its actuarial or quantitative use by those newer neuropsychologists, or by those neuropsychologists who only consider interesting and productive the quantitative neuropsychology). However, at the same time, for clinical neuropsychologists with a broad experience and theoretical framework that guides their professional interventions, the tests that follow will be of great use in achieving a qualitative neuropsychological diagnosis capable of guiding comprehensive neuropsychological rehabilitation.

The BNS tests or tasks obviously do not assess the entire human neuropsychological spectrum. They focus on the assessment of attention, vigilance, inattention, perception, cognitive interferences, reasoning, problem solving, and executive functioning. These functions are central to the assessment of human neuropsychological coherence. The qualitative use of these tests and tasks will complement and enrich their quantitative aspects.

ASSESSMENT OF ATTENTIONAL MECHANISMS

The assessment of attentional mechanisms is one of the challenges of neuropsychologists. This challenge is associated with the difficulty in obtaining an acceptable neuropsychological definition of attention.

On one hand, then, attention cannot be assessed with a single test. The "attention cannot be caught in a single definition, and attention cannot be related to a single cerebral structure." The problem of the present chapter could even be formulated more strongly with this statement: *there are no tests of attention.*[1]

However,

> *although attention concentration and tracking can be differentiated theoretically, in practice they are difficult to separate....Clarifying the nature of an attention problem depends on observations of the patient's general behavior as well as performance on tests involving concentration and tracking, for only by comparing these various observations can the examiner begin to distinguish the single global*

defects of attention from the more discrete, task-specific problems of concentration and tracking. Further, impaired attention is not always a global disability but may involve one receptive or expressive modality more than others. [2]

Recently, an attempt has been made to offer some attentional neuropsychological models that contain the difficulties mentioned above. One of these models has been proposed by Mirsky (1989, p. 85). Attention is not a unitary phenomenon but includes a series of elements or stages supported by different brain regions specialized for this purpose but not organized into a system. More recently, Posner and Petersen (1990, p. 260) made a new proposal for an attentional system:

First, the attention system of the brain is anatomically separate from the data processing systems that perform operations on specific inputs even when the attention is oriented elsewhere. In this sense, the attention system is like other sensory and motor systems. It interacts with other parts of the brain, but maintains its own identity. Second, attention is carried out by a network of anatomical areas. It is neither the property of a single center, nor a general function of the brain operating as a whole (Mesulan, 1981; Rizzolatti et al., 1985). Third, the areas involved in attention carry out different functions, and this specific competence can be specified in cognitive terms (Posner et al., 1988).

For them, attention is composed of two separate although related subsystems: the **posterior attention system,** which orients the individual to objects in the external world and which generates perceptual awareness, and the **anterior attention system,** which orients to the meaning of perceptions and which guides the selection of action. They proposed a possible hierarchy of attention systems in which the anterior system can pass control to the posterior system when it is not occupied with processing other material.

Posner and Petersen's model has been tested by León-Carrión, Rodriguez-Duarte, Barroso y Martín et al. (1995) in patients with traumatic brain injury. They analyzed a series of neuropsychological tests administered to the patients after they were discharged from the hospital. The results of these analyses are characterized by four factors that accounted for 85.4% of the variance. According to their data, factor 1 (perceptual and motor speed) and factor 2 (vigilance and alertness) represent Posner's posterior attention system (PAS). Factor 3 (encoding) and factor 4 (shifting) represent Posner's anterior attentional system (AAS), although they consider that the AAS is not only attention but is shared by other cognitive processes. Their results suggest that the attentional system could be stable and could be defined independently from the type of patient and type of illness.

The tests proposed in BNS to assess attention are those related to factor 1 and factor 2 (i.e., with perceptual and motor speed and vigilance and alertness more related to the posterior attentional system than to the anterior attentional system). They are computerized versions of the old "letter cancellation tasks." The letter to cancel is the "O." The author chooses the "O" because it could be easily confused with "Q," "D," "C," and "G," and the process of alertness needs to be stronger than when the letter to cancel is "A" or "E."

This test is composed of five subtests:

1. Test of attention—Simple cancellations test.
2. Test of vigilance—Conditioned cancellations test.
3. Tachistoscopic attention test for both eyes.
4. Tachistoscopic measure of visual attention of left eye.
5. Tachistoscopic measure of visual attention of right eye.

Test of Attention (Simple Cancellation Test)

The design of this test is as follows. Letters will appear in the center of the screen one by one. The patient has to press the space bar each time the letter "O" appears. The normal administration of the test lasts five minutes.

A possible interpretation of this test is the classic approach. The task measures the simple attentional capacity. In its performance, visual selectivity, motor speed, and the ability to put into action simple attention mechanisms are implied. Low scores indicate impairment or lesion of these mechanisms and could reflect some type of dysfunction at a brainstem level, a diffuse lesion of the brain, or a response to an acute condition of the brain (e.g., a drug or alcohol intoxication, etc.).

When the scores obtained in this test are low or pathological, it's expected that other cognitive tests administered to the patient will also show deficits. Our point of departure is that attention is at the base of all the cognitive processes (see León-Carrión, 1995a). All cognitive processes consume and need attention. If the attention, for whatever reason, deteriorates, all the remaining processes will be affected. Therefore, before assessing and interpreting the results obtained from the patient in other cognitive tests, the current level of attentional processing must be verified. As Posner (1978) pointed out, attention prepares to process high priority signals. But he suggests that alertness does not affect the accumulation of information in the sensory or memory system; it affects the rate at which attention can respond to that stimulus.

Test of Vigilance (Conditioned Cancellation Test)

This test is a variant of the former. The subject has to press the spacebar only if the letter "O" comes after the letter "X." The task lasts five minutes.

This test assesses the vigilance capacity of a person. Therefore, it shows the capacity of sustained attention, the resistance capacity before boring tasks, the capacity for selective motor activation and inhibition, and the capacity of silent activation. Lower scores should indicate a deficit in the vigilance capacity and of the fronto-reticular circuits involved in this process. Following Posner and Petersen (1990, p. 38),

> *alertness involves a specific subsystem of attention that acts on the posterior attention system to support visual orienting and probably also influences other attentional subsystems. Physiologically, this system depends upon the norepinephrine (NE) pathways that arise in the Locus Coeruleus and that is more strongly lateralized in the right hemisphere. Functionally, activation of NE works through the posterior attention system to increase the rate at which high priority visual information can be selected for further processing. This more rapid selection is often at the expense of lower quality information and produces a higher error rate.*

ASSESSMENT OF INATTENTION AND HEMIANOPSIA

These tasks introduced by BNS are related to the assessment of hemispatial neglect and hemi-inattention. Symptoms usually classified as neglect phenomena cannot be explained by a single theoretical model. Instead, there is a multiplicity of neglects that, although phenomenologically different, all share the same basic spatial characteristic (Berti & Rizzolatti, 1994, p. 111). It was Poppelreuter (1917) who introduced the term "inattention" to refer to the neglect syndrome, which was later supported by Brain (1941) and Critchley (1949). In any case, hemi-inattention is correlated with the presence of a visual field defect but is not synonymous with it because some individuals exhibit one without the other (Diller & Weinberg, 1977).

Following Heilman, Valenstein, and Watson (1994, p. 133) neglect could have two underlying mechanisms: inattention (sensory neglect), and disorders of attention and intention (motor neglect) and representational disorders. The inattention or sensory neglect is a deficit in awareness defined by its distribution (personal or spatial) and modality (tactile, visual, or auditory) and may be associated with an attentional bias that usually favors ipsilesional space but can be contralesional. Inattention is also associated with an inability to disengage attention. Following Posner (1994, p. 185), although there is a major organization of the visual-spatial attention system based on visual field (hemisphere), it seems clear that each hemisphere operates to shift the index of attention in the opposite direction. Right hemisphere lesions would only influence left visual field targets, but can also influence left ward shifts of attention within the right visual field.

The tachistoscopic method has not been widely employed in neuropsychological assessment, but the potential for the fruitful application of such techniques is great. Most of the uses are restricted to research rather than clinical applications (McKeever, 1986). The BNS includes three tachistoscopic measures able to be used routinely in the assessment of the attention in patients as well as in normals:

1. Visual fields attention task (both eyes).
2. Visual field attention task (left eye).
3. Visual field attention task (right eye).

In these tests, the screen is imagined to be divided into four identical quadrants: two above and two below. The two left quadrants form the left visual hemifield, and the two to the right form the right visual hemifield. Similarly, the two lower quadrants form the inferior visual hemifield, and the two upper quadrants form the superior visual hemifield. The errors made by a subject may be interpreted as a function of the quadrants and the hemifields in which they are produced.

In the interpretation of the task, neuropsychologists have to remember that the presence of a visual field defect does not necessarily indicate neglect or hemi-inattention; some individuals could exhibit the hemi-visual field defect and not present neglect. Although the diagnosis of neglect or hemi-inattention has to be clinically corroborated by other behavioral signs, at least the following criteria can be associated with hemi-inattention performance on visual cancellation tasks (adapted from Diller & Weinberg, 1977).

1. Errors are always those of omission, never of commission.
2. Errors appear more frequently on the side of the screen contralateral to the brain damage rather than on the ipsilateral side.
3. Many bizarre responses occur. The patients could target any letter when doing the task; the patients move their heads and can't center their eyes on the central point of the screen, focusing on the ipsilateral side of the screen with the lesion.
4. A stimulus on the left side is more likely to be omitted than one of the right.
5. Hemi-neglect is more frequent in patients with right hemisphere lesions (Weinstein, 1994).
6. Attentional deficits that are not apparent with single stimuli may become manifest with multiple simultaneous stimuli (Heilman, Valenstein, & Watson, 1994).

The results a patient obtains in these tasks can be effective in diagnosing *hemianopsia* or *hemianopia* (i.e., in diagnosing a defective vision or blindness in one half of the visual field).[3] When the defective vision is in the right or left halves of the visual fields of the two eyes, there is a *homonymous hemianopsia,* as well as when there is a blindness of one entire visual field as a result of a severe lesion of the optic tract, the lateral geniculate body, or Brodman's area 17. Neither eye can see objects in the opposite field due to the denervation of the corresponding half of each retina in the same side of the lesion. The visual field affected is the same for each eye.

- *Lower Hemianopsia* is a defective vision in the lower half of each eye.
- *Upper Hemianopsia* is the defective vision in the upper half of the visual field.
- *Quadratic hemianopsia* or *Quadrantopia* is a defective vision in one fourth of the visual field in each eye. It could be caused by lesion or destruction of a function of the visual field as a result of a partial lesion of the optic tract, lateral geniculate body, Brodman's area 17, or a lesion of the opposite anterior temporal lobe.
- *Temporal Hemianopsia* is loss of vision in the temporal field of the same side produced by lesion in the optic nerve affecting the nasal retinal fibers on the affected side.
- *Heteronymous* or *Bitemporal Hemianopsia* occurs when the temporal fields of both eyes are affected or lost. It is produced by a lesion on the optic chiasm and the bilateral nasal retinal component of the optic nerves.

This tachitoscopic administration of the visual stimuli also offers a campimetric evaluation of neuropsychological patients.

Tachitoscopic Attention Test for Both Eyes

The tachitoscopic test for both eyes consists of recognizing the letter "O" by pressing the space bar. In the tachistoscopic modules, the letter's position on the screen changes during the test, and **it is necessary that the subject keep his/her eyes fixed on the white point which will remain in the center of the screen during the entire test.** The evaluator must be careful that the subject does not make ocular movements. The interpretation is a function of the hemifields and quadrants in which the patient has made the errors.

Tachistoscopic Measure of Visual Attention of the Left and Right Eyes

These tasks are a variation from the former only in the way they are administered. The left eye tachistoscopic attention test consists of detecting the letter "O" by pressing the space bar while having the right eye covered. The same procedure is followed for the left eye of the patient. Similarly, as when measuring the tachistoscopic visual attention of both eyes, the patient must keep his/her eyes fixed on the white point that remains in the center of the screen during the entire test. The evaluator must make sure the patient does not perform ocular movements. The interpretation of these two tests is based mainly on the perimetric chart or map of the visual field of each eye (Figures 3.2 and 3.3).

ASSESSMENT OF EXECUTIVE FUNCTIONING: THE TOWER OF HANOI-SEVILLA

While it is possible to come to an agreement about the concept of executive function, it is not as easy to arrive at an agreement about methods of assessment. Executive functions or executive system can be conceptualized, but how can they be assessed? The general consensus is that the use of the current psychometric instrument or standard intelligence test is not routinely successful or adequate to differentiate detective frontal lobe damage (Walsh, 1978). When different tests have been used, some different results

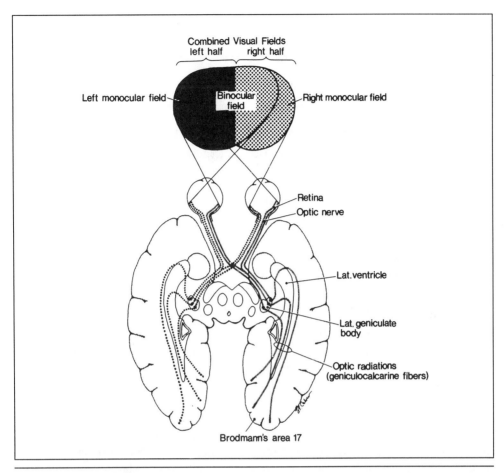

Figure 3.2: The visual pathway is structured so that the visual impulses from the right half of both retinas (representing the left half of the combined visual fields) are transmitted to the right occipital lobe, and all visual impulses from the left half of both retinas (representing the right half of the combined visual fields) are transmitted to the left occipital lobe. Lesions in the visual pathways normally produce complaints of visual deficits showing visual abnormalities. These abnormalities are the results of the lack of impulsive conductions in concrete areas of the visual pathway. (From Dunkerley, 1975.)

have been found. A task widely accepted is the Wisconsin Card Sorting Test (Grant & Berg, 1948; Milner, 1963; Welsh et al., 1991; Welsh & Pennington, 1988; Huber et al., 1992). Other tests that have been proposed are the Category Test (Halstead, 1947), the Tower of London Test (Levin et al., 1994; Shallice, 1992; Morris et al., 1990), the Maze Test (Lezak, 1995; Tow, 1995), and the Tinkertoy Test (Lezak, 1995).

For Lezak (op. cit.), the use of very structured tests may be not be sensitive to deficits of initiation and goal-directed behaviors, so she proposes using fewer structured tasks for the assessment of executive functioning. We propose using the Tower of Hanoi-Sevilla to assess the executive functional system associated with the frontal lobes.

The Tower of Hanoi-Sevilla is a computerized version of the Tower of Hanoi (Cagné & Smith, 1962; Hormann, 1965; Klix, 1971; Egan, 1973; Simon, 1975; León-Carrión et al., 1991; León-Carrión, 1995b). It was originally a game played by children in ancient times that recently has been included in psychological and neuropsychological test

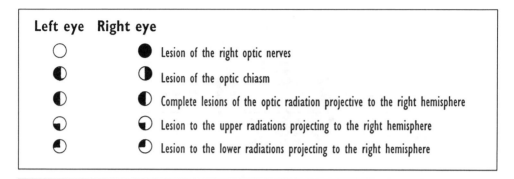

Figure 3.3: Damage to different parts of visual pathways could produce specific visual field deficits.

batteries due to the requirements of the task. These requirements include the abilities of reasoning and problem solving, and the capacity of learning (Anzay & Simon, 1979; Karat, 1982; Simon & Reed, 1976). It is easy to apply, evaluate, and interpret. The task belongs to a transformation problem class, which involves reaching a goal state through the execution of a series of moves using planning and strategies (Karat, op. cit.).

Administration and Procedures

The task is administered through a personal computer (IBM compatible) with a color screen and a normal keyboard. After filling out personal data, subjects receive instructions. There are two kinds of administration: A and B.

We suggest using the administration A of the computerized Tower of Hanoi-Sevilla (León-Carrión, 1996) because this version has obtained higher reliability and validity in assessing functional frontal lobe deficits (León-Carrión, Machuca et al., 1995). The task consists of three choices involving different colored beads and three different pegs that are displayed on the computer screen. The beads are placed in a starting configuration, and subjects must move them onto the third peg using the minimum number of movements and using the minimum amount of time, as well as making the minimum number of errors. The subjects must complete the task knowing some rules. The subjects in this administration (A) are not told they are not permitted to put a large bead over a smaller bead. They are told that it is possible to move the bead placed on the top of the tower, moving only one bead each time. When the patient attempts the task, the computer emits a beeping sound to indicate a mistake and refuses to allow the larger bead to be put over the smaller ones.

The minimum number of moves needed to solve the task is indicated in the formula $(2^n) - 1$, where "n" is the number of beads on peg number one at the beginning. When using three beads, the minimum number of moves is $(2^3) - 1 = 7$. Increasing the number of beads increases the difficulty of the task.

Errors are movements subjects make that computers do not allow, indicated by a beeping noise. There are three types of errors: type 1, type 2, and type 3 errors. Type 1 occurs when the subject tries to move a bead from an empty peg; type 3 occurs when the subject tries to move a larger bead over a smaller one, and type 2 happens when subjects try to move from one peg to the same peg.

Interpretation

The interpretation is made in the framework of the current knowledge about executive functioning and frontal areas of the brain. There are different kinds of people with different executive functioning. Some people could obtain low scores in solving the task. This means that the system needs to operate as a simple network. It seems as if nature could give humans a system capable of solving elementary problems and most importantly, the ability to learn.

A person may have the executive system intact, but the system may not be sophisticated or complex. Cohen (1984) and Cohen et al. (1985) suggested that the Tower of Hanoi might be the kind of task that could be done *procedurally* even by amnesic patients. Procedural learning could be an easy and natural way of building the human executive system, but declarative learning could be a more elaborate way. If education and the stimulating physical and social environment are associated with the former one, then a simple network becomes more complex.

The *total time* taken to complete the task is an index of the velocity of processing and of the integrity of the whole system. The lower the scores, the better the integrity and effectiveness of the system. Subjects need the capacity to begin an activity, as well as the capacity to plan and monitor the appropriate order of subgoals to reach the final goal.

The *total number of movements* can be seen as the use of learning strategies. The lower the scores, the better the uses of the strategies of the system, and the better the use of the feedback mechanisms involved. This may be the best score to indicate the integrity of prefrontal circuits.

The total number of errors can be associated with the mechanisms of monitoring or feedback of the executive system. The lower the scores, the higher the integrity of the mechanism.

Type 3 error scores are an index of learning capacity. They can also result from distraction, impulsivity, and confusion, and poor motor programs. The lower the scores, the higher the ability. *Type 1 and 2 error* scores are an index of the integrity of the system. The subjects do not understand the rules of the tasks. An alternative interpretation is that these two types of responses represent impulsivity.

We agree with Shallice (1982), when studying the Tower of London, that the nature of errors made by the frontal-lobe subjects indicates that they have difficulty in planning and that they could not establish an appropriate order of subgoals.

BNS administration could be a good tool to assess executive function associated with the frontal lobe, especially using administration A, which is a nonstructured task sensitive to deficits of initiation and goal-directed behavior.

ASSESSMENT OF NEUROCOGNITIVE INTERFERENCES

In the past, most neuropsychology was centered on neural and brain *activation* mechanisms. But now it is widely accepted that as important as the neural activation mechanisms are, so are the neural *inhibitory* mechanisms (i.e., at the same time some neural functional systems are activated, others have to be deactivated or inhibited). Each brain functional system is a neural network with a highly specialized and well-controlled balance between activation and inhibition. The integrity of this equilibrium is fundamental for the accuracy and efficacy of the cognitive processes (see Houghton & Tipper, 1994; Zacks & Hasher, 1994), and it is central in neurocognitive and mental disorders (Doyon

& Milner, 1991; David, 1992; Vakil, Weisz, Jedwad, Groswasser, & Aberbuch, 1995; Lobel, Swanda, & Losonczy, 1994).

BNS includes as a task a new computerized version of one of the most widely cited examples for automatic response and uncontrollableness: the Stroop effect (see MacLeod, 1991, for a revision). Certain subtasks indicate how inhibitory processes take place when information goes to the left eye or to the right eye.

The assessment of neurocognitive interferences with BNS is done by the following subtasks:

- Identification of monochromatic words.
- Identification of colors.
- Identification of the color of the words while ignoring the meaning of the words.
- Identification of the meaning of the word while ignoring the color of the words.
- Identification of the color of the word ignoring the meaning of the words—Right eye presentation.
- Identification of the color of the words ignoring the meaning of the words—Left eye presentation.
- Identification of the meaning of the words ignoring the color of the words—Right eye presentation.
- Identification of the meaning of the words ignoring the color of the words—Left eye presentation.

INTERPRETATION

The computer calculates four scores for each of the eight subtests that make up the test, including the number of congruencies, the number of noncongruencies, the mean time of response, and the total time used in taking the test. In the analysis of the test results, one can obtain the interference index, task index, correction index, and efficacy index. Different studies have shown that this test is indicated to assess frontal and prefrontal functioning (Perret, 1974; Regard, 1981; Stuss & Benson, 1986; Vendrell, Junqué, Pujol et al., 1995). Studies using Positron Emission Tomography (PET) have implicated the anterior cingulate gyrus in selecting information in a Stroop task (Pardo, Pardo, Janer, & Reichle, 1990). At the same time, using the mean time score the patient obtains, one can infer the speed of the process of activation/inhibition. Scores on monocular vision tasks offer important information for research purposes.

ENDNOTES

1. Van Zomeren & Brouwer, 1994, p. 249.
2. Lezak, 1995, p. 352.
3. The visual field of each eye has both temporal (lateral) and nasal (medial) sides. The nasal site is projected to the temporal part of the retina and the temporal site is projected to the nasal part of the retina. The binocular vision is produced by the overlapping of the nasal sites of both left and right visual field.

REFERENCES

Anzay, Y., & Simon, H.A. (1979). The theory of learning by doing. *Psychological Review, 86,* 124–140.
Berti, A., & Rizzolatti, G. (1994). Is neglect a theoretical coherent unit? In P.W. Halligan & J.C. Marsall (Eds.), *Spatial neglect: positions papers on theory and practise* (pp. 111–114). Mahwah, NJ: Lawrence Erlbaum Associates.

Brain, W.R. (1941). Visual disorientation with special reference to lesions of the right cerebral hemisphere. *Brain, 64,* 244–272.

Cohen, N.J. (1984). Preserved learning capacity in amnesia: Evidence for multiple memory systems. In L.R. Squire & N. Butters (Eds.), *Neuropsychology of memory* (1st ed.) (pp. 83–103). New York: Guilford Press.

Cohen, N.J., Eichenbaum, H., DeAcedo, H., & Corkin, S. (1985). Different memory systems underlying acquisition of procedural and declarative knowledge. *Annals of the New York Academy of Sciences, 444,* 54–71.

Critchley, M. (1949). The phenomenon of tactile inattention with special reference to parietal lesions. *Brain, 72,* 583–561.

David, S. (1992). Stroop effects within and between the cerebral hemispheres: Studies in normal and acallosals. *Neuropsychologia, 30,* 161–175.

Diller, L., & Weinberg, J. (1977). Hemi-inattention in rehabilitation: Devolution of a rational remediation program. In E.A. Weinstein & R.P. Friendland (Eds.), *Advances in neurology* (p. 18). New York: Raven Press.

Doyon, J., & Milner, B. (1991). Right temporal-lobe contribution to global visual processing. *Neuropsychologia, 29,* 343–360.

Egan, D.E. (1973). The structure of experience acquired while learning to solve a class problem. Unpublished doctoral thesis. Michigan University.

Gagné, R.M., & Smith, E.C. (1962). A study of the effects of verbalization on problem solving. *Journal of Experimental Psychology, 63,* 12–18.

Grant, P.B., & Berg, E.A. (1948). Behavioral analyses of degree of reinforcement and case of shifting to new response in a Weigl-type card-sorting problem. *Journal of Experimental Psychology, 38,* 404–411.

Halstead, W.C. (1947). *Brain and intelligence: A quantitative study of the frontal lobes.* Chicago: University of Chicago Press.

Heilman, K., Valenstein, E., and Watson, R. (1994). The what and how of neglect. In P.W. Halligan & J.C. Marsall (Eds.), *Spatial neglect: Position papers on theory and practice* (pp. 133–139). Mahwah, NJ: Lawrence Erlbaum Associates.

Hormann, A.M. (1965). Gaku: An artificial student. *Behavior Science, 10,* 88–107.

Houghton, G., & Tipper, S.P. (1994). A model of inhibition mechanisms in selective attention. In D. Dagenbach & T.H. Carr (Eds.), *Inhibitory processes in attention, memory and language* (pp. 53–112). San Diego: Academic Press.

Huber, S.I., Bornstein, R.A., Ranoham, K.W., & Christy, A. (1992). Magnetic resonance imaging correlates of executive function: Impairment in multiple sclerosis. *Neuropsychiatry, Neuropsychology and Behavioral Neurology, 5,* 33–36.

Karat, J. (1982). A model of problem solving with incomplete constraint knowledge. *Cognitive Psychology, 14,* 538–559.

Klix, F. (1971). *Information und verhalten.* Berlin: VEB Deustcher Verlag der Wissenschaften.

León-Carrión, J. (1986). Tratamiento psicológico de personas con daño cerebral. *Apuntes de Psicología, 18/19,* 26–32.

———. (1995a). *Handbook of human neuropsychology.* Madrid/Mexico: Siglo XXI Ed.

———. (1995b). *Sevilla Computerized Neuropsychological Test Battery (BNS).* Orlando: G.R. Press.

León-Carrión, J., Dominguez-Morales, M.R., Rodriguez-Duarte, R., Barroso-Martin, J.M., & Machuca, F. (in press). The attention system in brain injury survivors. *International Journal of Neuroscience.*

León-Carrión J., Machuca, F. et al. (1995). *Fiabilidad y validez de la torre de Hanoi-Sevilla: Datos preliminares.* Paper presented at the third symposium of the Spanish Society of Neuropsychology. September, Oviedo, Spain.

León-Carrión, J., Morales, M., Forastero, P., Dominguez, M.R., Murillo, F., Jimenez, R., & Gordón, P. (1991). The computerized Tower of Hanoi: A new form of administration and suggestions for interpretation. *Perceptual and Motor Skills, 73,* 63–66.

Levin, H.S., Mendelson, D., Lilly, M., Fletcher, J., Culhane, K., Chapman, S., Hardward, H., Kusnerik, L., Bruce, D., & Eisenberg, M. (1994). Tower of London in relation to magnetic resonance imaging following closed head injury in children. *Neuropsychology, 8,* 171–179.

Lezak, M.D. (1995). *Neuropsychological assessment* (3rd ed.). New York: Oxford University Press.

Lobel, D.S., Swanda, R.M., & Losonczy, M.F. (1994). Lateralized visual-field inattention in schizophrenia. *Perceptual and Motor Skills, 79,* 699–702.

Luria, A.R., & Majovski, L.V. (1977). Basic approaches used in American and Soviet clinical neuropsychology. *American Psychologist, 32,* 959–968.

MacLeod, C.M. (1991). Half a century of research on the Stroop effect: An integrative review. *Psychological Bulletin, 109,* 103–203.

McKeever, W.F. (1986). Tachistoscopic methods in neuropsychology. In H.J. Hannay (Ed.), *Experimental techniques in human neuropsychology* (pp. 167–211). New York: Oxford University Press.

Mesulan, M.M. (1981). A cortical network for directed attention and unilateral neglect. *Ann. Neurol., 10,* 309–325.

Milner, B. (1963). Effects of different brain lesions on card sorting. *Archives of Neurology, 9,* 90–100.

Mirsky, A.F. (1989). The neuropsychology of attention: Elements of a complex behaviour. In E. Perecman (Comp.), *Integrating theory and practice in clinical neuropsychology.* Mahwah, NJ: Lawrence Erlbaum Associates.

Morris, R., Downes, J., & Robbins, T. (1990). The nature of disexecutive syndrome in Parkinson's disease. In K. Gilhooly, W. Keave, R. Loge, & G. Erdos (Eds.), *Diseases of thinking.* New York: Wiley and Sons.

Pardo, J.V., Pardo, P.J., Janer, K.W., & Mesulam, M.M. (1990). The anterior cingulate cortex mediates processing selection in the Stroop attentional conflict paradigm. *Proceedings of the National Academy of Sciences USA, 87,* 256–259.

Perret, E. (1974). The left frontal lobe of man and the suppression of habitual responses in verbal categorical behavior. *Neuropsychologia, 12,* 323–330.

Poppelreuter, W.K. (1917). *Die Psychischen Schadigungen durch Kopfschuss im Krieg 1914-1916: Die Störungen der niederen und höheren Leistungen durch Veletzungen des Ikzipitalhirns. Vol. I.* Leipzig: Leopold Voss.

Posner, M.I. (1978). *Chronometic explorations of mind.* Hillsdale, NJ: Lawrence Erlbaum Associates.

———. (1994). Neglect and spatial attention. In P.W. Halligan & J.C. Marsall, *Spatial neglect: Position papers on theory and practise* (pp. 111–114). Mahwah, NJ: Lawrence Erlbaum Associates.

Posner, M.I., & Petersen, S.E. (1990). The attention system of the human brain. *Annual Review of Neuroscience, 13,* 25–42.

Posner, M.I., Petersen, S.E., Fox, P.T., & Raichle, M.E. (1988). Localization of cognitive operations in the human brain. *Science, 240,* 1627–1631.

Rizzolatti, G., Gentilucci, M., & Matelli, M. (1985). Selective spatial attention: One center, one circuit or many circuits. In M. Posner and O.S.M. Marin (Eds.), *Attention and Perfomance XI* (pp. 251–265). Hillsdale, NJ: Lawrence Erlbaum Associates.

Shallice, T. (1982). Specific impairment of planning. In D.E. Broadbent & L. Weiskrantz (Eds.), *The neuropsychology of cognitive function.* London: The Royal Society.

Shallice, T. (1992). *Neuropsychological investigation of supervisory processes: Attention, awareness, and control. A tribute to Donald Broadbent.* Oxford: Oxford University Press.

Shapiro, K.L., & Raymond, J.E. (1994). Temporal allocation of visual attention: Inhibitory or interference? In D. Dagenbach & T.H. Carr (Eds.), *Inhibitory processes in attention, memory and language* (pp. 151–188). San Diego: Academic Press.

Simon, H.A. (1975). The functional equivalence of problem solving skills. *Cognitive Psychology, 7,* 268–288.

Simon, H.A., & Reed, S.H. (1976). Modeling strategies in a problem solving task. *Cognitive Psychology, 8,* 86–87.

Smith, A. (1975). Neuropsychological testing in neuropsychological disorders. In W.J. Friendlander (Comp.), *Advances in neurology* (Vol. 7). New York: Raven Press.

Stuss, D.T., & Benson, D.F. (1986). *The frontal lobes.* New York: Raven Press.

Tow, P.M. (1955). *Personality changes following frontal leucotomy.* London: Oxford University Press.

Vakil, E., Weisz, H., Jedwab, L., Groswasser, Z., & Aberbuch, S. (1995). Stroop color-word task as a measure of selective attention: efficiency in closed head-injured patients. *Journal of Clinical Experimental Neuropsychology, 17,* 335–342.

Van Zomeren, A.H., & Brouwer, W.H. (1994). *Clinical neuropsychology of attention*. New York: Oxford University Press.

Vendrell, P., Junqué, C., Pujol, J., Jurado, M.A., Molet, J., & Grafman, J. (1995). The role prefrontal regions in the stroop task. *Neuropsychologia, 33*, 341–352.

Walsh, K.W. (1978). Frontal lobe problems. In G.V. Stanley & K.W. Walh (Eds.), *Brain impairment: Proceedings of the 1976 Brain Impairment Workshop*. Parkville, Victoria, Australia: Neuropsychology Group, Department of Psychology, University of Melbourne.

Weinstein, E.A. (1994). Hemineglect and extinction. In P.W. Halligan & J.C. Marsall (Eds.), *Spatial neglect: Position papers on theory and practise* (pp. 221–224). Mahwah, NJ: Lawrence Erlbaum Associates.

Welsh, M.C., Pennington, B.F., & Groisser, D.B. (1991). A normative- developmental study of executive function: A window on prefrontal function in children. *Developmental Neuropsychology, 7*, 131–149.

Welsh, M.C., & Pennington, B.F. (1988). Assessing frontal lobe functioning in children: Views from developmental psychology. *Developmental Neuropsychlogy, 4*, 199–230.

Zacks, R., & Hasher, L. (1994). Directed ignoring: iInhibition regulation on working memory. In D. Dagenbach & T.H. Carr (Eds.), *Inhibitory processes in attention, memory and language* (pp. 241–264). San Diego: Academic Press.

4 The Design of Neuropsychological Rehabilitation: The Role of Neuropsychological Assessment

Carla Caetano and Anne-Lise Christensen

Center for Rehabilitation of Brain Injury
Copenhagen University, Denmark

INTRODUCTION

Neuropsychological rehabilitation coexists with neuropsychological assessment, but the nature of the relationship may differ widely. This is due to the complex historical developments that both assessment procedures and rehabilitation approaches have taken. Initially, neuropsychological assessment was used to diagnose "organicity." However, with recent advances in neurological radiology, neuropsychological assessment outside of a rehabilitation context has increasingly moved away from localizing brain impairment to, for example, differentiating between two behaviorally similar disorders and/or evaluating the underlying causes of neuropsychological complaints (Bauer, 1995).

In assessments pertaining to neuropsychological rehabilitation, besides identifying deficits, there should also be an evaluation of the individual in a broader context. Historically, Boake (1991) notes that World War I marked the first time that there was significant survival from severe brain trauma due to improved medical care. Initially, treatment emphasized individualized management of physical difficulties and the treatment of specific cognitive deficits such as aphasia (e.g., in Germany and the United States). During World War II, however, treatment centers developed in the United States, in the Soviet Union, and in Great Britain that covered the acute stages through community re-entry. Although combined forms of therapy were used in treatment in the United States (e.g., occupational therapy, vocational services, and speech and language therapy, etc.), it was only in 1975 that Ben-Yishay and Diller established a holistic treatment program for patients with head injury near Tel Aviv, which came to serve as a guideline for current programs. As such, treatment goals in brain injury rehabilitation have also come to reflect these aspects of behavior, and emphasis has shifted from specific impairment training to holistic rehabilitation programs that integrate cognitive retraining with psychosocial and vocational goals, as may be seen in programs such as those found at the Center for Rehabilitation of Brain Injury in Denmark.

As a result of the development of such holistic programs, increasing emphasis has been on the psychosocial changes that occur after brain injury and the consequences this has on significant others. For example, Thomsen (1984) reports that with a 10- to 15-year follow-up of severe (PTA > 1 month) head-injured patients, although physical and cognitive impairments persist, permanent changes in personality and emotion are reported as the most serious problem by significant others. Similarly, Brooks, Campsie, Symington, Beattie, and McKinlay (1986) report that both at one- and five-year post-injury follow-ups (PTA>two days), psychosocial factors such as personality change and mood changes continue to exist along with the cognitive sequelae. Significant others again report having particular difficulty in dealing with the psychosocial changes, such that the greater the personality and behavioral changes in the brain-injured person, the greater the distress to relatives. Gainotti (1993) provides a thorough discussion of the predominant factors underlying the emotional and psychosocial problems after brain injury and the reasons why these aspects of brain injury sequelae have largely been ignored to date.

Current neuropsychological assessment and rehabilitation procedures, therefore, attempt to incorporate not only the cognitive sequelae of brain injury but also the broader psychosocial concerns of the brain-injured individual and family members. The program of the Center for Rehabilitation of Brain Injury (CRBI), Copenhagen University, Denmark, will now be presented to illustrate the manner in which these various aspects of assessment and rehabilitation interact to provide comprehensive post-acute rehabilitation of the brain-injured adult.

THE CENTER FOR REHABILITATION OF BRAIN INJURY

Theoretical Foundations

The CRBI is a comprehensive day treatment program for brain-injured adults, which was established by the founder of the Center (the second author) in 1985. The work of Luria (1966) has provided the theoretical foundation for the Center's assessment and rehabilitation approach, with his emphasis on a qualitative, individualized, hypothesis-testing approach. Equally important has been the work of Goldstein (1942, 1952), who emphasized a psychosocial rather than medical model in the understanding and treatment of brain injury. He was also influential in stressing the existential needs of brain-injured individuals rather than only the cognitive dysfunctions caused by brain injury. Furthermore, the development of group-based rehabilitation programs in the United States, particularly those of Ben-Yishay and associates (Ben-Yishay et al., 1978–1983) and Prigatano (Prigatano et al., 1986) have also provided the means by which a comprehensive approach could be achieved.

The location of the CRBI at the University of Copenhagen, rather than in a medical setting, is consistent with a psychosocial model of rehabilitation that stresses the principles of education and learning in active collaboration with the patients (at the CRBI, termed "students") in the recovery process. For treatment to be consistent with the individualized and qualitative approach of Luria, as well as comprehensive in orientation as stressed by a psychosocial model, all aspects of the brain-injured individual's functioning must be addressed (i.e., the cognitive, psychosocial, and physical needs of the individual). This has to be done in an individualized manner, and broader issues such as changes in levels of awareness and self-identity must be addressed. The needs of significant others and broader quality of life issues must also be considered.

The CRBI Program

The program is structured in the following manner. Typically 15 patients attend the program Tuesdays through Fridays from 9:00 A.M. until 3:00 P.M. (although the students frequently socialize outside of these hours) over approximately a 4-month period. Table 4.1 indicates the weekly structure of each of the activities.

Table 4.1: Day Program Activities (does not include follow-up activities)

Individual Activities		Group Activities	
Type	**Hours per week**	**Type**	**Hours per week**
Cognitve Training	1–2	Morning Meeting	4
Psychotherapy	2–3	Cognitve Training	3
Family Therapy	varies as needed	Psychotherapy	1.5
Voice Training	1–2	Project Groups	1.5
Speech & Language Therapy	1–3	Speech & Language Therapy	1
Physical Therapy	3	Significant Others	4 hours per month
Special Education	1–2		

The program is based on assessment and rehabilitation procedures that interact in a dynamic process through the process of feedback. Feedback occurs through two primary means: (1) formalized assessment that is quantitative and qualitative in nature and (2) through behavioral observations during program participation. The feedback may be from the therapists, from other students in the program, and/or by self-evaluation.

At the CRBI, formalized assessment and behavioral assessments are intrinsic to an individualized, hypothesis-testing, rehabilitation approach. Although it is in the individual sessions with each student's primary therapist that much of the feedback and integration of the rehabilitation process occurs, the group activities are equally important in providing the necessary contexts for behavior to be observed, ongoing assessments to be made, hypotheses to be generated, and treatment to be influenced. Because of the manner in which the program elements are structured, all the activities include the three possibilities for feedback previously mentioned—therapists, program peers, or self-evaluation.

1. *Individual activities* include cognitive training and psychotherapy with a psychologist, as well as language therapy for aphasics and voice training typically for dysarthric conditions with a speech and language therapist and voice therapist, respectively. A special education teacher provides training for those patients who require assistance in basic academic skills. Individualized physical training in groups is also provided.

2. *Group-based activities,* which include all the students participating together, consist of the daily morning meetings and the lecture series that is provided once a week. The morning meeting is built around a series of activities that serve to facilitate orientation and interaction, as well as requiring individual responsibili-

ties, and is typically facilitated by two staff members. The lecture series consists of a variety of topics related to brain injury, as well as topics of broader interest, and include visiting speakers, musicians, or previous students. One weekly group activity that includes all the students along with most of the treatment staff is the Friday "Joint Meeting," which allows for students and staff to evaluate and provide feedback on any aspect of the week's activities or occurrences.

Other group activities that typically occur with the overall group being subdivided into two smaller groups focus on (1) group cognitive training, (2) project groups, (3) group psychotherapy, and (4) physical training activities. With the exception of the physical training, all other groups are run by psychologists in collaboration with the speech and language therapist and/or special education teacher.

Thus, throughout the program period, feedback occurs based initially on (1) *formalized assessment,* which consists of qualitative and quantitative measures used by the therapists, and (2) *analysis of interpersonal interactions* by therapists, the participants themselves, and other program participants, all of which is incorporated throughout the program.

A discussion of the various evaluation procedures and some of the program activities will be provided to illustrate the manner in which these various feedback processes occur.

Formalized Assessment Procedures

Prior to program entry, qualitative evaluations are made by use of Luria's Neuropsychological Investigation (LNI) (Christensen, 1984) and the use of self and family report questionnaires to describe psychosocial functioning. The LNI is administered at the intake evaluation and integrated with the intake interviews of the student and family members (General Patient Inventory) as well as the medical records. The questionnaires are administered with the more psychometrically oriented cognitive evaluations used as pre-, post-, and one- and three-year follow-ups.

Qualitative Measures: The LNI

Luria's evaluation method is based on an individualized, qualitative methodology that reflects a Russian rather than Western tradition (Luria, 1979). Intrinsic to this phenomenological and interactive approach is the trusting, therapeutic relationship between patient and psychologist, where emphasis is placed on a collaborative, problem-solving, working relationship. Thus, task modification is important in the evaluation process and may include giving the patient more time or explanations to complete a task, allowing the patient to copy certain tasks, or asking patients to give their perception of the task, etc., so as to constantly obtain feedback on the unique nature of the patient's abilities (i.e., in terms of existing compensatory strategies and/or identifying alternate problem-solving strategies).

Luria (1966) describes the evaluation process as the analysis of disturbances in the hierarchically constructed motor, tactile-kinesthetic, visual, and auditory analyzers in terms of "syndrome analysis," where the general signs among the results of the assorted tests are grouped together into a unified syndrome composed of externally heterogenous but internally interrelated symptoms. The exact process through which the evaluation procedure should be conducted is comprehensively described in *Luria's Neuropsychological Investigation* (Christensen, 1984).

Based on observations of Luria's working method in his laboratory, Christensen (1989) notes that the evaluation process begins with history taking of the status of the patient where the state of consciousness and level of orientation of the patient is established (providing information on the functioning of subcortical structures). Thereafter, the premorbid level of the patient is ascertained (which also allows for an evaluation of the patient's memory), and an evaluation is made of the patient's awareness and self-evaluation of his/her situation in the discussion of the patient's subjective complaints. During the second phase of testing, a series of simple and short preliminary tests are performed to provide a comprehensive overview of the motor, auditory, visual, and tactile areas. The third phase consists of a more selective process of testing, where a more detailed evaluation is made of complex activities (e.g., language, memory) by varying the manner in which information is presented so as to establish the circumstances under which patients function best and where they encounter difficulties. This allows the neuropsychologist, therefore, not only to identify areas of strength and weakness but also to generate hypotheses about why a complex psychological task has failed. A comprehensive understanding of the functioning and organization of the nervous system is, therefore, essential to identifying the nature and extent of the brain injury.

This rich, qualitative analysis of functioning of the LNI provides the background on which additional information derived from the sources below are incorporated.

Quantitative Measures: Questionnaires to Evaluate Psychosocial Functioning

A semi-structured interview is used to obtain information from the patients and their significant others on past and present medical and psychosocial situations. Additional information is obtained by questionnaires that are administered to both patients and relatives. These include the specially devised questionnaire for brain-injured patients, the European Brain Injury Questionnaire (EBIQ). The questionnaire was developed by the Integration Subgroup of the EU-sponsored program ESCAPE (European Standardized Computerized Assessment Procedure for the Evaluation and Rehabilitation of Brain-Damaged Patients). Previously used measures such as the SCL90-R and the Katz-R were found to be of limited value in the evaluations of brain-injured patients (see Rattock, Ross, & Ohry, 1994; Teasdale & Caetano, [in press] for examples of such difficulties regarding the SCL-90). As such, the EBIQ has been used instead of these measures. An adapted version of an ADL questionnaire is also included.

Additional psychological information may be obtained from nonquestionnaire measures such as the Rorschach or the Thematic Apperception Test (TAT).

Quantitative Measures: Cognitive Neuropsychological Tests

The following measures are regarded as complementary to the information obtained from the LNI and the intake interview information and medical records. While the LNI is constructed to provide an individualized measure of cognitive functioning, the measures described here provide an opportunity for normative comparisons. Qualitative observations are, nonetheless, stressed in interpreting results even on these measures. For the sake of clarity, the normative measures will be described under specific cognitive categories, although they obviously overlap with other categories of cognitive functioning. Unless otherwise specified, detailed information about the particular tests may be found in Lezak (1995).

- *General intellectual functioning*: Evaluations are made using two subtests of the Danish normed Weschler Adult Intelligence Scale-Revised (WAIS-R). These include the Information Subtest, which provides data on the knowledge of general culture and the Vocabulary Subtest, which provides an indication of general mental ability. The twelve item Ravens Advanced Progressive Matrices is also used as a screening measure, as well as for evaluating problem solving strategies.

- *Attention/concentration*: A series of measures is used (i.e., two subtests from the WAIS-R, two paper-and-pencil tests, computerized reaction times, and an adaptation of the original PASAT). The WAIS-R subtests include Digit Symbol, which also evaluates visual motor coordination (dexterity) and the ability to learn a new task, and the Digit Span Subtest, which is particularly useful in evaluating immediate auditory recall as well as freedom from distractibility. The paper-and-pencil tests include the d2 (Brickenkamp, 1981), which is primarily a cancellation test that also requires attention to detail and visual scanning and that evaluates sustained attention as well (Spreen & Strauss, 1991). The Trail Making Test A & B is the other paper-and-pencil test that also evaluates visual-conceptual and visual-motor tracking components. Two elements of the computerized Memory Assessment Clinic (MAC) batteries are also used to evaluate visual reaction times and divided attention. For a description of the battery, refer to Larrabee, West, and Crooke (1991). Finally, there is the Danish version of the Paced Auditory Serial Addition Test (PASAT), with norms provided by Gade and Mortensen (1984), where the main variant is that the test is not "paced" (i.e., the examiner proceeds at the pace at which the patient is able to comply with the requirements). In the Danish version, a series of randomized digits is initially only asked to be repeated. In the second part of the test, each digit is added to the digit immediately preceding it in a series.

- *Visual spatial functioning*: WAIS-R subtests are primarily used, namely the Picture Completion Subtest, which evaluates attention to visual detail. The Block Design Subtest is also used to measure visual motor coordination, perceptual organization, spatial visualization, nonverbal reasoning, and analytical thinking, while the Picture Arrangement Subtest obtains information on perception, analysis, and synthesis of socially depicted events.

- *Memory:* The primary measure of memory is the computerized MAC battery that has American norms. It was developed as a result of limitations in current memory tests (i.e., the need for repeated measures and, therefore, alternate forms and for ecological validity in relation to everyday life). It consists of various verbal and nonverbal subtests, such as locating misplaced objects, facial recognition (delayed nonmatching to sample), reaction time (i.e., a lift and travel component) without interference (information processing), with interference (divided attention), name/face association (delayed), selective reminding of a grocery list, and first/last name learning. In addition, the Weschler Memory Scale Logical Memory Subtest (translated into Danish) is also used to evaluate free recall of a short story following an auditory presentation, and a 30-minute delayed recall is included.

- *Language:* Language functioning is measured by a Danish translation of selected subtests of the Boston Diagnostic Aphasia Examination (BDAE) (Goodglass & Kaplan, 1972).

- *Additional Measures:* A variety of other neuropsychological measures in the various cognitive domains may be included to provide additional information to the above measures.

The second form of evaluation that takes place, namely behavior observation, will now be discussed in greater detail to illustrate the manner in which it is used as feedback and, therefore, also as a means of integrating the corresponding changes in treatment that occur as a result of this feedback.

Analysis of Interpersonal Interactions in Program Participation

Feedback is based on an analysis of interpersonal interactions of the program participants in individual and group activities. The feedback process, as previously stated, may be generated by therapists, fellow program participants, and/or self-evaluation. Some examples of individual and group-based activities will now be discussed to show how this feedback process occurs.

Individual Treatment

The participants in the program may be seen individually by any of the staff, depending on the nature of their difficulties. The psychologist, however, serves as the primary therapist for a maximum of two students. In the individual hours with the psychologist, the emphasis is on providing a sense of continuity for the program participant. Thus, during this time, all the sources of feedback that the student has been given need to be integrated into a meaningful rehabilitation plan that addresses all aspects of the brain injury.

Group Treatment

- *Cognitive Training Group:* There are approximately five patients per group, selected for elements of cognitive homogeneity (e.g., premorbid intellectual functioning, level of language impairment, and speed of information processing). This information is obtained not only from the qualitative and quantitative test results but also from analysis of interpersonal interactions during a first week "program trial" period of participation in various group activities. Premorbid intellectual functioning is primarily deduced from past educational or occupational activities. Once established, the group serves to create awareness of specific areas of strength and weakness, as well as demonstrating ecologically valid relationships between the tasks completed in the training and external to the training hours. The tasks selected are dependent on the predominant difficulties of the individuals within the group. Thus, certain tasks may be excluded/amplified. Typically, the group is structured as follows. There is an introductory session where various cognitive functions are discussed, and group members are typically encouraged to identify their cognitive strengths and difficulties. Training begins with attentional tasks that are given in increasing complexity similar to those described by Sohlberg and Mateer (1989). Memory tasks may include development of a standardized calender and visualization techniques, etc. Study techniques may also be included (e.g., the use of mindmaps, the PQRST technique (Wilson, 1987), problem-solving tasks based on the principles of the Six Elements Test (Shallice & Burgess, 1991), and various inductive and deductive reasoning tasks).

  As there are two or three staff members present, the approximate 2:1 student/staff ratio allows for each patient to be monitored individually. Task requirements, therefore, are individually tailored within the group context as much as possible, so that the use of inappropriate tasks is minimized and individualized feedback can be given by the therapist.

The group context, however, is important in that it provides a more realistic working environment where susceptibility to distractions can be monitored. It provides the opportunity for feedback from peers, which gives social support, and allows patients to benefit from others' difficulties and coping strategies.

Self-evaluation is encouraged by the students keeping a "Cognitive File," which consists of categorizing the completed tasks, keeping a record of ongoing performance on a summary sheet, and creating graphs to monitor performance. Thus, approximately once a week, each student is asked to provide a summary of their week's performance to the group by means of graphs presented on overheads. Emphasis is placed on self-comparison and not on comparisons with other members of the group.

- *Project Group:* Essentially, the rationale is to create a context in which ecologically valid tasks can *only* be completed with the cooperative interaction of all participants. Thus, this process ensures that various elements of rehabilitation (e.g., cognitive training, individual psychotherapy, social interaction, etc.) become integrated in a meaningful manner. The students are divided into two groups and are similarly selected for elements of behavioral homogeneity (e.g., premorbid intellectual level, level of language impairment, and speed of information processing). What is more important, however, is that group members are matched as much as possible on past educational or occupational activities, as well as on their future plans in these areas. Group activities may include collaboration on the completion of "mini-projects" during the semester and/or joint collaboration on a "final project" presented to all students/staff at the end of the semester. The groups are structured as follows. Initially, the staff may provide specific short-term, problem-solving tasks that are to be completed. Thereafter, group members are encouraged to select "real life" tasks that are of particular interest to them. This process typically involves brainstorming, selection of one idea, group planning of task completion, and the initiation and completion of a task at a given deadline. Some examples of mini-projects are planning outings for the group (e.g., an informational visit to the parliament, which also requires the preparation of questions to ask the Ministers) and brief video presentations (e.g., 5 min. per student on a selected topic of common interest). Some examples of final projects are a video film about the rehabilitation process, a brochure on aphasia, a presentation of a Danish tourist attraction, and a memorabilia booklet on the staff and students based on a questionnaire.

As emphasis is placed on the development of a collaborative teamwork approach and problem-solving skills/strategies, this group activity provides not only an excellent opportunity for the individuals to self-evaluate strengths and deficits in this regard but also their potential to empathically and appropriately respond to others in the group. Peer and staff feedback also serve to fulfill this function.

- *Group Psychotherapy:* Once again the larger group of 15 patients is divided into 2 groups of approximately 6 patients per group. In this group activity, diversity in terms of sex, level of language impairment, and speed of information processing is preferred. This permits a balanced exchange of this predominantly verbally oriented group, where emphasis is on the communication of psychosocial status (i.e., attitudes, feelings, and relational concerns on a wide variety of subjects related to brain injury). The primary rationale of such a group is to create a context for peer discussion that develops awareness of each individual's psychosocial status and also allows for peer feedback and support. This also provides an opportunity for patients to minimize social isolation by interacting with others on a more personal level in that there is acknowledgment of psychosocial needs, and an empathic understanding of oneself and others is encouraged.

The group is structured for peer discussion with two therapists serving as facilitators. The group topics are generated from previous discussion either by the students or by the therapists and typically include an introductory session where potential topics are raised. The group discussion is usually summarized at the beginning and end of each session to facilitate continuity, particularly for those students with concentration and memory problems. Participation may be spontaneous or further encouraged by each student being asked to "take a turn" when discussing various topics. Topics that have been dealt with have included themes of the difficulties in acceptance of oneself after injury, as well as acceptance by others, changes in identity, the expectations and disappointments of the rehabilitation process, and the future—plans, fears, hopes, etc.

Each group, therefore, can be seen as providing the various elements of feedback requirements that are integrated not only in these groups but also in the individual treatment hours with the psychologist. As such, an individually designed rehabilitation program such as the CRBI is consistently influenced by these two broad-based treatment approaches to provide effective treatment. Ultimately, however, assessment and rehabilitation have to prove to be effective in terms of a complex interplay of factors, such as premorbid qualities, the injury type, and the specific sequelae of injury, as well as the type of measure used to evaluate such factors.

Future research should focus on the best manner in which to evaluate the effectiveness of treatment. Bearing in mind the complexity of the process described above, it may be argued that traditional experimental designs with emphasis on control groups and the effects of specific independent variables on groups of individuals may not be possible to establish. Similarly, it could be argued that measures of cognitive functions, such as traditional neuropsychological tests, may not be sophisticated enough to provide the necessary information on the complex interactions of emotion and behavior. Alternate approaches need to be found to adequately address an understanding of brain injury and its consequences. For example, with regard to research design, single case studies could be considered (Yin, 1994), or should group studies be used, variations in the elements of rehabilitation treatment could be studied with regard to effectiveness (Diller & Ben-Yishay, 1987).

Outcome measures that have better ecological validity may be questionnaires and/or other interpersonal measures that allow for evaluations made not only by therapists but by significant others and brain-injured persons themselves.

In this way, it may be possible not only to more fully integrate assessment and rehabilitation but also to address the real-life concerns of brain-injured individuals and their families.

REFERENCES

Bauer, R.M. (1994). The flexible battery approach to neuropsychological assessment. In R.D. Vanderploeg (Ed.), *Clinician's guide to neuropsychological assessment* (pp. 259–290). Hillsdale, NJ: Lawrence Erlbaum Associates.

Ben-Yishay, Y., et al. (1978–1983). Working approaches to remediation of cognitive deficits in brain damaged persons. *Rehabilitation Monograph, 59–61,* 65.

Boake, C. (1991). History of cognitive rehabilitation following head injury. In J.F. Kreutzer & P.H. Wehman, *Cognitive rehabilitation for persons with traumatic brain injury* (pp. 3–12). Baltimore: P.H. Brooks.

Brickenkamp, R. (1981). *Test d2: Aufmerksamkeits-Belastungs-Test.* (Handanweisung, 7th ed.) (Test d2: Concentration-Endurance Test Manual, 5th ed.). Göttingen: Verlag für Psychologie.

Brooks, N., Campsie, L., Symington, C., Beattie, A., & McKinlay, W. (1986). The five-year outcome of severe blunt head injury: A relative's view. *Journal of Neurology, Neurosurgery, and Psychiatry, 49,* 764–770.

Christensen, A.-L. (1984). *Luria's neuropsychological investigation* (2nd ed.). Copenhagen: Munskgaard.

———. (1989). The neuropsychological investigation as a therapeutic and rehabilitative technique. In D.W. Ellis & A.-L Christensen (Eds.), *Neuropsycholgical treatment after brain injury* (pp. 127–156). Boston: Kluwer Academic.

Diller, L., & Ben-Yishay, Y. (1987). Outcomes and evidence in neuropsychological rehabilitation in closed head injury. In H.S. Levin, J. Grafman, & H.M. Eisenberg (Eds.), *Neurobehavioral recovery from head injury.* Oxford: Oxford University Press.

Gade, A., & Mortensen, E.L. (1984). The influence of age, education and intelligence on neuropsychological test performance. Paper presented at the 3rd Nordic Conference in Behavioral Toxicology, December, 1994, Aarhus, Denmark.

Gainotti, G. (1993). Emotional and psychosocial problems after brain injury. *Neuropsychological Rehabilitation, 3,* 259–277.

Goldstein, K. (1942). *Aftereffects of brain injuries in war: Their evaluation and treatment.* London: Heinemann.

———. (1952). Effects of brain damage on personality. *Psychiatry, 15,* 245.

Goodglass, H., & Kaplan, E. (1983). *The assessment of aphasia and related disorders* (2nd ed.). Philadelphia: Lea & Febiger.

Larrabee, G.J., West. R. L., & Crook, T.H. (1991). The association of memory complaint with computer-simulated everyday memory performance. *Journal of Clinical and Experimental Neuropsychology, 13,* 466–478.

Lezak, M.D. (1995). *Neuropsychological assessment* (3rd ed.). Oxford: Oxford University Press.

Luria, A.R. (1966). *Higher cortical functions in man* (rev. ed.), (Basil Haigh, Trans.). New York: Basic Books.

———. (1979). The making of mind. In M. Cole & S. Cole (Eds.), *The making of mind: A personal account of Soviet psychology.* Cambridge: Harvard University Press.

Prigatano, G.P., Fordyce, D.J., Roueche, J.R., Pepping, M., & Case Wood, B. (1986). *Neuropsychological rehabilitation after brain injury.* Baltimore: John Hopkins University Press.

Rabbock, J., Ross, B., & Ohry, A. (1994). The use of SCL-90-R with the traumatically head injured. *Journal of the Neuropsychological Society, 7,* 213–216.

Shallice, T., & Burgess, P.W. (1991). Deficits in strategy application following frontal lobe damage in man. *Brain., 114,* 727–741.

Sohlberg, M.M., & Mateer, C.A. (1989). *Introduction to cognitive rehabilitation: Theory and practice.* New York: Guilford Press.

Spreen, O., & Strauss, E. (1991). *A compendium of neuropsychological tests: Administration norms and commentary.* Oxford: Oxford University Press

Teasdale, T.W., & Caetano, C. (1995). Psychopathological symptomatology in brain-injured patients before and after rehabilitation. *Applied Neuropsychology, 2,* 116–123.

Thomsen, I.V. (1984). Late outcome of very severe blunt head trauma: A 10–15 year second follow-up. *Journal of Neurology, Neurosurgery and Psychiatry, 47,* 260–268.

Wilson, B. (1987). *The rehabilitation of memory.* New York: Guilford.

Yin, R.K. (1994). *Case study research: Design and methods* (2nd ed.). London: Sage.

5 Neuroimaging Assessment in TBI and Stroke: Relevance for Acute and Post-Acute Treatment

Irith Reider-Groswasser,[1] Alex K. Ommaya,[2] and Andres M. Salazar[2]

[1]Section of Neuroradiology, Tel-Aviv Elias Sourasky Medical Center, Tel-Aviv, and Sackler Faculty of Medicine, Tel-Aviv University, Tel-Aviv
[2]Defense and Veterans Head Injury Program, Henry M. Jackson Foundation, Rockville, MD

INTRODUCTION

The aims of imaging are (1) the diagnosis of medical or surgically treatable disease, (2) the study of early alterations in tissue parameters and of late residua, (3) the assessment of prognosis, and (4) the study of structure-function relationships.

Neuroimaging, using modern modalities such as Computerized Tomography (CT), Magnetic Resonance Imaging (MRI), Magnetic Resonance Angiography (MRA), Ultrasonography (US) that includes color Doppler flow imaging, Digital Subtraction Angiography (DSA), and the less common modalities of MR phase imaging, functional MRI (fMRI), water-diffusion MRI (dMRI), MRI spectroscopy (sMRI), Magnetization Transfer-MRI, has played a major role in early and accurate diagnosis of traumatic brain injury (TBI) and stroke (CVA) and in their follow-up (Nadel et al., 1991; Wong et al., 1995). The combined use of these different modalities enables quick and accurate assessment of the morphological changes that occur in the brain during trauma and stroke and increased understanding of the basic intravascular, extra cellular, and intracellular events that occur in these conditions (Steinke, Kloetzsch, & Hennerici, 1990; Hajnal et al., 1991; Naidich & Righi, 1995; Le Bihan et al., 1988; Vardiman et al., 1995).

The complexity of the expanding clinical and laboratory assessment and the possible differential diagnoses support the notion that the optimal use of modern neuroimaging may be correctly approached only if a "team" that represents the various subspecialties comprises the basic functioning unit. Exchange of knowledge between clinicians and scientists (physicists, chemists, data analysts) should become a part of everyday work (Wolpert, 1995).

Thus, decisions regarding the choice of diagnostic modalities and the appropriate timing of imaging studies should be carefully chosen, preferably by a common clinical and radiological decision in which the neuroradiologist and the interventional-neuroradiologist play a central role (Wolpert, 1995; Lindgren & Greitz, 1995; Huckman, 1993). Standard protocols that are tailored for each hospital, taking into consideration the available clinical staff and technical equipment, may be very helpful. However, the clinical condition of each patient will ultimately influence imaging decisions.

The use of standardized parameters and terminology are crucial for delineation of pathology, for comparison of results from different studies, and for a basic mutual understanding. Interpretation of findings should be based on quantitative, semiquantitative, and subjective parameters, the usefulness of which has been shown through preliminary experience and studies.

Although TBI and CVA are caused by different etiologies, a similar diagnostic approach describing lesions (hematoma and contusion for TBI and infarction for CVA), CSF spaces (ventricles, basal, and other cisterns), brain tissue characteristics, vascular structures, and flow characteristics should be used for basic interpretation. In this chapter, a diagnostic approach using standard parameters that have been evaluated in various pilot studies will be delineated.

TRAUMATIC BRAIN INJURY

General

Trauma to the brain has become a major problem in modern society because of its impact on the individual and its influence on society in terms of human disability and suffering. It has been called a "silent epidemic" (Goldstein, 1990). Every year about 2 million Americans suffer injuries to the head (HHS, 1989). Approximately 500,000 Americans are hospitalized annually, and estimates of deaths due to head injury range from 40,000 to 100,000 annually (Sosin, Sacks, & Smith, 1989). Additionally, approximately 90,000 persons suffer life long disability as a result of head injuries each year. The total cost of head injuries estimated by Max et al. for 1985 was $37.8 billion, of which $4.5 billion was for direct costs (acute hospital care, nursing home costs, physician services, drugs, and other related goods and services) and $33.3 billion was for indirect costs (morbidity cost was estimated at $20.6 billion and mortality cost was estimated at $12.7 billion) (Max, MacKenzie, & Rice, 1991). In 1985, head injuries accounted for 29% of total injury cost and 25% of the injury death rate, while representing only 13% of the injury incidence rate (Rice, MacKenzie, & Associates, 1989). Studies of the U.S. population have estimated the crude head injury rate to be 200 cases per 100,000 individuals, but there is considerable variation in rates between geographic regions (Kraus, 1993). Generally, head injury rates are much higher in younger individuals, and overall injury rates of males are twice those of females. The majority of head injuries are caused by motor vehicle crashes (50%), followed by falls (25%) and sports/recreational injuries (10–15%), with assaults and other causes forming the remainder (Ibid.).

Primary and Secondary Damage

Trauma to the brain is a complex and continuous event that starts after a physical-mechanical injury to the skull, brain tissue, blood vessels, and adjacent structures. Primary injury includes hemorrhagic or nonhemorrhagic contusion, intra- or extra-cerebral hemorrhage, diffuse axonal injury (DAI), and pressure signs if bleeding is significant. Secondary damage includes brain swelling with increased intracranial pressure, herniation, ischemia, and/or infarction, as well as additional changes including alteration of vessel diameter and blood flow within large or small vessels, release of different toxic metabolites such as glutamate, production of oxygen free radicals, changes in interstitial fluid composition, and delayed cell death (Teasdale & Hadley, 1990).

DAI results from shearing of axons, especially at the gray/white matter junction, during acceleration-deceleration injury. It is probably a combination of primary shearing injury and at a later stage, secondary damage resulting from microscopic microfilament malalignment and/or ischemic changes with degraded axonal flow and delayed axonal disruption (Povlishock, 1993; Choi, 1995). Detailed pathological descriptions of DAI have been documented by Adams et al. (1977, 1982, 1984) and Gennarelli et al. (1985).

Imaging of Trauma

Imaging Modalities in TBI

Conventional skull X-rays play basically no role in the evaluation of head injury and may even delay diagnosis and treatment (Hackney, 1991; Moseley, 1995). The main imaging modalities for the evaluation of TBI are CT and MRI. There are a number of advantages to using CT during the acute stage of trauma:

1. It is available in most hospitals.
2. It can be quickly performed.
3. Its performance is not associated with contraindications such as presence of metallic foreign bodies.
4. It enables diagnosis of acute bleeding.
5. It is optimal for the diagnosis of very subtle fractures, particularly at the skull's base.
6. It is the modality of choice for evaluation of diffuse trauma that includes other organs.
7. It is relatively inexpensive and may serve as a base line for follow-up studies.

MRI is important for the overall assessment of brain damage and prognosis because of its superior ability to delineate brain lesions and late parenchymal alterations (Levin, 1993; Groswasser et al., 1987). The use of different MR sequences such as dMRI, MRA, MRs, Echo-planar MRI, fMRI, Magnetization Transfer MR imaging, etc. is a source of extensive additional information that will have a profound impact on the understanding, treatment, and the assessment of TBI in the future (Wong et al., 1995; Le Bihan et al., 1988; Warach et al., 1995).

Angiography may be indicated when injury to blood vessels is suspected, including dissection, pseudoaneurysm formation, occlusion, and formation of traumatic arteriovenous fistulae (Bar & Gean, 1994; Reider-Groswasser et al., 1993). Digital Subtraction Angiography (DSA) may have a role in selected cases of trauma, especially if dissection or vasospasm are suspected (Vardiman et al., 1995; McCullough, Nelson, & Ommaya, 1971; Higashida et al., 1989; Morgan et al., 1987). The use of noninvasive imaging of blood vessels, including color Doppler, MRI, and MR Angiography (MRA), may increase the diagnosis of vascular injury in TBI patients.

The distinction between primary and secondary injury is helpful in understanding the main processes in trauma. However, this approach has limitations in that the temporal distinction between primary and secondary events is not always clear. For example, acute brain swelling, which is a part of secondary damage, can also occur very early after TBI (Kobrine et al., 1977). As such, there may not be clear distinction between imaging findings and pathological processes.

The main goals of imaging are different during the acute-subacute phase and the late phase of trauma. During the acute-subacute phase, the main goal is to *quickly* obtain clear descriptions that will diagnose or rule out certain key conditions for acute therapeutic purposes. These include the findings shown in Table 5.1.

Table 5.1: Neuroradiological Findings for Trauma (acute phase)

Primary ("surgical") findings
- Extracerebral bleeding—subarachnoid, subdural, extradural
- Intracerebral bleeding ("discrete mass," "spotty")
- Intraventricular bleeding
- Brainstem bleeding
- Intraparenchymal changes
- Deformity of basal cisterns (quadrigeminal, suprasellar)
- Deformity of ventricles
- Enlarged ventricles, including temporal horns
- Midline shift
- Herniations (at levels of falx, tentorium, and foramen magnum)

Secondary ("other") findings
- Fractures—linear, comminuted, depressed
- Intracranial air
- Foreign body
- Site and size of extracerebral bleeding
- Size of extracerebral bleeding—maximal length and width in mm
- Site and size of supratentorial bleeding
- Other posterior fossa bleeding
- White matter hypodensity or altered signal
- Grey matter hypodensity or altered signal
- Grey-white matter junction abnormality
- "Small" ventricles
- Visible sulci
- Involvement of vascular structures, arteries, or veins
- Involvement of facial structures and upper cervical spine
- Presence of change on follow-up studies
- Impressions and remarks
- Recommendations

Intracerebral bleeding can be discrete, occurring as a result of tear in a blood vessel, or "spotty and diffuse," as a part of hemorrhagic cerebral contusion. Contusions that represent bruising of brain tissue at points of impact are probably the most common traumatic brain lesions. Most intracerebral hemorrhages are located in the frontal and temporal lobes, and rarely are they deep in the basal ganglia (Barr & Gean, 1994).

Intracerebral bleeding occurs 3–4 times more often after the age of 50 than with patients under 30 (Ibid.). It has to be stressed that only 29% of intracerebral hemorrhages are visible on imaging studies within the first 3 hours after brain injury, whereas 35% and 46% will be diagnosed 3–24 hours and over 24 hours after the injury, respectively (Soloniuk et al., 1986). The delayed development of intracerebral hematomas (termed by Bollinger "Spät" apoplexy) in intra- and extra-cerebral locations is caused by a chain of events that start as brain softening, edema, and injury to small arteries (Caplan, 1994). Deep, basal ganglionic hemorrhages occur rarely in TBI (3%), but they are more common in the pediatric age group and in adolescents (Caplan, 1994; Katz et al., 1989).

Brainstem bleeding has been classified by Gentry et al. (1989) as primary or secondary. The primary form may be a direct superficial laceration (rare) or contusion usually located in the dorsolateral aspect of the brainstem. Brainstem DAI is usually associated with the presence of similar lesions in the corpus callosum and in the deep cerebral white matter (Gentry, 1991). Thus the spread and the location of abnormal signal may be helpful in suggesting the possible diagnosis of DAI. Differential diagnosis from ischemia and infarction may be suggested by location; the latter are usually located in the central tegmentum of the brainstem (Ibid.). Delayed and secondary injuries include Duret's hemorrhages, which occur as result of stretching of the perforating branches of the basilar artery by transtentorial herniation. These hemorrhages are usually located in the midline and are often linear (Gentry, Godersky, & Thompson, 1989; Gentry, 1991; Holland, Brant-Zawadzki, & Pitts, 1986).

Intraventricular bleeding may be caused by different mechanisms, including tears of ependymal veins and retrograde flow of CSF from the subarachnoid space. According to Barr and Gean (1994), it is very common in TBI, but according to Cordobes et al. (1983) and Holland et al. (1986), rather rare (3%). In any case, it is usually associated with diffuse brain injury and a high mortality rate. The increased use of MR studies in trauma will help to establish the importance of intraventricular bleeding.

Intracerebral parenchymal abnormalities, such as gray or white matter hyper/hypo intensity, cannot establish by themselves the pathogenesis of the injury. Thus, the use of imaging characteristics such as location (degree of involvement of gray/white matter or at the junction site), density/intensity, and other imaging or clinical parameters may be helpful in the overall assessment of the contribution of DAI, contusions, and ischemic processes in TBI. The importance of location, lateralization, and size of these abnormalities has been described in various studies (Levin, 1993; Levin et al., 1993; Grattan et al., 1994).

Parenchymal changes on CT include areas of altered density or intensity (on CT and MR, respectively) that present as hypodensity with or without scattered hyperdense foci representing small hemorrhages. This may be evident as hypointensity on MRI T1WI and hyperintensity on T2WI, again with foci of bleeding. Small bleeding is best seen on heavily weighted T2WI or on the GRE sequences and remains visible as characteristic deposits of hypointense hemosiderin even years after trauma has occurred ((Barr & Gean, 1994; Gentry, 1991; Osborn, 1994). It has to be stressed that neither these changes by themselves nor any other imaging parameter are specific for DAI or contusion. The imaging diagnosis of DAI is suggested by a number of factors among which corpus callosal atrophy, involvement of the posterior part of the corpus callosum, and involvement of the gray/white matter junction area may be most valuable (Mendelsohn et al., 1992; Levin et al., 1990; Reider-Groswasser et al., 1995). The junction area may also be affected by ischemia that is either global, associated with hypoperfusion, or local, resulting from altered regional metabolic processes (Kjos, Brant-Zawadzki, & Young, 1983). The white matter hypodensity/abnormal signal and the gray-white matter junction (GWJ) abnormality may be caused by different underlying mechanisms that include contusion, DAI, ischemia, and others. Significant correlation between indices of corpus callosal atrophy, the chronicity of injury, and the amount of lateral ventricular enlargement might point to the severity of DAI (Levin et al., 1990).

The four main anatomical locations of DAI are lobar white matter, corpus callosum, the dorsolateral aspect of the upper brainstem, and the gray-white junction (Gennarelli et al., 1985; Gentry, Godersky, & Thompson, 1989; Gentry, 1991; Gentry, Thompson, & Godersky, 1988). Hypodensity or changes in intensity may be visible immediately or few hours following injury; thus, the distinction between DAI and contusion may not be possible even when temporal changes occur. The exact relationship between DAI and loss of consciousness (LOC) in TBI patients remains to be elucidated; the centripetal theory of deep injury connecting DAI to LOC suggested by Ommaya and Generelli (1974) should be reassessed on MR studies.

The importance of "perimesencephalic cisterns" and "midline shift" on early CT studies as markers of generalized brain swelling and of outcome was stressed in the studies of Marshall et al. (1991), Liu & Su (1995), and of Eisenberg et al. (1990). Marshall et al. (Ibid.) suggested a classification of diffuse head injury based on CT findings as follows: subgroup I—no visible pathology; II—cisterns present, midline shift <5 mm, and lesions are <25 cc; III—compressed or absent cistern, midline shift <5 mm, and lesions <25 cc; and IV—midline shift of >5 mm, and lesions >25 cc.

The size of the ventricular system is usually appreciated subjectively in acute studies. Detailed measurements (see below) are part of assessment of the late studies. It is important to comment on any change in size on follow-up studies, whether this involves a part of or the entire ventricular system and whether it is accompanied by concomitant changes in the cerebral subarachnoid spaces. These changes may indicate performance of additional studies such as CSF flow studies. According to preliminary results, these might be especially valuable in TBI patients who have sustained a closed or penetrating injury (Reider-Groswasser et al., 1995). The correlation between clinical parameters and ventricular size is outlined elsewhere (Levin, 1993; Reider-Groswasser et al., 1993; Gale et al., 1994). The diagnosis of small ventricles is very subjective. Thus, conditions such as diffuse brain swelling (with or without sinus thrombosis) should be based on additional imaging parameters.

Visibility of cerebral sulci or asymmetry of cerebral sulci may be the only signs of localized superficial subarachnoid bleeding. Lack of visibility of sulci may be within normal range for young persons or may be an early sign of brain swelling or altered CSF dynamics. Thus, visibility of sulci is not a reliable single sign of abnormality on a study; a change on subsequent studies may be more meaningful.

Involvement of facial structures and the upper cervical spine (gross fractures) are readily visible on CT studies. Subtle fractures are diagnosed with increased frequency when thin cuts, bone algorithms, and reformatting in coronal, sagittal, and 3D are performed. These should be performed only if a fracture is suggested on an axial cut by findings such as a laterally tilted dens or a clinical problem suggesting a blow-out fracture and entrapment of orbital contents, optic canal fracture, rhinorrhea, or other relevant complaints (Thomeier, Brown, & Mirvis, 1990; Lloyd, Kimber, & Burrows, 1994).

Involvement of vascular structures through the dissection of arteries, presence of infarcts, post-traumatic arteriovenous fistulae, and venous sinus thrombosis may occur in

TBI and are suggested on CT, MR, and on additional studies (see also Part II) (Morgan et al., 1987; Osborn, 1994; Lewin et al., 1994).

Optic pathway sections should reflect a rough correlation between the clinical condition of the patient and imaging findings. An example of this is the presence of a visual problem that might be secondary to the involvement of anterior or posterior optic pathways. The posterior pathways are readily assessed by MR of the brain. The assessment of the anterior optic pathways might necessitate performance of additional "tailored" CT and MR studies using thin slices, slices along the planes of the optic nerves, the use of "bone algorithms" viewed with appropriate window settings, and/or special MR sequences. Thus, the presence of "visual problems" as a clinical problem should be approached primarily on the brain study and only subsequently, by the use of the above-mentioned, additional diagnostic procedures. Even contusions of the optic nerves and post-traumatic cataract and fluctuating visual loss secondary to intraorbital emphysema can be confirmed by imaging diagnosis (Breslau et al., 1995; Segev et al., 1995; Carter & Nerad, 1987; Mauriello et al., 1986). The choice of additional imaging studies should be inserted in "recommendations."

The *late phase of TBI* should be evaluated when changes associated with the initial injury are completed, including the process of the anterograde degeneration of axons secondary to proximal axonal injury or death of the cell body (Wallerian degeneration). Wallerian degeneration occurs 5–12 weeks following injury and may be visible during this period as high signal on T2WI along pyramidal tracts, whereas ipsilateral atrophy may be visible only after a few months (Orita et al., 1991; Inoue, Matsumura, & Fukuda, 1990). Therefore, the imaging assessment of the late stage of TBI should be performed some 3 months following the trauma or later.

During the "late phase," the main purpose is to assess tissue loss, whether local (encephalomalacia) or diffuse (ventricular and sulcal widening—atrophy), and alteration in cerebral tissue parameters such as density on CT and intensity on MRI. In addition, widening of the ventricular system should be further assessed as to whether it reflects tissue loss only or is associated with altered CSF dynamics. The diagnosis of post-traumatic normal pressure hydrocephalus (NPH) may be made only after change of CSF spaces on subsequent imaging studies or after elucidation of CSF dynamics by additional studies such as cisternography or dMR. A description of measurements of CSF spaces and of brain structures is given below.

STROKE (CVA)

Stroke is the third leading cause of death and a major cause of disability in the United States (Goldstein, 1993). There are approximately 500,000 new strokes reported annually, with a recurrence rate of 20–50% within 5 years, and an estimated survival rate after second stroke of 40% (Naidich & Righi, 1995; Zwiebel, 1992). Stroke is a dynamic process in which the location and degree of cerebral ischemia and resultant infarction change with time (ter Penning, 1992). The capability of the imaging modalities to assess vascular structures, blood flow, and metabolic processes within brain tissue on the one hand, and medical and surgical treatments on the other hand, have had a major impact on management of cerebrovascular disease (Naidich & Righi, 1995; NASCET, 1991a, b).

There are various different etiologies that present as a stroke—either ischemic or hemorrhagic. The most common cause of CVA is ischemic atherosclerotic vascular disease presenting as infarction (80%). Other causes of ischemic CVA include other vasculopathies and blood disorders (Bryan, Whitlow, & Levy, 1991). Primary intracranial hemorrhage accounts for about 15% of CVA patients and is caused mainly by hypertensive bleeding. Nontraumatic subarachnoid hemorrhage and venous sinus thrombosis are rare causes of CVA. The clinical presentation of CVA is typified by focal neurological deficits with acute onset. However, different clinical presentation such as vascular dementia (VD), depression, mood disorders, or asymptomatic presence are also recognized (Liu et al., 1992; Herdescheé et al., 1992; Fujikawa, Yamawaki, & Touhouda, 1993; Nusbaum, Reider-Groswasser, & Korczyn, 1989; Aharon-Peretz, Cummings, & Hill, 1988; Dupont, Cullum, & Jeste, 1988; Feinberg et al., 1990). The neuroanatomy of the biogenic amine-containing pathways in the cerebral cortex might help explain the relationship between the intracerebral location of stroke and mood disorder (Robinson et al., 1984).

The common risk factors for stroke are hypertension, heart disease, diabetes, hyperlipidemia, coagulopathy, drug abuse, history of surgery, and the presence of antiphospholipid antibodies (APLA). History of surgery as a risk factor associated with the presence of lacunar infarcts in the thalami was suggested in the studies of Amarenco et al. (1993) and Hirshenbein (1993) and was found to be of importance in nonhypertensive patients. The presence of APLA is important in young patients with cerebrovascular disease and in demented patients (Levin & Welch, 1987; Inzelberg et al., 1992). The suggested imaging approach to CVA is similar to the one used for TBI, using different parameters for the acute/subacute phases and the late phase.

Epidemiology and CVA

In a cardiovascular multicenter study, the analysis of MR studies of the brain performed in adults age 65 and older indicated that identification of cerebrovascular disease is feasible, that the interpretative results are reproducible, and that MR evidence of stroke is more prevalent than reported clinical history of stroke (Bryan et al., 1994).

The Acute/Subacute Phase of CVA

During the acute phase, the injured cerebral tissue comprises the irreversibly damaged central core and the still viable but "at risk" tissue in the periphery. The main effort at this phase is aimed, therefore, at promptly starting salvage therapy for the rescue of the "at risk" tissue (Osborn, 1994; Marshall & Mohr, 1993). The main imaging modality in the hyperacute phase remains CT, and the initial aim of the study is to distinguish between ischemic infarction and other types of stroke, mainly hemorrhage. However, MRI is the most sensitive and accurate modality, especially when it includes specialized sequences and various MR techniques such as diffusion weighted MRI, MRA, and DSA angiography (Naidich & Righi, 1995; Warach et al., 1995; NASCET, 1991; NASCET, 1991; Bryan, Whitlow, & Levy, 1991; Mori et al., 1992; Barnwell et al., 1994; Tsai et al., 1994; NASCET, 1993). Ischemic infarction can be subdivided according to the location of infarct and the difference in involvement of gray and white matter (Table 5.2). The distinction between small (<3 mm) and large (>3 mm) infarcts has been suggested Bryan et al. (1994). Templates for classifications of infarcts according to site, size, swelling, and hemorrhagic transformation were described by Wardlaw and Sellar (1994).

The Late Phase of CVA

At this stage the infarct has sharp margins and density and intensity values on CT and MR that are close to CSF values. The ipsilateral ventricle may be enlarged focally, and generalized atrophy and abnormal signals on MRI in the surrounding tissue may be

Table 5.2: Ischemic Infarction—Imaging Parameters

1. Type of infarct
   - Cortical infarct
   - Lacunar infarct
   - Watershed infarct
   - Laminar necrosis or neuronal necrosis
   - White matter changes
2. Blood vessel involvement
   Arteries:
   - Main vascular territory:
     Carotid circulation, Vertebro-basilar circulation
   - Cervical carotid artery and vertebral arteries
   - Cortical branches of internal carotid and basilar arteries:
     ACA, MCA, PCA, SCA, AICA, PICA
   - Involvement of all the cortical branch's territory, or partial
   - Perforating branches: Lenticulo-striate, Thalamo-perforators.
   Veins:
   - Venous sinuses, Cortical veins
3. Location
   - In cerebral hemispheres: Cortical location or deep location
   - In midbrain
   - In pons
   - In cerebellar hemispheres
   - In medulla oblongata
   - Multiple locations
4. Changes in adjacent brain
   - Presence of edema, local pressure signs
   - Presence of local atrophy

visible. Quantitative assessment of tissue loss was performed by Skriver et al. (1990) in large and medium size infarcts using linear measurements.

Cortical Infarcts (CI)

The most common CI occur in middle cerebral artery (MCA) territory (Osborn, 1994; Bryan, Whitlow, & Levy, 1991), which supplies the anterolateral portions of the temporal lobes and the lateral convexity of frontal, temporal, and parietal lobes. The blood supply of the cortex and the underlying white matter differ, and since the cortex is supplied by short arterioles and has a dense capillary bed, it is at risk for hypoperfusion and anoxia at watershed (Moody, Bell, & Challa, 1986). The vascular territories and the clinical features of CI are summarized by different authors (Osborn, 1994; Bryan, Whitlow, & Levy, 1991; Wardlaw & Sellar, 1994; Bamford, Sandercock, & Dennis, 1991; Greenberg, Aminoff, & Simon, 1993; Berman, Hayman, & Hinck, 1980; Berman, Hayman, & Hinck, 1984; Hayman, Berman, & Hinck, 1981).

CI occurring in MELAS (mitochondrial encephalomyopathy with lactic acidosis and stroke-like episodes) may be accompanied by generalized cerebral hyperperfusion persisting for several months (Gropen et al., 1994). The presence of CI and the absence of arterial occlusions in MELAS may be attributed to the metabolic etiology of infarction in this entity, similar to the "metabolic stroke" attributed to toxic organic acid metabolites in patients with methylmalonic acidemia (Gropen et al.; Heindenreich et al., 1988). The

Table 5.3: Imaging Signs Relevant for the Diagnosis of CVA

<u>CT signs</u>
- Dense middle cerebral artery sign (Bastianello et al., 1991; Leys et al., 1992; Tomsick et al., 1990; Rauch et al., 1993).
- Obscuration of the Lentiform nucleus sign (Tomura et al., 1988).
- Insular ribbon sign (loss of GWMD along lateral insula (Truwit et al., 1990).
- The reversal sign (Kim Han et al., 1989; Vergote, Vandeperre, & DeMan, 1992).
- Cord sign (Anderson, Chah, & Murtagh, 1987).
- Empty delta sign (Virapongse et al., 1989).
- Fogging effect (Osborn, 1994; Asato, R. et al., 1991).

<u>MR signals and signs</u>
- Absence of normal flow-void sign and arterial enhancement (Mueller et al., 1993; Elster, & Moody, 1990).
- Brain swelling sign (Osborn, 1994).
- Hyperintense signal on T2WI (acute subacute CVA) (Osborn, 1994; Yuh et al., 1991).
- Hypointense signal on T1WI (subacute CVA)
- Subcortical low intensity in early cortical ischemia on T2WI (Ida et al., 1994).
- Fogging effect sign (Osborn, 1994). 138]
- Meningeal enhancement sign (Osborn, 1994; Asato, Okumura, & Konishi, 1991).
- Hemorrhagic transformation sign
- Gyral enhancement pattern sign
- Post infarct wallerian degeneration (Kuhn et al., 1989).

<u>Angiographic signs</u>
- Vessel occlusion (with or without meniscus sign)
- Change in arterial flow
- Retrograde filling by collaterals
- "Bare" nonperfused areas
- Early appearing draining veins
- Mass effect, varying degrees

<u>Positron Emission Tomography (PET) signs</u>
- Low perfusion with increased oxygen extraction fraction (important risk factor for development of hemodynamic infarction)

---

metabolic changes could account for the extensive basal ganglia calcifications described in these entities. The imaging features of CI are summarized in Table 5.3. Quantitative measurements of CI, of CSF compartments, and of the brain, including gray and white matter, may be important for the assessment of prognosis (Liu et al., 1992). Silent CI are less frequent than silent lacunar infarcts (LI) and are not significantly related to risk factors such as the presence of widespread vascular disease (Ricci et al., 1993).

The principal CT findings in CI are diminished density of brain, particularly of gray matter and the gray-white matter junction area. Mass effect occurs usually during the first days and may not be apparent unless a comparison is performed. Skriver et al. (1990) found that mass effect occurred in 81% of patients with large infarcts and in 38% of patients with medium-size infarcts. The occurrence of late atrophic changes was found in 58% of patients with large infarcts and in 45% of the medium-size infarcts. Large hemispheric (particularly frontal) infarcts may be accompanied by atrophy of the ipsilateral cerebral peduncle (due to Wallerian degeneration) and contralateral cerebellar atrophy due to altered cerebellar blood flow and metabolism (crossed cerebellar diaschisis) (Martin & Raichle, 1983).

Lacunar Infarcts (LI)

Lacunar infarcts occur in the territory of perforating branches of the carotid and the basilar circulation (Osborn, 1994; Bryan, Whitlow, & Levy, 1991; Fisher, 1965; Bogousslavsky, Regli, & Uske, 1988; Ghika, Bogosslavsky, & Regli, 1989; Graff-Radford, Damasio, & Yamada, 1988). LI are diagnosed in about 25% of CVA patients, but they are much more common in patients with hypertension, episodes of TIA or minor ischemic stroke, nonvalvular atrial fibrillation, and patients with coronary artery disease (Osborn, 1994; Herderscheé et al., 1992; Hirshenbain, 1993; Regli et al., 1993; Tanaka et al., 1993). LI are the most common infarcts in the group of "silent" brain infarction (Ricci et al., 1993; Chodosh et al., 1988). They are diagnosed on both CT and MR studies, but Gadolinium enhancement on MR improves the rate of precise clinico-anatomic correlation (Regli et al., 1993). LI, most common in the striatum, are caused by occlusion of the long, medial, and lateral lenticulostriate arteries branches of the anterior and middle cerebral arteries, respectively (Osborn, 1994; Moody, Bell, & Challa, 1990; Fisher, 1965). Parkinsonism and stroke were found in 38% and 31% of the patients with LI on their CT scans respectively, and a causal link was confirmed in patients with unilateral LI who had Parkinsonism on the contralateral side (Reider-Groswasser, Bornstein, & Korczyn, 1995). Patients with Parkinsonism associated with basal ganglia lacunes showed tremor less frequently than other idiopathic Parkinson's disease patients; otherwise, clinical features and the course of the disease were indistinguishable from idiopathic Parkinson's disease (Inzelberg et al., 1994).

Galynker et al. (1995) showed that basal ganglia stroke, especially in the striatum, has an etiologic role in "negative psychiatric symptoms" as measured by the positive and negative symptom scale (PANSS) and the scale for the assessment of negative symptoms (SANS), which are in turn related with decreased dopaminergic activity. Damage to the basal ganglia was also found to correlate with neurobehavioral problems by Bahtia & Marsden (1994). LI in the thalami are located in four main areas. The most common is in the anterior and dorsolateral regions supplied by the tuberothalamic branch originating in the posterior communicating artery and by the inferolateral branch, which originates from the posterior cerebral artery, respectively (Hirshenbain, 1993; Bogousslavsky, Regli, & Uske, 1988). Medial thalamic infarcts are bilateral in about 30% of cases. The medial thalamic areas are often supplied by one stem artery, the paramedian pedicle, which originates in the basilar artery (Graff-Radford, Damasio, & Yamada, 1988). Patients with LI in the medial thalamic areas are older and have higher values of cerebral atrophy than patients with LI in other parts of the thalami (Hirshenbain, 1993). Hirshenbain found significant correlations between vascular anatomy and the morphometric parameters. LI in the midbrain and in the pons are caused by occlusion of perforating branches of the basilar arteries, and their accurate etiology may be difficult to determine (Regli et al., 1993).

Watershed Infarcts (WI)

These involve both gray and white matter in the border areas of cortical and perforating branch territories. They may be caused by hypotensive episodes, by hypoxic-ischemic events, in conditions with low perfusion with increased oxygen extraction fraction ("misery perfusion syndrome," hemodynamic infarction), or by embolic phenomena (Osborn, 1994; Yamauchi et al., 1992). They are diagnosed owing to their density/intensity parameters, anatomic location, and absence or lack of significant mass effect. They may also be suggested by clinical presentation (Osborn, 1994; Bryan,

Whitlow, & Levy, 1991; Amarenco et al., 1993; Skriver, Skyhoi, & McNair, 1990; Skriver, & Olsen, 1981). The parieto occipital area is the most frequent and severely affected watershed area at the confluence of the ACA, MCA, and PCA territories (Osborn, 1994). The high frequency of very small cerebellar infarcts (26-43% in a series of cerebellar strokes) has been described by Amarenco et al. (1993).

Laminar Necrosis (LN)

This is the result of a selective vulnerability of certain neural cells (such as hippocampal cells, or striatal cells) to hypoxia and of the type and severity of anoxia to which the patient was exposed (Liwnich, Mouradian, & Ball Jr., 1987; Sawada et al., 1990). LN may show temporarily as a "gyral blush" of the gray matter on post-contrast CT or MR studies (Liwnich et al.). Cortical laminar necrosis comprises ischemic neuronal changes and glial reaction that is accompanied by laminar deposition of fat-laden macrophages (Sawada et al.). According to Sawada et al., gliosis that results in high spin intensity and the accumulation of the fat-ladden macrophages may explain the high intensity signal on MR—T1WI in LN. It is possible that LN is underestimated, since it may be diagnosed during the acute-subacute stages and missed during the late stage. Awareness of this entity might influence the diagnosis. Late cortical atrophy after CVA may result from LN.

White Matter Involvement in Vascular Disease

The periventricular white matter surrounding the frontal horns and in the parieto occipital area is the watershed for the anterior, middle, and posterior cerebral arteries and is most vulnerable to ischemia (Osborn, 1994; Sawada et al., 1990). This white matter can show abnormal signals in different conditions, such as cerebral edema, elevated venous or CSF pressure, immunological reactions, and as an early sign of primary or secondary cerebral malignancy. A delayed and progressive post-ischemic white matter encephalopathy was described by Sawada et al. (1990).

Sinus Thrombosis (ST)

This may occur as an isolated phenomenon or as part of other underlying disorders, including trauma (Osborn, 1994; Zimmerman & Ernst, 1992; Taha et al., 1993; Mokri, Jack, & Petty, 1993). ST most commonly affects the superior sagittal sinus, followed by the transverse, sigmoid, and cavernous sinuses (Osborn, 1994). Thrombosis of the deep cerebral veins, the internal cerebral veins, and/or the vein of Galen are a relatively rare but clinically devastating event that leads to venous infarcts in the deep structures, including the thalami and the upper midbrain (Osborn, 1994; Ur-Rahman & Al-Tahan, 1993). In most instances, the thrombosis is subacute and presents as high intensity signal on all the sequences of conventional MRI. However, in the acute stage or when a small segment is involved, distinction between thrombosis and slow flow may not be possible (Zimmerman & Ernst, 1992). Conventional spin-echo and gradient echo MRI in conjunction with phase imaging are simple to perform and reliable for the diagnosis of thrombosis and its distinction from flow phenomena (Nadel et al., 1991). The use of oblique-acquisition, time-of-flight MR venography was suggested as a useful adjunct to parenchymal MR in the evaluation of suspected veno-occlusive disease (Lewin et al., 1994). The different MR technologies are thus considered the method of choice in the noninvasive diagnosis of dural sinus thrombosis during the acute and the subacute stages (Nadel et al., 1991; Naidich & Righi, 1995; Lewin et al., 1994; Zimmerman & Ernst, 1992; Sze et al., 1988). In the acute stage the thrombus is isointense on T1WI and hypointense on T2WI, and during the subacute stage, it is hyperintense on both. During the late or chronic period the thrombus is isointense on T1WI and hyperintense on T2WI (Sze et al., 1988).

MR Angiography (MRA)

The two fundamental MR techniques used for MRA are time of flight (TOF) and phase contrast (PC) angiography. The TOF angiography is based on the difference between signals in static tissue and flowing blood, has a higher intrinsic contrast, and is more sensitive to slow flow, but fine detail is limited by poor signal to noise ratio. The PC angiography is based on the interaction between flowing blood and magnetic gradients and enables flow measurements (Naidich & Righi, 1995; Sheppard, 1995). The combined use of PC and TOF angiographic techniques or the use of MOTSA (multiple overlapping thin slab acquisition), which is a technology that appears to combine the advantages of both 2D and 3D TOF, could be necessary for diagnosis (Naidich & Righi; Blatter et al., 1992). Detailed specific protocols for the evaluation of cerebrovascular disease with MRA of the head and the neck are described by Naidich and Righi (1995).

MEASUREMENTS

Linear Measurements

Advantages of linear measurements include simplicity of performance, ability to be performed on old studies that are not suitable for computer analysis, and a high interreader reliability. Disadvantages are that they are not suitable for volume analysis of structures such as amygdala and hippocampus. Linear measurements are most valuable in the late stage, strongly correlate with volume measurements, and have been associated with clinical outcome (Reider-Groswasser et al., 1993). Linear measurements performed on axial CT studies, using a transparent ruler, in a variety of clinical conditions showed a significant relationship between motor and cognitive impairment and cella media or ventricular indices; caudal measurements and mental deterioration; and frontal indices, the width of the third ventricle, and the number of sulci (but not their width), and indicated the degree of motor incapacity in demented patients with Parkinson's disease (Inzelberg et al., 1987). The correlation between cognitive decline and the width of the third ventricle has been found in various studies of different clinical conditions such as Parkinson's disease, Alzheimer's disease, and TBI (Reider-Groswasser et al. 1993; Inzelberg et al., 1987; Korczyn et al., 1986; De Leon, Ferris, & Georg, 1980; Reider-Groswasser et al., 1995; Sroka et al., 1981; Reider-Groswasser et al. 1993; Inzelberg et al., 1994).

The distinction between primary and secondary linear measurements (Table 5.4) is based on correlations with other radiological parameters and clinical outcome measures (Reider-Groswasser et al., 1995, 1993, 1995). Linear measurements also aide in the standardized assessment of tissue loss and its localization in TBI, CVA, and other diseases (Hirshenbain, 1993; Korczyn et al., 1986; Inzelberg et al., 1994; Reider-Groswasser et al., 1988). These parameters have significantly correlated with injury severity and return to work (Reider-Groswasser et al., 1995). Additionally, these parameters might be helpful in distinguishing between different underlying mechanisms for ventricular enlargement. Different correlations between supratentorial ventricles, fourth ventricle ratio and cerebral sulci were seen in closed vs. penetrating head injuries (Reider-Groswasser et al., 1995). These parameters may eventually prove to be valuable in selection of patients for CSF flow studies.

Table 5.4: Linear Measurements (CT and MR)

<u>Primary Parameters</u>	<u>Secondary Parameters</u>
• Septum caudate distance—SCD	• Frontal horn width—FHW
• 3rd ventricle's width—3V	• Cella media width—CMW
• Interuncal distance—IUD	• Cerebro-ventricular index—CVI-1
• 4th ventricle ratio—4th VR	• Cerebro-ventricular index—CVI-2
• Width of the genu of corpus callosum—WGCC	• Ventricular score—VS
• Midbrain's length—ML	• Temporal horn width—THW
	• Cistern-brainstem ratio—CBR
	• Sucal width—SW
	• Optic nerve width—ONW
	• Pituitary gland's height—PGH

Most of these measurements have been previously described (Reider-Groswasser et al., 1993; Gyldensted & Kostelijanetz, 1976; Gyldensted & Kostelijanetz, 1977; Koller et al., 1981; Hahn & Rim, 1976; Hughes & Gado, 1981; Doraiswamy et al., 1992, 1993; Early et al., 1993; Raininko et al., 1994; LeMay et al., 1986; Dahlbeck et al., 1991) and were measured with a transparent ruler in our previous studies described (Reider-Groswasser et al. 1995, 1993; Inzelberg et al., 1987; Reider-Groswasser et al., 1995; Inzelberg et al., 1994; Reider-Groswasser et al., 1988).

The interuncal distance was described mainly on MR studies and was used by us on CT studies as well (Reider-Groswasser et al. 1995; Inzelberg et al., 1994). IUD was found to be a useful parameter for estimation of atrophy by LeMay et al. (1986).

The optic nerve width was measured using a transparent ruler and/or a computerized program on CT studies with patients with different disorders and on a group of patients with symptomatic carotid artery stenosis (the optic nerve research tool) (Reider-Groswasser et al., 1993; Friedland et al., 1992).

The *frontal horn* parameters, *maximal width* and *septum-caudate distance, CVI-1 and CVI-2,* are measured on axial CT cuts at the level of the basal ganglia and the third ventricle near or at the foramen of Monro or on T1W axial MR cuts at the level of the upper part of the third ventricle, which best shows the course of the internal cerebral veins (Figures 5.1 and 5.2).

The width of the third ventricle measurements are performed on the axial CT cut best showing the third ventricle and the foramen of Monro (Figure 5.3). The width is measured on the middle third of the third ventricle. The 3VW can also be measured on a TW1 coronal cut at the level of the dorsum sellea (Figure 5.4).

On MR studies the third ventricle is measured on the cut that shows the upper part of the anterior commissure on T1W image. If the massa intermedia is very large, the measurement can be performed just behind this structure.

Cella media distance (necessary also for calculation of VS) is measured as the minimal distance between the bodies of the lateral ventricles just above the internal cerebral veins (Figure 5.3).

The *interparietal distance* (necessary for calculation of the VS) is measured at the level of the bodies of the lateral ventricles, between the inner tables of skull on CT cuts (Figure 5.3) and between the outer brain surface margins on axial T1W MR cuts.

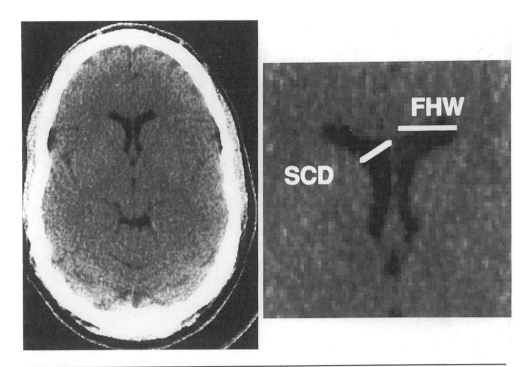

Figure 5.1: Frontal horn parameters. FHW—Frontal horn width; SCD—Septum caudate distance.

Ventricular score is calculated by adding left and right septum caudate distances, bi caudate measurement, third ventricle and cella media width all divided by interparietal distance (Figure 5.3) (Reider-Groswasser et al., 1993; Inzelberg et al., 1987; Hughes & Gado, 1981).

Fourth ventricle ratio is obtained by dividing the maximal width of the fourth ventricle by the skull width at the same level (note, skull width is outer skull to outer skull) as suggested by Koller et al. (1981) (Figure 5.5).

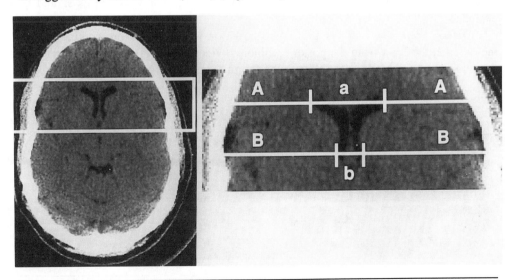

Figure 5.2: Cerebro-ventricular indexes. CVI 1—a/A bifrontal index at maximal width of frontal horns; CVI 2—b/B bicaudate index measured just in front of foramen of Monro.

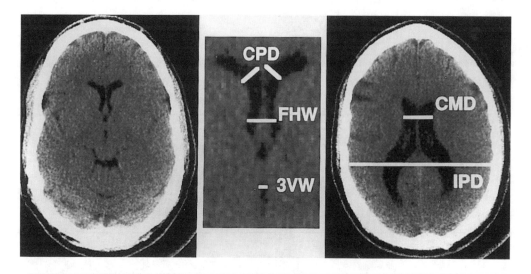

Figure 5.3: Ventricular score (VS). CPD—Caudate pellucidum distance; FHW—Frontal horn width; 3VW—Third ventricular width; CMD—Cella media distance; IPD—Inter-parietal distance (inner to inner bone margin).

The *temporal horn width (THW)* refers to the antero-posterior size of the temporal horns at the level of the suprasellar cistern on axial CT or T1W MR cuts (Figure 5.5). The THW was measured at the maximal convexity of the horn. THW (latero-lateral) can also be measured on a coronal T1W MRI cut at level of the dorsum sellae. The width of the temporal horn is measured at its maximal convexity or at the maximal convexity of the hippocampus on this cut (Figure 5.4)

The interuncal distance is measured at the level of the suprasellar cistern at the same cut on which THW measurements are performed (Figure 5.5). IUD measurement is also performed on T1W coronal MR cut between the maximal convexities of the unci (Figure 5.4). It should be noted that adjacent blood vessels in the Circle of Willis should be excluded.

Cistern brainstem ratio is the antero-posterior width of the pre-pontine cistern measured at the front from the posterior clinoid divided by the distance measured from the same point on the dorsum sellae to the fourth ventricle (Figure 5.6) (Ibid.).

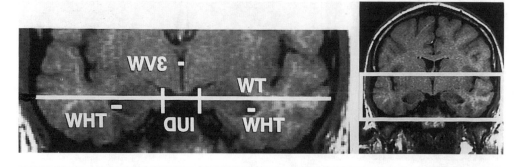

Figure 5.4: Temporal lobe and 3VW. 3VW—Third ventricular width; THW—Temporal horn width; TH—Temporal width; IUD—Inter-uncal distance.

Sulcal Width (SW) can be obtained as mean values or as a score measuring the four largest sulci on the highest supra ventricular axial cuts (Inzelberg et al., 1987; Gyldensted & Kostelijanetz, 1977; Hughes & Gado, 1981).

Genu of the corpus callosum antero-posterior width is measured on the midsagittal T1W MR cut from the maximal convexity of the inner surface of the genu of the corpus callosum to its outer surface. The connecting line should be horizontal (Figure 5.7) (Laissy et al., 1993).

Midbrain, anteroposterior length, is performed on the midsagittal T1W MR cut, from anterior midbrain (a point at the level of upper pons) to a midpoint between upper and lower colliculus as suggested by Raininko et al. (1994) (Figure 5.7). Dimensions of the midbrain can also be evaluated on axial MR cuts as suggested by Doraiswamy et al. (1992).

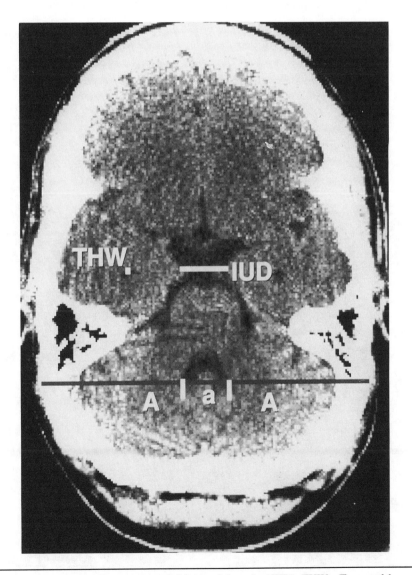

Figure 5.5: Temporal lobe parameters and 4th ventricle ratio (4VR). THW—Temporal horn width; IUD—Inter-uncal distance; 4VR—a/A (A=outer to outer bone margin).

Pons, anteroposterior length, is performed on the midsagittal T1W MR cut. The anterior landmark is at the maximal anterior convexity of the pons (also usually at the level of the highest point of the sphenooccipital synchondrosis, as suggested by Raininko et al. (1994)) to a posterior landmark located on the floor of the fourth ventricle at the level of the festigium (Figure 5.7). This measurement is slightly different from the one performed by Raininko et al., who took as a landmark a line perpendicular to the long axis of the pons (Ibid.).

In the *Pituitary gland's height* on sagittal T1W, the MR cut is from midpoint of the lowest boundary to the upper border of the gland. Pituitary dysfunction as a consequence of TBI was described by Klingbeil et al. (1985) (Figure 5.7).

Linear measurements may also be performed on coronal MR cuts. These are especially useful for the evaluation of temporal lobe parameters and for the third ventricle. These measurements have been performed on a T1W cut on which the clivus dorsum sellae, including the posterior clinoid, are best seen (it is the first cut where the pituitary

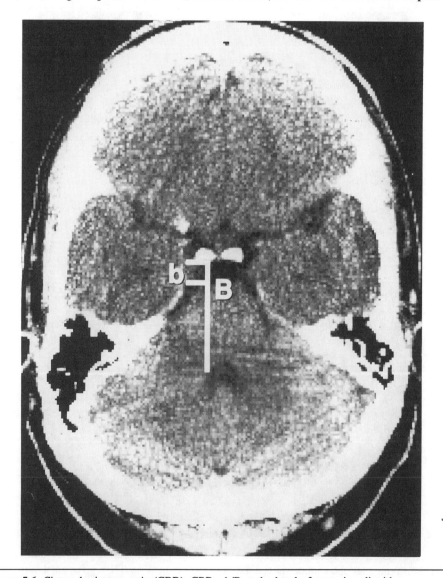

Figure 5.6: Cistern brainstem ratio (CBR). CBR—b/B at the level of posterior clinoid.

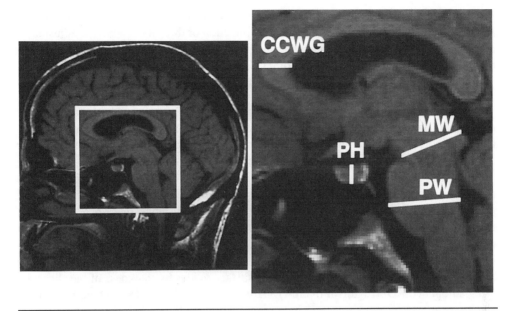

Figure 5.7: Measurements performed on mid-sagittal cut. CCWG—Corpus Callosum width of Genu; MW—Midbrain width; PQ—Pontine width; PH—Pituitary gland's height.

gland is not visible). They include (1) *interuncal distance*, measured between maximal convexities of the unci; *(2) temporal width,* measured from brain surface on the one side to the other at the level of the interuncal distance; *(3) width of the third ventricle,* measured at the middle third of this ventricle; and *(4) temporal horn size,* measured from side to side or the maximal convexity of the temporal horns (Figure 5.4).

Optic nerve widths, both right and left, are usually measured on the axial CT or MR cut where the whole nerve is visible. The measurement is taken perpendicular to the long axis of the optic nerve at a site where uniform width of the nerve and it's sheath are seen (usually in the middle third of the optic nerve).

Linear measurements can be performed either directly on the radiograph film or using computer programs such as MEDVISION, NIH Image, or others.

Image Analysis and Measurement Parameters

Images can be analyzed using radiographic films or digitized data. Digitized images can be viewed or analyzed on the console, or using computer programs such as NIH Image, ANALYZE, MEDVISION, etc. This method enables magnification and adjustment of images so that measurements can be performed more easily and accurately. The recording of results can be automated, and calculations can be automatically performed by spreadsheets. By this method, intensity/density measurements of gray and white matter in various parts of the brain can be measured, offering information about subtle changes in tissue characteristics that may not be appreciated by inspection (see below). In addition, the analysis of high resolution images enables acquisition of volumetric and structural information that is not obtained by other methods and may be the single best parameter for diagnosis in various pathologies (e.g., early Alzheimer's disease and mesial temporal sclerosis). The use of digitized data also allows for the analysis of data at remote locations by experts.

Window settings should be set with a mean value of gray and white matter and a range of about 200 units. Values of intensity are not dependent on the window level settings.

For separation of CSF, brain tissue, and gray and white matter, the use of threshold values for automatic quantization is valuable. The application of threshold should be adjusted by measurement of CSF in the lateral ventricles. The threshold level width is set by adjusting the level to separate or distinguish by color CSF in the ventricles and subarachnoid spaces.

Volumetric Measurements

ADVANTAGES: measurements are accurate, can be performed using automatic computer programs and are thus accurately reproducible, have high interreader reliability, and can indicate pathology that is otherwise not suspected (such as damage to the hippocampus or local atrophic processes).

DISADVANTAGES: the imaging study (CT, MR) on which the measurements are performed has to be specially "tailored" using thin (1–3 mm) contiguous slices, and the patient has to be motionless throughout the whole study since motion or change of position during the study (mainly CT) *prevent* the whole volume calculation (whereas, at the same time, some of the linear measurements can still be performed). The same is true for metallic artifacts. Volume measurements can be obtained by delineation of surface areas on contiguous cuts and multiplying the surface values by thickness of the slices, by using automated ROI (region of interest) analysis, or by segmentation techniques that use pixel intensity histograms to determine separation between anatomical regions (Kohn et al., 1991; Tanna et al., 1991; Blatter et al., 1995; Killiany et al., 1993). The interactive 3D segmentation of MRI and CT volumes may also require human judgement and knowledge, but can be very helpful for delineation of anatomical structures for measurements (Heinz & Hanson, 1992). The very high interreader reliability (.97) makes these findings very useful for diagnosis (Kohn et al., 1991).

Automatic techniques for segmentation allow rapid calculation of volume and may thus allow regular use for certain clinical indications such as epilepsy, Alzheimer's disease, late TBI, schizophrenia, stress disorders, etc. (Cascino et al., 1991; Cendes et al., 1993; Deweer et al., 1995; Shenton et al., 1992; Lehéricy et al., 1994; Kesslak, Nalcioglu, & Cotman, 1991; Zentner et al., 1995; Bremner et al., 1995; Jack et al., 1992; Rusinek et al., 1991; Cook et al., 1992; Jackson et al., 1993; Jackson, Kuzniecky, & Cascino, 1994; Bronen et al., 1995; Soininen et al., 1994). Volumes of specific brain structures such as the hippocampi and the amygdala that have a major role in memory (verbal and visual), or the basal ganglia that regulate behavior in different diseases, have become very popular (Bhatia & Marsden, 1994; Soininen et al., 1994; Squire & Zola-Morgan, 1991). Normative values are shown in Table 5.5 (Blatter et al., 1995; Lehéricy et al., 1994; De Carli & Murphy, 1994; Filipek et al., 1989; Jack et al., 1989).

Other Abnormalities

Small hyperintense areas beyond values selected by threshold option are often numerous in practice, and we suggest a classification ranging 0–2 that is based on the number of these lesions rather than on their volume. Thus, 0 = none, 1 = <5 abnormalities, and 2 = >5 abnormalities, as selected by inspection.

Hypointense areas are apparent on inspection as discrete or diffuse areas. Discrete lesions within the presence of a widespread lesion are identified as diffuse lesions, and volume measurements are not performed. The clear definition of lesion character, location, and volume is necessary for structure-function relationship studies (Levin, 1993; Grattan et al., 1994; Robinson et al., 1984; Grafman et al., 1988; Salazar et al., 1986; Lopez et al., 1995).

Table 5.5: Selected Normal Volume Measurement Values (MRI studies)

Structures	Measurement cc^3	Reference
Whole brain volume	1180–1730	(Blatter et al., 1995; Rusinek et al., 1991; De Carli & Murphy, 1994; Filipek et al., 1989)
Total grey matter	580–760	(Blatter et al., 1995)
Total white matter	400–750	(Blatter et al., 1995; Filipek et al., 1989)
Total ventricular volume	15–30	(Blatter et al., 1995; Filipek et al., 1989)
Third ventricular volume	0.06–2.20	(Blatter et al., 1995; De Carli & Murphy, 1994)
Fourth ventricular volume	1.3–2.1	(Blatter et al., 1995)
Left temporal horn	0.0–0.16	(De Carli et al., 1992; De Carli & Murphy, 1994)
Right temporal horn	0.07–0.13	(De Carli et al., 1992; De Carli & Murphy, 1994)
Ventricular/brain ratio	1.20–2.10	(Blatter et al., 1995)
Right lateral ventricle	3.4–22.4	(De Carli et al., 1992)
Left lateral ventricle	3.7–22.0	(De Carli et al., 1992)
Left temporal horn	0.0–1.6	(Gale et al., 1994; De Carli et al., 1992)
Right temporal horn	0.07–1.6	(Gale et al., 1994; De Carli et al., 1992)
Total cerebral CSF	79–250	(De Carli et al., 1992)
Total cerebral subarachnoid CSF	71–256	(De Carli et al., 1992)
Right temporal lobe volume	47–83	(De Carli et al., 1992; De Carli & Murphy, 1994; Jack et al., 1988)
Left temporal lobe volume	44–82	(De Carli et al., 1992; De Carli & Murphy, 1994; Jack et al., 1988)
Right hippocampus	2.7–3.83	(Lehéricy et al., 1994; Soininen et al., 1994; Jack et al., 1989)
Left hippocampus	2.3–3.47	
Right amygdala	1.74–2.29	(Lehéricy et al., 1994; Soininen et al., 1994)
Left amygdala	2.05–2.43	

Volume of the brain can be expressed as a volume or as a ratio that takes into account the size of the skull. Blatter et al. found a significant difference in total brain volume between men and women, which disappeared after correction for skull size. The effect of age was similar on both sexes, and the brain's volume decreases in size during aging (Blatter et al., 1995).

Volumes of the temporal lobes are important considerations. The right temporal lobe is significantly bigger than the left in most normal subjects (De Carli & Murphy, 1994; Jack et al., 1989, 1988; Lencz et al., 1992). DeCarli et al. (1994) found that these differences were not age-related in healthy adults. Lench et al. (1992) found a significant correlation between left temporal lobe size and the verbal selective reminding test scores in epileptic patients. Temporal lobe morphometric analysis in psychiatric and behavioral studies is increasingly important (Inzelberg et al., 1994; Killiany et al., 1993; Shenton et al., 1992;, Young, et al., 1991; Leonard et al., 1993).

Temporal lobes are usually measured on coronal cuts in a slightly different way by various groups. The anterior pole is easy to visualize on the first cut on which the temporal lobe is seen. The anterior medial end of the temporal lobe is the entorhinal sulcus and the lateral border at the level of the Sylvian fissure, excluding the frontal operculum. The line connecting these borders passes through the temporal stem and separates the frontal from the temporal lobes. The posterior border of the temporal lobe is at the temporo-occipital incisura, at which the vertical anterior occipital sulcus separates the temporal from occipital lobes (Damasio, 1995). Since this anatomical landmark is difficult to assess on the coronal cuts, the posterior border of the temporal lobes was set arbitrarily by Jack et al. (1988) at the level of the internal auditory canal and the vestibule, by de Carli et al.

(1994) at the cut on which the aqueduct of Sylvius was seen, by Bremner et al. (1995) at the cut anterior to the superior colliculus, and by Lencz et al. (1992) at the cut that was 15 mm posterior to the basilar artery. Detailed descriptions of measurement of the temporal lobes volume are in the above-mentioned studies and in Levin et al. (1995). The volumes of the frontal, parietal, and occipital lobes may be of importance in the investigation of neurological or psychological disorders and MRI-based regional analysis of the cerebral lobes and of the posterior fossa in the axial plane described by Rusinek et al. (1991).

Volume measurements of gray and white matter were performed on CT, MRI studies using either manual tracing or interactive threshold and provide very important information in patients with brain damage of various etiologies (Rusinek et al., 1991; Filipek et al., 1989; Levin et al., 1995; Schwartz et al., 1985).

Volumes of specific brain structures such as the hippocampus, amygdala, caudate nuclei, and other basal ganglia, corpus callosum, etc. are powerful tools for individually assessing the relationship of these structures to clinical and neurobehavioral findings.

Volumes of the hippocampus and amygdala—the memory system includes structures located in the medial temporal lobe, mainly the hippocampus and the amygdala (Squire & Zola-Morgan, 1991). The hippocampus itself appears to be intimately involved with recent memory; bilateral destruction of the hippocampus or the fimbriae causes profound, persistent disturbance in recent and declarative memory (Naidich et al., 1987; Alper, 1986; Woolsey & Nelson, 1975; Mishkin, Ungerleider, & Macko, 1983). The hippocampal formation and related structures are demonstrated well on MRI studies (Naidich et al., 1987; Mark, Daniels, & Naidich, 1993; Mark et al., 1995). Severe hippocampal damage was found in patients with history of anoxia and TBI (Lévesque et al., 1991). Volumetric measurements of the hippocampus and amygdala were performed mainly for the investigation of epilepsy and the early stages of Alzheimer's disease (Cascino et al., 1991; Lehéricy et al., 1994; Zentner et al., 1995; Cook et al., 1992; Jackson et al., 1993; Bronen et al., 1995; Jack et al., 1989, 1988; Lencz et al., 1992; Levin et al., 1995; Achten et al., 1995; Tien & Felsberg, 1995; Watson et al., 1992). These studies may be important for the evaluation of post-traumatic or post-CVA memory disturbances and serve in the choice of appropriate treatment and in the assessment of prognosis in TBI patients and possibly in Post-Traumatic Stress Disorder (Bremner et al., 1995). Ideally, they should be performed in conjunction with a neuropsychological evaluation (Deweer et al., 1995). Soininen et al. (1994) found a correlation between volumes of amygdala and the performance on visual memory tests, but not with scores on the verbal memory test, and Loring et al. (1993) showed significant correlations between Wada memory asymmetries and hippocampal volume asymmetries in patients with complex partial seizures who did not have structural lesions other than atrophy on radiological evaluation. Lencz et al. (1992) found significant correlations between the size of the left hippocampus and the Wechsler logical memory percent retention scores. These authors stress the fact that asymmetry in normal structures was found for the size of *temporal lobes,* but not for *hippocampi.*

The amygdala is almond-shaped, composed of a number of nuclei, has a heterogenous structure, and is continuous with the periamygdaloid cortex. It is part of the basolateral circuit of Yakovlev and plays a major role in regulating emotion. It has been suggested that the right amygdala influences the arousal and activation of negative emotions, and the left may be important for positive emotions. Amygdala contributes to memory and, in particular, to visual memory and has close connections with the orbitofrontal the hippocampus from the amygdala, each using slightly different definitions (Cendes et al., 1993; Watson et al., 1992).

The hippocampal formation includes the hippocampus proper, the dentate gyrus, and the subicular complex. It is part of the Papez circuit and is closely associated with memory and particularly with verbal memory (Soininen et al., 1994). Selective damage to CA1 cells of the hippocampus or to the perforant pathway may result in memory loss in Alzheimer's disease (Hyman et al., 1986). Since different disease processes, such as temporal lobe epilepsy, TBI, Alzheimer's disease, cerebrovascular disease, and others have symptoms that are related to the anatomical structures that are involved, it is important to assess the volumes of the amygdala and the hippocampus separately. Other conditions that are associated with altered memory processes and/or damage to the medial temporal lobes or to the CA1 cell population (like TBI or severe hypotensive states) should be investigated using this technique.

In *delineation of the hippocampus*, anterior and superior margins provide the most reliable landmark in the temporal horn. When it is obliterated, a line is drawn connecting the temporal horn to the surface of the uncus or to the sulcus at the inferior margin of the semilunar gyrus. Distinction of the hippocampal head from the amygdala can be aided by recognizing the undulating contour of the digitations and by the fact that the alveus provides a high signal intensity (white matter) marker that defines the superior border of the hippocampus (Jack et al., 1992). The inferior margin of the hippocampus includes the subicular complex and the uncal cleft, which separates the hippocampus from the parahippocampal gyrus or the entorhinal cortex. The posterior margin is where the crus of the fornix clearly separates from the hippocampus or on a plane intersecting the posterior commissure (Killiany et al., 1993; Lehéricy et al., 1994; Soininen et al., 1994; Jack et al., 1989; Watson et al., 1992). Bremner et al. (1995) used slightly different landmarks for the delineation of the hippocampus that included the anterior border on a slice anterior to the superior colliculus and the posterior border at the level of bifurcation of the basilar artery. A protocol based on previous and newly accumulated experience that includes detailed descriptions of volumetric measurements of the hippocampus and the amygdala is referenced in Levin et al. (1995).

The measurements of Soininen et al. (1994) showed significant volume difference (p< 0.001) between the left and right sides, the amygdala being larger on the left side and the hippocampus being larger on the right side. The volumes of the amygdala obtained by other authors were larger than in Soininen's study (Cook et al., 1992; Soininen et al., 1994; Watson et al., 1992). The relation of age and the volume of the amygdala was shown in the study of Coffey et al. (1992). Normal volumes of the amygdala and the hippocampi are shown in Table 5.5.

Volume of the corpus callosum and corpus callosum/brain ratio—these measurements are performed on a midsagittal T1W MRI cut where best visualization of the corpus callosum is obtained (Laissy et al., 1993). The different measurements of the corpus callosum enable assessment of white matter damage in different pathologies including TBI and cerebrovascular disease (see section on imaging of trauma) (Levin et al., 1990; Laissy et al., 1993).

In determining the *volume of CSF* (produced by the choroid plexus mainly within the cerebral ventricles), total CSF volume depends on several factors: the rate of production and absorption of CSF; the patency of narrow passages such as Foramina of Monro, Magendie, and Luschka, and of the aqueduct of Sylvius; cerebral tissue loss; the cerebral interstitial fluid characteristics; and various additional factors such as elongation and tortuousity of blood vessels. The computerized quantification of total CSF within the different compartments in the brain and skull was proven to be accurate and reliable and thus serve for correlations with clinical parameters in various neuropsychiatric disorders (Kohn et al., 1991). Total ventricular volume, the ventricle brain volume ratio (VBR), volumes of the third and fourth ventricles, and of the frontal and temporal horns on the left and on the right may be of importance for the assessment of patient's findings, especially as a part of structure-function analysis. Volume can be measured using the threshold option and different segmentation techniques (Kohn et al., 1991; Tanna et al., 1991; Blatter et al., 1995; De Carli et al., 1992; Jack et al., 1992). Normative volume values are listed in Table 5.5. The VBR obtained from CT studies in 78 control subjects was 5.2 (a median value) which was significantly lower in comparison with TBI patients (Levin, 1993; Levin et al., 1981).

Ventricular enlargement in closed head injury was assessed using CT and MR studies by Levin et al. and by others, and correlated with residual disturbance in cognition and memory, which was more marked when it occurred gradually (Levin, 1993; Gale et al., 1994; Levin et al., 1981). In Gale's study, temporal horn's volume was an indication of local temporal lobe damage and disruption of memory performance. The lateralization of visual and verbal memory tasks suggested in the study of Nasrallah et al. (1982) and by Levin (1993) was not supported in Gale's study (1994). Tanna et al. (1991) found that patients with Alzheimer's disease had higher total CSF (total ventricular, third ventricular, total extraventricular) and lower brain volumes than the controls. Enlarged ventricles (expressed as ventricle-brain ratio) were found in chronic schizophrenia (especially in the paranoid subgroup) (Uzzell et al., 1979).

TISSUE CHARACTERISTICS

The use of CT and of MRI as the main diagnostic modalities in neuroradiology enabled tissue recognition, differentiation, and characterization using density as a parameter in CT and the intensity as a parameter on MR (Brooks, Di Chiro, & Keller, 1980; Armitsu et al., 1977; Maravilla, Pastel, & Kirkpatrick, 1978; Weinstein, Duchesneau, & MacIntyre, 1977). Normal intensities and volumes of cerebral gray and white matter were measured and calculated and serve as a control for normal aging and for the assessment of diseases of various etiologies even at their preclinical presentations (Table 5.5) (Blatter et al., 1995; Armitsu et al., 1977; Meguro et al., 1990; Zatz, Jernigan, & Ahumada Jr., 1982). The increased use of modern MR technologies and sequences enable tissue and fluid characterization by additional parameters, such as diffusion, perfusion, magnetization transfer, etc. advancing the diagnostic capabilities (Hajnal et al., 1991; Le Bihan et al., 1988; Warach et al., 1995; Sheppard, 1995).

In *altered tissue*, MR is especially sensitive in depicting *density/intensity* characteristics, and these are readily seen as abnormal signals on T2W studies. These changes may occur either due to tissue loss or as part of demyelination.

The appearance of abnormal density or signal intensity in the *gray matter of the cortex or the basal ganglia* usually signifies cerebrovascular, metabolic, or tumoral etiology of disease (Kjos, Brant-Zawadzki, & Young, 1983; Gropen et al., 1994; Heindenreich et al., 1988; Baganz & Dross, 1994). Abnormal signal of the *gray matter of the hippocampus* is one of the findings in mesial temporal sclerosis and may be assessed by T2 relaxometry (T2 values greater than 116 ms) (Jackson, Kuzniecky, & Cascino, 1994; Bronen et al., 1995; Bronen, 1994; Grunewald et al., 1994; Ylikoski et al.,

1993). Since the biological factors that are the basis for T2 prolongation and for the atrophic changes may be independent, relaxometry and volumetry cannot substitute each for the other at the present stage. In fact, it was shown in different studies that atrophy occurred more frequently than signal changes, but signal changes were independent of atrophy (Jackson, Kuzniecky, & Cascino, 1994; Bronen et al., 1995; Damasio, 1995).

Post-traumatic cortical "lesions" are compatible with cortical contusions, may show hypointense signal on T2WI (hemosiderin), and are often accompanied by the presence of irregular brain margins and by decreased Gray-White Discrimination (GWD) (Groswasser et al., 1987). On subacute T1W images, these lesions may be mainly hyperintense. Presence of areas of hypodensity on a CT study or a hyperintense signal in *white matter* on T2W MR images occurs in aging, in cerebrovascular diseases, and in tumoral, toxic, metabolic, and other processes. The presence of white matter changes in healthy elderly persons correlates with attention and with speed of mental processing and with frontal lobe abilities (Ylikoski et al., 1993; Hunt et al., 1989).

The presence of signal abnormality on post-traumatic MRI studies was especially common in the frontal and temporal lobes (Levin, 1993; Groswasser et al., 1987; Levin et al., 1992). Levin et al. reported on the correlation between the disappearance of the abnormal signals on MR studies in mild and moderate closed head injuries and the parallel improvement of cognitive and memory functions of the patients. However, the relationship between neuroanatomic localization of abnormal signals and the most salient deficits was inconsistent (Levin et al., 1992). Levin et al. found that cognitive impairment was more consistently present in children who were 6–10 years old than in older children and adolescents (Levin et al., 1993). Presence of frontal lobe MRI lesions in children was associated with greater disability than children who sustained a diffuse injury (Mendelsohn et al., 1992). Depth of location of parenchymal abnormalities was related to the level of consciousness and outcome after closed head injury, confirming the centripetal model of progressive brain injury suggested by Ommaya and Gennarelli (Levin, 1993; Ommaya & Gennarelli, 1974; Levin et al., 1988).

Quantitative assessment of tissue densities and intensities was also performed in Alzheimer patients and in MS patients (Reider-Groswasser et al., 1988; George et al., 1981). The quantitative data in these studies offered additional tissue characterization that could not be obtained by visual inspection. In addition, correlation between tissue parameters, such as quantity of abnormal signal in white matter, showed a significant relationship to tissue loss as expressed by some of the linear measurements (Reider-Groswasser et al., 1988). The volumetric assessment of certain brain structures, such as the gray matter of the amygdaloid-hippocampal complex and the white matter of the corpus callosum, are powerful tools in the assessment of normal brain development and of certain conditions such as TBI, hypoxic-ischemic events, and temporal lobe epilepsy (mesial temporal sclerosis) (Levin et al., 1990; Laissy et al., 1993; Soininen et al., 1994). This subject is discussed in more detail in the previous section on volume measurements. The explosion in the use of quantitative MR using T2 relaxometry and MR-based volumetrics raises the question as to what extent these are clinical or research tools (Bronen, 1994).

Gray/white matter junction characterization using a gray/white matter discriminability scale ranging 0–3 was used for the evaluation of late CT studies of 111 head-injured Vietnam war veterans (Reider-Groswasser et al., 1995a, b). This scale is rated in the following manner: 0–normal, 1–hazy junction, 2–hazy and partially missing white matter digitations, and 3–diffuse changes (Figure 5.8). High correlations between GWD and the

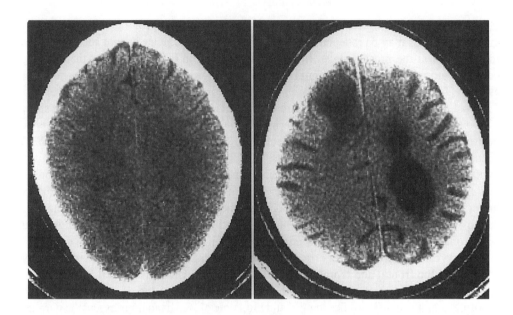

Figure 5.8: Gray White Matter Discriminability (GWMD). Left—Supra ventricular CT cut demonstrates haziness of gray white junction many in frontal lobe. Note widening of adjacent sulci. GWMD=Grade 1. Right—Bilaterial encephalomalacic areas, lack of gray white discriminability, and marked widening of sulci. GWMD=Grade 3.

width of the third ventricle in both closed and penetrating lesions indicated probably diffuse DAI and/or ischemia (Reider-Groswasser et al., 1995a, b; 1993). Loss of GWD was also described by George et al. (1981) in CT studies of patients with Alzheimer's disease and was referred to in CT studies of patients with global hypoperfusion by Kjos et al. (1983).

The subcortical low intensity in early cortical ischemia on T2- and proton-density MR images was attributed to disruption of the axonal transportation and continuous production of free radicals and iron accumulation by Ida et al. (1994). These authors stressed the distinction between hypointensity that was the result of a local metabolic process as distinguished from a similar appearance that may be caused by minute hemorrhages at the gray/white matter junction. Iron deposition in the basal ganglia after a cortical ischemic hypoxic episode has been described by Dietrich and Bradley (1988).

Tissue characterization using MR spectroscopy (when MR imaging is normal) may offer additional information that might be useful for determining when to operate on patients with chronic subdural hematomas and for the assessment of the efficacy of treatment (Yoshida et al., 1994).

CONCLUSIONS AND RECOMMENDATIONS

We suggest a diagnostic approach to imaging in early and late phases of TBI and CVA. The subjective, quantitative, and semiquantitative parameters (such as the width of the third ventricle and GWD), which were shown to be significant for the assessment of TBI and of vascular disease, are described. The contribution of a standardized quantitative approach is stressed, and the importance of additional subjective impressions with special attention for individual clinical complaints and problems are noted. The suggested protocols will enable clinicians and researchers to estimate brain damage caused by lesions and by the diffuse process of tissue injury with the concomitant loss that accompanies the local processes. The data from these protocols may suggest the efficient use of additional studies for further elucidation and may contribute to standardized multicenter clinical/ imaging correlations.

REFERENCES

Achten, E., et al. (1995). An MR protocol for presurgical evaluation of patients with complex partial seizures of temporal lobe origin. *American Journal of Neuroradiology, 16*, 1201–1213.

Adams, J. (1984). Head injury. In J.H. Adams, J.A.N. Corsellis, & L.W. Duchen (Eds.), *Greenfield's neuropathology* (4th ed.) (pp. 85–124). New York: John Wiley & Sons.

Adams, J., et al. (1977). Diffuse brain damage of immediate impact type: Its relationship to primary brain stem damage in head injury. *Brain, 100*, 489–502.

———. (1982). Diffuse axonal injury due to non-missile head injury in humans: an analysis of 45 cases. *Annals of Neurology, 12*, 557–563.

Aharon-Peretz, J., Cummings, J.L., & Hill, M.A. (1988). Vascular dementia, and dementia of the Alzheimer type: Cognition, ventricular size and leuko-araiosis. *Archives of Neurology, 45*, 719–721.

Alper, J. (1986). Our dual memory. *Science, 7*, 44–49.

Amarenco, P., et al. (1993). Very small (border zone) cerebellar infarcts. Distribution, causes, mechanisms and clinical features. *Brain, 116*, 161–186.

Anderson, S.C., Chah, C.P., & Murtagh, F.R. (1987). Congested deep subcortical veins as a sign of dural venous thrombosis. *Journal of Computer Assisted Tomography, 11*, 1059–1061.

Armitsu, T., et al. (1977). White-gray matter differentiation in computed tomography. *Journal of Computer Assisted Tomography, 1*, 489–491.

Asato, R., Okumura, R., & Konishi, J. (1991). "Fogging effect" in MR of cerebral infarct. *Journal of Computer Assisted Tomography, 15*, 160–62.

Baganz, M.D., & Dross, E. (1994). Valproic acid-induced hyperammonemic encephalopathy. *American Journal of Neuroradiology, 15*, 1779–1781.

Bamford, J., Sandercock, A.G., & Dennis, M.S. (1991). Classification and natural history of clinically identifiable subtypes of cerebral infarction. *Lancet, 337*, 1521–1526.

Barnwell, S.L., et al. (1994). Safety and efficacy of delayed intraarterial urokinase therapy with mechanical clot disruption for thromboembolic stroke. *American Journal of Neuroradiology, 15*, 1817–1822.

Barr, R., & Gean, A.D. (1994). Craniofacial trauma. In W. Brant (Ed.), *Fundamentals of diagn,ostic radiology* (pp. 52–84). Baltimore: Williams & Wilkins.

Bastianello, S., et al. (1991). Hyperdense middle cerebral artery CT sign. *Neuroradiology, 33*, 207–211.

Becker, H., et al. (1979). CT fogging effect with ischemic cerebral infarcts. *Neuroradiology, 18*, 185–192.

Berman, S.A., Hayman, L.A., & Hinck, V.C. (1980). Correlation of CT cerebral vascular territories with function. I. Anterior cerebral artery. *American Journal of Roentgenology, 135*, 253–257.

———. (1984). Correlation of CT cerebral vascular territories with function: 3. Middle cerebral artery. *American Journal of Neuroradiology, 5*, 161–166.

Bhatia, K.B., & Marsden, C.D. (1994). The behavioural and motor consequences of focal lesions of the basal ganglia in man. *Brain, 117*, 859–876.

Blatter, D.D., et al. (1992). Cerebral MR angiography with multiple overlapping thin slab acquisition. Part II. Early clinical experience. *Radiology, 183*, 379–389.

———. (1995). Quantitative volumetric analysis of brain MR: Normative database spanning 5 decades of life. *American Journal of Neuroradiology, 16*, 241–245.

Bogousslavsky, J., Regli, F., & Uske, A. (1988). Thalamic infarcts: Clinical syndromes, etiology and prognosis. *Neurology, 38*, 837–847.

Bremner, J.D., et al. (1995). MRI-based measurement of hippocampal volume in patients with combat-related posttraumatic stress disorder. *American Journal of Psychiatry, 152*, 973–981.

Breslau, J., et al. (1995). Phased-array surface coil MR of the orbits and optic nerves. *American Journal of Neuroradiology, 16*, 1247–1251.

Bronen, R.A. (1994). Quantitative MRI for epilepsy: A clinical and research tool? (commentary). *American Journal of Neuroradiology, 15*, 1157–1160.

Bronen, R.A., et al. (1995). Regional distribution of MRI findings in hippocampal sclerosis. *American Journal of Neuroradiology, 16*, 1193–1200.

Brooks, R.A., Di Chiro, G., & Keller, M.R. (1980). Explanation of cerebral white-gray contrast in computed tomography. *Journal of Computer Assisted Tomography, 4*, 489–491.

Bryan, R.N., et al. (1994). A method for using MR to evaluate the effects of cardiovascular disease on the brain: The Cardiovascular Health Study. *American Journal of Neuroradiology, 15*, 1625–1633.

Bryan, R.N., Whitlow, W.D., & Levy, L.M. (1991). Cerebral infarction and ischemic disease. In S.W. Atlas. (Ed.), *Magnetic resonance imaging of the brain and spine* (pp. 411–437). New York: Raven Press.

Carter, K.D., & Nerad, J.A. (1987). Fluctuating visual loss secondary to orbital emphysema. *American Journal of Ophthalmology, 104*, 664–665.

Cascino, G.D., et al. (1991). Magnetic resonance imaging-based volume studies in temporal lobe epilepsy: Pathological correlations. *Annals of Neurology, 30*, 31–36.

Cendes, F., et al. (1993). Early childhood prolonged febrile convulsions, atrophy and sclerosis of mesial structures, and temporal lobe epilepsy: An MRI volumetric study. *Neurology, 43*, 1083–1087.

Chodosh, E.H., et al. (1988). Silent stroke in the NINCDS stroke data bank. *Neurology, 38*, 1674–1679.

Choi, D. (1995). Secondary neuronal injury after head trauma: Role of excitixicity. *Journal of Neurologic Rehabilitation, 9*, 61–64.

Coffey, C., et al. (1992). Quantitative cerebral anatomy of the aging human brain: A cross-sectional study using magnetic resonance imaging. *Neurology, 42*, 527–536.

Cook, M.J., et al. (1992). Hippocampal volumetric and morphometric studies in frontal and temporal lobe epilepsy. *Brain, 115*, 1001–1015.

Cordobes, F., et al. (1983). Intraventricular hemorrhage in severe head injury. *Journal of Neurosurgery, 58*, 217–222.

Dahlbeck, S.W., et al. (1991). The interuncal distance: A new MR measurement for the hippocampal atrophy of Alzheimer's disease. *American Journal of Neuroradiology, 12*, 931–932.

Damasio, H. (Ed.). (1995). *Human brain anatomy in computerized images.* New York: O.U. Press.

De Carli, C., & Murphy, D.G.M. (1994). Lack of age-related differences in temporal lobe volume of very healthy adults. *American Journal of Neuroradiology, 15*, 689–696.

De Carli, C., et al. (1992). Method for quantification of brain, ventricular, and subarachnoid CSF volumes from MR images. *Journal of Computer Assisted Tomography, 16*, 274–284.

De Leon, M.J., Ferris, S.H., & Georg, A.E. (1980). Computed tomography evaluation of brain-behaviour relationship in senile dementia of the Alzheimer type. *Neurobiology of Aging, 1*, 69–77.

Deweer, B., et al. (1995). Memory disorders in probable Alzheimer's disease: The role of hippocampal atrophy as shown on MRI. *Journal of Neurology, Neurosurgery, and Psychiatry, 58*, 590–597.

Dietrich, R.B., & Bradley, W.G., Jr. (1988). Iron accumulation in the basal ganglia following severe ischemic-anoxic insults in children. *Radiology, 168*, 203–206.

Doraiswamy, P., et al. (1992). Morphometric changes of the human midbrain with normal aging: MR and stereologic findings. *American Journal of Neuroradiology, 13*: 383–386.

———. (1993). Interuncal distance as a measure of hippocampal atrophy: Normative data on axial MR imaging. *American Journal of Neuroradiology, 14*, 141–143.

Dupont, R., McCullum, M., & Jeste, D.V. (1988). Post-stroke depression and psychosis. *Psychiatric Clinics of North America, 11*, 133–149.

Early, B., et al. (1993). Interuncal distance in healthy volunteers and in patients with Alzheimer's disease. *American Journal of Neuroradiology, 14*, 907–910.

Eisenberg, H.M., et al. (1990). Initial CT findings in 753 patients with severe head injury: A report from the Traumatic Coma Data Bank. *Journal of Neurosurgery, 73*, 688–698.

Elster, A.D., & Moody, D.M. (1990). Early cerebral infarction: Gadopentetate dimeglumine enhancement. *Radiology, 177*, 627–632.

Feinberg, W.M., et al. (1990). Epidemiologic features of asymptomatic cerebral infarction in patients with nonvalvular atrial fibrillation. *Archives of Internal Medicine, 150,* 2340–2344.

Filipek, A., et al. (1989). Magnetic resonance imaging-based brain morphometry: Development and application to normal subjects. *Annals of Neurology, 25,* 61–67.

Fisher, C.M. (1965). Lacunes: Small deep cerebral infarcts. *Neurology, 15,* 774–784.

Friedland, S., et al. (1992). *The thickened optic nerve: A CT study.* Paper presented at The Brommelschlager Conference and Postgraduate Course on Head and Neck Imaging, October 18–23, Jerusalem, Israel.

Fujikawa, T., Yamawaki, S., & Touhouda, Y. (1993). Incidence of silent cerebral infarction in patients with major depression. *Stroke, 24,* 1631–1634.

Gale, S.D., et al. (1994). Traumatic brain injury and temporal horn enlargement: Correlates with tests of intelligence and memory. *Neuropsychiatry, Neuropsychology, and Behavioral Neurology, 7,* 160–165.

Galynker, I.I., et al. (1995). Negative symptoms in patients with basal ganglia strokes. *Neuropsychiatry, Neuropsychology, and Behavioral Neurology, 8,* 113–117.

Gennarelli, T., et al. (1985). Diffuse axonal injury and traumatic coma in the primate: In R.G. Dacey Jr., H.R. Winn, R.W. Rimel, & J.A. Jane (Eds.), *Trauma of the central nervous system* (pp. 169–193). New York: Raven Press.

Gentry, L.R. (1991). Head trauma. In S.W. Atlas (Ed.), *Magnetic resonance imaging of the brain and spine* (pp. 439–466). New York: Raven Press.

Gentry, L.R., Godersky, J.C., & Thompson, B.H. (1989). Traumatic brainstem injury: MR imaging. *Radiology, 171,* 177–187.

Gentry, L.R., Thompson, B., & Godersky, J. (1988). Trauma to the corpus callosum: MR features. *American Journal of Neuroradiology, 9,* 1129–1138.

George, A.E., et al. (1981). Parenchymal CT correlates of senile dementia (Alzheimer's disease): Loss of gray-white matter discriminability. *American Journal of Neuroradiology, 2,* 205–213.

Ghika, J., Bogosslavsky, J., & Regli, F. (1989). Infarcts in the territory of the deep perforants from the carotid system. *Neurology, 39,* 507–512.

Goldstein, M. (1990). Traumatic brain injury: A silent epidemic (editorial). *Annals of Neurology, 27,* 327.

———. (1993). Decade of the brain: National Institute of Neurological Disorders and Stroke. *Neurosurgery, 32,* 297.

Graff-Radford, N.R., Damasio, A.R., and Yamada, T. (1988). Nonhemorrhagic infarction of the thalamus: Behavioral, anatomic and physiologic correlates. *Neurology, 34,* 14–23.

Grafman, J., et al. (1988). Intellectual function following penetrating head injury in Vietnam veterans. *Brain, 111,* 169–184.

Grattan, L.M., et al. (1994). Cognitive flexibility and empathy after frontal lobe lesion. *Neuropsychiatry, Neuropsychology, and Behavioral Neurology, 7,* 251–259.

Greenberg, D.A., Aminoff, M.J., & Simon, R.P. (1993). Stroke. In *Clinical neurology* (2nd ed.) (pp. 250–280). Englewood Cliffs, NJ: Prentice-Hall International.

Gropen, T.I., et al. (1994). Cerebral hyperemia in MELAS. *Stroke, 25,* 1873–1876.

Groswasser, Z., et al. (1987). Magnetic resonance imaging in head injured patients with normal late computed tomography scans. *Surgical Neurology, 27,* 331–337.

Grunewald, R.A., et al. (1994). MR detection of hippocampal disease in epilepsy: factors influencing T2 relaxation time. *American Journal of Neuroradiology, 15,* 1149–1156.

Gyldensted, C., & Kostelijanetz, M. (1976). Measurements of normal ventricular system with computer tomography of the brain a preliminary study on 44 adults. *Neuroradiology, 11,* 204–213.

———. (1977). Measurements of normal ventricular system and hemispheric sulci of 100 adults with computed tomography. *Neuroradiology, 14,* 183–192.

Hackney, D. (1991). Skull radiography in the evaluation of acute head trauma: A survey of current practice. *Radiology, 181,* 711–714.

Hahn, F., & Rim, K. (1976). Frontal ventricular dimensions on normal computed tomography. *American Journal of Roentgenology, 126,* 593–596.

Hajnal, J.V., et al. (1991). MR imaging of anisotropically restricted diffusion of water in the central nervous system: Technical, anatomic, and pathological considerations. *Journal of Computer Assisted Tomography, 15*, 1–18.

Hayman, L.A., Berman, S.A., & Hinck, V.C. (1981). Correlation of CT cerebral vascular territories with function. II. Posterior cerebral artery. *American Journal of Roentgenology, 137*, 13–19.

Heindenreich, R.E., et al. (1988). Acute extrapyramidal syndrome in methymalonic acidemia "metabolic stroke" involving the globus pallidus. *Journal of Pediatrics, 113*, 1022–1027.

Heinz, K., & Hanson, W.A. (1992). Interactive 3D segmentation of MRI and CT volumes using morphological operations. *Journal of Computer Assisted Tomography, 16*, 285–294.

Herderscheé, D., et al. (1992). Silent stroke in patients with transient ischemic attack or minor ischemic stroke. *Stroke, 23*, 1220–1224.

HHS. (1989). *Interagency head injury task force report.* Bethesda, MD: DHHS, PHS, NIH, NINDS.

Higashida, R.T., et al. (1989). Transluminal angioplasty for treatment of intracranial arterial vasospasm. *Journal of Neurosurgery, 71*, 648–653.

Hirshenbain, A. (1993). Lacunar infarcts in the thalamus: A retrospective study of computerized tomography and its correlation to other CT findings and to clinical observations. Unpublished dissertation. Tel-Aviv University: Haifa.

Holland, B.A., Brant-Zawadzki, M., & Pitts, L.H. (1986). Computed tomography in the evaluation of trauma. In M.P. Federle & M. Brant-Zawadzki (Eds.), *The role of CT in evaluation of head trauma* (pp. 1–63). Baltimore: Williams & Wilkins.

Huckman, M.S. (1993). The lessons of history (editorial). *American Journal of Neuroradiology, 14*, 1–2.

Hughes, C.P., & Gado, M. (1981). Computed tomography and aging of the brain. *Radiology, 139*, 391–396.

Hunt, A.L., et al. (1989). Clinical significance of MRI white matter lesions in the elderly. *Neurology, 39*, 1470–1474.

Hyman, B.T., et al. (1986). Perforant pathway changes and the memory impairment of Alzheimer's disease. *Annals of Neurology, 20*, 472–481.

Ida, M., et al. (1994). Subcortical low intensity in early cortical ischemia. *American Journal of Neuroradiology, 15*, 1387–1393.

Inoue, Y., Matsumura, Y., & Fukuda, T. (1990). MR imaging of the Wallerian degeneration in the brainstem: Temporal relationships. *American Journal of Neuroradiology, 11*, 897–902.

Inzelberg, R., et al. (1987). Computed tomography brain changes in Parkinsonian dementia. *Neuroradiology, 29*, 535–539.

———. (1992). The lupus anticoagulant and dementia in non-SLE patients. *Dementia, 3*, 140–145.

———. (1994). Dementia in Parkinson's disease. In A.D. Korczyn (Ed.), *Evaluation of temporal lobe changes in Parkinson's disease in relation to dementia* (pp. 195–221). Bologna: Monduzzi Editore.

———. 1994. Basal ganglia lacunes and Parkinsonism. *Neuroepidemiology, 13*, 108–112.

Jack, J.C.R., et al. (1988). Temporal lobe volume measurement from MR images: Accuracy and left-right asymmetry in normal persons. *Journal of Computer Assisted Tomography, 12*, 21–29.

———. (1989). Anterior temporal lobes and hippocampal formations: Normative volumetric measurements from MR images in young adults. *Radiology, 172*, 549–554.

———. (1992). MR-based hippocampal volumetry in the diagnosis of Alzheimer's disease. *Neurology, 42*, 183–188.

Jackson, G.D., Kuzniecky, R.I., & Cascino, G.D. (1994). Hippocampal sclerosis without detectable hippocampal atrophy. *Neurology, 44*, 42–46.

Jackson, G.D., et al. (1993). Detection of hippocampal pathology in intractable partial epilepsy: Increased sensitivity with quantitative magnetic resonance T2 relaxometry. *Neurology, 43*, 1793–1799.

———. (1993). Optimizing the diagnosis of hippocampal sclerosis using MR imaging. *American Journal of Neuroradiology, 14*, 753–762.

Katz, D.I., et al. (1989). Traumatic basal ganglia hemorrhage: Clinico-pathologic features and outcome. *Neurology, 39*, 897–904.

Kesslak, J.P., Nalcioglu, O., & Cotman, C. (1991). Quantification of magnetic resonance scans for hippocampal and parahippocampal atrophy in Alzheimer's disease. *Neurology, 41*, 51–54.

Killiany, R.J., et al. (1993). Temporal lobe regions on magnetic resonance imaging identify patients with early Alzheimer's disease. *Archives of Neurology, 50*, 949–954.

Kim Han, B., et al. (1989). Reversal sign on CT: Effect of anoxic/ischemic cerebral injury in children. *American Journal of Neuroradiology, 10*, 1191–1198.

Kjos, B., Brant-Zawadzki, M., and Young, R. (1983). Early CT findings of global central nervous hypoperfusion. *American Journal of Radiology, 141*: 1227–1232.

Klingbeil, G.E.G., & Cline, P. (1985). Anterior hypopituitarism: A consequence of head injury. *Archives of Physical Medicine and Rehabilitation, 66*, 44–46.

Kobrine, A., et al. (1977). Demonstration of massive traumatic brain swelling within 20 minutes after injury. *Journal of Neurosurgery, 46*, 256–258.

Kohn, M.I., et al. (1991). Analysis of brain and cerebrospinal fluid volumes with MR imaging: Part I. Methods, reliability, and validation. *Radiology, 178*, 115–122.

Koller, C., et al. (1981). Cerebellar atrophy demonstrated by computed tomography. *Neurology, 31*, 404–412.

Korczyn, A.D., et al. (1986). Dementia in Parkinson's disease. In M.D. Yahr and K.J. Bergmann (Eds.), *Advances in neurology* (Vol. 45). New York: Raven Press.

Kraus, J.F. (1993). Epidemiology of head injuries. In P. Cooper (Ed.), *Head injury* (pp. 1–26). Baltimore: Williams and Wilkins.

Kuhn, M.J., et al. (1989). Wallerian degeneration after cerebral infarction. *Radiology, 172*, 170–182.

Laissy, J.P., et al. (1993). Midsaggital MR measurements of the corpus callosum in healthy subjects and diseased patients: A prospective study. *American Journal of Neuroradiology, 14*, 145–154.

Le Bihan, D., et al. (1988). Separation of diffusion and perfusion in intravoxel incoherent motion MR imaging. *Radiology, 168*, 497–505.

Lehéricy, S., et al. (1994). Amygdalohippocampal MR volume measurements in the early stages of Alzheimer's disease. *American Journal of Neuroradiology, 15*, 929–937.

LeMay, M., et al. (1986). Statistical assessment of perceptual CT scan ratings in patients with Alzheimer-type dementia. *Journal of Computer Assisted Tomography, 10*, 802–809.

Lencz, T., et al. (1992). Quantitative magnetic resonance imaging in temporal lobe epilepsy: Relationship to neuropathology and neuropsychological function. *Annals of Neurology, 31*, 629–637.

Leonard, C.M., et al. (1993). Anomalous cerebral structure in dyslexia revealed with magnetic resonance imaging. *Archives in Neurology, 50*, 461–469.

Lévesque, M.F., et al. (1991). Surgical treatment of limbic epilepsy associated with extrahippocampal lesions: The problem of dual pathology. *Journal of Neurosurgery, 75*, 364–370.

Levin, H.S. (1993). Neurobehavioral sequelae of closed head injury. In E. Cooper (Ed.), *Head injury* (pp. 525–551). Baltimore: Williams and Wilkins.

Levin, H.S., & Welch, K.M.A. (1987). Cerebrovascular ischemia associated with lupus anticoagulant. *Stroke, 18*, 257–263.

Levin, H.S., et al. (1981). Ventricular enlargement after closed head injury. *Archives of Neurology, 38*, 623–629.

———. (1988). Relationship of depth of brain lesions to consciousness and outcome after closed head injury. *Journal of Neurosurgery, 69*, 861–866.

———. (1990). Corpus callosum atrophy following closed head injury: Detection with magnetic resonance imaging. *Journal of Neurosurgery, 73*, 77–81.

———. (1992). Serial magnetic resonance imaging and neurobehavioral findings after mild to moderate closed head injury. *Journal of Neurology, Neurosurgery and Psychiatry, 55*, 255–262.

———. (1993). Cognition in relation to magnetic resonance imaging in head-injured children and adolescents. *Archives of Neurology, 50*, 897–905.

———. (1995). Unpublished data.

Lewin, J.S., et al. (1994). Time-of-flight intracranial MR venography: Evaluation of the sequential oblique section technique. *American Journal of Neuroradiology, 15*, 1657–1664.

Leys, D., et al. (1992). Prevalence and significance of hyperdense middle cerebral artery in acute stroke. *Stroke, 23*, 317–324.

Lindgren, E., & Greitz, T. (1995). The Stockholm school of neuroradiology. *American Journal of, Neuroradiology, 16*, 351–360.

Liu, C.K., et al. (1992). A quantitative MRI study of vascular dementia. *Neurology, 42*, 138–143.

Liu, H.M., Tu, Y.K., & Su, C.T. (1995). Changes of brainstem and perimesencephalic cistern: Dynamic predictor of outcome in severe head injury. *The Journal of Trauma: Injury, Infection and Clinical Care, 38*, 330–333.

Liwnicz, B.H., Mouradian, M.D., & Ball, J.B., Jr. (1987). Intense brain cortical enhancement on CT in laminar necrosis verified by biopsy. *American Journal of Neuroradiology, 8*, 157–159.

Lloyd, M.N.H., Kimber, M., & Burrows, E.H. (1994). Post-traumatic cerebrospinal fluid rhinorrhea: Modern high-definition computed tomography is all that is required for the effective demonstration of the site of leakage. *Clinical Radiology, 49*, 100–103.

Lopez, O.L., et al. (1995). Computed tomography—but not magnetic resonance imaging—identified periventricular white-matter lesions predict symptomatic cerebrovascular disease in probable Alzheimer's disease. *Archives of Neurology, 52*, 659–664.

Loring, D.W., et al. (1993). Wada memory testing and hippocampal volume measurements in the evaluation for temporal lobectomy. *Neurology, 43*, 1789–1793.

Maravilla, K.R., Pastel, M.S., & Kirkpatrick, J.B. (1978). White matter of the cerebellum demonstrated by computerized tomography: Normal anatomy and physical principles. *Journal of Computer Assisted Tomography, 2*, 156–161.

Mark, L.P., Daniels, D.L., & Naidich, T.P. (1993). The fornix. *American Journal of Neuroradiology, 14*, 1355–1358.

Mark, L.P., et al. (1995). Linbic connections. *American Journal of Neuroradiology, 16*, 1303–1306.

Marshall, L.F., et al. (1991). A new classification of head injury based on computerized tomography. *Journal of Neurosurgery, 75*, S14–S 20.

Marshall, R., & Mohr, J. (1993). Current management of ischemic stroke. *Journal of Neurology, Neurosurgery and Psychiatry, 56*, 4–46.

Martin, W.R.W., & Raichle, M.E. (1983). Cerebellar blood flow and metabolism in cerebral hemisphere infarction. *Annals of Neurology, 14*, 168–176.

Mauriello, J.A., et al. (1986). *Diagnostic imaging in radiology* (pp. 323–341). New York: Springer-Verlag.

Max, W., MacKenzie, E.J., & Rice, D.P. (1991). Head injuries costs and consequences. *Journal of Head Trauma Rehabilitation, 6*, 76–91.

McCullough, D., Nelson, K.M., & Ommaya, A.K. (1971). The acute effects of experimental head injury on the vertebrobasilar circulation: angiographic observations. *Journal of Trauma, 11*, 422–428.

Meguro, K., et al. (1990). Cerebral circulation and oxygen metabolism associated with subclinical periventricular hyperintensity as shown by magnetic resonance imaging. *Annals of Neurology, 28*, 378–383.

Mendelsohn, D.B., et al. (1992). Corpus callosum lesions after closed head injury in children: MRI, clinical features and outcome. *Neuroradiology, 34*, 384–388.

————. (1992). Late MRI after head injury in children: Relationship to clinical features and outcome. *Child's Nervous System, 8*, 445–452.

Mishkin, M., Ungerleider, I.G., & Macko, K.A. (1983). Object vision and spatial vision: Two cortical pathways. *Trends in Neuroscience, 6*, 414–417.

Mokri, B., Jack Jr., C.R., & Petty, C.R. (1993). Pseudotumor syndrome associated with cerebral sinus venous occlusion and antiphospholipid antibodies. *Stroke, 24*, 469–472.

Moody, D.M., Bell, M.A., & Challa, V.R. (1990). Features of the cerebral vascular pattern that predict vulnerability of perfusion or oxygenation deficiency: An anatomic study. *American Journal of Neuroradiology, 11*, 431–439.

Morgan, M.K., et al. (1987). Intracranial carotid artery injury in closed head trauma. *Journal of Neurosurgery, 66*, 192–197.

Mori, E., et al. (1992). Intravenous recombinant tissue plasminogen activator in acute carotid artery territory stroke. *Neurology, 42*, 976–982.

Moseley, I. (1995). Imaging the adult brain. *Journal of Neurology, Neurosurgery and Psychiatry, 58*, 7–21.

Mueller, D.P., et al. (1993). Arterial enhancement in acute cerebral ischemia: clinical and angiographic correlation. *American Journal of Neuroradiology, 14*, 661–668.

Nadel, L., et al. (1991). Intracranial vascular abnormalities: Value of MR phase imaging to distinguish thrombus from flowing blood. *American Journal of Neuroradiology, 11*, 1133–1140.

Naidich, T.P., & Righi, A.M. (1995). Imaging. *Radiologic Clinics of North America, 33*, 115–166.

Naidich, T.P., et al. (1987). Hippocampal formation and related structures of the limbic lobe: Anatomic-MR correlation. Part I. Surface features and coronal sections. *Radiology, 162*, 747–754.

———. (1987). Hippocampal formation and related structures of the limbic lobe: Anatomic-MR correlation. Part II. Sagittal sections. *Radiology, 162*, 755–761.

NASCET. (1991). Beneficial effect of carotid endarterectomy in symptomatic patients with high grade carotid stenosis. *New England Journal of Medicine, 325*, 445–453.

———. (1991). Methods, patient characteristics, and progress. *Stroke, 22*, 711–720.

Nasrallah, H.A., et al. (1982). Cerebral ventricular enlargement in subtypes of chronic schizophrenia. *Archives of General Psychiatry, 39*, 774–777.

Nusbaum, M., Reider-Groswasser, I., & Korczyn, A.D. (1989). A differential diagnosis between primary senile dementia (PDD) and multi infarct dementia (MID) using computed tomography. Paper presented at Alzheimer's Meeting, Kyoto, Japan.

Ommaya, A.K., & Gennarelli, T.A. (1974). Cerebral concussion and traumatic unconsciousness: Correlation of experimental and clinical observations on blunt head injuries. *Brain, 97*, 633–654.

Orita, T., et al. (1991). Coronal MR imaging for visualization of Wallerian degeneration of the pyramidal tract. *Journal of Computer Assisted Tomography, 15*, 802–804.

Osborn, A.G. (1994). *Diagnostic neuroradiology* (pp. 330–397). St. Louis: Mosby.

Povlishock, J. (1993). Pathobiology of traumatically induced axonal injury in animals and man. *Annals of Emergency Medicine, 22*, 980–986.

Raininko, R., et al. (1994). The normal brain stem from infancy to old age. A morphometric MRI study. *Neuroradiology, 36*, 364–368.

Rauch, R.A., et al. (1993). Hyperdense middle cerebral arteries as identified on CT as a false sign of vascular occlusion. *American Journal of Neuroradiology, 14*, 669–674.

Regli, L., et al. (1993). Magnetic resonance imaging with gadolinium contrast agent in small deep (lacunar) cerebral infarcts. *Archives of Neurology, 50*, 175–180.

Reider-Groswasser, I., Bornstein, N.M., & Korczyn, A.D. (1995), Parkinsonism in patients with lacunar infarcts of the basal ganglia. *European Neurology, 35*, 46–49.

Reider-Groswasser, I., et al. (1988). MRI parameters in multiple sclerosis patients. *Neuroradiology, 30*, 219–223.

———. (1993a). Late CT findings in brain trauma: Relationship to cognitive and behavioral sequelae and to vocational outcome. *American Journal of Radiology, 160*, 147–152.

———. (1993b). *Optic nerve thickening: CT and angiographic findings in patients with cerebrovascular diseases.* Paper presented at the International Congress on "Advances in Brain Revascularization," April 18–22, Eilat, Israel.

———. (1993c). Spontaneous posttraumatic thrombosis of traumatic cavernous sinus fistula. *Brain Injury, 7*, 547–550.

———. (1995a). Application of neuroimaging for the evaluation of brain trauma. Paper presented at Polish-Israeli Neurological Conference, May, 1995, Warsaw, Poland.

———. (1995b). *Neuroradiologic assessment in traumatic brain injury and stroke.* Paper presented at the Congress on Rehabilitation Medicine, Istanbul, May, 27–31.

Ricci, S., et al. (1993). Silent brain infarction in patients with first-ever stroke: A community-based study in Umbria, Italy. *Stroke, 24*, 647–651.

Rice, D.P., & E.J. MacKenzie Associates. (1989). *Cost of injury in the United States: A report to Congress.* San Francisco, CA: Institute for Health and Aging, University of California and Injury Prevention Center, The Johns Hopkins University.

Robinson, R.G., et al. (1984). Mood disorders in stroke patients. Importance of location of lesion. *Brain, 107*, 81–93.

Rusinek, H., et al. (1991). Alzheimer's disease: Measuring loss of cerebral gray matter with MR imaging. *Radiology, 178*, 109–114.

Salazar, A.M., et al. (1986). Penetrating war injuries of the basal forebrain: Neurology and cognition. *Neurology, 36*, 459–465.

Sawada, H., et al. (1990). MRI demonstration of cortical laminar necrosis and delayed white matter injury in enoxic encephalopathy. *Neuroradiology, 32*, 319–321.

Schwartz, M., et al. (1985). Computed tomographic analysis of brain morphometrics in 30 healthy men, aged 21 to 81 years. *Annals of Neurology, 17*, 146–157.

Segev, Y., et al. (1995). CT appearance of a traumatic cataract. *American Journal of Neuroradiology, 16*, 1174–1175.

Shenton, M., et al. (1992). Abnormalities of the left temporal lobe and thought disorder in schizophrenia: A quantitative magnetic resonance imaging study. *The New England Journal of Medicine, 327*, 604–612.

Sheppard, S. (1995). Basic concepts in magnetic resonance angiography. *Radiologic Clinics of North America, 33*, 91–113.

Skriver, E.B., & Olsen, T.S. (1981). Transient disappearance of cerebral infarcts on CT scanning, the so-called fogging effect. *Neuroradiology, 22*, 61–65.

Skriver, E.B., Skyhoi, O., & McNair, P. (1990). Mass effect and atrophy after stroke. *Acta radiologica, 31*, 431–438.

Soininen, H.S., et al. (1994). Volumetric MRI analysis of the amygdala and the hippocampus in subjects with age associated memory impairment: Correlation to visual and verbal memory. *Neurology, 44*, 1660–1668.

Soloniuk, D., et al. (1986). Traumatic intracranial hematomas: timing of appearance and indications for operative removal. *Journal of Trauma, 26*, 787–794.

Sosin, D.M., Sacks, J.J., & Smith, S. (1989). Head injury associated deaths in the United States from 1979 to 1986. *Journal of American Medical Association, 262*, 2251–2255.

Squire, L.R., & Zola-Morgan, S. (1991). The medial temporal lobe memory system. *Science, 253,* 1380–1386.

Sroka, H., et al. (1981). Organic mental syndrome and confusional states in Parkinson's disease. *Archives of Neurology, 38*, 339–342.

Steinke, W., Kloetzsch, C., & Hennerici, M. (1990). Carotid artery disease assessed by color Doppler flow imaging: Correlation with standard Doppler sonography and angiography. *American Journal of Neuroradiology, 11*, 259–266.

Sze, G., et al. (1988). Dural sinus thrombosis: Verification with spin-echo techniques. *American Journal of Neuroradiology, 9*, 679–686.

Taha, J.M., et al. (1993). Sigmoid sinus thrombosis after closed head injury in children. *Neurosurgery, 32*, 544–546.

Tanaka, H., et al. (1993). Silent brain infarction and coronary artery disease in Japanese patients. *Archives of Neurology, 50*, 706–709.

Tanna, N.K., et al. (1991). Analysis of brain and cerebrospinal fluid volumes with MR imaging: Impact on PET data correction for atrophy: Part II. Aging and Alzheimer's dementia. *Radiology, 178*, 123–130.

Teasdale, E., & Hadley, D.M. (1990). Radiodiagnosis of brain injury. In P.J. Vinken, G.W. Bruyn, & H.L. Klawans (Eds.), *Handbook of Clinical Neurology: Head injury* (Vol.13) (pp. 143–179). Amsterdam: Elsevier.

ter Penning, B. (1992). Pathophysiology of stroke. *Neuroimaging Clinics of North America, 2*, 389–408.

Thomeier, W.C., Brown, D.C., & Mirvis, S.E. (1990). The laterally tilted dens: A sign of subtle odontoid fracture on plain radiography. *American Journal of Neuroradiology, 11*, 605–608.

Tien, R.D., & Felsberg, G.J. (1995). The hippocampus in status epilepticus: Demonstration of signal intensity and morphologic changes with sequential fast spin-echo MR imaging. *Radiology, 194*, 249–256.

Tomsick, T.A., et al. (1990). Hyperdense middle cerebral artery sign on CT: Efficacy in detecting middle cerebral artery thrombosis. *American Journal of Neuroradiology, 11*, 473–477.

Tomura, N., et al. (1988). Early CT finding in cerebral infarction: Obscuration of the lentiform nucleus. *Radiology, 168*, 463–467.

Truwit, C.L., et al. (1990). Loss of the insular ribbon: Another CT sign of acute middle cerebral artery infarction. *Radiology, 176*, 801–806.

Tsai, F.Y., et al. (1994). Percutaneous transluminal angioplasty adjunct to thrombolysis for acute middle cerebral artery rethrombosis. *American Journal of Neuroradiology, 15,* 1823–1829.

Ur-Rahman, N., & Al-Tahan, A.R. (1993). Computed tomographic evidence of an extensive thrombosis and infarction of the deep venous system. *Stroke, 24,* 744–746.

Uzzell, B.P., et al. (1979). Lateralized psychological impairment associated with CT lesions in head injured patients. *Cortex, 15,* 391–401.

Vardiman, A.B., et al. (1995). Treatment of traumatic arterial vasospasm with intraarterial papaverine infusion. *American Journal of Neuroradiology, 16,* 319–321.

Vergote, G., Vandeperre, H., & DeMan, R. (1992). The reversal sign. *Neuroradiology, 34,* 215–216.

Virapongse, C., et al. (1989). The empty delta sign: frequency and significance in 76 cases of dural sinus thrombosis. *Radiology, 162,* 779–785.

Warach, S.M., et al. (1995). Acute human stroke studied by whole brain echo planar diffusion-weighted magnetic resonance imaging. *Annals of Neurology, 37,* 231–241.

Wardlaw, J.M., & Sellar, R. (1994). A simple practical classification of cerebral infarcts on CT and its interobserver reliability. *American Journal of Neuroradiology, 15,* 1933–1939.

Watson, C., et al. (1992). Anatomic basis of amygdaloid and hippocampal volume measurement by magnetic resonance imaging. *Neurology, 42,* 1743–1750.

Weinstein, M.A., Duchesneau, M., & MacIntyre, W.J. (1977). White and gray matter of the brain differentiated by computed tomography. *Radiology, 122,* 699–702.

Wolpert, S.M. (1995). Neuroradiology in Boston: Historical beginnings. *American Journal in Neuroradiology, 16,* 1093–1098.

Wong, K.T., et al. (1995). Magnetization transfer imaging of periventricular hyperintense white matter in the elderly. *American Journal of Neuroradiology, 16,* 253–258.

Woolsey, R.M., & Nelson, J.S. (1975). Asymptomatic destruction of the fornix in man. *Archives of Neurology, 32,* 566–568.

Yamauchi, H., et al. (1992). Significance of low perfusion with increased oxygen extraction fraction in a case of internal carotid artery stenosis. *Stroke, 23,* 431–432.

Ylikoski, R., et al. (1993). White matter changes in healthy elderly persons correlate with attention and speed of mental processing. *Archives of Neurology, 50,* 818–824.

Yoshida, K., et al. (1994). Dynamics of cerebral metabolism in patients with chronic subdural hematoma evaluated with Phosphorous 31 MR spectroscopy before and after surgery. *American Journal of Neuroradiology, 15,* 1681–1686.

Young, A., et al. (1991). A magnetic resonance imaging study of schizophrenia: Brain structure and clinical symptoms. *British Journal of Psychiatry, 158,* 158–164.

Yuh, W.T.C., et al. (1991). MR imaging of cerebral ischemia: findings in the first 24 hours. *American Journal of Neuroradiology, 12,* 621–629.

Zatz, L.M., Jernigan, T.L., & Ahumada, A.J., Jr. (1982). White matter changes in cerebral computed tomography related to aging. *Journal of Computer Assisted Tomography, 6,* 19–23.

Zentner, J., et al. (1995). Surgical treatment of temporal lobe epilepsy: clinical, radiological, and histopathological findings in 178 patients. *Journal of Neurology, Neurosurgery, and Psychiatry, 58,* 666–673.

Zimmerman, R.D., & Ernst, R.J. (1992). Neuroimaging of cerebral veins: Thrombosis. *Neuroimaging Clinics of North America, 2,* 463–485.

Zwiebel, W.J. (1992). Duplex sonography of the cerebral arteries: Efficacy, limitations and indications. *American Journal of Roentgenology, 158,* 29–36.

6 Evaluation of Neuropsychological Rehabilitation Programs[1]

Manuel Morales

University of Seville
Seville, Spain

INTRODUCTION

Recent years have seen a growing interest in neuropsychological assessment and the development of rehabilitation programs to improve the quality of life of people who have suffered some kind of brain damage (Boake, 1989; Mateer & Sohlberg, 1989). The result of this has been recognition of the need for evaluation of the effectiveness of the different intervention programs proposed (León-Carrión, 1995).

Evaluating the effectiveness of a neuropsychological intervention program involves ascertaining whether the rehabilitative strategies introduced produce improvements in subjects' cognitive and behavioral functioning. Put another way, the aim is to demonstrate that the changes occurring in the behavior of a certain group of subjects (or in just one subject) are exclusively the result of the program's characteristics.

Ideally, when carrying out an intervention, the neuropsychologist aims to obtain an improvement in the patients as a result of the implementation of the rehabilitation program. This involves finding a covariation between the program and the subjects' behavior (i.e., finding significant differences between the performance of the subject before undergoing the rehabilitation program and his/her general state following the intervention). However, finding covariation between two variables does not always mean the existence of a causal relationship between them. It may be that subjects recuperate at that time without the need of treatment or that the treatment is not effective with alcoholic patients while it does work with those who have suffered head injuries, etc.

Therefore, in order to evaluate the effectiveness of a treatment, it is necessary to measure the covariation existing between the rehabilitation program and the performance of the subject in certain conditions that guarantee the validity of the relation. This means that changes in performance are strictly the result of the introduction of the program and are not the result of extraneous variables that may confound the effect of the treatment. Essentially, the idea is to establish a causal relationship between program and behavior.

However, to be assured of the existence of a causal relation means it is vital to elaborate a suitable design that would take into account all the extraneous variables which may be affecting the subjects' behavior. The main objective of any design is to determine the conditions during which the data collection that is used to measure the covariation existing between the variables takes place (Judd & Kenny, 1982).

There is a wide range of criteria for classifying the different research designs whose suitability will depend on whether the design is being used for basic or applied research (Keppel, 1983; Arnau, 1986; Mead, 1988; Anguera, 1995). In relation to neuropsychological intervention, there are two main types: synchronic and diachronic designs (Tupper, 1991).

SYNCHRONIC DESIGNS

Although different levels of complexity exist, the simplest strategy consists of studying two groups of subjects. One group undergoes the treatment while the other is given a placebo. However, there are occasions when the placebo group is substituted by a group receiving another type of treatment in order to find out whether one program is better than another. There are also cases in which various treatments are studied simultaneously using as many groups as there are treatments being tested (Clark, 1986).

An example of this type of study is the research done by Antonucci, Guariglia, Judica, Magnotti, Paolucci, Pizzamiglio, and Zoccolotti (1995), who studied two randomly selected groups of patients with brain damage in the right hemisphere. The aim was to evaluate the effectiveness of a new treatment with patients who showed chronic and persistent unilateral neglect. The patients were randomly assigned to one of the groups (immediate or delayed intervention) depending on whether their beds were evenly or unevenly numbered. The immediate intervention group was evaluated on admission and then at the end of the intervention, eight weeks later. The delayed intervention group was studied three times: on admission, at eight weeks, and at the end of the general cognitive intervention that started eight weeks after being admitted. The immediate intervention group began the rehabilitation procedure straight after the initial assessment, and it continued for the following eight weeks. The subjects of the delayed intervention group were told that they would receive an unspecific cognitive stimulation program and later the specific training program for neglect. At eight weeks, the subjects of both groups were evaluated with the aim of comparing them; in this comparison, the delayed intervention group was used as the control group. The results showed the effectiveness of the neglect rehabilitation.

CONTROL TECHNIQUES IN SYNCHRONIC DESIGNS

The main advantage of this type of design is that it is very easy to plan. However, there are some drawbacks, as its validity is closely linked to the manipulation of the independent variable (the intervention program in our case) and to the use of randomization. Depending on the extent to which these two requisites can be met, it will be possible to guarantee that there are no other extraneous variables that would vary at the same time as the treatment.

Manipulating the independent variable means that the researcher may decide which of the program's values each subject is to receive. Thus, the researcher may determine, for example, the specific treatment that each subject is to receive. Of the two above-mentioned requisites, manipulation is the easiest to achieve, and it is vital to be able to guarantee equivalence between the groups.

Randomization is the main control technique of the extraneous variables in this type of design. It consists of randomly selecting the subjects that are going to take part in the study and randomly assigning each of the treatments. So, for example, in the study by Gabriella Antonuci et al. (1995), the subjects were put into groups on the basis of whether their beds were evenly or unevenly numbered.

Obviously, the random selection of the sample that is going to take part in the research is not easy to achieve and is sometimes even undesirable. For instance, suppose that we want to evaluate a new rehabilitation treatment for patients with brain damage. It would be logical for us to want to make this as extensive as possible and use all those suffering from this and not just a small sample, however representative it might be. Because it is not always possible to have available all those with brain damage, it is more likely that we will have to make do with those being treated by a certain institution.

With randomization failing, the equivalence of the different groups evaluated cannot be guaranteed and, as a result, if differences appear between the groups, it cannot be said that these are solely the result of the differential treatment (Browers & Mohr, 1991). It may be, for example, that the subjects who received a certain treatment were those who showed less serious symptoms. Similarly, interactions may occur between subject variables (age, socioeconomic level, etc.) and the treatment that are the actual causes for the changes found.

Finally, it would be a good idea to point out that randomization in itself is not an absolute guarantee for obtaining equivalent groups. There is always a probability (albeit small) that in spite of using randomization, the groups do not end up equivalent. That is what happened to Antonucci et al. (1995) who, despite randomly assigning subjects to groups, ended up with nonequivalent ones. In the first assessment, the group that was to receive an immediate treatment was found to perform better before the treatment had started. In these cases, the randomization technique would best be replaced by more restrictive designs using the blocking technique (Browers & Mohr, 1991).

Blocking consists of creating groups that are homogeneous with respect to a series of extraneous variables such as age, sex, socioeconomic level, seriousness of injuries, etc. Within each block, the treatments are randomly assigned to the subjects.

The main advantage of this strategy is that it allows the elimination of possible distortioning effects of the variables that have been chosen to match the subjects. However, its main drawback is that as we increase the number of blocking variables, the more difficult it becomes to find subjects that present the specific value of each of the controlled variables. It is much easier to find subjects ages 30–35 than if we have to find subjects ages 30–35 who are also male. If we add another variable, the localization of the injury, there will be more complications, as the subjects will have to be 30–35, male, and have injuries, for example, to the frontal lobe.

Although it is more convenient to design the research taking into account beforehand the blocking variables (Parsons & Prigatano, 1978), sometimes the relevance of certain variables is not discovered until the data have been collected. In these cases, the only option is to rework the research so that the unforeseen blocking variable may be included.

Another option may be to use statistical procedures such as covariance analysis (ANCOVA) to guarantee the control of the variable (Adams, Brown, & Grant, 1985).

There are several advantages to using ANCOVA as a statistical control technique (Tupper & Rosenblood, 1984). The first of these is that it increases the accuracy of the randomized experiments when the extraneous variable is statistically independent of the treatment. The ANCOVA increases the sensibility of the analysis by extracting the variance owing to the extraneous variable that correlates with the dependent variable. The second is that this technique may also be used to find out the effects of the treatment when this is correlating with an extraneous variable. However, this second use has come under question (Games, 1976; Tupper & Rosenblood, 1984).

One example of the use of ANCOVA may be found in the work of Brandt, Butters, Ryan, and Bayog (1983), who used this technique to match three groups of alcoholics (short-term abstinence, long-term abstinence, and prolonged abstinence). The subjects differed in age, in years of abstinence, and in the scores on the WAIS vocabulary subtests. Thanks to the use of ANCOVA, these researchers were able to isolate the effects of these three variables and determine that the performance deficiencies found were attributable to alcohol.

Finally, it should be pointed out that the randomization technique, the blocking technique, and ANCOVA are only possible in those designs where the independent variable has been manipulated. In the case of the treatments not being randomly assigned, it is very likely that correlations will exist between the dependent variable and certain extraneous variables (age, sex, socioeconomic level, etc.). Therefore, control of the extraneous variables will be low, and this will mean an inability to meet the supposed orthogonality necessary in order to apply the classical statistical tests of ANOVA and ANCOVA (Appelbaum & Cramer, 1974). In these cases, the researcher must resort to techniques such as the multiple regression, path analysis, or causal models (Anderson, 1984; Van de Geer, 1986; Jóreskog & Sórbom, 1986).

SYNCHRONIC DESIGN PROBLEMS

Using the group strategy for investigating the effectiveness of a treatment has various drawbacks. First, by focusing on the average effects of a group, we are forgetting individual differences. The average is a measurement that is highly sensitive to extreme scores (Hoaglin, Mosteller, & Tukey, 1983), and it may be that the treatment has only been effective with certain patients. To avoid this, it is advisable to provide information about the percentage of subjects who have undergone significant change (Graves, 1991).

Second, there are difficulties in obtaining homogeneous groups (Wilson, 1987). In many cases, it is not possible to use randomization, as patients suffer very diverse complications, nor is it possible to use the blocking technique.

A third problem with the synchronic designs is that they attribute greater importance to statistical than to clinical significance, with there often being an unsatisfactory synchronization between the two. Statistical significance may be important in basic research, but in clinical and applied research, the changes may be so insignificant that they lack any clinical relevance whatsoever. Although the results of clinical investigations should be evaluated with statistical techniques, it is vital not to lose track of the criteria of utility and clinical relevance.

Similarly, this type of design is inadequate for studying syndromes which, because of their very nature, do not occur frequently. This makes the possibility of forming groups of subjects more difficult. As Wilson points out (1987), "visual-object agnosia and ideational apraxia are syndromes which would never get treated if we had to wait for large group studies to be completed." Another disadvantage with this type of design is that it does not allow the studying of the subjects' development. As a result of obtaining few measurements for each subject, it is not possible to observe the pattern of change during the treatment. Similarly, with so few observations per subject, it is not possible to study the behavioral stability of the subject, relapses, etc. (Singer & Willett, 1995). Finally, group designs have the ethical drawback of leaving the control group without intervention.

All these problems have led many authors to defend the use of other types of designs in neuropsychological research, with frequent calls for the use of diachronic designs (Gianutsos & Gianutsos, 1987; Gordon & Hibbard, 1992; Wilson, 1993).

DIACHRONIC DESIGNS

This type of design may assume different formats. We may find an intrasubject experimental design, a case study, or a single case experimental design.

The intrasubject experimental design is a generalization of the group design in which the blocking technique has been used at its optimum level, as only one subject per block is used. It is not often used in neuropsychological evaluation, so it will not be discussed here. A more detailed account of these designs may be found in any handbook on experimental designs (see Keppel, 1983; Mead, 1988).

Case studies are used frequently in neuropsychological research (Shallice, 1991; Prigatano, O'Brien, & Klonoff, 1993), although the pioneering work carried out before World War II was heavily criticized for the lack of rigor in the criteria used. However, over the last 15 years, there has been a resurgence of this methodology (Shallice, 1991). The main reason for this change in approach on the part of researchers is due largely to the richness and depth of the data collected using this technique and the methodological improvements that have been recently incorporated (Yin, 1987).

Generally, case studies give a detailed description of a patient's characteristics in special conditions, describing his/her subsequent development as a consequence of therapeutic intervention. Seen in this light, studying cases is a methodology of great value for the description of symptoms linked to a particular syndrome and for the elaboration of hypotheses about the possible causal agents of the illness.

Unfortunately, case studies are not very useful for the contrasting of hypotheses, because they do not include a control group for comparison. Nor do they carry out evaluations before continued introduction of the treatment. They thus require a series of methodological refinements which, when put into practice, give rise to the so-called single case experimental designs, designs N of 1, and also intrasubject replication experimental designs. As these are the designs that have been most widely accepted in the field of neuropsychological intervention (Gianutsos & Gianutsos, 1987; Gordon & Hibbard, 1992; Wilson, 1993), we will discuss them at length.

GENERAL CHARACTERISTICS OF SINGLE CASE EXPERIMENTAL DESIGNS

The main characteristic of these designs is the repeated measuring of the patient both before the introduction of and during the treatment. In general, each of the observation periods is called a *phase*. So, for example, the basic model structure of this type of design is as follows:

$$O_1 \; O_2 ... \; O_n \; I \; O_{n+1} \; O_{n+2} ... \; O_{2n}$$

This design is made up of two clearly differentiated phases. In a first phase (phase A or observational baseline), different measurements of a behavior are taken ($O_1 \; O_2 ... \; O_n$), until a level of stability is noted in the observations (stable baseline). Next, treatment (I) is introduced, and measurements of the behavior continue to be taken until a specific pattern in the observations is obtained ($O_{n+1} \; O_{n+2} ... \; O_{2n}$). The new pattern shown by the behavior is considered to be the result of the treatment. This phase is labelled experimental baseline or phase B.

The intervention in a design of this type may affect the series of observations in very different ways. There may be changes in level, changes in trend, or changes in both. The change in level refers to the changes existing between the last score of the observational baseline (OBL) and the first of the following experimental baseline (EBL). Some authors have highlighted the importance of the temporal criterion for delimiting the different changes in level (Glass, Wilson, & Gottman, 1975; Arnau, 1994). With regard to these two criteria, three different types can be distinguished: (1) no level change, (2) stable level change, and (3) transitory level change.

A second type of change may appear in the trend. The concept of trend is defined as "the developmental curve the data follow in the temporal series" (Martínez Arias, 1987), providing the possibility that it will stay constant in all the phases or change from one to the other.

CLASSIFICATION OF THE DESIGNS OF N=I

Two criteria have been put forward for classifying the intrasubject replication designs, which depend on the basic components of the design and on the meaning of the comparison for inferring the effect of the interventions (Hayes, 1981; Kratochwill, 1992). In relation to these criteria, we have intra-series designs, inter-series designs, and combined designs.

Intra-Series Designs

This type of design is characterized by evaluating the dependent variable over different phases. The simplest model is the design A-B. First, in this design, an observational baseline (OBL) of the studied behavior is obtained; then, after the introduction of the treatment, the experimental baseline (EBL) is obtained. As a result, its structure will be as follows:

$$O_1 \; O_2 ... \; O_n \; I \; O_{n+1} \; O_{n+2} ... \; O_{2n}$$

$$A \qquad\qquad B$$

Although this design has advantages over the previously mentioned case studies, it still has problems of internal validity as it confuses the effects of the treatment with possible effects due to, for example, the spontaneous improvement that patients can experience. This occurs more frequently in those cases in which tendencies appear in phase A, so that for their correct use, it is necessary to achieve stability in the baseline scores.

The problems of control of extraneous variables that the design A-B presents are solved by withdrawing the treatment and registering what happens to the behavior from that point on (*reversal designs*). If a change is produced in the response variable measurement when the program is applied and a regression to the initial level or the baseline occurs when it is withdrawn, then there is a powerful argument for concluding that the response controlling variable has been the treatment. This basic reversal design presents various possibilities:

1. **Design A-B-A:** This consists of adding a third phase in which the behavior is recorded, again having eliminated the action of treatment. Its structure is as follows:

$$O_1 \; O_2 \ldots \; O_n \; I \; O_{n+1} \; O_{n+2} \ldots \; O_{2n} \; O_{2n+1} \; O_{2n+2} \ldots \; O_{3n}$$

$$\text{A} \qquad\qquad\qquad \text{B} \qquad\quad \text{A}$$

2. **Design A-B-A-B:** The only difference here is that of introducing a fourth phase in which the behavior is again observed under the treatment.
3. **Design B-A-B:** The main characteristic here is that the researcher acts when the treatment is already underway and it is necessary to evaluate its effectiveness. There is a temporary interruption in the treatment to find out whether some kind of discontinuity or change occurs in the behavioral pattern generated by the subject under the action of the therapeutic intervention or for any other reason.

An example of these intra-series designs may be found in Wilson (1987), who describes the procedure of an A-B-A-B design to teach the name of a clinical psychologist to a young boy who had suffered head injuries two years earlier. The baselines were drawn up by telling the patient the name of the psychologist and asking him to remember the name after a period of between 5 seconds and 3 minutes had passed. During this time, a conversation with the patient took place. The patient always remembered the name if the time interval was 30 seconds or less, while he made mistakes if the interval was greater. The baseline lasted one hour, with a timer being introduced to model the subject's behavior. The timer was programmed initially to sound every 30 seconds during his one-hour daily sessions. Each time the alarm sounded, the boy was asked to say the name of the psychologist, with the time interval being increased by 5 seconds every time the patient gave four consecutive correct responses. After 3 weeks of intervention, the subject was able to remember the name of the psychologist up to $10\frac{1}{2}$ minutes after having been told it. To ascertain that the timer treatment was responsible for the improvement, the program reverted to the conditions of the baseline. As in the initial baseline sessions, the patient was asked the name of the psychologist at random intervals. After 2 weeks, the performance of the subject had worsened to the extent of making mistakes $1\frac{1}{2}$ minutes after having been told the psychologist's name. The second phase B introduced the timer again, and the subject's performance began to improve once more.

The main advantage of adding new phases in the intra-series designs is that it increases its internal validity. As a result, it increases the guarantee of concluding that the return of the subject's behavior to the initial levels are a result of the treatment. However, this type of design presents us with the drawback that it does not allow the evaluation of certain treatments nor those treatments that produce an irreversible effect (Poling & Grossett, 1986), which happen to be those of greatest interest in neuropsychology. So, for example, a person who has been instructed to remember the way from the ward will not forget that. Similarly, it would be hard to ethically justify this type of design in situations in which eliminating the treatment might mean a serious risk to the patient. For example, Wilson (1987) recalls the case of a patient who was taught to check that he had turned the gas-tap off, and then he is no longer reminded to check it. For these sorts of reasons, it is perhaps sometimes wiser to use other types of designs.

To study two or more treatments, more complex intra-series designs are normally used; they have the advantage of offering information about the interaction between the treatments introduced. In general, the effects are additive, with some treatments being more effective than others. To establish the effect of each of these treatments, the researcher needs to test, first and separately, each of the components of the treatment and then compare them in a combined form. In addition, between each phase, it is not advisable to change more than one treatment at a time, from one phase to another (Hersen & Barlow, 1976). There are several possibilities:

1. **Multilevel designs:** In the simplest case, it would be characterized as a four-phase design A-B-A-C where B and C are different treatments. They have the advantage of allowing the testing of hypotheses about the relative efficiency of two or more treatments. They may also be used in those cases in which a first intervention has not managed to attain the desired objectives and a new treatment is to be applied. On the other hand, they have the drawback of not offering information about the possible interaction between treatments.

2. **Interaction designs:** They form the most complex research strategy and are analogous to the factorial designs of the synchronic approach of the design. This type can be seen as a natural extension of the multiple treatment design. The structure of the basic model would be as follows:

$$O_1 \ldots O_n \qquad I_1\, O_{n+1} \ldots O_{2n} \qquad O_{2n+1} \ldots O_{3n}$$

$$I_1\, O_{3n+1} \ldots O_{4n} \quad I_1\, I_2\, O_{4n+1} \ldots O_{5n} \qquad I_1\, O_{5n+1} \ldots O_{6n}$$

$$I_1\, I_2\, O_{6n+1} \ldots O_{7n}$$

This type of design poses the problem of the possible effect of the order of introduction of the interventions. For example, in a 2 x 2 factorial analysis, there are $4! = 24$ possible orders for presenting two interventions and the noninterventions. It is possible that sometimes the changes observed in the series of data may reveal the effect of the different orders of introduction.

Before its application, three basic points have to be considered. First, considerable attention must be paid to the baseline data in order to ensure that possible changes later on have not come about spontaneously; this is normal procedure in all designs using the baseline. Second, it is important to achieve stability in each phase before moving on to another, as each phase will in turn act as the baseline for the following one. Third, to evaluate the changes in the dependent variable, it is necessary to examine the variability of the data; if this is large, then broad criteria and long-lasting phases are required.

The main drawback with the interactive designs is that it is not always clear when the behavior observed follows the changes of criteria. In these cases, researchers or therapists may manipulate the length, depth, and direction of the changes of criteria as they go along.

Inter-Series Designs

There are many situations in which the withdrawal of the treatment is impossible, thus allowing the use of nonreversion strategies. Kratochwill et al., (1984) describes three classes: multiple schedule designs, concurrent schedule designs, and changing criterion designs.

1.   **Multiple schedule designs:** Their main feature is studying the same behavior under different conditions. It represents a similar situation to that of animal conditioning in the laboratory, where it is possible to reinforce the response of key pressing in the presence of a light or sound. Its schematic representation would be as follows:

Condition 1: $I_1\ O_1\ ...\ O_n$ $I_2\ O_{n+1}\ ...\ O_{2n}$

$I_1\ O_{2n+1}\ ...\ O_{3n}$ $I_2\ O_{3n+1}\ ...\ O_{4n}$

Condition 2: $I_2\ O_1\ ...\ O_n$ $I_1\ O_{n+1}\ ...\ O_{2n}$

$I_2\ O_{2n+1}\ ...\ O_{3n}$ $I_1\ O_{3n+1}\ ...\ O_{4n}$

There are two advantages with this design strategy. First, when the behaviors present great variability, the designs of change between phases are unable to detect the action of the treatments. As a result, when the treatments produce considerable changes, their effects can be inferred more easily. Second, they are more effective structures, and they permit a quicker inference of the treatment.

2.   **Concurrent schedule designs:** In this design, the subject is submitted simultaneously to the different conditions of the first term. This design starts with a first behavior observation baseline (phase A of the design). Following this, two or more interventions are then applied simultaneously under the same stimulus conditions that were used in the baseline recordings. These conditions of stimulus or observation periods may be, for example, in or outside the treatment room, in the morning or afternoon, with members of the center present or not, etc. It is not very frequently used in clinical practice.

3.   **Changing criteria designs:** This design starts with a baseline phase on a certain study behavior. Next, the corresponding reinforcement contingency or treatment is applied in such a way that the intervention is programmed over a successive series of phases. In each one, the subject is required to reach a certain level of performance in order to attain the reinforcement. The subject may be set a certain behavior until meeting a criteria. When the criteria has been reached with the necessary regularity, the experimenter introduces a new phase in which the criteria is more restrictive. This way, the subject is set increasingly limited levels in relation to the response in question. The criteria to which the subject has to adapt change little by little over the different phases until finally reaching the ultimate objective of the program. The treatment's possible effect is demonstrated

by the behavior adjusting to the criteria (a change in criteria is accompanied by a corresponding change in behavior). Its diagrammatical representation is as follows:

$$O_1 \ldots O_n \qquad I_1 \, O_{n+1} \ldots O_{2n}$$

$$I_1 \, O_{2n+1} \ldots O_{3n}$$

$$I_1 \, O_{3n+1} \ldots O_{4n}$$

Combined Series Designs

Combined series designs involve comparisons that are both intra-series and inter-series. Their logical bases attempt to correct the main deficiencies of the basic A-B design and the ethical problems linked to intra-series designs.

These designs are also known by the name of multiple baseline designs. A feature of the most widely used model is to study different behaviors, one at a time, with the same treatment. The research plan will start by identifying and recording a quantity of responses over time to provide baselines against which it will be possible to evaluate changes. Once this baseline is established, the researcher applies an experimental variable to one of the behaviors, produces a change in it, and perhaps notes little or no change in the other baselines. Then, the same treatment is given to a second behavior, and the rate of change in this is also recorded. This procedure continues until each of the behaviors selected has been subjected to the treatment (Hersen & Barlow, 1976).

There are three basic modalities of multiple baseline designs: multiple baseline across behaviors, multiple baseline across subjects, and multiple baseline across situations design. The basic structure of the first of these is as follows:

$$\text{Cd A: } O_1 \ldots O_n \qquad I_1 \, O_{n+1} \ldots O_{2n} \qquad O_{2n+1} \ldots O_{3n} \qquad O_{3n+1} \ldots O_{4n}$$

$$\text{Cd B: } O_1 \ldots O_n \qquad I_1 \, O_{n+1} \ldots O_{2n} \qquad O_{2n+1} \ldots O_{3n} \qquad O_{3n+1} \ldots O_{4n}$$

$$\text{Cd C: } O_1 \ldots O_n \qquad I_1 \, O_{n+1} \ldots O_{2n} \qquad O_{2n+1} \ldots O_{3n} \qquad O_{3n+1} \ldots O_{4n}$$

An example of multiple baseline across behaviors is presented by Wilson (1987) to treat T.B., a 43-year-old male suffering from the Korsakov syndrome. The behaviors treated were (1) learning short routes around the rehabilitation center, (2) recalling newspaper articles, and (3) learning the names of the hospital staff. During the baseline phase, no improvement occurred in the reading of newspapers or in recalling the names of staff members, while an improvement did occur in learning some of the routes inside the hospital. Following this, a treatment was introduced to improve recall of articles read in newspapers based on the PRQST strategy (Preview, Read, Question, State, and Test). One week later, the treatment was introduced for the recognition of the staff members that was based on a procedure associating the face with the name. The results indicated that the learning of different paths inside the center improved with practice, the PRQST helped considerably with the newspaper articles, and the procedure associating the face with the name enabled the patient to learn the names of all the staff.

For multiple-baseline-across-subjects design, the structure will be the same, but behaviors A, B, and C will be replaced by subjects 1, 2, and 3. The same applies to the multiple-baseline-across-situations design.

Another mode of combined design is the so-called multiple test design, which add to the logic of the multiple-baseline-design test procedures for evaluating the effects of the interventions. They are highly useful in those situations in which the aim is to install a new behavior through successive approximations. After an observational baseline phase, the treatment is applied to the first behavior in the chain. When this reaches a certain criteria, additional test data continue to be recorded for the remaining behaviors in the sequence. These test data constitute the true baseline for the second response, which is subsequently treated.

Data Analysis in the Designs of N=1

Data analysis in single case experimental designs has received a lot of attention from authors, with a wide variety of opinions existing. While some authors have defended the ideal nature of the analyses using visual inspection (Baer, 1977; Ballard, 1983; Parsonson & Baer, 1992), other authors have argued about the inconsistency of this type of analysis and have proposed the use of statistical procedures (Gottman & Glass, 1978; Kazdin, 1984).

The main advantage of visual analysis is that it is very easy to use, and it does not require a great knowledge of statistics. The researchers only have to undergo the training necessary to identify the changes of level and/or trend that have occurred between phases.

However, graphic analysis has various drawbacks. First, it has been demonstrated that the evaluators who use this type of technique are not consistent. De Prospero and Cohen (1979) found a level of agreement between observers of 0.61; Jones, Weinrott, and Vaught (1978) only 0.39, etc. It seems that these judgements depend on the size of the effect, the variance existing in the data, the level of autocorrelation existing in the sample, and even on the type of training received by the subjects (Morales, 1991; Parsonson & Baer, 1992). A second problem is that the analysis of the effectiveness of a treatment using graphic techniques is not consistent with the inferences derived from the application of the statistical tests.

These findings have led to the questioning of the suitability of graphic techniques for the analysis of single-case experimental designs. On the other hand, these are considered to be a good back-up to statistical analyses.

There are a great number of statistical tests that can be applied to intrasubject replication designs. In the literature, we find proposals varying from the classic t-test, ANOVA, or regression analysis (Gentile, Roden, & Klein, 1972), through the most sophisticated time series techniques (Gottman & Glass, 1978; Gottman, 1981), through the relatively simple randomization tests (Edginton, 1984, 1992).

Neither is the application of these statistical tests free of difficulties. For example, inferences through the classic t-test, ANOVA, or regression are rendered invalid if autocorrelation exists between the scores, increasing the possibility of committing type I errors. The authors have tried to resolve these problems using different strategies (Shine & Bower, 1971; Gentile, Roden, & Klein, 1972) that have not turned out to be sufficiently satisfactory. Only the regression procedure corrected by autocorrelation has been valued positively by researchers (Lewis-Beck, 1986).

Time series techniques have the advantage of allowing the modeling of a temporal sequence of observations in terms of the process that has generalized them. More specifically, it is thought that the temporal series is the result of a series of stationary random impulses that may generate some correlated or serially dependent residuals. So it is a question of modeling the structure of the series, taking into consideration that the dependence of the data may be autoregressive (AR), moving average (MA), or a combination of the two (ARMA). The aim of the analysis will be to identify which of these possible structures is the one that is present in the data. Once identified, it can be eliminated from the data, and then the effectiveness of the treatment can be evaluated.

The main drawback with these techniques is that they require a great number of observations in order to be applied. Box and Jenkins (1970) point out a minimum of 50 observations and an optimum number of 100. As a result, it is increasingly frequent not to recommend this type of technique for analyzing data coming from clinical practice, since Huitema and Mckean (1991) have demonstrated that, with few observations, it is not possible to make a balanced estimate of the autocorrelation existing between the scores.

All of these problems have led the authors to defend with greater conviction the use of nonparametric tests for the data analysis of these designs (Morley & Adams, 1989; Edginton, 1992), most importantly the randomization test, the signed-rank test, the test for serial dependency (the Dufour test), the test for the average trend (Kendall's tau), and finally, the test for the trend in the average and the variance.

CONCLUDING REMARKS

Evaluating the effectiveness of a neuropsychological intervention program involves ascertaining whether the rehabilitation strategies introduced produce improvements in subjects' cognitive and behavioral functioning. Put another way, the aim is to demonstrate that the changes occurring in the behavior of a certain group of subjects (or in just one subject) are exclusively the result of the program's characteristics. There are two main types of designs to study the effectiveness of the treatment in neuropsychological intervention: synchronic and diachronic designs.

The simplest synchronic strategy consists of studying two groups of subjects. One group undergoes the treatment while the other is given a placebo. The main advantage of this type of design is that it is very easy to plan. However, there are some drawbacks, as its validity is closely linked to the manipulation of the independent variables and to the use of randomization. Another possibility is the use of blocking designs, ANCOVA techniques, or other strategies of data analysis.

Single-case experimental designs have been defended by several authors in neuropsychological research. The main characteristic of these designs is the repeated measurement of the patient both before the introduction of and during the treatment. In general, each of the observation periods is called a phase.

The intervention in a design of this type may affect the series of observations in very different ways. There may be changes in level, changes in trend, or changes in both. The change in level refers to the changes existing between the last score of the observational baseline (OBL) and the first of the following experimental baseline (EBL). Some authors have highlighted the importance of the temporal criteria for delimiting the different changes in level (Glass, Wilson, & Gottman, 1975; Arnau, 1994). With regard to these two criteria, three different types can be distinguished: (1) no level change, (2) stable level change, and (3) transitory level change. A second type of change may appear in the trend.

Two criteria have been put forward for classifying the intrasubject replication designs depending on the basic components of the design and on the meaning of the comparison for inferring the effect of the interventions (Hayes, 1981; Kratochwill, 1992). In relation to these criteria, we have intra-series designs, inter-series designs, and combined designs.

ENDNOTES

1. This research was conducted in part with financing from the Dirección General de Investigación Científica y Técnica (DGICYT) under project PB93-1173.

REFERENCES

Adams, K.M., Brown, G.G., & Grant, I. (1985). Analysis of covariance as a remedy for demographic mismatch of research subject groups: Some sobering simulations. *Journal of Clinical and Experimental Neuropsychology, 7,* 445–462.

Anderson, T.W. (1984). *An introduction to multivariate statistical analysis.* New York: John Wiley & Sons.

Anguera, M.T. (1995). Diseños de investigación. In R. Fernández Ballesteros (Ed.), *Evaluación de programas* (pp. 149–172). Madrid: Síntesis.

Antonucci, G., Guariglia, C., Judica, A., Magnotti, L., Paolucci, S., Pizzamiglio, L., & Zoccolotti, P. (1995). Effectiveness of neglect rehabilitation in a randomized group study. *Journal of Clinical and Experimental Neuropsychology, 17,* 383–389.

Appelbaum, M.I., & Cramer, E.M. (1974). Some problems in the nonorthogonal analysis of variance. *Psychological Bulletin, 81,* 335–343.

Arnau, J. (1986). *Diseños experimentales en Psicología y Educación. Vol I.* México: Trillas.

Baer, D.M. (1977). Perhaps it would be better not to know everything. *Journal of Applied Behavior Analysis, 10,* 166–172.

Ballard, K.D. (1983). The visual analysis of time series data: Issues affecting the assessment of behavioural interventions. *New Zealand Journal of Psychology, 12,* 69–73.

Boake, C. (1989). A history of cognitive rehabilitation of head-injured patients, 1915 to 1980. *Journal of Head Trauma Rehabilitation, 4,* 1–8.

Box, G.E.P., & Jenkins, G.M. (1970). *Time series analysis: Forecasting and control.* San Francisco: Holden Day.

Brandt, J., Butters, N., Ryan, C., & Bayog, R. (1983). Cognitive loss and recovery in chronic alcohol abusers. *Archives of General Psychiatry, 40,* 435–442.

Browers, P., & Mohr, E. (1991). Design of clinical trials. In E. Mohr & P. Browers (Eds.), *Handbook of clinical trials: The neurobehavioral approach* (pp. 45–66). Amsterdam: Swets and Zeitlinger.

Clark, C.M. (1986). Statistical models and their application in clinical neuropsychological research and practice. In S.B. Filskov & T.J. Boll (Eds.), *Handbook of clinical neuropsychology* (Vol. 2) (pp. 577–605). New York: John Wiley & Sons.

De Prospero, A., & Cohen, S. (1979). Inconsistent visual analysis of intrasubject data. *Journal of Applied Behavior Analysis, 12,* 573–579.

Edginton, E.S. (1984). Statistics and the single case. In M. Hersen, R.M. Eisler, & P.M. Miller (Eds.), *Progress in behaviour modification* (Vol. 16). New York: Academic Press.

———. (1992). Nonparametric tests for single-case experiments. In T.R. Kratochwill & J.R. Levin (Eds.), *Single-case research design and analysis.* Hillsdale, NJ: Lawrence Erlbaum Associates.

Games, P.A. (1976). Limitations of analysis of covariance on intact group quasi-experimental designs. *Journal of Experimental Education, 44,* 51–53.

Gentile, J.R., Roden, A.H., & Klein, R.D. (1972). An analysis of variance model for the intrasubject replication design. *Journal of Applied Behavioral Analysis, 15,* 415–421.

Gianutsos, R., & Gianutsos, J. (1987). Single-case experimental approaches to the assessment of interventions in rehabilitation. In B. Caplan (Ed.), *Rehabilitation psychology desk reference* (pp. 453–470). Rockville, MD: Aspen Publishers.

Glass, G.V., Wilson, V.L., & Gottman, J.M. (1975). *Design and analysis of time-series experiments.* Boulder: University of Colorado Press.

Gordon, W.A., & Hibbard, M.R. (1992). Critical issues in cognitive remediation. Special section: Neuropsychology and rehabilitation. *Neuropsychology, 6,* 361–370.

Gottman, J.M. (1981). *Time series analysis: A comprehensive introduction for social scientists.* Cambridge: Cambridge University Press.

Gottman, J.M., & Glass, G.V. (1978). Analysis of interrupted time-series experiments. In T.R. Kratochwill (Ed.), *Single-subject research: Strategies for evaluating change.* New York: Academic Press.

Graves, R.E. (1991). The use of experimental techniques in clinical trials. In E. Mohr & P. Browers (Eds.), *Handbook of clinical trials: The neurobehavioral approach* (pp. 121–130). Amsterdam: Swets and Zeitlinger.

Hayes, S.C. (1981). Single case experimental design and empirical clinical practice. *Journal of Consulting and Clinical Psychology, 49,* 193–211.

Hersen, M., & Barlow, D.H. (1976). *Single case experimental designs: Strategies for studying behavior change.* New York: Pergamon Press.

Hoaglin, D.C., Mosteller, F., & Tukey, J.W. (1983). *Understanding robust and exploratory data analysis.* New York: John Wiley & Sons.

Huitema, B.E., & McKean, J.W. (1991). Autocorrelation estimation and inference with small samples. *Psychological Bulletin, 11,* 291–304.

Jöreskog, K.G., & Sörbom, D. (1986). *LISREL VI: Analysis of linear structural relationships by the method of maximum-likelihood.* Chicago: National Educational Resources.

Judd, C.M., & Kenny, D.A. (1982). Research design and research validity. In D. Brinberg & L.H. Kidder (Eds.), *Forms of validity research* (pp. 23–39). San Francisco: Jossey-Bass.

Kazdin, A.E. (1984). Statistical analysis for single-case experimental designs. In D.H. Barlow & M. Hersen (Eds.), *Single case experimental designs* (2nd ed.). New York: Pergamon Press.

Keppel, G. (1983). *Design and analysis: A researcher's handbook* (2nd ed.). Englewood Cliffs, NJ: Prentice-Hall Inc.

Kratochwill, T.R. (1992). Single-case research design and analysis: An overview. In T.R. Kratochwill & J.R. Levin (Eds.), *Single-case research design and analysis.* Hillsdale, NJ: Lawrence Erlbaum Associates.

Kratochwill, T.R., Mott, S.E., & Dodson, C.L. (1984). Case study and single-case research in clinical and applied psychology. In A.S. Bellack & M. Hersen (Eds.), *Research methods in clinical psychology.* New York: Pergamon Press.

León-Carrión, J. (1995). *Manual de neuropsicología.* Madrid: Siglo XXI.

Lewis-Beck, M.S. (1986). Interrupted time series. In W.D. Berry & M.S. Lewis-Beck (Eds.), *New tools for social scientists.* Beverly Hills, CA: Sage.

Martínez Arias, M.R. (1987). Diseños experimentales y cuasi-experimentales con sujeto único en modificación de conducta. In J. Mayor & F.J. Labrador (Eds.), *Manual de modificación de conducta* (pp. 123–154). Madrid: Alhambra.

Mateer, C., & Solhberg, K. (1989). *Introduction to cognitive neuropsychology.* New York: Guilford Press.

Mead, R. (1988). *The design of experiments: Statistical principles for practical applications.* Cambridge, MA: Cambridge University Press.

Morales, M. (1991). Factores que influyen en la inspección visual de diseños de series de tiempo. *Revista Española de Terapia del Comportamiento, 9,* 146–166.

Morley, S., & Adams, M. (1989). Some simple statistical tests for exploring single-case time-series data. *British Journal of Clinical Psychology, 30,* 95–115.

Parsons, O.A., & Prigatano, G.P. (1978). Methodological considerations in clinical neuropsychological research. *Journal of Consulting &Clinical Psychology, 46,* 608–619.

Parsonson, B.S., & Baer, D.M. (1992). The visual analysis of data, and current research into the stimuli controlling it. In T.R. Kratochwill & J.R. Levin (Eds.), *Single-case research design and analysis.* Hillsdale, NJ: Lawrence Erlbaum Associates.

Poling, A., & Grossett, D. (1986). Basic research designs in applied behavior analysis. In A. Poling & R.W. Fuqua (Eds.), *Research methods in applied behavior analysis. Issues and advances.* New York: Plenum.

Prigatano, G.P., O'Brien, K.P, & Klonoff, P.S. (1993). Neuropsychological rehabilitation of young adults who suffer brain injury in childhood: Clinical observations. (Special issue: Issues in the neuropsychological rehabilitation of children with brain dysfunction). *Neuropsychological Rehabilitation, 3*, 411–421.

Shallice, T. (1991). Case study approach in neuropsychological research. In B.P. Rourke, L. Costa, D.V. Cicchetti, K.M. Adams, & K.J. Plasterk (Eds.), *Methodological and biostatistical foundations of clinical neuropsychology* (pp. 55–83). Amsterdam: Zeitlinger B.V.

Shine, L.C., & Bower, S.M. (1971). A one-way analysis of variance for single-subject designs. *Educational and Psychological Measurement, 31,* 105–113.

Singer, J.D., & Willet, J.B. (1995). Modeling the days of our lives: Using survival analysis when designing and analyzing longitudinal studies of duration and the timing of events. *Psychological Bulletin, 110*, 268–290.

Tupper, D.E. (1991). Clinical trials of cognitive rehabilitation. In E. Mohr & P. Browers (Eds.), *Handbook of clinical trials: The neurobehavioral approach* (pp. 307–327). Amsterdam: Swets and Zeitlinger.

Tupper, D.E., & Rosenblood, L.K. (1984). Methodological considerations in the use of attribute variables in neuropsychological research. *Journal of Clinical Neuropsychology, 6*, 441–453.

van de Geer, J.P. (1986). *Introduction to linear multivariate data analysis* (2 vols.). Leiden, The Netherlands: DSWO.

Wilson, B.A. (1987). Single-case experimental designs in neuropsychological rehabilitation. *Journal of Clinical and Experimental Neuropsychology, 9*, 527–544.

———. (1993). How do we know that rehabilitation works? *Neuropsychological Rehabilitation, 3*, 1–4.

Yin, R.K. (1987). *Case study research.* Beverly Hills, CA: Sage.

PART II:

BRAIN INJURY TREATMENTS

7 Interventions in the Acute Phase of Severe Brain-Injured Patients

José Maria Domínguez-Roldán, Francisco Murillo-Cabezas, and María Angeles Muñoz-Sánchez

Hospital Universitario Virgen del Rocío
Seville, Spain

INTRODUCTION

The incidence of brain injury is very high in developed countries. In the United States the rate of deaths related to cranioencephalic injuries is approximately 19.3/100,000 people annually. Most of these traumas affect patients in the second and third decades of their lives. The medical repercussions of this fact also have significant social repercussions.

The brain injuries that occur in the peritraumatic period could be developed either as a consequence of the trauma itself, which we could refer to as *primary traumatic brain injury*, or as a result of systemic or intracranial conditions associated with the trauma, which we could refer to as *secondary brain injury* (Tables 7.1 and 7.2).

Table 7.1: Secondary Brain Insults of Extracranial Origin

1.	Arterial hypotension
2.	Hypoxia
3.	Anemia
4.	Hyperthermia
5.	Hypercapnia
6.	Hydroelectrolytic disorders
7.	Hyperglycemia
8.	Systemic inflammatory response syndrome

Table 7.2: Secondary Brain Insults of Intracranial Origin

1.	Intracranial hypertension
2.	Mass lesions
3.	Cerebral edema
4.	Vasospasm
5.	Hydrocephaly
6.	Cerebrospinal fluid infection
7.	Convulsions
8.	Other

Primary Brain Injury

A primary brain injury is conditioned on the mechanism that produced the impact. Traumatic intracranial injuries have a different prognosis depending on their location and extent. When the brain of a patient who has died as a result of brain injury is examined, contusive injuries in the grey matter make up the most evident injuries on the surface of the injured brain. These intraparenchymatous injuries show a certain degree of leakage of blood, which could extend itself in the form of a subpial or subarachnoid hemorrhage. At times, we may observe the confluence of several near hemorrhagic foci that could be considered authentic intracranial hematomas. When the cranial impact has been sufficiently important, the hemorrhagic contusions will be seen in its underlying cerebral regions. In other cases lacking the evidence of a direct impact, the injuries appear in the temporal and frontal lobes. This is due, among other reasons, to the irregular nature of the adjacent cranial surface in these areas. Thus, impacts to the occipital region tend frequently to produce contralateral injuries (frontal and temporal), a situation that occurs less frequently when the impact is frontal. When the brain injury has been severe, the brain contusions usually are multiple and bilateral.

Other major injuries with great clinical relevance due to their intracranial location are the extradural hematomas and the subdural hematomas. Extradural hematomas, caused as a result of the breaking of a vessel (frequently the middle meningeal artery) in the epidural space, usually carry with them a serious prognosis if they are numerous and are not evacuated quickly. The mechanisms implicated in their severity are, first, the increase of the intracranial pressure due to the rapid development of the injury occupying the space. The second mechanism is the sudden compression of the encephalic structures of great functional importance (mesencephalon, brainstem) with the resulting risk for the life of the patient. Their prevailing location is the tempoparietal region. They are less frequently noted in the vertex or posterior fossa; in the genesis of these cases, an injury of the sagital or lateral sinus is implicated. Their association to intraaxial injuries is less than 15%.

Subdural hematomas are due usually to disruption of superficial bridging cerebral veins that cross the subdural space, and frequently the production mechanism is a sudden desacceleration of the brain. Although their location is variable, they usually affect the frontal and occipital poles. In over 80% of cases, they are associated with severe brain injuries, often underlying and which, at times, participate as a hemorrhagic focus of the subdural hematoma. The prognosis of subdural hematomas is usually more serious than for the epidural ones and is determined by the mass effect that a hematoma develops as evidenced by the frequent existence of associated brain injuries that contribute frequently to the development of intracranial hypertension, shifting of centroencepahlic structures, etc.

In 1956, Strich (1956) described an extensive degeneration of the white brain substance of patients surviving head injury but who had remained in a coma for months. Since then, several studies have pointed out the relation between direct injury to the white brain matter and the poor recovery of patients. Small hemorrhagic foci in the corpus callosum, thalamus, basal ganglia, superior cerebellar peduncle, and brainstem, associated or not with hemorrhage in the subarachnoid spaces, are injuries frequently associated with a poor clinical evolution (represented by a low level of consciousness, a tendency toward the rigidity of the extensor muscles, and a certain vegetative disautonomy). There are several microscopic findings linked to the diffuse injury of the white matter in patients who have suffered brain injury. Retraction spheres appear in the period immediately after the trauma. Marked microglia stars, which represent hypertrophied microglia accumulations, appear early and last for months after the trauma. The degeneration of the long tracts are also frequent, degeneration that goes from the brainstem paths to the hemispheres, which serves to suggest that this injury is not the result of a direct trauma but rather is part of a disseminated injury.

Secondary Brain Injury

The brain injury may be caused not only as a result of the direct impact to the brain of an external agent, but it could also be due to the development of a series of systemic and intracranial insults resulting from the trauma (Tables 7.1 and 7.2). Among these, the increase of intracranial pressure and brain ischemia are the two most important factors that condition the development of significant modifications in the brain structure. The necropsic study of the brains of patients who have developed intracranial hypertension before death shows certain signs, such as flattening of the circumvolutions; shift of midline, tentorial and supracallosum hernias; and a certain degree of distortion of the brainstem, hemorrhage, or ischemia. Adams and Graham (1976) have established morphologic traits that may be considered indicative of an intracranial hypertensive episode. The most consistent trait is the presence of a necrotic area along the line of the border of the tentorium in one or both parahippocampic curves. In some cases, we can also observe a necrotic area due to pressure in the curve of the cingulum and infarction of the middle occipital cortex.

The episodes of decrease of the cerebral perfusion due to intracranial hypertension, systemic arterial hypotension, or direct compression of the intracranial arteries by pressure wedges determine whether brain ischemia is either global or in certain cerebral areas with a greater tendency toward the same. The focal ischemia in the vicinity of contusions and the calcarine infarction secondary to the occlusion of the posterior cerebral artery due to a transtentory hernia are the most macroscopically frequent ischemic injuries. The systematic study of the brain of patients who have died as a result of cranioencephalic trauma shows ischemic injuries that reach a 90% rate. The hippocampus and the basal ganglia are the areas that most frequently present signs of ischemic damage. In over 45% of patients, we observe signs of cortical ischemia. If the middle occipital cortex is excluded, the most common place for the injuries of the neocortex is in the areas bordering the major arterial territories. It is not uncommon to find multiple ischemic foci in the brain of these patients.

CURRENT BASES FOR MANAGING PATIENTS WITH SEVERE BRAIN INJURY IN THE ACUTE PHASE

Physiological Bases

It is believed that there are two basic functions for the adequate functioning of neuronal activity: the maintenance of the neuronal integrity and the possibility of establishing electrocommunication between the neurons. For this to occur, it is necessary that an important amount of enegetics and nutritional elements flow to the brain that will allow the performance of these functions.

The cerebral blood flow is the conducting link between the contribution of substrata to the brain and the neuronal function. The blood flow to the brain in an awake adult is approximately 50 ml/100 grams of brain tissue per minute. The oxygen content of the internal jugular vein is 7.7 ml/dl. Under normal conditions, the brain's consumption of oxygen is around 3.5 ml for each 100 grams of brain tissue per minute. Since the weight of a normal brain in an adult is around 1,200–1,400 grams, its consumption is approximately 40 ml of oxygen per minute (i.e., 15% of the total amount of oxygen consumed by the organism). In order to maintain this level of consumption, 35% of the oxygen content of the arteries that is carried through the arteries at the base of the brain is extracted in the course of its intracranial circulation, which determines that the venous saturation in the internal jugular bulb will be placed at around 65% on average.

Approximately 55% of the oxygen consumed by the brain is used in the maintenance of the integrity of the cells (normal ionic gradient, neurotransmitter synthesis, cell proteins, nucleic acids, etc.). The remaining 45% is used in the so-called "activation metabolism," necessary energy for the neuronal functioning consisting of the synaptic transmission of nervous action potentials, electrical activity that may be detected by means of an electroencephalogram.

The importance of the maintenance of an adequate delivery of oxygen to the brain is seen through the phenomenon of the joining of the cerebral blood flow and the cerebral use of oxygen. As seen in Figure 7.1, there is a coupling between both so that when the oxygen demands of the brain are increased, there is a parallel increase in the flow of blood to the brain. As a cerebral protection mechanism, when there is a drop in the flow of blood to the brain, the brain's oxygen consumption may be maintained due to an increase in the cerebral extraction of oxygen. The cerebral extraction of oxygen reaches its limit when the venous content drops below 1 ml/dl, and the artery-jugular oxygen difference rises to 13 ml/dl. However, a drop in the blood flow to the brain greater than 50% cannot be compensated, resulting in a brain ischemia and a cessation of the neuronal functions. A brain blood flow below 23 ml/100 grams per minute seriously compromises neuronal functions; when the drop in brain blood flow goes over 18 ml/100 grams per minute, the infarct phenomena are evident. However, this level of flow may have its consequences modified if previously the synaptic functions have been suppressed by means of the use of barbiturates or hypothermia.

The transcendence of the maintenance of the optimum blood flow to the brain is also evidenced by the large number of autoregulatory mechanisms that have been shown. The factors that govern the blood flow to the brain are (in physical terms) cerebral perfusion pressure, vessel diameter (both directly proportional), blood viscosity, and the length of the vessel (both inversely proportional to the flow of blood to the brain). In physiological conditions, the diameter of the vessel is the most important factor of the cerebrovascular

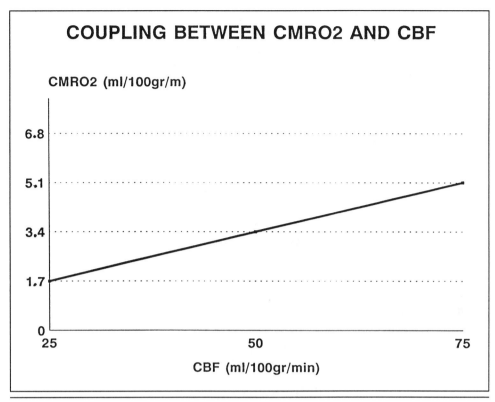

Figure 7.1: "Coupling" phenomena between cerebral metabolic rate for oxygen and cerebral blood flow. Cerebral blood flow and cerebral metabolic rate for oxygen rises or falls to a similar extent.

resistance. This is partly due to the fact that modifications in the arterial pressure or in the blood's viscosity are counterbalanced by changes in the diameter of the arterioles. This phenomenon, called "autoregulation" (apparently produced by vessel relaxing or constricting factors derived from the vascular endothelium), makes it possible for the usual modifications in the systemic arterial pressure to not correspond in a lineal manner with the modifications of the blood flow to the brain. This vasoregulating is capable of maintaining the constant brain blood flow, despite the changes in the arterial pressure (within certain limits of the latter) (Figure 7.2) or the changes that take place in the brain blood flow, before changes of certain modifications in the internal medium (e.g., the arterial concentration of carbon dioxide, oxygen, etc.) are known. All these mechanisms are aimed at preserving the delivery of oxygen to the brain.

It is important to consider the reactivity of the cerebral vessels to carbon dioxide, a powerful vasodilator of the cerebral arterioles. High levels of carbon dioxide cause vasodilation, while low levels of $PaCO_2$ cause vasoconstriction. The response of the brain blood flow to carbon dioxide is somewhat proportional to the level of blood flow to the brain at rest. In areas of the brain with greater neuronal activity and with greater blood flow, the response to CO_2 is more pronounced than in areas with a lesser flow. The reaction to the CO_2 is usually expressed as a percentage of change of the flow of blood to the brain induced by a change in the $PaCO_2$ of 1 torr—the normal value being 3%/torr.

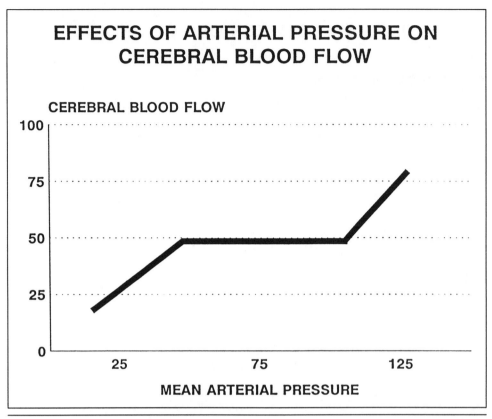

Figure 7.2: Cerebral autoregulation. Changes in arterial pressure produce little change in cerebral blood flow over a broad range of pressures.

Physiopathologic Aspects of the Brain Injury

In cases of cerebral catastrophes such as acute brain injury, important brain blood flow changes have been detected. Thus, while in children an initial increase in the blood flow to the brain is noted, among adults, a high percentage of patients experience a reduction of the flow. It is important to stress, however, that comatose patients with reduced brain metabolism may tolerate the decrease in the brain blood flow. This reduction may reflect the normal adjustment of the brain flood flow and the cerebral metabolism.

The majority of studies on the flow of blood to the brain in patients with head injury rarely reflect values below the ischemia level. In a study conducted by Bouma (1991), it was noted that in the first 4–6 hours after the trauma, the levels of blood flow to the brain were significantly decreased in comparison with those observed hours later. Simultaneous studies of the arteriojugular oxygen difference showed that in those patients with lower levels of brain blood flow, the arteriojugular oxygen difference was pathologically elevated, indicating cerebral ischemia. It is also important to note that the cerebral ischemia concept must take into account important regional variations; it is possible that ischemic cerebral areas exist next to others with a sufficient brain blood flow. This phenomenon has appeared during postmortem examinations that have demonstrated the presence of ischemic cell changes in some regions of the brain taking place after the trauma.

PRINCIPLES OF MANAGING PATIENTS WITH SEVERE HEAD INJURY

Table 7.3 shows the current general guidelines for managing the trauma in its severe stage for patients with head injury. It lists some of the interventions directed toward the rapid diagnosis of the physiopathologic conditions that accompany the trauma, as well as those concerning the primary brain injury and the prevention of the secondary brain injury.

Table 7.3: General Directives in the Management of a Patient with Brain Trauma

1.	Diagnosis of the brain injuries
2.	Optimum delivery of oxygen to the brain
3.	Prevention of secondary brain damage
4.	Prevention of infectious complications
5.	Maintenance of the nutritional state

Diagnosis of Brain Injuries

The brain damage resulting from the trauma is something that cannot be changed. Nevertheless, it is important that it be diagnosed as soon as possible, for several reasons. First, the existence of injuries taking a large volume of space may require evacuation, which in many patients means an emergency intervention. A second reason is the diagnosis of intracranial injuries compatible with intracranial hypertension. A third indication for the quick diagnosis is the need to establish a prediction on the evolution, as well as knowing the intracranial risks that might be anticipated.

Optimum Delivery of Oxygen to the Brain

Getting oxygen to the brain is the main objective of the treatment of a patient with a brain injury. To achieve this goal, we must obtain an adequate perfusion in all cerebral regions to which an adequate amount of oxygen and cell nutrients must be carried. The development of intracranial post-traumatic hypertension frequently compromises cerebral perfusion by decreasing the cerebral perfusion pressure, which in turn may also occur by a lowering of the mean arterial pressure. The normalization of the physiological parameters also implicated in carrying oxygen to the brain, such as the plasma hemoglobin levels, hypoxia, hypercapnia, etc., will also help in the normalization of getting oxygen to the brain.

Prevention of Secondary Brain Damage of Extracranial Origin

Of the extracranial factors mentioned in Table 7.1, hypoxia and hypotension are clearly determining signs of poor evolution of patients favoring the increase of the brain injury. This is more evident when we analyze the development of the secondary brain injury in the early stage. The influence of the hypotension on the prognosis is even greater than that of the hypoxia, as shown in the study of the Traumatic Coma Data Bank. The latter not only determines the worsening of the cerebral perfusion pressure in the pre-hospital period, but it has also been shown that the frequency and magnitude of the uncontrolled intracranial hypertension are increased when the hypotension is present in the pre-hospital period (Lobato, 1988; Seelig, 1986; Narayan, 1982).

Prevention of Infectious Complications

The development of infectious complications is very frequent in patients with brain trauma. The rate of infections, especially pulmonary ones, is very high. The deleterious effect of the hyperthermia and of the sepsis on the central nervous system is well known; therefore, the prevention of infections and their quick treatment, if they appear, is also a priority.

Maintenance of an Adequate Nutritional State

The hypercatabolic and hypermetabolic effect of the severe brain injury forces making optimum use of nourishing the patient so that it will be enough to defray the energy-protein needs of the patient. This together with the frequent incidence of sepsis and the difficulty of keeping the enteral path of nourishing requires establishing a specific nutritional strategy.

MONITORING AND DIAGNOSTIC TECHNIQUES

Computed Tomography

General Points on Computed Tomography and Severe Head Injury

Computed tomography is one of the neurodiagnostic techniques that has contributed most to the management of patients with critical severe cerebral pathology, especially traumatic pathology. Computed tomography is an indispensable study for all those patients who, as a result of a trauma, have suffered a decrease in their consciousness level or present any of the situations reflected in Table 7.4. Based on the basic principles of conventional radiology and backup by computer technology for the reconstruction of images in several planes, computed tomography allows for the construction of plane images and for the identification of different anatomical structures based on the different degrees of absorption of X-rays.

Table 7.4: Indication of the Performance of a Brain -Computed Tomography during the Acute Phase of Brain Injury

1.	Decrease of the level of consciousness below 14 points on the Glasgow Scale
2.	Otorrhagia
3.	Leakage of cerebrospinal fluid
4.	Open skull fracture
5.	Motor asymmetry in the clinical exploration
6.	When as a consequence of another injury, sedation and muscular relaxation of the patient is necessary

The various intracranial structures present a degree of absorption of the radiation that places them on a spectrum ranging from 0 to +50 Hounsfield Units. Besides these structures, it is important to the diagnosis of hemorrhagic injuries represented as hyperdense, which, in turn, fall between +50 and +200 Hounsfield Units. It is also important to the diagnosis of the existence of radiologically less dense areas than the normal brain (placed between +4 and +24 Hounsfield Units), which would correspond to edematous or ischemic brain structures.

Performing a computed tomography during the severe phase of the head injury must be aimed at the diagnosis of those injuries most frequently present after brain trauma. Toward this end, there are a series of technical recommendations for tomographic study that will increase its diagnostic sensitivity. These conditions are shown in Table 7.5.

Table 7.5: Recommendations for the Performance of a Computed Tomography during the Acute Phase of a Brain Injury

1.	10 mm-thick slices
2.	Window: 100 HU amplitude
3.	Center: +45 HU
4.	Nonroutine use of intravenous contrast
5.	Axial plane: cantomeatal inclination

The first great contribution of computed tomography to the management of patients suffering from head injury was the rapid diagnosis of lesions that occupied large volumes of space, which required immediate surgical evacuation. Subsequent technological developments have made possible better viewing of the intracranial structures in such a way that now it is possible to establish a diagnosis of small volume structural injuries, as well as establish the probability of the presence of certain pathological intracranial conditions of great clinical transcendence for the evolution of the patient. In Table 7.6, there are some physiopathologic conditions that may be inferred from viewing the computed tomography of patients who have suffered a severe head injury.

Table 7.6: Some Physiopathologic Intracranial Conditions which May Be Inferred from the Visualization of the Computed Tomography

1.	Intracranial hypertension
2.	Disturbance of structures with clinical relevance
	Signs of uncal herniation
	Signs of subfacial herniation
	Compression of mesencephalon and brainstem
	Diencephalic affectation
	Corpus callosum injury
	Brainstem injury
	Other
3.	Compression of vascular structures
	Anterior cerebral artery (subfacial herniation)
	Posterior cerebral artery (uncal herniation)
	Other

The information gathered through the viewing the cerebral computed tomography must be aimed at establishing the diagnosis of structural injuries, as well as to confirming the suspicion of changes in the intracranial fluid dynamics. Intracranial hypertension, compression of the arteries of the base of the brain (anterior cerebral, posterior cerebral, etc.), and obstruction of the flow of the cerebrospinal fluid, etc. may be suspected through the images obtained from the computed tomography. Table 7.7 presents a protocol that may be useful in reading these injuries. Such a scheme allows, on the one hand, the establishment of a diagnosis of primary intra- and extra-axial injuries resulting directly from the trauma. A second level of analysis allows for the establishment of possible changes in the intracranial fluid dynamics described in three separate sections: increase of the cerebral volume, signs of intracranial hypertension, and compression of relevant intracranial vascular structures. Finally, we analyze whether the pathological signs present in the computed tomography affect a structure of recognized clinical relevance.

Table 7.7: Protocol to Analyze the Computed Tomography

Vascular compression
    Of the anterior cerebral artery
    Of the posterior cerebral artery
    Other
Disturbance of clinically significant structures
    Uncal hernia
    Subfacial hernia
    Midline shift
    Bilateral injuries
    Centroencephalic injuries
    Diffuse axonal injury
Signs of intracranial hypertension
    Injury occupying large volume space
    Signs of increase of cerebral volume
Increase of the cerebral volume
    Compression of base cisternae
    Compression of fourth ventricle
    Compression of third ventricle
    Decrease in size lateral ventricles
Signs of diffuse axonal injury
    Corpus callosum injury
    Mesencephalon-brainstem injury
    Injury to basal ganglia
    Subarachnoid hemorrhage
    Intraventricular hemorrhage
Hypodense occupying space lesions
    Simple contusion
    Hemispheric swelling
    Hypodense vascular distribution
Hyperdense occupying space lesions, with potential evacuation
    Subdural hematoma
    Extradural hematoma
    Intraparenchimatous hematoma

This systematic approach to the reading of the image of the computed tomography post-severe brain injury allows, on the one hand, the completion of a therapeutic approximation, surgical as well as medical, and on other hand, the establishment of an initial prognosis, something of great transcendence for the patient that his/her relatives frequently demand.

The identification of the intracranial injuries by means of the computed tomography in patients with a severe brain injury has made possible the identification of pathological groups that present common physiopathological conditions and prognosis. The classification of the Traumatic Coma Data Bank (Table 7.8), developed with a large number of patients, analyzes, on the one hand, radiologic elements clearly related to the intracranial hypertension (compression of the cerebrospinal fluid spaces, shift of midline, injuries taking up large volumes of space), and, therefore, is a classification with a predicting capability of the final evolution of the patients, not only from the point of view of survival but also from the point of view of long-term neurological recovery of the patient (Table 7.9).

Table 7.8: Traumatic Coma Data Bank Diagnostic Categories

Diffuse Injury Type I
    No Visible Pathology on Computed Tomography
Diffuse Injury Type II
    Cisterns Are Present with Shift < 0–5 mm
    No High or Mixed Density Lesions > 25 ml
    May Include Bone Fragments and Foreign Bodies
Diffuse Injury Type III
    Cisterns Compressed or Absent
    Shift 0–5 mm
    No High Or Mixed Lesion > 25 ml
Diffuse Injury Type IV
    Shift > 5 mm
    No High or Lesion > 25 ml
Evacuated Mass Lesion
    Any Lesion Surgically Evacuated
Non-Evacuated Mass Lesion, High or Mixed Density Lesion > 25 ml Non-Surgically Evacuated

Table 7.9: Classification of Patients (%) by Glasgow Outcome Scale (GOS) and Intracranial Diagnosis (Traumatic Coma Data Bank)

	Good	Moderate	Severe	Veg. State	Dead
Total	7.0	18.5	28.0	14.0	32.5
Type I	27.0	34.6	19.2	9.6	9.6
Type II	8.15	6.0	40.7	11.3	13.5
Type III	3.3	13.1	26.8	22.9	34.0
Type IV	3.1	3.1	18.8	18.8	56.2
Evacuated Mass	5.1	17.7	26.1	12.3	38.8
Non-Evacuated Mass	2.8	8.3	19.4	16.7	52.8
Others	--	5.9	33.0	--	--

The Significance of Various Injuries Visible in Computed Tomography of Patients with Head Injury

The frequency of intracranial hypertension in patients who have suffered a severe brain injury is more than 50%. It is also well accepted that the monitoring of the intracranial pressure is the best method for the diagnosis and management of said hypertension. However, one of the uses of computed tomography is the ability to do an estimate of the risk of intracranial hypertension derived from the findings. The Traumatic Coma Data Bank develops a classification of the patients (Table 7.9) according to the findings of computed tomography, considering, among other aspects, the changes produced in the brain volume after the trauma, from which one can deduce that the categories mentioned try to be an early indicator of intracranial hypertension. There are several signs in this classification that relate more directly to the existence of intracranial hypertension: compression or absence of the cisternae of the base of the brain, the existence of mass injuries of over 25 ml in volume, and the shift of midline over 5 mm. Thus, for example,

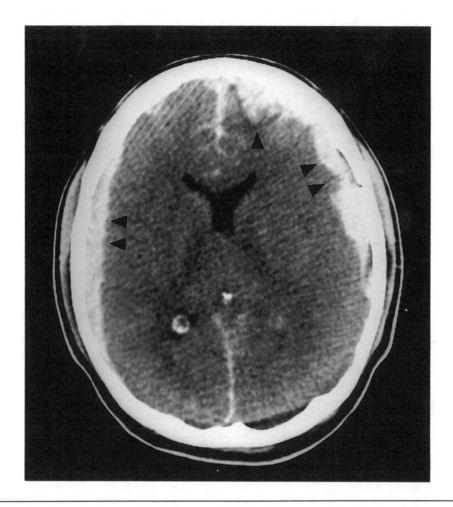

Figure 7.3: Computed tomography that shows a bilateral subdural hematoma and a frontal intracerebral hematoma.

Eisenberg (1990) showed how, in patients with abnormal cisternae, the incidence of intracranial hypertension is three times greater than in the group of patients with normal cisternae in the computed tomography. In addition to the radiologic signs, there are others that have been associated with the existence of intracranial hypertension: absence of the third ventricle, decrease in size of the lateral ventricles, shift of the cerebrospinal fluid from the subarachnoid hemispheric spaces, or dilatation of the occipital contralateral horn to an injury occupying a large volume of space that shifts midline. Some studies present as nonexistent the incidence of intracranial hypertension in patients with brain injury and normal computed tomography, or present only when there are extracranial factors that complicate the patient's evolution. Nevertheless, not all authors agree with this data; in a series done by the authors, in which a first generation scanner was used and in which 8.5% of the studies were considered normal, the incidence of intracranial hypertension of these patients was 9% (Murillo et al., 1986). Narayan (1982) places this percentage at 13%, and Eisenberg (1990) between 10% and 15%.

Although their location might suggest a similar prognosis, hyperdense injuries with extra-axial location (epidural or subdural) in practice show that they vary in severity. The most important risk that can be derived from the extradural hematomas is the quick development of intracranial hypertension and the rapid compression of the intracranial structures with functional relevance. The risks accompanying a subdural severe traumatic hematoma (Figure 7.3) are due not only to the mass effect generated by the increase of the intracranial volume but also to their frequent association with severe intracerebral injuries, both with the hemorrhagic type and with the swelling of the underlying cerebral tissue.

Small hemorrhagic lesions accompanying the diffuse axonal damage have special prognosis interest. These injuries, whose prevailing localizations are in the lobar subcortical white matter, the corpus callosum, and the dorsolateral mesencephalon (Figures 7.4 and 7.5), are difficult to identify in the computed tomography. In less than 30% of cases, the diffuse axonal injuries are accompanied by a visible hemorrhagic component in the computed tomography (this is not the case in nuclear magnetic resonance, which presents a greater capability of diagnosis). The degree of vascularization of the injured areas is the

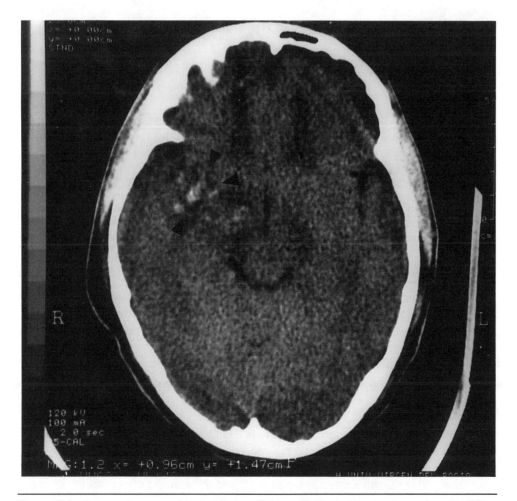

Figure 7.4: Computed tomography showing small hemorrhagic lesions accompanying the diffuse axonal damage.

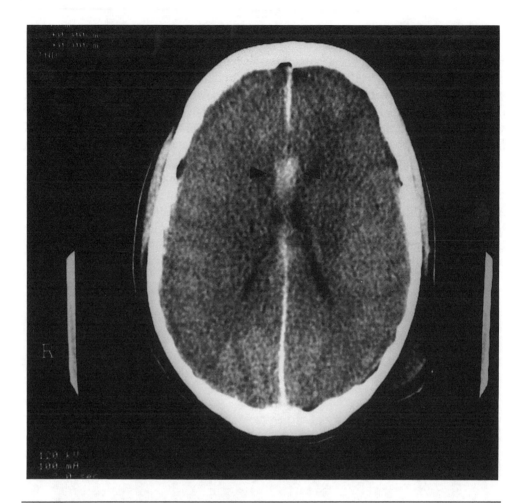

Figure 7.5: Computed tomography of a patient who had suffered a brain injury, showing a hematoma in the corpus callosun and a subaracnoid hemorrhage.

main determining factor for the presence of hemorrhagic images accompanying the diffuse axonal damage. As mentioned above, the presence in the computed tomography of suspicious signs of diffuse axonal injury neccessitate a more detailed study with a nuclear magnetic resonance, since in a significant number of patients, the functional recovery of these patients depends on diagnosis of these injuries.

Monitoring of the Intracranial Pressure

Measuring Systems

The increase of the intracranial pressure is a phenomenon present in 30–70% of the patients who have suffered severe cranioencepahlic trauma. The importance of the increase of the intracranial pressure is due mainly to two phenomena: the shifting of the brain mass within the intracranial compartments and the negative effect that the increase of the intracranial pressure has on the cerebral perfusion.

There are three mechanisms more frequently implicated in the increase of the intracranial pressure after a brain injury: (1) the appearance of injuries that take up space, especially hemorrhagic injuries; (2) the increase of the water content of the brain tissue (edema or brain swelling); and (3) the increase of the intravascular blood brain volume. These three mechanisms may be present separately or combine among themselves. The final consequence is the increase of the usual intracranial volumes contained in an unenlargeable box, the skull. As a result, the intracranial pressure rises.

For an estimate of this increase in the intracranial pressure, there is presently no better method than the direct measurement. Several technical methods have been developed in recent years to measure intracranial pressure. Hydrostatic, pneumatic, or fiberoptic systems have been developed recently. Discussions have also occurred regarding what is the most appropriate intracranial compartment for measuring intracranial pressure. Intraventricular, intraparenchymatous, subarachnoidal, subdural, and epidural locations have been used. Discussions have also focused on the location of the sensor and also on the exactness required for the measurement, the stability of the sensors, and the complications that each measuring system generates. Historically, the intraventricular location has been the one most frequently used as a reference for comparing the exactness of the measurement of the intracranial pressure with that of other compartments. The greatest equivalence with the intraventricular pressure has been found with the intraparechymatous transductors and with the subdural ones. The factors complicating the intracranial pressure monitoring are infection, hemorrhage, obstruction, and bad positioning. The intraventricular systems are the ones most often affected by infections. However, the link between the contamination of the system and true infection is not completely clear. However, it is true that the risk of bacterial contamination increases significantly after the fifth day of the implant, and, therefore, the risk of the associated clinical infection does as well.

It has not been clearly established yet what the best system is for monitoring the intracranial pressure of patients with brain injury. The combination of four variables—exact measurement, the experience of the physician in the interpretation of the values measured, cost, and morbidity—allows each group to choose the most adequate method in each hospital.

How Measuring Intracranial Pressure Influences the Management of Patients Suffering Brain Injury

As was mentioned before, there are two relevant aspects in the changes of the intracranial pressure: (1) the pressure gradient generated from the encephalic regions with greatest hypertension, with the consequent shift of the brain structures within the skull (herniation, shifting of the centroencephalic structures, or compression of the vascular structures are their main consequences); and (2) the negative influence the cerebral perfusion pressure has on the increase of intracranial pressure. The latter, derived from the difference between the pressure of the middle artery and the intracranial pressure, is directly related to the brain blood flow. The decreases in the cerebral perfusion pressure determines cerebral ischemia with important clinical consequences.

Various studies have shown that the probability of a good evolution is inversely proportional to the time that the intracranial pressure has remained over 20 mmHg (value considered pathologic) (Johnston et al., 1970; Marshall et al., 1979; Miller et al., 1981). The beneficial effect over mortality of treatment of intracranial hypertension has been demonstrated in the study by Saul (1982), which showed that patients whose treatment of the intracranial hypertension was begun when the latter was at levels around 15 mmHg had a lower mortality rate than if the treatment had been started when the intracranial pressure was above 20 mmHg. The study done by Eisenberg (1988) also showed that there are beneficial effects derived from the control of the intracranial pressure and that in a group of patients in which the intracranial pressure was controlled with barbiturates, the mortality rate was significantly lower than in the group of patients whose pressure was not modified after being given the barbiturates.

Electrophysiologic Monitoring of Patients with Severe Brain Injury

The use of neurodepressing medication may lower the need of the clinical exploration in the follow-up of the evolution of patients who have suffered brain injury. The use of neurophysiologic monitoring techniques such as the encephalogram and the evoked potentials eases the neuromonitoring in these situations.

Electroencephalogram

The electroencephalogram has been used very much for the follow-up of patients with brain injury and has shown good results in the prediction of poor evolution of the patients. Patients with encephalographic registries with low amplitude and low rhythms have a significantly worse prognosis than those whose registries show a prevailing alpha rhythm. The prediction of the positive evolution of the patient is less exact than the prediction of the negative evolution. This is due, among other reasons, to the fact that the encephalogram does not present specific patterns for situations relevant for the negative evolution of the patient. There are no encephalographic registries characteristic of the effect of the cerebral perfusion pressure by the increase of the intracranial pressure. The electroencephalogram is a late detector of the changes of the cerebral perfusion when compared with other methods of neuromonitoring. Nevertheless, there are some registries that allow an increase in the capability of prediction of a positive prognosis of the encephalogram. The reactivity of the electroencephalogram to stimuli such as auditory stimuli has been identified as an indicator of good prognosis in patients with brain injury. A similar significance is given to the periodic registry of sleep in the encephalogram.

The computer analysis of the condensed electroencephalogram registry, called "compressed spectral array," converts the information provided by the classic encephalogram into a registry of dominant frequencies in time. Some authors affirm that the compressed spectral array (Karnaze et al., 1982) has increased the diagnostic and prognosis sensitivity for a good evolution of the electroencephalogram in patients with brain injury.

Evoked Potentials

The sensitive responses evoked are small electrical responses generated in sensory paths as a reaction to certain stimuli. The three stimuli most frequently used clinically in order to register the potentials evoked are somesthetic stimuli (electrical stimuli applied to the nerves of the extremities), auditory stimuli, and visual stimuli.

The somesthetic stimulus explores the various sections through which the electrical stimulus is transmitted; a first wave, generated in the brachial plexus (if the stimulus has been done over the upper extremity) is followed by those generated in the superior cervical column, dorsal nuclei, and primary sensitive parietal cortex. In the case of auditory potentials, the stimulus is a "click" sound that stimulates the eighth cranial pair and travels through the cochlear nucleus, superior olivary complex (low pons), the lateral lemniscus (high pons), and the inferior coliculus (midbrain). The presence of wave I ensures the integrity of the peripheral auditory apparatus. Visual evoked potentials test the integrity of the retina, optic nerve, optic chiasm, and the occipital cortex. They are usually measured when the other types of evoked potentials are monitored, and in general, the visual evoked potentials have not been as useful as brainstem auditory-evoked responses or somatosensory-evoked responses. The major advantage of evoked potentials monitoring is that signals are resistant to alteration by pharmacologic agents such as barbiturates. Consequently, changes observed in evoked potentials registers can be attributed to genuine functional disintegration.

In patients with brain injury, the predictive value of the somatosensory-evoked potentials may be superior to the electroencephalogram because many of the extraneurologic factors that influence an electroencephalogram have a markedly reduced effect on the somatosensory-evoked potentials. Many studies have shown that the existence of significantly pathologic somesthetic potentials are correlated with a negative clinical evolution. Discordant results regarding the predictive capability of the auditory evoked responses have been found. While some studies have found a good correlation between auditory responses and the patient's prognosis with brain injury, this correlation has not been found in others (Karnaze et al., 1985; Becker et al., 1990; Dauch, 1991; Alters et al., 1993). Comparative studies between the somesthetic potentials and the auditory potentials have demonstrated the superiority of the former over the latter. This is probably due to the fact that the somesthetic potentials evoked present several components, which include from the peripheric nerve to the cerebral cortex, while the superior level of the processing of the auditory signal is the brainstem.

Estimating Methods for the Cerebral Blood Flow

The modifications of the cerebral blood flow that develop during the acute phase of the brain injury generate relevant quantifications of the cerebral delivery of oxygen. Therefore, the quantification of the cerebral blood flow is an important contribution in the management of the patient suffering from severe brain injury. However, the precise technological requirements for the direct measurement of the cerebral blood flow (nitrous oxide method, Xenon 133) do not, at the present time, allow for the continuous bedside monitoring of the cerebral blood flow. For this reason, in most neurologic intensive care units, indirect estimates of the cerebral blood flow are done with techniques such as the doppler transcranial sonogram or the monitoring of the saturation of oxygen in the bulb of the internal jugular vein.

Transcranial Doppler Sonography

The transcranial doppler sonogram, discovered by Aaslid in 1982 and based on the Doppler effect, shows the velocity of the flow of blood in the arteries at the base of the skull. It also facilitates registering the time of those velocities, which may be represented by a graph called a "sonogram." In order to carry out these studies, a 2 MHz bidirectional flowmeter is used that emits pulsating signals through a piezoelectric device. To access sonographically the arteries of the circle of Willis, the so-called "sonic windows" are used—cranial areas which, due to their structural characteristics, present a greater transparency for ultrasounds. The most frequently used windows are the temporal window, the ophthalmic window, and the foramen magnum window. Three characteristics help identify the arteries explored: (1) the depth of the artery, (2) the existence of the anterograde flow (the arterial flow approaches the probe) or retrograde flow (distances itself from the probe), and (3) the response that the arterial flow presents after the compression of the two carotids.

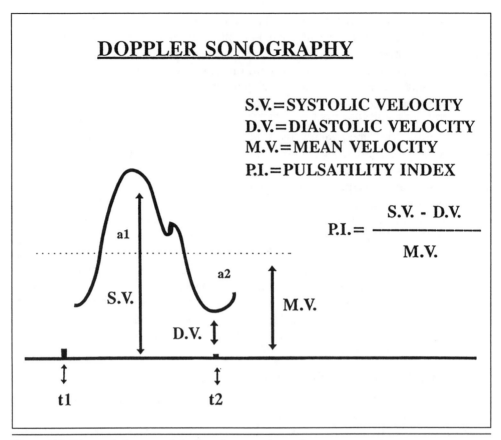

Figure 7.6: Diagnostic features of the Doppler spectral waveform.

The sonographic signal shows (Figure 7.6) (1) the morphology of the sonogram, (2) the values (in cm/sec) of the systolic (SV), diastolic (DV), and mean (MV) velocities, and (3) an estimate of the cerebrovascular resistance by means of the pulsatility index or Gosling index ((SV-DV)/MV) and the resistance index or Pourcelot index (SV-DV/SV). After a brain injury, the increase in intracranial pressure determines changes in the cerebrovascular resistance, which, when accompanied by changes in the cerebral blood flow, produce changes in the velocity of the flow of blood in the arteries at the base of the skull. In addition to the intracranial pressure, other factors also determine changes in the velocity of the blood—the changes of the cerebral metabolic rate for oxygen, changes in the vascular response to carbon dioxide, vasospasm due to subarachnoid hemorrhage, etc. In patients with a severe brain injury, it is frequent that during the first 24 hours after the trauma, a sonographic registry may contain low velocities. This may be due to various factors: hypovolemia secondary to the trauma, lowering of the cerebral metabolic rate for oxygen, intracranial hypertension, etc. This sonographic pattern, especially when it is due to intracranial hypertension and continues with an increment of the pulsatility index beyond the normal limits, usually corresponds to a condition of cerebral hypoperfusion. The increase in mean velocity and the decrease in the pulsatility index on the days following the trauma usually indicate a favorable prognosis.

In a certain percentage of patients with brain injury, it is possible to find an increase in velocities. When this happens, it is difficult to know if it is due to a vasospasm or to a hyperemia. The hyperemia exhibits as differential traits: it is frequently bilateral, it appears 24 hours later, its presence is rare after the fifth day, and the dicrotic notch disappears in the sonogram. On the other hand, the following data may indicate a vasospasm: velocity greater than 120 cm/sec and a pulsatility index < 1, a unilateral increase in the mean velocity, and an appearance on the second day and persistence beyond the tenth day of cranioencephalic post-trauma.

Generally, the existence of low velocity in the intracranial arteries after a brain injury is due either to a decrease in the cerebral metabolism or to an increase in the intracranial pressure. An inverse correlation between the severity of the trauma and the mean velocity of the middle cerebral artery has been shown (Chan et al., 1992). Nevertheless, the mean velocity does not usually indicate a significant decrease until the cerebral perfusion pressure has begun to descend below normal limits. The pulsatility index maintains a close correlation with the intracranial pressure. Increases in the latter determine parallel increases in the pulsatility index due to the decrease of the diastolic velocity.

When the intracranial pressure rises in an uncontrollable manner, a sonographic systolized pattern is registered. This pattern registers a decrease of the mean velocity and an increase of the pulsatility index. When the value of the cerebral perfusion pressure approaches the value of the mean arterial tension, the anterograde flow ceases in the diastolic phase, producing then a retrograde flow. This sonographic pattern is known as "reverberating flow" and is indicative of the cessation of the cerebral blood flow. In more advanced stages of cerebral circulatory cessation, the diastolic wave disappears with only the systolic component remaining. The final phase of the cerebral circulatory cessation is accompanied by the impossibility of registering any signal at the level of the arteries at the base (Dominguez et al., 1995a, b).

Jugular Oxygen Saturation

If we assume that arterial oxygen content, haemoglobin concentration, and the position of the oxyhemoglobin dissociation curve are largely constant (or changing slowly), then the ratio of cerebral metabolic rate for oxygen to cerebral blood flow will vary with the venous oxygen content and with the jugular venous haemoglobin oxygen saturation. Therefore, the monitoring of oxygen saturation in the internal jugular (SJO2) vein becomes a useful element for purposes of estimating the balance between the cerebral metabolic rate for oxygen and cerebral blood flow.

It has not been possible to decide which side is the most appropriate to place the catheter in the jugular vein. Some authors favor its placement in the hemisphere where the injuries are more obvious according to the computed tomography. Others suggest that a compliance test should be done in order to estimate the side with the greater venous flow, while still others propose, especially in patients for whom the compliance test results were doubtful, the insertion in the right jugular vein. The end of the catheter should be placed in the internal jugular vein's bulb to minimize extracranial contamination proceeding from the pterygoid and facial veins. The catheter's position should be checked by means of a lateral X-ray, confirming that the tip of the catheter is located above the lower edge of the first cervical vertebra.

There are several ways of using the data reported from placing a catheter in the internal jugular vein. The direct measurement of the venous saturation is one of these. The normal limits are placed around 50–55% as a lower limit and 75% as an upper limit. When the saturation exceeds 75%, it is thought that the patient presents a relative hyperemia (high cerebral flow in relation to the extraction of oxygen, which in turn may be normal or low). In those patients where a high extraction determines a low jugular saturation, it is thought that there is a low cerebral blood flow in relation to consumption.

Some authors prefer the arteriojugular difference in oxygen content (AJDO2) to calculate the amount of oxygen extracted from the cerebral circulation by the brain. The formula for its computation is as follows:

$$AJDO2 = Hb \times 1.34 \times (SaO2 - SJO2)/100 + (0.03 (PaO2 - PvO2))$$

Another way of expressing the extraction of oxygen from the brain using the data provided by the jugular saturation of oxygen is the formula of *Oxygen Extraction Ratio* (OER):

$$OER = (SaO2 - SJO2)/SaO2$$

Other parameters have also been used, such as the Lactate/Oxygen Index, the cerebral consumption of glucose, etc. Nevertheless, currently the SJO2 is still the parameter more widely used for the management of the patient with severe brain injury. The possibility of continuous monitoring and direct reading makes it possible to use as an effective method for detecting episodes of jugular desaturation (compatible with episodes of cerebral hypoperfusion) or saturation above the normal range (compatible with low perfusion or hyperemia).

THERAPEUTIC STRATEGY IN PATIENTS WITH SEVERE BRAIN INJURY

The Resuscitation Phase

Basically, the initial assistance to a patient with severe head injury does not differ basically from that which should be done to any other type of severe trauma patient. The scheme proposed by the Advanced Trauma Life Support of the American College of Surgeons is a valid application scheme for these patients. It is based on the administering of a series of evaluation and assistance techniques to the traumatized patient in which the assistance priorities are established. In the first evaluation phase, the following scheme is followed:

1. Airway maintenance with C-Spine control
2. Breathing
3. Circulation with hemorrhage control
4. Disability: neurologic status
5. Exposure: completely undress the patient

The sequence of these interventions allows for the initial assistance to those organic functions whose involvement may threaten the life of the patient, such as aiding breathing and circulation, in order to later develop a more detailed study of other possible injuries associated with the trauma.

There are several phenomena frequently present in the moments after the head injury that could become in an element of added cerebral aggression to the primary injury. The depression of the breathing function often occurs and is accompanied by hypoxemia and hypercapnia with the consequent deterioration of the delivery of oxygen to the brain, cerebral vasodilation, and possible intracranial hypertension. Arterial hypotension (accompanied or not by absolute or relative hypovolemia) is also usually associated with severe trauma. The frequent disorder of the cerebral autoregulation in these patients, together with arterial hypotension, determines a decrease of the cerebral perfusion that also becomes a secondary insult to the brain. Thus, in patients with severe brain injury, a endotracheal tube must be placed when the consciousness level ≤ 8 points, when there are signs of severe neurologic focalization (signs of cerebral hernia), when there is breathing difficulty (obstruction of the airway or as a result of other factors), and when there is significant arterial hypotension. The placing of the endotracheal tubes must address, initially, correcting the hypercapnia or maintaining a moderate hyperventilation, as well as normalizing the oxygen content of the blood.

All patients with severe brain injury must have one or more high flow veins canalized to permit a vigorous reanimation with fluids and to allow the administration of medication. The relation between low values of mean arterial pressure during the first hours of the brain injury and a greater rate of mortality has been clearly demonstrated, as well as worse functional results and a greater incidence of systemic complications. On the other hand, a high percentage of patients with severe brain injury present intracranial hypertension during the first hours following the trauma. If the mean arterial pressure remains low, the cerebral perfusion pressure will be compromised. Hypertonic fluids are being used more and more in the resuscitation of this type of patient (e.g., a saline solution at 3–7%). These solutions have been used successfully for the control of intracranial hypertension and for the treatment of hemorrhagic shock (Todd et al., 1985; Gunnar et al., 1988; Shacford et al., 1992). The infusion of hypertonic saline serum manages to quickly restore the intravascular volume, improve the myocardial contractility, and decrease the intracranial pressure in traumatized patients. The final objective of this therapy is to assure the patient a normal intravascular volume with a normal mean arterial pressure.

The third step in the management of the patient with severe brain injury, once adequate breathing has been assured and adequate venous paths for the infusion of fluids have been established, is the urgent neurological evaluation. The neurological evaluation must determine the level of consciousness, pupils' reaction to light, and alterations in motor reactions. In order to evaluate the level of consciousness, the Glasgow Scale (Table 7.10) is used. It has several advantages: it can be applied easily, it is objective, and it provides for close correlation with the patient's prognosis. Assessment of the pupils provides invaluable information about cranial nerves II and III and the brainstem. The responses of the pupils to light in terms of both shape and reactivity is controlled by the nucleus of III cranial nerve and reflects an interaction of sympathetic and parasympathetic nervous supply to the muscles controlling the pupils. The pupillary pathways are quite resistant to metabolic insults. Consequently, the presence or absence of the light reflex is an extremely important physical sign that can be used to distinguish structural from metabolic or systemic coma. The direct light response refers to the direct constriction of the pupil in the eyes stimulated by light. A dilated and unreactive pupil following a brain injury is an ominous finding. Often accompanying pupillary abnormality are the others signs of transtentorial herniation: changes in the level of consciousness and abnormal motor responses.

Table 7.10: Glasgow Coma Scale

Eyes Open
>   Spontaneously (eyes open, does not imply awareness) 4
>   To Speech (any speech, not necessarily a command) 3
>   To Pain (should not use supraorbital pressure for pain) 2
>   Never 1

Best Verbal Response
>   Oriented (to time, person, place) 5
>   Confused Speech (disoriented) 4
>   Inappropriate (swearing, yelling) 3
>   Incomprehensible Sounds (moaning, groaning) 2
>   None 1

Best Motor Response
>   Obeys Commands 6
>   Localizes Pain (deliberate or purposeful movement) 5
>   Withdrawal (moves away from stimulus) 4
>   Abnormal Flexion (decortication) 3
>   Extension (decerebration) 2
>   None (flaccidity) 1

Total Score _____

Specific Treatment of the Intracranial Injury

Once the resuscitation has been done, the specific treatment of the intracranial injuries must be considered. Surgical evacuation of the mass injuries, treatment of the intracranial hypertension, and optimum delivery of oxygen to the brain become the three fundamental pillars of the treatment.

Surgical Evaluation of the Intracranial Masses

Over a third of all the patients in the United States who suffer from severe brain injury undergo surgical evacuation of a intracranial hematoma. Nevertheless, the surgical criteria in this type of patient are not firmly established, and the surgical intervention depends on the criteria of the medical team in charge at the moment. However, there are general norms that support the surgical decision. Thus, the following are considered to be possible to evacuate surgically: extra-axial injuries (subdural or epidural hematomas) that cause a midline shift > 5 mm, severe subdural hematomas > 30 ml in size, and, in general, those hematomas surgically accessible that justify an important increase in the intracranial pressure or decrease of the cerebral perfusion pressure.

Management of the Intracranial Hypertension

The intracranial hypertension is the most important secondary insult of all those factors involved in the secondary brain injury. There are two goals of the treatment of the intracranial hypertension: normalization of the intracranial pressure and maintenance of the cerebral perfusion pressure at values above 70 mmHg. There are a series of general measures (Table 7.11) in the routine treatment of patients with brain injury that try to prevent increases in the intracranial pressure.

Table 7.11: General Measures for Treatment of Patients with Severe Brain Injury

1.	Place Head 30° above the Horizontal Line
2.	Effective Analgesic
3.	Normothermia
4.	Pa02 > 70 mmHg
5.	Mean Arterial Pressure 80–100 mmHg
6.	Normovolemia
7.	Hemoglobin > 10 gr/dl
8.	Plasma Osmolarity > 290 mOsm/l
9.	Glucemia < 200 mg/dl
10.	Seizures Profilaxis

Except for patients in a state of shock, it is proper to keep the head of the patient who has suffered brain injury in a neutral and elevated 30° position above the horizontal line. This measure helps decrease the volumes of intracranial as the cerebrospinal fluid is shifted toward the perispinal spaces; it also helps with the venous drainage. Proper analgesics limit the neurovegetative responses of the patient toward the pain, as well as limit the agitation and anxiety that it produces. Keeping a body temperature below 37° C also becomes a useful treatment mechanism. Hyperthermia is accompanied by an increase in the brain oxygen consumption and by an increase of the brain blood volume with the corresponding increase of the intracranial pressure. Control of the glucemia is also considered an important goal, since a correlation has been found between high levels of glucemia with an increase of the lactate in the cerebrospinal fluid. The remaining measures listed in Table 7.11 are aimed at improving the delivery of oxygen to the brain (oxemia and mean arterial pressure control and normal hemoglobin), limiting the brain edema (control of the osmolarity), and preventing the increase of cerebral metabolic rate for oxygen and, therefore, of cerebral blood flow.

Table 7.12 presents some therapeutic elements that have been used for the control of the intracranial pressure in patients with brain injury. Steroids in high doses have been used in various studies. However, the steroids have not shown any positive effect in the control of the intracranial hypertension nor in the positive clinical evolution of the patients. The secondary effects of this medication, such as the elevation of the levels of glucemia, risk of gastrointestinal hemorrhage, and the increase in infections, are additional factors which, together with their demonstrated lack of effectiveness, have resulted in discontinued use of steroids as useful medication in the treatment of brain injury.

Table 7.12: Some Therapeutic Elements Used in the Treatment of Intracranial Hypertension

1.	Mannitol
2.	Steroids
3.	Hypertonic Solutions
4.	Sedatives
5.	Muscle Relaxants
6.	Analgesics
7.	Barbiturates in High Doses
8.	Evacuation of the Cerebrospinal Fluid

The ideal sedative for patients with brain trauma has not been established. Nevertheless, there are medications that ease the patient's adapting him/herself to the mechanical breathing, reduce the need for analgesics, limit the high intracranial pressure levels, and generally ease the care of the patients with brain injury. Benzodiazepines, especially Midazolam and Propofol, are the medications used most often. Although muscle relaxing medications ease the control of the intracranial pressure, they are associated, especially if used for a prolonged period of time, with the development of a series of adverse effects (prolonged neuromuscular weakness, autonomic dysfunction, etc.), which makes them of limited use in the management of these patients. Pancuronium and Atracurium have been the relaxants used most often. A new group of muscle relaxants is being developed, although their effects on the intracranial pressure in patients with brain injury have not been sufficiently evaluated.

Hyperventilation has been used for years as one of the cornerstones in the treatment of intracranial hypertension. Hyperventilation is very useful in reducing blood flow to the brain. Some classic protocols have established values of 25–30 mmHg optimum values of $PaCO_2$ for patients with brain injury. Recent studies have shown that those patients with brain injury who have been kept on a standard hyperventilation protocol for five days presented a worse clinical evolution. That could be justified by an excessive cerebral vasoconstriction, which produces a cerebral ischemia and secondary brain damage. Presently it seems appropriate to use hyperventilation together with the monitoring of the jugular saturation in order to limit the global cerebral ischemia.

Mannitol has been a medication classically used in the control of intracranial hypertension. The effects of mannitol are an osmotic effect and an increase in the brain blood volume (initially), and it probably unleashes a vasoconstrictory cascade. Mannitol is more useful in bolus than as a continuous infusion. It is a useful medication in the reanimation stages of hypovolemic patients with associated brain injury. Its usefulness has also been demonstrated in situations such as with rapid increase of the intracranial pressure, with patients who develop pupil dilation or sudden neurological deterioration, and during certain therapeutic maneuvers or when transferring the patient for explorations (e.g., computed tomography). However, its adverse effects (excessive dehydration and secondary hypovolemia and its toxic renal action) must be controlled in order to avoid their deleterious effects on the patient.

An alternative to mannitol is hypertonic sodium at 3%. Several researchers have shown an increase of the cerebral perfusion pressure, of the intravascular volume, of the microcirculation, and, consequently, of the intracranial pressure. Our experience with hypertonic sodium is satisfactory. Presently we prefer to use it over mannitol when plasma sodium is < 145 mEq/l and when an endocraneal hypertension coexists with a deficit in the volume of effective circulation.

Barbiturates in high doses are not first choice medications in the treatment of patients with brain injury. Their known effects on intracranial structures (decrease of the blood flow to the brain, decrease of the cerebral metabolic rate for oxygen) could be useful in the management of the intracranial hypertension of patients with brain injury, but they are accompanied by undesirable systemic effects, such as the decrease of the mean arterial pressure (especially in patients with hypovolemia or previous cardiovascular disease) with a decrease of the cerebral perfusion pressure. Presently, barbiturates in high doses have shown their efficacy in the control of intracranial hypertension in a third of the patients who present intracranial hypertension resistant to standard therapy. High doses of barbiturates are more effective in controlling intracranial pressure in the following circumstances: (1) intracranial hypertension secondary to a brain swelling, (2) high amplitude to the vascular component of the pulse wave, (3) jugular saturation of oxygen in the internal jugular vein > 75%, and (4) when hyperventilation has been shown to be effective in reducing the intracranial pressure.

The drainage of cerebrospinal fluid is a useful measure to control rises in the intracranial pressure. However, we know that it has two limitations; first, it induces the overproduction of cerebrospinal fluid, and second, its efficacy in controlling intracranial hypertension is limited when the latter reaches or surpasses 30 mmHg since at this level of intracranial hypertension, a compression around the catheter's tip is produced, which obstructs it and prevents the cerebrospinal fluid from coming out.

Guidelines for the Treatment of Intracranial Hypertension

There are several schemes and algorithms that have been proposed for the management of intracranial hypertension of the patient with brain injury. Although the development of the monitoring techniques of the intracranial pressure presents the normalization of the values of the intracranial pressure as the key objective of the treatment of brain injury, subsequent knowledge about intracranial physiopathology, as well as technological developments, has allowed us to know, more importantly than in the normalization of the intracranial pressure, how to maintain cerebral perfusion pressure within normal limits. But it is also known that it is important not only to keep intracranial pressure but also that cerebral ischemia must be avoided, for which reason the maintenance of a SJO2 within a normal limit is also a priority. The transcranial Doppler sonography permits an estimate of the brain blood flow; consequently, normal velocities with a normal pulsatility index also become basic treatment goals.

The conjunction of these four elements—cerebral perfusion pressure, SJO2, intracranial pressure, and velocities registered in the Doppler—present a range within which to establish an adequate therapeutic strategy. Frequently, the normalization of one of the parameters mentioned above carries with it the normalization of the others, since we must not forget that they are different perspectives of one single objective—the normalization of the delivery of oxygen to all brain areas.

Other Therapeutic Measurements

Brain injury is accompanied by a marked metabolic response. Hypermetabolism, hypercatabolism, and hyperglycemia are frequent phenomena in these patients. Therefore, the maintenance of adequate nutritional support (via enteral and, if necessary, parenteral) will be of great value in the maintenance of the corporal configuration of the patient.

Infections frequently develop in patients with brain injury. Pneumonia, sinusitis, meningitis, ventriculitis, sepsis related to catheter, etc. are frequently observed. Factors that encourage these infections are the need for breathing assistance for several days, facial trauma, base skull fractures, etc. The maintenance of an adequate prophylactic strategy for the infections, as well as an aggressive therapeutic protocol, become a fundamental element in the management of patients with brain injury.

REFERENCES

Adams, J.M., & Graham, D.I. (1976). The relationship between ventricular fluid pressure and the neuropathology of raised intracranial pressure. *Neuropathol. Appl. Neurobiol., 2,* 323–332.

Alster, J., Pratt, H., & Feinsod, M. (1993). Density spectral array, evoked potentials, and temperature rhythms in the evaluation and prognosis of the comatose patient. *Brain Inj., 7,* 191–208.

Bouma, G.J., Muizelaar, J.P., Choi, S.C., Newlon, P.G., & Young, M.F. (1991). Cerebral circulation and metabolism after severe traumatic brain injury: The elusive role of ischemia. *J. Neurosurg., 75,* 685–693.

Becker, D.P., Gade, G.F., & Miller, J.D. (1990). Prognosis after head injury. In J.R. Youmas (Ed.), *Neurological surgery* (3rd ed.) (pp. 2194–2229). Philadelphia: WB Saunders.

Chan, K.H., Miller, J.D., & Dearden, N.M. (1992). Intracranial blood flow velocity after head injury: Relationship to severity of injury, time, neurological status and outcome. *J. Neurol. Neurosurg. Psychiatry, 55,* 787–791.

Dauch, W.A. 1991. Prediction of secondary deterioration in comatose neurosurgical patients by serial recording of multimodality evoked potentials. *Acta Neurochir. (Wien,) 111,* 84–91.

Dominguez, J.M., Murillo, F., Muñoz, A., Santamaria, J.L., & Villen, J. (1995). Changes in the doppler waveform of intracranial arteries in patients in brain death status. *Transplantation Proc., 27,* 2391–2392.

Dominguez, J.M., Murillo, F., Muñoz. A., Santamaria, J.L., Villen. J., & Barrera, J.M. (1995). Study of blood flow velocities in the middle cerebral artery using transcranial doppler sonography in brain-dead patients. *Transplantation Proc., 27,* 2395–2396.

Eisenberg, H.M., Frankowski, R., Contant, C., Marshall, L.F., & Walker, M.D. (1988). High-dose barbiturate control of elevated intracranial pressure in patients with severe head injury. *J. Neurosurg., 69,* 15–23.

Eisenberg, H.M., Gary, H.E., Aldrich, E.F., Saydjari, C., Turner, B., & Foulkes, M.A. (1990). Initial CT findings in 753 patients with severe head injury: A report from the NIH Traumatic Coma Data Bank. *J. Neurosurg., 73,* 68–698.

Gunnar, W., Jonasson, O., Merlotti, G., Stone, J., & Barret, J. (1988). Head injury and hemorrhagic shock: Studies of the blood brain barrier and intracranial pressure after resuscitation with normal saline solution 3%, saline solution and dextran-40. *Surgery, 103,* 398–407.

Johnston, I.H., Johnston, J.A., & Jennet, B. (1970). Intracranial pressure changes following head injury. *Lancet, 2,* 433–436.

Karnaze, D.S., Marshall, L.F., & Bickford, R.G. (1982). EEG monitoring of clinical coma: The compressed spectral array. *Neurology, 32,* 289–292.

Karnaze, D.S., Weiner, J., & Marshall, L.F. (1985). Auditory evoked potentials in coma after close head injury: A clinical-neurophysiologic coma scale for predicting outcome. *Neurology, 35,* 1122–1126.

Lobato, R.D., Sarabia, R., Cordobes, F., Castro, S., & Muñoz, M.J. (1988). Post-traumatic cerebral hemispheric swelling. Analysis of 55 cases studied with computerized tomography. *J. Neurosurg., 68,* 417–423.

Marshall, L.F., Smith, R.W., & Shapiro, R. (1979) The outcome with aggressive treatment in severe head injuries. Part II: Acute and chronic barbiturate administration in the management of severe head injury. *J. Neurosurg., 50,* 26–30.

Murillo, F., Dominguez, J.M., Monreal, C., Ruano, J., & Muñoz, A. (1986). Traumatismo craneoencefalico grave ¿Cuando monitorizar la PIC? *Med. Intensiva, 10,* 113–116.

Miller, J.D., Butterworth, J.F., Gudeman, S.K., & Faulkner, J.E. (1981). Further experience in the management of severe head injury. *J. Neurosurg., 54,* 289–299.

Narayan, R., Kishore, P., Becker, D., Ward, J.D., Enas, G.G., & Greenberg, G. (1982). Intracranial pressure: To monitor or not monitor? A review of our experience with head injury. *J. Neurosurg., 56,* 650–659.

Saul, T.G., & Ducker, T.B. (1982). Effect of intracranial pressure monitoring and aggressive treatment on mortality in severe head injury. *J. Neurosurg., 56,* 498–503.

Seelig, J.M., Klauber, M.R., & Toole, B.M. (1986). Increased ICP and systemic hypotension during the first 72 hours following severe head injury. In J.D. Miller, G.M. Teasdale, & J.O. Rowan (Eds.), *Intracranial pressure VI* (pp. 675–679). Berlin: Springer-Verlag.

Shacford, S.R., Zhuang, J., & Schmokers, H. (1992). Intravenous fluid tonicity: Effect of intracranial pressure cerebral blood flow, and cerebral oxygen delivery in focal brain injury. *J. Neurosurg., 76,* 91–98.

Strich, S.J. (1956). Diffuse degeneration of the cerebral white matter in severe dementia following head injury. *J. Neurol. Neurosurg. Psychiatry, 19,* 163–185.

Todd, M.M., Tomasino, C., & Moore, J.J. (1985). Cerebral effects of isovolemic hemodilution with a hypertonic saline solution. *J. Neurosurg., 63,* 944–948.

8

Definitions, Assessment, and Treatment of the Comatose Patient: A Neuropsychological Perspective

David W. Ellis,[1] Christopher D. Royer,[1] and Kenneth B. Goldberg

[1]Independence Rehab Services
Widener University, Cherry Hill, NJ

INTRODUCTION

The evaluation and treatment of the patient in an altered state of consciousness has presented one of the greatest challenges to rehabilitation clinicians. Many professionals have not had the clinical training to perform evaluations or treatment with those patients who are not responsive or are in altered states (i.e., disoriented or not responsive to people, place, or time). However, the diagnostic and treatment decisions during this phase of recovery may affect the final outcome of the survivor's life. The decision of whether a person is brain dead, in a coma, in a vegetative state, an emerging state, or some other altered state of consciousness affects the delivery or use of services available to that person.

In the United States, clinical and financial treatment decisions rest almost exclusively on the aforementioned diagnostic decisions. In most countries, the care and treatment of the comatose or vegetative patient is usually handled either in the acute care hospital, a nursing facility, or the home of the survivor. The distinction is that the use of resources does not appear to be the same across societies. Regardless of the political structure of the specific country's healthcare system, the balance between treatment benefits and costs remains critical.

The research on these issues over the last ten years has shown that it is almost impossible to predict outcome based upon identification of predictive factors after admission of a comatose patient. The treatment team is left with several questions:

1. What is the chance of recovery?
2. What is the appropriate treatment?

3.   When should treatment be stopped?
4.   What type of outcome can be expected after prolonged coma?
5.   What are the realistic goals of treatment?

This chapter will examine methods of intervention with comatose patients. In order to provide a background, we will first discuss the pathophysiological mechanisms underlying the process of coma. Then, we will outline outcomes and prognosis, predictors of outcome, behavioral manifestations of altered consciousness, assessment procedures, and bio-behavioral treatments. In conclusion, research that evaluates the effectiveness of treatment methodologies is examined in an attempt to evaluate the aforementioned questions.

PATHOPHYSIOLOGICAL MECHANISMS OF TRAUMATIC COMA

The pathological mechanisms of traumatic coma may be more reliably characterized as resulting from either diffuse damage to large areas of the brain or severe focal damage to a localized area of the brain or from both mechanisms. While diffuse injuries involve large amounts of neuronal tissue, focal injuries are restricted to circumscribed areas of the brain. Among focal injuries, primary brainstem lesions account for a large proportion of comatose patients (McLellan, 1990; Adams & Victor, 1993). These types of lesions can result in herniation and compression of the brainstem reticular activating system, as well as thalamic involvement. Case studies (e.g., Karen Ann Quinlan) have identified lesions of the thalamus as important in regulating the level of arousal (Kinney et al., 1994). These pathological mechanisms are known as *primary* mechanisms of damage. Both types of injury can contribute to *secondary* mechanisms of damage such as cerebral edema or the release of free radicals. Secondary mechanisms of damage can also include neurotoxic events such as glutamate abnormalities in anoxic brain injury (Carlson, 1994).

Diffuse Brain Injury

Diffuse axonal injury (DAI) has been described as the most common cause of persisting coma. DAI represents "widespread damage to axons in the cerebral hemispheres, cerebellum, and brainstem" (McLellan, 1990; Adams & Victor, 1993). In histological specimens, DAI is visible microscopically in the form of axonal bulbs, which are evident when cytoplasmic material collects at the ends of severed axons. Demyelinization of the Wallerian type occurs in these areas, as well as microglial scarring. DAI has been described as occurring throughout the brain parenchyma; however, it is most often observed in the areas of the corpus callosum and rostral brainstem. Three levels or grades of DAI have been identified: (1) microscopic evidence of DAI with no focal lesions, (2) microscopic evidence of DAI with focal lesions in the corpus callosum, and (3) microscopic evidence of DAI with focal lesions in the corpus callosum and the brainstem. Not surprisingly, higher mortality rates have been found to be related to the severity of DAI (McClellan, 1990).

Other causes of diffuse brain damage include hypoxic injury and brain edema. Hypoxia is the result of an interruption in the flow of oxygen to the brain (Victor & Adams, 1993). Brain edema can be caused by a number of processes (e.g., vascular disorders and trauma). Although edema accompanies and is often a result of primary injury, a large percentage of cases in which there is brain swelling occur with an absence of any apparent cause (McLellan, 1990). Brain edema can cause damage to the cortex through swelling of the ventricles, which forces brain matter to compress against the skull. A typical cause of coma results when the brainstem is forced against the foramen magnum, thus disrupting the activity of the reticular activating system.

Neurological and Clinical Manifestations of Coma

Over the past decade, a general consensus has been reached that depth of coma exists along a continuum. At the deepest level, corneal, pupillary, pharyngeal, and plantar reflexes are absent (Adams & Victor, 1993; Cohen, 1993). At a "lighter" level, plantar and brainstem reflexes and ocular movements may remain intact. Decerebrate posturing (e.g., arched back, increased tone in the antigravity muscles) might be exhibited in the deepest coma, whereas in less deep levels of coma, there may be evidence of resistance to passive flexion of the neck. Vocalization does not occur in deep coma, although it may occur in a lighter state.

The level of coma is not necessarily fixed. Approximately 2–4 weeks post-injury, a patient's status may change (Bricolo, Turazzi, & Feriotti, 1980; Plum & Posner, 1982; Sandel & Ellis, 1990; Wilson, Powell, Elliott, & Thwaites, 1991). Patients either begin to become responsive (i.e., begin to emerge from coma) or transition into a vegetative state. Death may occur in some cases (Jennett & Plum, 1972).

Coma may not occur immediately following traumatic injury. In some instances, the injured patient may show signs of ongoing deterioration consequent to progressive intracranial pathology (Stein & Schraeder, 1990). On other occasions, patients may appear aroused and awake and then lapse into coma due to the secondary complications (e.g., DAI, hematomas) (Lobato et al., 1991).

BEHAVIORAL MANIFESTATIONS OF ALTERED CONSCIOUSNESS

The behavioral features of an altered state have been clearly described for years. This section will describe the behavioral characteristics of altered states, as well as the behavioral features of the more severe conditions.

States of Consciousness

According to Plum and Posner (1982), consciousness is "the state of awareness of the self and the environment." Consciousness is defined by two components: content and arousal. The content of conscious behavior is created by cognitive and affective mental functions. For example, reading involves cognitive functions such as language, processing, comprehension, and memory. These functions may also involve affective states such as enjoyment or pleasure. Arousal represents an appearance of wakefulness, which is a primitive function related to the functioning of the reticular activating system (RAS). The level of an individual's arousal "can be defined operationally by the intensity of stimulation required to elicit a response from the patient" (Weintraub & Mesulam, 1985).

These two functions, content and arousal, are separate; a patient may be aroused, yet may not be able to perform cognitively (Plum & Posner, 1982). Characteristics of comatose patients include: (1) physiological unresponsiveness to the environment (i.e., arousal and awareness are absent), (2) immobility, and (3) a lack of the ability to open their eyes (Jennett & Plum, 1972; Berral, 1990; Multi-Society Task Force on PVS, 1994; American Congress of Rehabilitation Medicine, 1995). Consciousness exists along a continuum in which patients may display a variety of levels of arousal and behavior. The following will illustrate several of the common states of consciousness that can be observed in a clinical setting.

Inattention, Confusion, and Clouding of Consciousness

Inattention, confusion, and clouding of consciousness represent conditions in which "the patient does not take into account all elements of his environment" (Adams & Victor, 1993). In these conditions, the patient demonstrates an element of imperceptiveness, distractibility, or sensorial clouding. These patients have difficulty attending to stimuli and are often unable to carry out simple commands. In addition, memory of events that occur during a confused state is typically impaired. The defective process in their memory is in encoding or registration, not in their retention (Ibid.). These patients also appear to be drowsy, especially in the daytime, while at night they may appear hyperactive (Plum & Posner, 1982). In addition, they may be disoriented to time and place.

Stupor

Stupor represents another more severe degree of impaired consciousness in the continuum. A stuporous patient is in a state of "deep sleep" or behavioral unresponsiveness and can be aroused only by vigorous and repeated stimuli (Ibid.). When stimulated, these patients do not appear to be conscious and may react to a stimulus in a delayed or slowed manner. However, once the stimulus is removed, the patient returns to the previous baseline functioning level (Adams & Victor, 1993; Plum & Posner, 1982).

Delirium

The *Diagnostic and Statistical Manual of Mental Disorders* (DSM-IV) characterizes delirium as "a disturbance of consciousness and a change in cognition that develop over a short period of time" (DSM IV, 1994). The patient may also demonstrate signs of autonomic hyperactivity, including trembling and convulsions (Plum & Posner, 1982; Adams & Victor, 1993). Due to the patient's inability to accurately perceive his/her environment, the patient frequently appears to be in a "dreamlike" state in which he/she is unreachable by the examiner or environment. The delirious state typically has a rapid onset and usually lasts less than seven days (Plum & Posner, 1982).

There is no consistent and distinct pathology that represents delirium; however, alterations in the temporal lobes possibly give rise to the complex hallucinations found in delirium. Other areas potentially responsible for states of delirium include the subthalamic nuclei and midbrain (Adams & Victor, 1993). Delirium is most evident in toxic and metabolic disorders such as (1) atropine poisoning, (2) alcohol or barbiturate withdrawal, (3) acute porphyria, (4) uremia, (5) acute hepatic failure, (6) encephalitis, and (7) the collagen vascular diseases (Plum & Posner, 1982). From a clinical standpoint, an accurate diagnosis is crucial due to the potential reversibility of many toxic and metabolic etiologies (Adams & Victor, 1993).

Obtundation

Obtundation represents a state of mental blunting in which the patient demonstrates a mild to moderate reduction in alertness. This situation is accompanied by slowed responses to environmental stimulation, increase in drowsiness and sleep, and an apparent reduction of interest in the environment (Plum & Posner, 1982).

Akinetic Mutism

Akinetic mutism, also known as coma vigil, represents a state in which the patient retains some level of altered consciousness but is unable to perform voluntary movements of the trunk and limbs despite intact sensory and motor systems (Adams & Victor, 1993; Multi-Society Task Force on PVS, 1994). The condition is characterized by severely diminished neurologic drive, while movement and speech are markedly deficient. However, meaningful responses can be elicited inconsistently after sensory or pharmacologic stimulation (American Congress of Rehabilitation Medicine, 1995). Lesions that sever the cortex from the reticular activating system (RAS) appear to be responsible for this condition. These lesions are typically found in the posterior diencephalon and the midbrain, but bilateral lesions of the cingulate gyri or frontal lobes may also be responsible for this condition (Pryse-Phillips & Murray, 1982; Adams & Victor, 1993).

Locked-In Syndrome

In contrast to akinetic mutism, patients in the locked-in syndrome maintain an unimpaired awareness of both internal and external stimuli, despite motor paralysis of all four extremities and, usually, muscles innervated by the cranial nerves (Ibid.). In this condition, corticospinal and corticobulbar motor de-efferentation occurs with a lesion in the ventral portion of the basis pontis (American Congress of Rehabilitation Medicine, 1995; Adams & Victor, 1993; Toly, personal communication, 1995). These patients are unable to communicate by words or through body movement but can respond to stimuli with either vertical eye movements or through eye blinks. The locked-in syndrome is typically a result of a vascular disease; however, severe peripheral neuropathies, myasthenia gravis, or poliomyelitis may be responsible for a similar appearing condition (Plum & Posner, 1982; Pryse-Phillips & Murray, 1982). Despite the severity of this condition, some patients recover (Ibid.).

Dementia

Dementia is "characterized by the development of multiple cognitive deficits (including memory impairment) that are due to the direct physiological effects of a general medical condition, to the persisting effects of a substance, or to multiple etiologies (e.g., the combined effects of cerebrovascular disease and Alzheimer's disease)" (DSM-IV, 1994, p. 133). Unlike the other conditions that have been previously mentioned, dementia does not result in a reduction in consciousness. However, because of the cognitive changes associated with dementia, these syndromes must be differentially ruled out when working with confused, inattentive, or unresponsive patients.

Coma

Coma is defined by the patient's inability to be aroused (with the absence of sleep-wake cycles on an electroencephalogram) and the inability to interact with the environment (i.e., open the eyes, follow commands, or communicate) (American Congress of Rehabilitation Medicine, 1995; Plum & Posner, 1982; Sazbon & Groswasser, 1991). It is characterized by an inability to sense or respond to external stimuli and internal needs. Among the many causes of coma, traumatic brain injury, stroke, toxic/metabolic causes, and infectious processes account for the vast majority of cases (Adams & Victor, 1993; The Multi-Society Task Force for PVS, 1994).

Vegetative State

The Multi-Society Task Force on PVS (1994, p. 1499) defines vegetative state as a "clinical condition of complete unawareness of the self and the environment, accompanied by sleep-wake cycles, with either complete or partial presentation of hypothalamic and brainstem autonomic functions." The term "vegetative state" has been used because of the continuance of the vegetative functions (sleep-wake cycles, autonomic control, and ventilation) coupled with the absence of awareness (cognitive and emotional functioning) (Jennett & Plum, 1972; Kinney & Samuels, 1994). The length of time in the vegetative condition has been considered a good prognostic indicator.

The persistence of this syndrome beyond 12 months for post-traumatic patients, three months for non-traumatic patients, and several months for metabolic or congenital malformations is indicative of a poor prognosis for emergence (The Multi-Society Task Force on PVS, 1994; Sazbon & Groswasser, 1991). These findings hold for both children and adults. However, several authors have described cases in which patients emerge from persistent vegetative state with varied levels of recovery, including several patients who achieved functional independence (Sazbon, Zagreba, Ronen, Solzi, & Costeff, 1993; Andrew, 1993).

The American Congress of Rehabilitation Medicine (1995) differs from the Multi-Society Task Force on PVS (1994) on the nomenclature used when describing vegetative states. The American Congress of Rehabilitation Medicine (1995) has taken the position that the terms "persistent" or "permanent," used to describe a vegetative state, should be avoided because they imply that the condition is absolutely refractory to rehabilitation treatment. The designation of PVS implies that there is a 100% certainty that the person beyond a certain time period in a vegetative state, will not recover, yet research supports the opposite position (American Congress of Rehabilitation Medicine, 1995; Sazbon, Zagreba, Ronen, Solzi, & Costeff, 1993; Andrew, 1993). The American Congress of Rehabilitation Medicine (1995) instead supports the use of the term "vegetative state" because of the potential for recovery of these patients.

Brain Death

Brain death is an irreversible condition in which brain function has ceased but in which pulmonary and cardiac functions can be artificially maintained (Adams & Victor, 1993). The hallmark findings in brain death are the lack of cerebral and brainstem activity, and the irreversibility of the condition (Walker, 1985; Adams & Victor, 1993). Clinical findings such as spontaneous movements and responses to external stimulation support the diagnosis. Spontaneous eye movements, pupillary changes (including dilation and fixed position), paralysis of bulbar musculature, absence of decerebrate responses to noxious stimuli, and cessation of spontaneous respiration are used to determine brainstem death (Adams & Victor, 1993). Electroencephalogram, cerebral blood flow, and metabolic criteria have also been described for diagnosing brain death (Walker, 1985). In an effort to provide standard diagnostic criteria, the Multi-Society Task Force on PVS (1994) has identified the following indicators of brain death: (1) absence of self-awareness, (2) absence of sleep-wake cycles, (3) no motor function or only reflex spinal movements, (4) no suffering, (5) absence of respiratory function, (6) electrocerebral silence, (7) absence of cerebral metabolism, and (8) no chance of recovery.

PREDICTORS OF OUTCOME

Age and Prognosis

The age of the individual has been found to be correlated to outcome after traumatic brain injury. Most reports indicate younger patients generally have a better prognosis, whereas older patients tend to have lower survival rates (Katz & Alexander, 1994; Braakman et al., 1988; Bricolo et al., 1980; Jennett et al., 1976; Overgaard et al., 1973). According to Becker et al. (1977), low survival rates in older patients result in part from systemic complications. However, the relationship between age and outcome has not been uniformly confirmed (Bates et al., 1977; Levy et al., 1985). Katz and Alexander (1994) found interactions between age and outcome at 6 and 12 months and suggested that the effects of age are complex and probably not linear. The effects of age on recovery were most evident in patients with severe injuries and for those who were above age 40 (Katz & Alexander, 1994).

Depth and Duration of Coma

Studies have indicated that longer coma duration correlates with poorer outcomes (Jennett et al., 1976; Anzell & Keenan, 1989; Carlson, von Essen, & Longren, 1968; Levy et al., 1985). Sazbon and Groswasser (1991b) reported that patients who experienced the greatest functional recovery emerged from coma by the second month post-injury. Once the patient was awake, level of awareness (i.e., cognition of self and environment) suggested better outcome. In addition, the time interval between injury and the ability to perform simple commands appeared to be related to outcome (Bricolo et al., 1980; Giacino, 1991). Markers of a favorable outcome after injury include verbal responsivity, eye opening, and withdrawal to pain (Bates et al., 1977; Levy et al., 1985).

Neuro-Ophthalmologic Signs

The absence of pupillary and/or oculocephalogyric responses suggests poor outcome (Bates et al., 1977; Becker et al., 1977; Braakman et al., 1988; Jennett, Teasdale, & Braakman, 1976; Levy et al., 1985; Facco et al., 1986; Sandel & Labi, 1990), whereas eye opening has been found to be an indicator of favorable outcome (Bates et al., 1977; Levy et al., 1985). Levy et al. (1985) determined, through a multivariate analysis, that the variable most predictive of outcome was pupillary light reflex assessed during the initial neurological evaluation. Spontaneous eye movements, eye opening, and oculocephalogyric responses were also found to be strong predictors of outcome, but not to the same degree as pupillary light response (Levy et al., 1985).

Motor Signs

Motor abnormalities, such as flexor and extensor posturing or the absence of response, also suggest poor outcomes (Bates et al., 1977). Lack of motor responses three days post-injury were identified as powerful predictors of a poor outcome. In contrast, the ability to withdraw from pain within the first 24 hours was a positive sign (Levy et al., 1985). Overgaard et al. (1973) stated that a normal motor response is strongly predictive of a positive outcome, especially in a younger patient. Motor-evoked potentials (MEPs), which provide information on upper motor neuron functioning, have also been investigated, and results demonstrated good prognostic value during the acute stages of coma (Facco et al., 1991).

Anatomic Variables

Poor prognosis has been associated with loss in forebrain function (Bates et al., 1977), specific focal pathology such as pressure from contusions (Katz, 1991), and indication of midline shift (Lobato et al., 1991). Katz (1992) has reported that the effects of focal lesions probably evolve faster and plateau earlier than those of diffuse lesions. In addition, there is consistent evidence of poorer outcome for anoxic patients (Groswasser, Cohen, & Costeff, 1989; Katz, 1992; Goldberg, in press). However, Lobato et al. (1991) reported that this effect may be specific only when the anoxia is causative in the coma, not merely when it is present post-injury.

OUTCOME AND PROGNOSIS

Because coma occurs in patients with a complex set of structural and physiological disruptions, outcome is difficult to predict (Katz, 1992). Some types of coma have a relatively predictable course of recovery (e.g., hypoxia-induced coma), whereas others have a highly unpredictable course (e.g., traumatically induced coma) because of multiple variables in an individual patient.

Vegetative State

A high rate of poor outcome has been reported in comatose patients, with death occurring in approximately 50% of cases (Bates et al., 1977; Cullen, 1977; Levin et al., 1991; Levy et al., 1985). Emergence from coma does not necessarily represent or indicate a complete recovery of functioning. On the contrary, such patients may remain relatively unable to interact with their environment. This "vegetative" condition can be long-term and is characterized by eye opening and sleep-wake cycles but, otherwise, is similar to behaviors that occur in coma (Multi-Society Task Force, 1994). According to Jennett and Plum (1972, p. 736), "The essential component of this syndrome is the absence of any adaptive response to the external environment and the absence of any evidence of a functioning mind which is either receiving or projecting information in a patient who has long periods of wakefulness." This syndrome has been identified as a "vegetative state" by Jennett and Plum (1972), as "prolonged coma" by Sazbon (1985), and as "post-comatose unawareness" by Sazbon and Groswasser (1991b). The persistence of this syndrome beyond six months has been said to indicate poor prognosis for emergence (Sazbon & Groswasser, 1991b). Andrews (1993) reported that 26% of a sample of severely brain-injured patients regained some level of awareness after four months in a "vegetative state" (Andrews, 1993).

Bricolo et al. (1980) and Berral (1990) have argued that the term "persistent vegetative state" (PVS) should only be used if this syndrome persists for one year post-injury. It should be noted that the terminology for describing patients who have emerged from coma but who have not regained any functional abilities has been called into question (American Congress of Rehabilitation Medicine, 1995; Multi-Society Task Force on PVS, 1994).

The Glasgow Outcome Scale (GOS) has been used to differentiate different outcomes (Jennett et al., 1976). "Good" recovery (i.e., outcome that does not include death, PVS, or severe disability) occurs fairy infrequently in long-term vegetative patients. At one year post-injury, Braakman, Jennett, and Minderhoud (1988) reported good recovery in only 10% of patients, and Bricolo et al. (1980) reported that just over 13% of patients demonstrated a good recovery. By contrast, a better rate of recovery at a three-year follow-up was reported by Levin et al. (1991). They reported that 58% showed an improvement in level of consciousness in contrast to 42% who remained vegetative or died. Presence of bilateral neuro-ophthalmologic abnormalities characterized patients who remained vegetative and those who died, as did the type of intracranial injury, the presence of shock, and a shift in midline brain structures.

Studies have shown that approximately 50% of patients emerge from a vegetative state within 3 years post-injury (Groswasser & Sazbon, 1990; Levin et al., 1991; Sazbon & Groswasser, 1991c), with most emerging within the first 6 months (Bricolo et al., 1980; Carlson, von Essen, & Lofgren, 1968; Jennett, Teasdale, Braakman, Minderhoud, & Knill-Jones, 1976; Levy et al., 1985). Bricolo et al. (1980) contend that 6 months is an important marker for neurological as well as general medical stabilization. This contention is based on the number of patient deaths that occur within this 6-month time frame. It is exceptional to find reports of patients who emerge from coma after 6 months, although such reports exist (Arts, Van Dongen, Van Hof-Van Duin, & Lammens, 1985).

In Sazbon and Groswasser's (1991a) study of 62 non-emergent patients, all died within 10 years post-injury. After one year, 69% of patients had died and 86% had died within 2 years. The most frequently cited cause of death was sepsis of pulmonary or urinary origin. This was closely followed by death due to generalized systemic failure. Whyte (1994) argues that aggressive medical management of non-emergent patients can increase life span and quality of life (Whyte, 1994).

One of the issues being debated in the study of rehabilitation and the prediction of outcome is the criteria used to define outcome. As noted, a frequently used measure of outcome is the Glasgow Outcome Scale (GOS) (Jennett & Bond, 1975). The GOS identifies five categories of recovery: death, persistent vegetative state, severe disability (conscious but disabled), moderate disability (disabled but independent), and good recovery. However, the GOS has been criticized for its inability to reflect more subtle changes in recovery (Hall et al., 1985). Neuropsychological assessment has been used in evaluating and tracking rehabilitation outcomes following severe brain injury, both in comatose patients as well as with those in altered states of consciousness. In general, neuropsychological assessment can provide a quantitative measure of a wide variety of cognitive, motor, and psychological domains. Dikmen et al. (1990) incorporated various neuropsychological measures to demonstrate more subtle recovery of severely brain- injured individuals over 1-, 12- and 24-month intervals. Functional measures such as psychosocial and vocational variables have also been used as measures of recovery (Dacey et al., 1991).

The debate surrounding outcome measures is confounded by the length of time post-injury at which the different measures are assessed. For example, neuropsychological evaluations, psychosocial scales, and coma emerging scales make use of information that is available following emergence and some return of cognitive function. These measures may have power for predicting future outcome, but they are usually not fully applied in an acute hospital setting (Katz, 1995).

ASSESSMENT PROCEDURES

The field of treatment of the comatose and vegetative patient remains controversial. Any treatment technique or practice must be placed in the context of the overall rehabilitation treatment program for this type of patient. Interventions have been framed around two aspects—assessment and treatment. The efficacy of different sensory stimulation/

regulation or enrichment programs has been a continuing question. Measures have been developed in an attempt to assess a patient on admission, follow-up, and discharge.

O'Dell and Riggs (1995) did a meta-analysis of the Behaviorally Based Assessment Instruments (BBAI) most often used for the evaluation of the minimally responsive patient. The authors reported that the use of BBAIs provided the following: (1) a "structured approach by which neurologic and cognitive recovery can be monitored and documented," (2) identification of "sensory, physical, and cognitive strengths and weaknesses," (3) a method for interdisciplinary communication, and (4) empirically reliable and valid measures of recovery (O'Dell & Riggs, in press). The four scales that O'Dell and Riggs analyzed were the (1) Sensory Stimulation Assessment Measure (Rader & Ellis, 1989), (2) Western Neuro Sensory Stimulation Profile (Ansell & Keenan, 1989), (3) the Coma / Near Coma Scale (Rappaport, Dougherty, & Kelting, 1992), and (4) Coma Recovery Scale (Giacino et al., 1991).

As outlined by O'Dell and Riggs (in press), several stimulation assessment protocols are currently being used clinically. The first approach to be described is the Sensory Stimulation Assessment Measure (SSAM) (Rader & Ellis, 1989). The SSAM uses a standard stimulation protocol, with a stimulator and rater. Stimulation is applied to all five sensory modalities by the stimulator. The rater scores the response of the patient on a 6-point scale ranging from no response to appropriate communicative responses (e.g., clear, intelligible answers) (Rader & Ellis, 1989). Rader & Ellis (1989) describe the following clinical uses of the measure: (1) to establish a pretreatment behavioral baseline; (2) to plan patient-specific treatment, including modality-specific pathways for early rehabilitation efforts; (3) to monitor the patient's progress; (4) to monitor the effectiveness of the patient's interventions (e.g., coma stimulation, medications, therapists); (5) to describe initial indications of neuropsychological deficits; and (6) to provide objective data to family members and treatment team members about progress to stimulate ideas for future treatment planning. Finally, Rader and Ellis (1989) also believe that family members should be trained to use the SSAM. Helwick (1994) agrees with the use of family members in a coma stimulation, believing that familiarity produces a higher likelihood of response (Helwick, 1994).

Another sensory stimulation assessment procedure is the Western Neuro Sensory Stimulation Profile (WNSSP) (Ansell & Keenan, 1989). The scale was developed to monitor the progress of patients who were slow to emerge from coma. The WNSSP covers auditory, tactile, and olfactory senses, as well as arousal, attention, and expressive language skills. The WNSSP takes about 20 to 40 minutes to administer and has been used to measure improvement across the time of rehabilitation treatment (Ansell & Keenan, 1989).

The Coma/Near Coma scale (CNS) (Rappaport, Dougherty, and Kelting, 1992) was designed to measure both the level of coma and the progress of the emerging patient. This scale consists of five severity levels, ranging from "No Coma" to "Extreme Coma" based on patients' responses to 11 sensory and physiological measures (Rappaport, Dougherty, & Kelting, 1992).

The Coma Recovery Scale (CRS) (Giacino et al., 1991) assesses seven domains, including arousal and attention, auditory response, visual response, motor response or motor skills, communication, and initiative. Each domain reflects a continuum from reflexive to spontaneous actions (Giacino et al., 1991). O'Dell (in press) reported that the Coma Recovery Scale was "an effective tool for predicting outcome in severely brain-injured patients." The Coma Recovery Scale has been used to measure depth of unresponsive-ness, as well as outcome.

In a comparative evaluation of three assessment scales (CNS, CRS, WNSSP), O'Dell found that the CNS and the CRS appeared to have a greater clinical usefulness. The study was confounded by a small sample size and needs to be replicated with a larger sample to include the SSAM (O'Dell, in press).

BIO-BEHAVIORAL TREATMENT OF MINIMALLY RESPONSIVE PATIENTS

The term bio-behavioral treatment is currently being used to describe the behavioral interventions used for the treatment of this condition. Neuropharmacological, medical, or surgical interventions have been thoroughly described elsewhere and will not be presented here (O'Dell, 1995; Andrews, 1990).

Historical Perspective

The earliest evidence of human interest in the treating of effects of post-traumatic brain injury were found in hieroglyphics in an Egyptian papyrus somewhere between 2500 and 300 B.C. (Breasted, 1930). This ancient papyrus includes the first reference to the word "brain" and describe the observation, understanding, and treatment of 48 cases that suffered traumatic injuries to the head and neck (Walsh, 1987). The present focus of this chapter, the arousal of comatose and vegetative patients, is, however, a relatively recent phenomenon. The primary reason for this is the recent advances in medical procedures and heroic measures that created a new population of survivors, comatose, and vegetative patients (Ellis & Rader, 1990). The final section will discuss some recently developed intervention techniques used with comatose patients. In a forthcoming book on rehabilitation after traumatic brain injury (Horn & Zasler, in press), O'Dell and Riggs provide a thorough review of the comprehensive rehabilitation medical management of the minimally responsive patient.

Behavioral Treatments of "Coma"

Treatment of the comatose patient includes providing stimulation through the usual and customary rehabilitation medical treatments. These would include (1) nursing, (2) physical therapy (PT), (3) occupational therapy (OT), and (4) other treatments. In some instances, informal stimulation from the environment is supplemented by carefully structured presentation of materials to the senses with the purpose of arousing the patient.

At present, there is no single "gold standard" for treatment of post-traumatic brain-injured comatose patients (Helwick, 1994; Pierce et al., 1990). Several treatment approaches are available, which are called "environmental" enrichment (LeWinn & Dimancescu, 1986), "sensory stimulation" (Aldridge, 1991; Rader, Alston, & Ellis, 1989; Hall, MacDonald, & Young, 1992; Johnson, 1987; Kater, 1989; Ellis & Rader, 1990; Mitchell, Bradley, Welsh, & Britton, 1990; Giacino et al., 1991; Helwick, 1994), and "sensory regulation" (Wood, 1991; Wood, Winkowski, Miller, Tierney, & Goldman, 1992). These techniques are essentially the same even though each technique appears to represent slight variations in approach and measurement of response.

Environmental Enrichment

Proponents of environmental enrichment (e.g., LeWinn & Dimancescu, 1986) hold that while in a coma or vegetative state, patients are in a state of sensory deprivation. As a result, the traditional early intensive provision of stimuli by emergency medical teams and subsequent routine hospital care are insufficient to adequately counter this deprivation. This deprivation, in turn, prevents the fullest recovery. These clinicians support a program of enhanced stimulation via enriched surroundings and input. La Puma, Schiedermayer, Gulyas, and Stiegler (1988) urge physicians to communicate verbally while treating and monitoring patients. Initial outcomes reported were favorable but not clearly documented by research protocols. Concerns remain about the effectiveness of sensory stimulation with comatose patients and the methods used to achieve it (Gianutsos, 1990). These methods appear to be focused on continuous stimulation.

Sensory Stimulation

The literature contains anecdotal reports documenting the spontaneous and sudden arousal of patients, who have been comatose for significant time periods, using some form of sensory stimulation or nontraditional methods (i.e., ritualized healing, prayer sessions, burning of incense). In the 1970s, case-study presentations regarding sensory stimulation of chronically ill patients began to appear in the popular press and medical literature as the medical community began to address the treatment of these patients (Ellis & Rader, 1990). LeWinn and Dimancescu (1978) were the first to publish results of their approach to environmental enrichment and/or sensory stimulation. Their dramatic results were viewed quite skeptically at the time. However, their work spawned a new era of research and exploration into this field of rehabilitation.

The results of these sensory stimulation techniques on patient outcomes still remains controversial as several studies have demonstrated the benefits of stimulation while others did not (Pierce, 1990; Rader, Alston, & Ellis, 1989; Hall, MacDonald, & Young, 1992). O'Dell (in press) noted that sensory stimulation procedures appear to have a significant temporal affect on vital signs and electrophysiological responses; however, there was no evidence of alteration of the course of recovery.

High-intensity sensory stimulation (Mitchell et al., 1990) was developed out of experimental and developmental psychology, which hold that stimulation from the environment is essential for the maintenance of arousal, decreased sensory deprivation, and increased synaptic growth. The goal of sensory stimulation is two-fold—to achieve arousal and to increase the patient's level of awareness (Ellis & Rader, 1990). This treatment approach adheres to the notion that sufficient input to cortical networks is necessary for maintaining optimal potential for awareness.

The hallmark of the sensory stimulation programs is the provision of an intensive and prolonged daily regimen of multisensory stimulation, preferably from familiar sources. According to Ellis & Rader (1990), stimulation should occur across all five sensory systems (i.e., visual, auditory, tactile, gustatory, and olfactory). In addition, several authors also have noted attempts to stimulate the vestibular or kinesthetic system (Helwick, 1994; Ellis & Rader, 1990).

Visual stimulation is performed when the patient is able to open his/her eyes spontaneously. Typically, visual tracking, as well as attention, is measured (Helwick, 1994; Rader & Ellis, 1989). Auditory stimulation involves attention to a sound or voice; of particular use is a family member's voice because of its familiarity to the patient (Ibid.). Tactile stimulation is the most primitive sensation (afferent fibers are myelinated early in development) and is used to elicit awareness of sensation. Clinician's touch, heat, and cold packs have been used to encourage a response (Ibid.). In gustatory stimulation, the clinician is attempting to stimulate lip smacking or salivation (Ibid.). The olfactory system is typically associated with the limbic and emotional systems. Olfactory stimulation may evoke emotions and memories (Ibid.). Finally, kinesthetic stimulation, which is designed to stimulate proprioception, can be achieved through various range of motion exercises (Helwick, 1994).

The stimulation treatment protocol can be performed by an interdisciplinary team including nurses, respiratory therapists, cognitive specialists, speech pathologists, physical therapists, and neuropsychologists (Ellis & Rader, 1990; Giacino et al., 1992; Helwick, 1994). When patient improvement is noted, stimuli of increased complexity and sophistication are substituted (Pierce et al., 1990), and more interdisciplinary team members can be included (Ellis & Rader, 1990). Several studies have reported positive results (Kater, 1989; Hall et al., 1992; Mitchel et al., 1990; Wilson et al., 1991). It has been suggested that vegetative patients may demonstrate a physiologic response to stimulation that indicates brainstem functioning even when the cortex is severely damaged (Davis, 1979). However, Pierce et al. (1990) found only a marginal trend towards greater impairment in patients who receive a program of coma arousal.

Sensory Regulation

A sensory regulation approach to stimulation has been reported by Wood (1991) based on an information-processing model that addresses the brain's ability to take in and process information in a meaningful manner. Wood et al. (1992) advocated structuring and limiting input while maintaining the salience of new information. Patients who have been in a vegetative state for approximately two months were studied, and positive results were reported (Wood et al., 1992).

Treatment Outcomes

Ellis et al. (1995) described a study in which a group of 59 patients were studied during their course of intensive rehabilitation. During the treatment period, approximately one-half (51%) of the patients emerged (defined as Rancho level IV or better), and 49% remained in the non-emerged (Rancho level III or less) group. The researchers noted that length of acute hospitalization, not severity of injury, was a significant predictor of whether or not the patient would improve during rehabilitation. At discharge from inpatient rehabilitation services, approximately 50% of the emerged patients were discharged to home, while only 6% of the non-emerged group went home. Two-year follow-up data indicated significantly higher levels of employability and personal independence in the group that had emerged during their rehabilitation stay. Two years following discharge, almost half of the non-emerged group were still considered totally dependent for self care (Ellis et al., 1995)

Intensity of treatment was measured in another study by Ellis et al. (1995). In this study, patients who were at Rancho level II or III during the first two months of rehabilitation were compared based on eventual emergence or non-emergence from coma. It was concluded that the emerged group retained the same intensity of treatment over two months, while the non-emerged group's level of treatment decreased significantly during the second month (Ellis et al., 1995). Both studies highlighted the important contributions of intensive medical rehabilitation services to eventuate levels of independent functioning free of secondary complications.

CONCLUSIONS

Sandel, Horn, and Bontke (1993) addressed the issues of whether sensory assessment, sensory stimulation, and/or coma management as part of brain injury rehabilitation programs should be supported by the rehabilitation community. A comprehensive, medically managed system of rehabilitation care was identified as critical. As Horn (1991) reported, "...to the newly sentient individuals, who awake in a nursing home contorted, incontinent, and in pain, and to their families," how they have been medically managed means a great deal.

Sandel (1991) reported her position in favor of the use of sensory stimulation. She reported that treatment considerations should include (1) the responsiveness of the individual, (2) the reaction of the family, and (3) the integration of the concepts of an enriched environment into the treatment regimen. Sandel discussed the indicators of a specific program: (1) the population served, type of injury, mechanisms of injury, and age; (2) time from trauma to the initiation of treatment; (3) protocols of treatment; (4) outcome and assessment measures; and (5) cost.

Bontke (1991) summarized her position by stating, "Sensory stimulation has a place in the overall management of the comatose patient. Nevertheless, it needs to be cost-contained, time limited, provided in the most humane way, and used primarily for the purpose of observation."

The controversy over sensory stimulation continues; however, the proper medical/ rehabilitation management of the comatose /vegetative patient is critical for the possible survival of the individual, the maximal response to treatment, and the reduction of the ultimate cost to society.

REFERENCES

Adams, R.D., & Victor, M. (1993). *Principles of neurology* (5th ed.). New York: McGraw-Hill.

Aldridge, D. (1991). Creativity and consciousness: Music therapy in intensive care. *The Arts in Psychotherapy, 18,* 359–362.

American Congress of Rehabilitation Medicine. (1995). Recommendations for use of uniform nomenclature pertinent to patients with severe alterations in consciousness. *Archives of Physical Medicine and Rehabilitation, 76,* 205–209.

Andrews, K. (1990). Medical management. In M. E. Sandel & D. W. Ellis (Eds.), *The coma-emerging patient* (pp. 389–409). Philadelphia: Hanley & Belfus, Inc.

———. (1993) Recovery of patients after four months or more in the persistent vegetative state. *British Medical Journal, 306,* 1597–1599.

Ansell, B.J., & Keenan, J.E. (1989). The western neurosensory stimulation profile: A tool for assessing slow-to-recover head-injured patients. *Archives of Physical Medicine and Rehabilitation, 70,* 104–108.

Arts, W., van Dongen, H., van Hof-van Duin, J., & Lammens, E. (1985). Unexpected improvement after prolonged post-traumatic vegetative state. *Journal of Neurology, Neurosurgery, and Psychiatry, 48,* 1300–1303.

Bates, D., Caronna, J.J., Cartlidge, N.E.F., Knill-Jones, R.P., Levy, D.E., Shaw, D.A., & Plum, F. (1977). A prospective study of nontraumatic coma: Methods and results in 310 patients. *Annals of Neurology, 2,* 211–220.

Becker, D.P., Miller, D., Ward, D., Greenberg, R.P., Young, H.F., & Sakalas, R. (1977). The outcome from severe head injury with early diagnosis and intensive management. *Journal of Neurosurgery, 47,* 491–502.

Berrol, S. (1986a). Considerations for the management of persistent vegetative state. *Archives of Physical Medicine and Rehabilitation, 67,* 283–285.

————. (1986b). Evolution and the persistent vegetative state. *Journal of Head Trauma Rehabilitation, 1,* 7–13.

————. (1990). Persistent vegetative state. *Physical Medicine and Rehabilitation: State of the Art Review, 4,* 559–567.

Bontke, C.F., Baize, C.M., & Boske, C. (1992). Coma management and sensory stimulation. *Physical Medicine and Rehabilitation: Clinical, 3,* 259–272.

Braakman, R., Habberno, J.F., & Helpke, H.J. (1986). Prognosis and prediction of outcome in comatose head-injured patients. *Acta Neurochir, 36* (Suppl.), 112–117.

Braakman, R., Jennett, W.B., & Minderhoud, J.M. (1988). Prognosis of the post-traumatic vegetative state. *Acta Neurochirurgica, 95,* 49–52.

Breasted, J. H. (1930). *Edwin Smith Surgical Papyrus.* Chicago: University of Chicago Press.

Bricolo, A., Turazzi, S., & Feriotti, G. (1980). Prolonged post-traumatic unconsciousness: Therapeutic assets and liabilities. *Journal of Neurosurgery, 52,* 625–634.

Carlson, C.-A., von Essen, C., & Lofgren, J. (1968). Factors affecting the clinical course of patients with severe head injuries. Part 1: Influence of biological factors. Part 2: Significance of post-traumatic coma. *Journal of Neurosurgery, 29,* 242–251.

Carlson, N.R. (1994). *Physiology of behavior* (5th ed.). Boston: Allyn and Bacon.

Cullen, D.J. (1977). Results and costs of intensive care. *Anesthesiology, 47,* 203–216.

Cummings, J. L. (1992). Neuropsychiatric aspects of Alzheimer's disease and other dementing illnesses. In S.C. Yudofsky & R.E. Hales (Eds.), *Textbook of neuropsychiatry.* Washington, DC: The American Psychiatric Press.

Dacey, R., Dikmen, S., Temkin, N., McLean, A., Armsden, G., & Winn, H.R. (1991). Relative effects of brain and non-brain injuries on neuropsychological and psychological outcome. *Journal of Trauma, 31,* 217–222.

Davis, H. (1979). United States-Japan seminar on auditory responses from the brain stem. *The Laryngoscope, 89,* 1336–1339.

Dikmen, S., Machamer, J., Temkin, N., & McLean, A. (1990). Neuropsychological recovery in patients with moderate to severe head injury: Two-year follow-up. *Journal of Clinical and Experimental Neuropsychology, 12(4),* 507–519.

Ellis, D.W., & Rader, M.A. (1990). Structured sensory stimulation. In M.E. Sandel & D.W. Ellis (Eds.), *The coma-emerging patient* (pp. 465–477). Philadelphia: Hanley & Belfus, Inc.

Facco, E., Baratto, F., Munari, M., Dona, B., Casartelli Liviero, M., Behr, A.U., & Giron, G.P. (1991). Sensorimotor central conduction time in comatose patients. *Electroencephalography and Clinical Neurophysiology, 80,* 469–476.

Facco, E., Zuccarello, M., Pittoni, G., et al. (1986). Early outcome prediction in severe head injury in childhood: Comparison between children and adults. *Child's Nervous System, 2,* 67–71.

Giacino, J.T., & Zasler, N.D. (1995). Outcome after severe traumatic brain injury: Coma, the vegetative state, and the minimally responsive state. *Journal of Head Trauma Rehabilitation, 10,* 40–56.

Giacino, J.T., Kezmarsky, M.A., DeLuca, J., & Cicerone, K.D. (1991). Monitoring rate of recovery to predict outcome in minimally responsive patients. *Archives of Physical Medicine and Rehabilitation, 72,* 897–901.

Giacino, J.T., Sharlow-Galella, M., Kezmarsky, M.A., McKenna, K., Nelson, P., King, M., Brown, A., & Cicerone, K.D. (1991). *JFK coma recovery scale.* JFK Medical Center.

Gianutsos, R. (1990). Response system analysis: What the neuropsychologist can contribute to the rehabilitation of individuals emerging from coma. *Neuropsychology Review, 1,* 21–30.

Goldberg, K. (in press). Anoxic encephalopathy: A study in rehabilitation.

Groswasser, Z., & Sazbon, L. (1990). Outcome in 134 patients with prolonged post-traumatic unawareness. Part 2: Functional outcome of 72 patients recovering consciousness. *Journal of Neurosurgery, 72,* 81–84.

Groswasser, Z., Cohen, M., & Costeff, H. (1989). Rehabilitation outcomes after anoxic brain damage. *Archives of Physical Medicine Rehabilitation, 70,* 186–188.

Haig, A.J., & Ruess, J.M. (1990). Recovery from vegetative state of six months' duration associated with Sinemey (levodopa/carbodopa). *Archives of Physical Medicine and Rehabilitation, 71,* 1081–1083.

Hall, K., Cope, N., & Rappaport, M. (1985). Glasgow outcome scale and the disability rating scale: Comparative usefulness in following recovery in traumatic head injury. *Archives of Physical Medicine and Rehabilitation, 66,* 35–37.

Hall, M.E., MacDonald, S., & Young, G.C. (1992). The effectiveness of directed multisensory stimulation versus non-directed stimulation in comatose CHI patients: Pilot study of a single subject design. *Brain Injury, 6,* 435–445.

Helwick, L.D. (1994). Stimulation programs for coma patients. *Critical Care Nurse, 14(4),* 47–52.

Higashi, K., Hatano, M., Abiko, S., et al. (1981). Five-year follow-up study on patients with persistent vegetative state. *Journal of Neurology, Neurosurgery and Psychiatry, 44,* 552–554.

Higashi, K., Sakata, M., Hatano, S., et al. (1977). Epidemiological studies on patients with a persistent vegetative state. *Journal of Neurology, Neurosurgery and Psychiatry, 40,* 876–885.

Jennett, B., & Bond, M. (1975). Assessment of outcome after severe brain damage: A practical scale. *Lancet,* March 1, 480–484.

Jennett, B., & Plum, F. (1972). Persistent vegetative state after brain damage: A syndrome in search of a name. *Lancet,* April 1, 734–737.

Jennett, B., Teasdale, G., Braakman, R., Minderhood, J., & Knill-Jones, R. (1976). Predicting outcome in individual patients after severe head injury. *Lancet,* May 15, 1031–1034.

Johnson, G.M. (1987). Hypnotic imagery and suggestion as an adjunctive treatment in a case of coma. *American Journal of Clinical Hypnosis, 29,* 255–259.

Johnstone, B., & Bouman, D.E. (1992). Anoxic encephalopathy: A case study of an eight-year-old male with no residual cognitive deficits. *International Journal of Neuroscience, 62,* 207–213.

Kacmarek, R.M., Mack, C.W., & Dimas, S. (1990). *The essentials of respiratory care* (3rd ed.). St. Louis: Mosby Year Book

Kanno, T., Kamel, Y., Yokoyama, et al. (1987). Neurostimulation for patients in vegetative state. *PACE, 10,* 207–208.

Kater, K.M. (1989). Response of head-injured patients to sensory stimulation. *Western Journal of Nursing Research, 11,* 20–33.

Katoyama, Y., Tsubokawa, T., Yamamoto, T., et al. (1991). Characterization and modification of brain activity with deep brain stimulation in patients in a persistent vegetation state: Pain-related late positive component of cerebral evoked potentials. *PACE, 14,* 116–120.

Katz, D.I. (1991). Neuropathology and neurobehavioral recovery from closed head injury. *Journal of Head Trauma Rehabilitation, 7,* 1–15.

Kazdin, A.E. (1982). *Single-case research designs.* New York: Oxford University Press.

Kinney, H.C., & Samuels, M. A. (1994). Neuropathology of the persistent vegetative state: A review. *Journal of Neuropathology and Experimental Neurology, 53,* 548–558.

Kinney, H.C., Korein, J., Panigrahy, A., Dikkes, P., & Goode, P. (1994). Neuropathological findings in the brain of Karen Ann Quinlan: The role of the thalamus in the persistent vegetative state. *The New England Journal of Medicine, 330,* 1469–1475.

Kolb, B., & Whishaw, I.Q. (1990). *Fundamentals of human neuropsychology* (3rd ed.). New York: W.H. Freeman and Co.

Kriel, R.L., Krach, L.E., & Jones-Saete, C. (1993). Outcome of children with prolonged unconsciousness and vegetative states. *Pediatric Neurology, 9,* 362–368.

Kumar, A., & Agarwal, M. (1988). Secondary affective disorder of cardiac arrest. *British Journal of Psychiatry, 153,* 836–839.

Lalonde, R. (1994). Cerebellar contributions to instrumental learning. *Neuroscience and Biobehavioral Reviews, 18,* 161–170.

LaPuma, J., Schiedermayer, D.L., Gulyas, A.E., & Siegler, M. (1988). Talking to comatose patients. *Archives of Neurology, 45,* 20–22.

Levin, H.S., Williams, D., & Crafford, M.J. (1988). Relationship of depth of brain lesions to consciousness and outcome after closed head injury. *Journal of Neurosurgery, 69,* 861–866.

Levin, H.S., Saydjari, C., Eisenberg, H.M., Foulkes, M., Marshall, L.F., Ruff, R.M., Jane, J.A., & Marmarou, A. (1991). Vegetative state after closed-head injury: A traumatic coma data bank report. *Archives of Neurology, 48,* 580–585.

Levitzky, M.G., Cairo, J.M., & Hall, S.M. (1990). *Introduction to respiratory care*. Philadelphia: W.B. Saunders Co.

Levy, D.E., Bates, D., Caronna, J.J., et al. (1981). Prognosis in non-traumatic coma. *Annals of Internal Medicine, 94,* 298–301.

Levy, D.E., Caronna, J.J., Singer, B.H., Lapinski, R.H., Fryman, H., & Plum, F. (1985). Predicting outcome from hypoxic-ischemic coma. *Journal of the American Medical Association, 253,* 1420–1426.

LeWinn, E.B., & Dimancescu, M.D. (1978). Environmental deprivation and enrichment in coma. *Lancet*, July 15, 156–157.

Lezak, M.D. (1995). *Neuropsychological assessment* (3rd ed.). New York: Oxford University Press.

Lobato, R.D., Rivas, J.J., Gomez, P.A., Castaneda, M., Canizal, J.M., Sarabia, R., Cabrera, A., & Munoz, M.J. (1991). Head-injured patients who talk and deteriorate into coma. Analysis of 211 cases studied with computerized tomography. *Journal of Neurosurgery, 75,* 256–261.

Malkmus, D., Booth, B., & Kodimer, C. (1980). *Rehabilitation of the head-injured adult: Comprehensive cognitive management*. Downey, CA: Rancho Los Amigos Hospital.

Martin, G.B., Paradis, N.A., Helpern, J.A., Nowak, R.M., & Welch, K.M. (1991). Nuclear magnetic resonance spectroscopy study of human brain after cardiac resuscitation. *Stroke, 22,* 462–468.

McLellan, D. R. (1990). The structural basis of coma and recovery: Insights from brain injury in humans and experimental animals. In M.E. Sandel & D.W. Ellis (Eds.), *The coma-emerging patient* (pp. 389–409). Philadelphia: Hanley & Belfus.

Mitchell, S., Bradley, V.A., Welch, J.L., & Britton, P.G. (1990). Coma arousal procedure: A therapeutic intervention in the treatment of head injury. *Brain Injury, 4,* 273–279.

Modell, J.H. (1993). Drowning. *The New England Journal of Medicine, 328,* 253–256.

Multi-Society Task Force on PVS. Medical aspects of the persistent vegetative state (Part 1). *New England Journal of Medicine, 330,* 1499–1508.

———. Medical aspects of the persistent vegetative state (Part 2). *New England Journal of Medicine, 330,* 1572–1579.

O'Dell, M.W. (in press). Standardized assessment instruments for minimally responsive, brain injured patients.

O'Dell, M.W., & Riggs, R.V. (in press). Management of the minimally responsive patient.

Overgaard, J., Christensen, S., Hvid-Hansen, O., Haase, J. Land, A., Hein, O., Pedersen, K.K., & Tweed, W.A. (1973). *Lancet*, September 22, 631–635.

Parkin, A.J., Miller, J., & Vincent, R. (1987). Multiple neuropsychological deficits due to anoxic encephalopathy: A case study. *Cortex, 23,* 655–665.

Petri, H.L., & Mishkin, M. (1994). Behaviorism, cognitivism and the neuropsychology of memory. *American Scientist, 82,* 30–37.

Pierce, J.P., Lyle, D.M., Quine, S., Evans, N.J., Morris, J., & Fearnside, M.R. (1990). The effectiveness of coma arousal intervention. *Brain Injury, 4,* 191–197.

Plum, F., & Posner, J.B. (1982). *The diagnosis of stupor and coma* (3rd ed.). Philadelphia: F.A. Davis Co.

Pryse-Phillips, W., & Murray, T. J. (1982). *Essential Neurology* (2nd ed.). Garden City: Medical Examination Publishing Co., Inc.

Putnam, S.H., & Adams, K.M. (1992). Regression-based prediction of long-term outcome following multidisciplinary rehabilitation for traumatic brain injury. *Clinical Neuropsychologist*.

Rader, M.A., & Ellis, D.W. (1989). *Sensory stimulation assessment measure: Manual for administration*. (Available from Independence Rehab Services, 1030 N. Kings Highway, Suite 210, Cherry Hill, NJ 08034).

Rader, M.A., Alston, J.B., & Ellis, D.W. (1989). Sensory stimulation of severely brain-injured patients. *Brain Injury, 3,* 141–147.

Rappaport, M., Doughety, A.M., & Kelting, D.L. (1992). Evaluation of coma and vegetative states. *Archives of Physical Medicine and Rehabilitation, 73,* 628–634.

Rappaport, M., Hall, K.M., Hopkins, K., Belleza, T., & Cope, D.N. (1982). Disability rating scale of severe head trauma: Coma to community. *Archives of Physical Medicine and Rehabilitation, 63,* 118–123.

Read, W., Nenov, V.I., & Halgren, E. (1994). Role of inhibition in memory retrieval by hippocampal area CA3. *Neuroscience and Biobehavioral Reviews, 18,* 55–68.

Reitan, R.M., & Wolfson, D. (1985). *Neuroanatomy and neuropathology: A clinical guide for neuropsychologists.* Tucson: Neuropsychology Press.

Rosenberg, G.A., Johnson, S.F., & Brenner, R.P. (1977). Recovery of cognition after prolonged vegetative state. *Annals of Neurology, 2,* 167–168.

Ross, E.D., & Stewart, M.D. (1981). Akinetic mutism from hypothalamic damage: Successful treatment with dopamine agonists. *Neurology, 31,* 1435–1439.

Sandel, M.E., & Labi, M.L.C. (1990). Outcome prediction: Clinical and research perspectives. In M.E. Sandel & D.W. Ellis (Eds.), *The coma-emerging patient* (pp. 409–420). Philadelphia: Hanley & Belfus.

Sandel, M.E., Horn, L.J., & Bontke, C.F. (1993). Sensory stimulation: Accepted practice or expected practice. *Journal of Head Trauma Rehabilitation, 7,* 116–120

Sargent, M.M. (1989). Residential treatment. In D.W. Ellis & A.L. Christensen (Eds.), *Neuropsychological treatment after brain injury* (pp. 183–219). Boston: Kluwer.

Sazbon, L. (1985). Prolonged coma. *Progress in Clinical Neurosciences, 2,* 65–81.

Sazbon, L., & Groswasser, Z. (1990). Outcome in 134 patients with prolonged post-traumatic unawareness. Part 1: Parameters determining late recovery of consciousness. *Journal of Neurosurgery, 72,* 75–80.

———. (1991a). Medical complications and mortality of patients in the postcomatose unawareness (PC-U) state. *Acta Neurochirurgica, 112,* 110–112.

———. (1991b). Prolonged coma, vegetative state, postcomatose unawareness: Semantics or better understanding? *Brain Injury, 5,* 1–2.

———. (1991c). Time-related sequelae of TBI in patients with prolonged postcomatose unawareness (PC-U) state. *Brain Injury, 5,* 3–8.

Sazbon, L., Costoff, H., & Groswasser, Z. (1992). Epidemiological findings in traumatic post-comatose unawareness. *Brain Injury, 6,* 359–362.

Sazbon, L., Fuchs, C., & Costeff, H. (1991). Prognosis for recovery from prolonged post-traumatic unawareness: Logistic analysis. *Journal of Neurology, Neurosurgery and Psychiatry, 54,* 149–152.

Scoville, W.B., & Milner, B. (1957). Loss of recent memory after bilateral hippocampal lesions. *Journal of Neurology, Neurosurgery, and Psychiatry, 20,* 11–21.

Segatore, M., & Way, C. (1992). The Glasgow Coma Scale: Time for a change. *Heart and Lung, 21,* 548–557.

Silver, B.V., Boake, C., & Cavazos, D.I. (1994). Improving functional skills using behavioral procedures in a child with anoxic brain injury. *Archives of Physical Medicine Rehabilitation, 75,* 742–745.

Spettell, C.M., Ellis, D.W., Ross, S.E., Sandel, M.E., O'Malley, K.F., Stein, S.C., Spivack, G., & Hurely, K.E. (1991). Time of rehabilitation admission and severity of trauma: Effect on brain injury outcome. *Archives of Physical Medicine and Rehabilitation, 72,* 320–325.

Spivack, G., Spettell, C.M., Ellis. D.W., & Ross, S.E. (1992). Effects of intensity of treatment and length of stay on rehabilitation outcomes. *Brain Injury, 6,* 419–434.

Squire, L. (1986). The neuropsychology of memory dysfunction and its assessment. In I. Grant & K. Adams (Eds.), *Neuropsychological assessment of neuropsychiatric disorders* (pp. 268–299). New York: Oxford University Press.

Stein, S., & Schraeder, P. (1990). Persistent vegetative state. In M.E. Sandel & D.W. Ellis (Eds.), *The coma-emerging patient.* (pp. 543–557). Philadelphia: Hanley & Belfus.

Takahashi, S., Higano, S., Ishii, K., Matsumoto, K., Sakamoto, K., Iwasaki, Y., & Suzuki, M. (1993). Hypoxic brain damage: Cortical laminar necrosis and delayed changes in white matter at sequential MR imaging. *Radiology, 189,* 449–456.

Teasdale, G., & Jennett, B. (1974). Assessment of coma and impaired consciousness: A practical scale. *Lancet,* July 13, 81–84.

Thompson, R.F. (1991). Brain substrates of learning and memory. In T. Boll & B.K. Bryant (Eds.), *Clinical neuropsychology and brain function: Research, measurement, and practice* (pp. 61–83+). Washington, DC: American Psychological Association.

Tsubokawa, T., Yamamoto, T., Katoyama, Y., et al. (1990). Prediction of outcome of prolonged coma caused by brain damage. *Brain Injury, 4,* 329–337.

———. Deep-brain stimulation in a persistent vegetative state: Follow-up results and criteria for selection of candidates. *Brain Injury, 4,* 315–327.

Vannucci, R.C. (1990). Current and potentially new management strategies for perinatal hypoxic-ischemic encephalopathy. *Pediatrics, 85,* 961–968.

Walker, A. E. (1985). *Cerebral death* (3rd ed.). Baltimore: Urban & Schwarzenberg.

Walsh, K. (1987). *Neuropsychology: A clinical approach* (2nd ed.). New York: Churchill Livingstone.

Weintraub, S., & Mesulam, M.M. (1985). Mental state assessment of young and elderly adults in behavioral neurology. In M.M. Mesulam (Ed.), *Principles of behavioral neurology.* Philadelphia: F.A. Davis Co.

Whyte, J. (1992). Individualized quantitative assessment of the minimally responsive patient. Paper presented at the 54th Annual Meeting of the American Academy of Physical Medicine and Rehabilitation, San Francisco, November.

Whyte, J., & Glenn, M.B. (1988). The care and rehabilitation of the patient in a persistent vegetative state. *Journal of Head Trauma Rehabilitation, 1,* 39–53

Wilson, S.L., Powell, G.E., Elliott, K., & Thwaites, H. (1991). Sensory stimulation in prolonged coma: Four single case studies. *Brain Injury, 5,* 393–400.

Wood, R.L. (1991). Critical analysis of the concept of sensory stimulation for patients in vegetative states. *Brain Injury, 5,* 401–409.

Wood, R.L., Winkowski, T.B., Miller, J.L., Tierney, L. & Goldman, L. (1992). Evaluating sensory regulation as a method to improve awareness in patients with altered states of consciousness: A pilot study. *Brain Injury, 6,* 411–418.

Yuen, H.K. (1993). Increasing medication compliance in a woman with anoxic brain damage and partial epilepsy. *American Journal of Occupational Therapy, 47,* 30–33.

———. Improved productivity through purposeful use of additional template for a woman with cortical blindness. *American Journal of Occupational Therapy, 47,* 105–110.

Zasler, N.D., Kreutzer, J.S., & Taylor, D. (1991). Coma stimulation and coma recovery: A critical review. *Neuro Rehabilitation, 1,* 33–40.

Zasler, N.D., Taylor, D., & Decker, M. (1991). Characteristics and outcome of coma following severe traumatic brain injury. *Archives of Physical Medicine and Rehabilitation, 71,* 783.

9 Gene Therapy Strategies for Treatment of Post-Acute Impairment Following Injury to the Central Nervous System

Ronald L. Hayes and Keyi Yang

Department of Neurosurgery
University of Texas, Houston Health Science Center

INTRODUCTION

Rehabilitation of the brain-injured and spinal-cord-injured patient poses special challenges. Unfortunately, few basic scientific investigations have addressed important questions related to the development of therapies useful for rehabilitating these patients. Recently, our laboratory devoted considerable effort to characterizing changes in neurotrophic factors following brain injury. Our studies have lead us to conclude that modulation of neurotrophic responses by transfecting cDNA for specific neurotrophins could significantly facilitate the recovery of chronic brain injury and spinal-cord-injury. Importantly, the therapeutic effect of neurotrophins may not necessarily be related to their ability to promote neuronal regeneration. As documented by much of the research outlined in this chapter, neurotrophins may provide important therapeutic benefits simply by enhancing the recovery of damaged cytoskeletal proteins in surviving neurons.

Derangements of the neuronal cytoskeleton are undoubtedly important pathological consequences of traumatic brain injury (TBI). While most investigators have long recognized that diffuse axonal injury (DAI) is an important derangement following trauma to the central nervous system (CNS), recent advances in our study of cytoskeletal derangements have shown that structural disturbances to neurons may be considerably more widespread, involving dendrites and cell bodies as well as axons. Most research interests have focused on understanding the acute pathological mechanisms mediating neuronal injury, including loss of important cytoskeletal proteins. However, it is also important to understand how to enhance recovery of critical structural proteins once they have been injured. Although not widely appreciated, neurotrophins could have important influences on the recovery of cytoskeletal proteins following damage. This chapter briefly reviews studies from our laboratory examining cytoskeletal derangements both in *in vivo* models of TBI and in *in vitro* models of depolarization injury to primary septo-hippocampal cultures. The chapter also summarizes data indicating that transfection of cDNA for brain-derived neurotrophic factor (BDNF) can rescue injury-induced neurofilament loss *in vitro*, thus suggesting the potential for neurotrophins either produced by gene transfection or administered exogenously to enhance recovery of cytoskeletal derangements following traumatic injury to the CNS.

CYTOSKELETAL DERANGEMENTS *IN VIVO* WITH TBI

Neurofilament (NF) proteins are primary components of the neuronal cytoarchitecture, including axons and dendrites (Shaw, 1986). Neurofilaments (NFs) consist of three separate protein elements collectively called the *neurofilament triplet proteins* (Hoffman & Lasek, 1975). These subunits have apparent molecular weights of 200 kilodaltons (kD) (NF-H), 150 kD (NF-M), and 68 kD (NF-L) as estimated by gel electrophoresis (Dautingy et al., 1988). The 68 kD subunit is an assembly protein found predominantly in the NF core, and the 150 kD and 200 kD subunits are cross-linking proteins found in the connecting branches. All NF triplet proteins exhibit significant sequence homology in the amino terminal, alpha helical domain. The 150 kD and 200 kD subunits possess highly repeating lysine-serine-proline (KSP) sequences that are heavily phosphorylated and contribute to anomalous electrophoretic mobilities (Julien & Mushynski, 1982; Nixon & Shiang, 1991). The assembly of NF proteins results in the formation of neurofibrils of approximately 10 mm in diameter in the axon hillock, which are transported down the axon. Although their function is primarily structural, NF proteins have been implicated in many disease processes such as Alzheimer's disease (Sternberger et al., 1985; Ulrich et al., 1987), amyotrophic lateral sclerosis (Troost et al., 1982), Pick's disease (Pietrini et al., 1993), and neurological insults such as stroke (Arai & Kessler, 1990; Arai et al., 1991; Inuzuka et al., 1990a, b; Kaku et al., 1993; Kudo et al., 1993; Lee et al., 1991; Nakamura et al., 1992).

Axonal injury has long been thought to be a primary pathological feature of TBI. Animal models of severe TBI and human post-injury pathology demonstrate axonal damage (Gennarelli et al., 1989; Yaghmai & Povlishock, 1992). A central polemic in TBI investigation is the relative roles of structural determinants vs. concurrent biochemical derangements as the crucial pathological events post-injury. In human studies, investigators have identified DAI as the key pathological feature responsible for the neurobehavioral deficits that accompany human TBI (Adams et al., 1983; Gennarelli et al., 1989; Yaghmai & Povlishock, 1982). To date, current studies investigating DAI after TBI have been predominantly pathomorphological and qualitative in nature. Recent investigations of the role of NF68 in DAI pathology are a noteworthy exception (Yaghmai & Povlishock, 1992). While axonal dysfunction may play an important role in TBI pathology, no causal relationship has been established as yet between DAI and post-injury neurobehavioral deficits. In fact, numerous studies have revealed that functionally normal neurotransmission can be preserved in pathways that have suffered significant loss of fibers (Beattie et al., 1988; Sautter et al., 1991). Thus, a comprehensive quantitative assessment of cytoskeletal alterations would contribute to the understanding of DAI and its role in TBI pathology.

Rodent models of TBI cause neurobehavioral deficits, including motor and memory disturbances, that resemble those seen in human patients (Lyeth et al., 1990; Hamm et al.,

1992). Today, little is known of the molecular events leading to post-injury pathology in these animal models. Recent laboratory studies have determined that TBI induces a significant decrease in the protein levels of key dendritic cytoskeletal elements (Taft et al., 1992, 1993), including microtubule-associated protein 2 (MAP2). Post-TBI excitotoxicity (Gorman et al., 1989; Hayes et al., 1992), loss of calcium homeostasis (Fineman et al., 1993), and pathological activation of calcium-dependent proteases (e.g., calpain) may be principal causes of cytoskeletal degradation (Taft et al., 1992, 1993). Although calpains are found in both axonal and dendritic environments (Perlmutter et al., 1988), previous examination of cytoskeletal pathology after TBI has focused on dendritic cytoskeletal elements (MAP2) (Taft et al., 1992, 1993). NF proteins (Kamakura et al., 1985; Schalepfer et al., 1985a, b), MAP2 (Johnson et al., 1991), spectrin (Siman et al., 1984), and other cytoskeletal proteins are substrates for calpain-dependent proteolysis.

We have examined the effect of lateral cortical impact injury on the levels of axonal cytoskeletal proteins in adult rats (Posmantur et al., 1994b). TBI causes a significant decrease in the protein levels of two prominent NF proteins, NF68 and NF200. We employed quantitative immunoreactivity measurements on Western blots to examine NF68 and NF200 levels in homogenates of hippocampal and cortical tissue taken at several intervals post-injury. Sham injury had no effect on NF protein levels. However, injury was associated with a significant loss of NF68 restricted to the cortex ipsilateral to the injury site. NF68 loss was detectable as early as three hours and lasted at least two weeks post-injury. Similarly, TBI induced a decrease in NF200 protein, although losses were observed both ipsilateral and contralateral to the injury site. No loss of NF68 or NF200 protein was detected in hippocampal samples obtained from the same injured animals. An increase in the presence of lower molecular weight (MW) NF68 immunopositive bands was associated with the decrease of NF68 in the ipsilateral cortex (Figure 9.1). This NF68 antigenicity pattern suggests the production of NF68 breakdown products caused by the pathological activation of neuronal proteases such as calpain. Putative NF68 breakdown products increase significantly until one day post-injury, suggesting that NF degradation may be ongoing until that time and indicating that a potential therapeutic window may exist within the first 24 hours post-injury. In summary, these data identified specific biochemical alterations of the neuronal cytoskeleton following TBI and laid the foundation for further investigation of post-injury cytoskeletal changes in neuronal processes.

Since Western blot analyses have showed reduction of levels of NF68 and NF200 (Posmantur et al., 1994a), as well as the exclusively dendritic protein MAP2 (Taft et al., 1992, 1993) as early as three hours post-TBI in cortical homogenates, we used antibodies NF68 (Sigma NR4), NF200 (Sigma N52), and MAP2 (Sigma AP-20) to conduct the first studies of the morphopathological characteristics of these cytoskeletal derangements in TBI (Posmantur et al., in press). These antibodies were specifically selected to examine axons as well as dendrites. The decision to focus on cortical regions three hours post-TBI was based on previous Western data showing NF68 and NF200 loss and associated NF proteolytic fragments in cortical homogenates but not in hippocampal samples at this early time (Posmantur et al., 1994a). This study employed a widely used model of experimental mechanical brain injury, lateral cortical impact injury (Dixon et al., 1991). TBI induced the most prominent alterations in NF68, NF200, and MAP2 immunolabeling within ipsilateral and contralateral contusion sites. Marked changes in immunolabeling were detected in brain regions within and beyond areas containing macroscopic subarachnoid vascular destruction but were reliably associated with the presence of dark shrunken

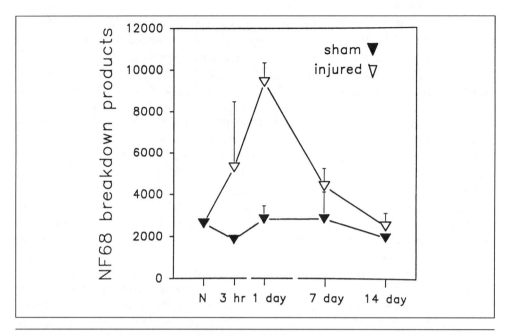

Figure 9.1: Quantification of the appearance of NF68 breakdown products. Immunoblots were analyzed quantitatively for total NF68 breakdown products by computer-assisted scanning densitometry. Ordinate values represent arbitrary densitometric units. The low MW immunoreactivity in sham (closed triangles) animals did not change with time, but a dramatic increase was seen in injured (open triangles) animals. The greatest amount of NF68 breakdown products appears at one day post-injury.

neurons labeled by hematoxylin and eosin staining. Light microscopic studies of NF200 immunofluorescence revealed a prominent fragmented appearance of apical dendrites within pyramidal neurons layer 3 and 5, as well as a loss of fine dendritic arborization within layer 1. Confocal microscopy detected varying degrees of NF200 disassembly associated with these areas of NF fragmentation. Light microscopic studies of NF68 immunofluorescence detected subtle and less severe ultrastructural changes, including smaller breaks and focal vacuolization of apical dendrites. Light microscopic immunofluorescence of MAP2 revealed changes similar to that of NF200. Acute axonal alterations detected with NF68 were minimal compared to immunofluorescence changes seen in dendritic regions. Since cytoskeletal proteins are structural proteins found abundantly in dendritic as well as axonal processes, diffuse injury to neuronal processes may be an important early morphological features of TBI.

DEPOLARIZATION OF PRIMARY SEPTO-HIPPOCAMPAL CULTURES AND LOSS OF NF PROTEINS

Potassium depolarization lasting for 24 hours or more enhances the developmental expression and maturation of the neuronal cytoskeleton in a number of systems (see Franklin & Johnson, 1992; Ghosh et al., 1994; Sambrook et al., 1989). Depolarization lasting from 4–20 hours produces a Ca^{++}-dependent neurite retraction in hippocampal neurons *in vitro* (Mattson et al., 1988; Nakamura & Araki, 1992). Recently, eight minutes of depolarization with 50mM K^+ has been shown to increase phosphorylation of cyclic adenosine monophosphate-responsive, element-binding protein (CREB) (Ghosh et al.,

1994), indicating that even brief depolarization may produce significant and measurable effects. Since brief periods of acute depolarization accompany injuries to the brain such as TBI (Katayama et al., 1991; Nixon & Marotta, 1984), ischemia (Liem, 1993; Taft et al., 1992), and epilepsy (Dietzel et al., 1986; Jensen & Chiu, 1990), investigations of brief depolarization could provide important insights into the pathophysiology of brain injury. However, the cytoskeletal and morphological effects of brief ($\leq$ 15 min.) potassium depolarization have not previously been examined.

As mentioned above, the NF triplet proteins—heavy (NF-H), middle (NF-M), and light (NF-L)—are major components of the mature neuronal cytoskeleton (Mattson et al., 1988; Ogata et al., 1989). Alterations in the levels and/or phosphorylation states of cytoskeletal proteins occur in numerous neurodegenerative disorders (Forno et al., 1986; Poltorak et al., 1988; Szatkowski & Atwell, 1994; Wang et al., 1994) including Alzheimer's disease (Cork et al., 1986; Sternberger & Sternberger, 1983). Alterations in cytoskeletal proteins have been documented following injuries associated with acute depolarization: MAP2 and NF-L, and NF-H are decreased in rat models of head trauma (Posmantur et al., 1994a; Posmantur et al., 1994b; Towbin et al., 1979); tubulin, MAP2 and NF-L, NF-M, and NF-H are decreased by ischemia (Katayama et al., 1990; Nilsson et al., 1993; Poltorak et al., 1988); and NF-L and NF-H levels drop after epileptic activity (Weiss et al., 1993).

In order to test the hypothesis that pathophysiologically relevant brief depolarization is capable of initiating disruption of the neuronal cytoskeleton and to determine the role played by calcium in that effect, we exposed mixed septo-hippocampal cultures to depolarization by 60 mM KCl for six minutes in the presence of various extracellular $CaCl_2$ concentrations (0-11.8 mM Ca^{++}) and examined the effect of this treatment on NF protein immunoreactivity by densitometric analyses of immunolabelled Western blots. Immunohistochemistry was also used to examine corresponding changes in neuronal morphology (Whitson et al., 1995). Twenty-four hours later, NF immunoreactivity in Western blots of depolarized cultures were decreased to 60% or less of control levels. Decreases were Ca^{++}-dependent, not due to cell loss, and affected both phosphorylated and nonphosphorylated proteins (Figure 9.2). The phosphorylation state of NF-M and NF-H influenced the degree of loss observed. Changes in the pattern of immunolabelling of neuritic processes were also associated with depolarization. Thus, brief potassium depolarization may contribute to cytoskeletal disruption following brain injury.

TBI AND NGF, BDNF, AND NT-3

Our laboratory has recently examined TBI-induced changes in nerve growth factor (NGF) (REF: regional and temporal profiles...) as well a BDNF and neurotrophin-3 (NT-3) (REF: increased expression of BDNF...). Administration of exogenous NGF has been reported to spare cholinergic neurons from death and degeneration following injury to the CNS. Many of these studies have focused on enhanced survival of septo-hippocampal neurons (Varon & Conner, 1994). There is also substantial evidence that disturbances in cholinergic neurotransmission, especially within the hippocampus, can contribute to chronic memory deficits following TBI in rats (see Hayes et al., 1992; Dixon et al., 1994, in review). Thus, an enhanced understanding of changes in the expression of neurotrophic factors such as NGF following TBI, as well as mechanisms regulating these changes, could provide critical insights into pathobiological responses to TBI.

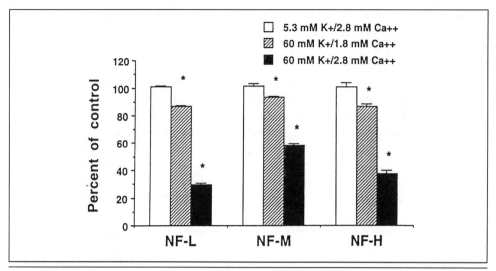

Figure 9.2: Neurofilament light (NF-L), middle (NF-M), and heavy (NF-H) immunoreactivity 24 hours after depolarization or control treatment (5.3 mM K^+ and 1.8 mM Ca^{++}). Levels were not altered by 6-min. exposure to media containing increased Ca^{++} and normal K^+, but were significantly decreased by 6-min. exposure to media containing increased K^+ and normal Ca^{++}. Increasing K^+ and Ca^{++} produced significantly greater loss than increased K^+ in the presence of normal Ca^{++}. Open bars, 5.3 mM (normal) K^+ and 2.8 mM Ca^{++}; Striped bars, 60 mM K^+ and 1.8 mM (normal) Ca^{++}; gray bars, 60 mM K^+ and 2.8 mM Ca^{++}. Values are mean ± SEM of samples (4 wells each) from three separate experiments expressed as a percentage of corresponding control (cultures exposed for 6 min. to normal media) values. *=values significantly different than control. ANOVA with post-hoc Sheffe, $p<0.05$, $n=3$.

We recently reported that lateral cortical impact injury produces transient increases of *c-fos* mRNA and AP-1 complex expression in the ipsilateral neocortex (Yang et al., 1994); however, the pathophysiological significance of this transient *c-fos* mRNA expression is still unresolved. Several studies suggest that *c-fos* may mediate NGF expression (Zheng & Heinrich, 1988; Mocchetti et al., 1989; Hengerer et al., 1990; Ballarin et al., 1991; Morgan & Curran, 1991; Ladenheim et al., 1993; Herrera et al., 1993; Gwag et al., 1994). Also, there is increased NGF expression in animals after experimental CNS insults such as ischemia (Lindvall et al., 1992; Hashimoto et al., 1992; Shozuhara et al., 1992), seizure (Gall & Isackson, 1989; Rocamora et al., 1992; Gall et al., 1991a, b), hippocampal damage induced by kainic acid injection (Ballarin et al., 1991), and cortical trauma (Dekosky et al., 1994). However, there is no direct evidence that *c-fos* induces NGF expression in the CNS.

Exogenous NGF administration does induce expression of the *c-fos* gene *in vitro* (Curran & Morgan, 1985; Greenberg et al., 1985; Kruijer et al., 1985) and *in vivo* (Sharp et al., 1989; Peng et al., 1993). However, the effects of endogenous NGF gene expression may differ from those resulting from the exogenous administration of NGF. Because there is a relationship between *c-fos* and NGF expression *in vitro*, researchers have posited that immediate early genes (IEGs) might induce neurotrophic factors (NTFs) presynaptically, while NTFs might induce IEGs postsynaptically (Morgan & Curran, 1991).

In view of the uncertainty as to the nature of the relationships between endogenous *c-fos* and NGF gene expression in the brain, it is important to determine the relationships between endogenous *c-fos* and NGF expression *in vivo*. Importantly, there are no published reports of systematic comparisons of *c-fos* and NGF expression following TBI. Thus, we examined the regional and temporal profiles of *c-fos* and NGF mRNA co-expression in rat brain after cortical impact injury as one component of the relationship between endogenous *c-fos* and NGF gene expression. Since the lateral cortical impact injury device employed in these studies produces prominent and reliable injury ipsilateral to the site of impact, we focused our studies of gene expression on brain regions ipsilateral to the injury.

Using alternate sections from the same rat brains, *in situ* hybridization studies showed that in the neocortex, *c-fos* mRNA transiently increased at 30 min., 1 hr., and 3 hrs. after injury, while there were no increases of NGF mRNA at these post-injury points. In the hippocampus, *in situ* hybridization showed that *c-fos* mRNA increased at 30 min., 1 hr., and 3 hrs. post-injury, while NGF mRNA increased at 1 hr. and 3 hrs. but not at 30 min. after injury. RT-PCR studies in hippocampus confirmed that *c-fos* mRNA increased as early as 5 min. after injury, peaked at 30 min. post-injury, and remained elevated 5 hrs. post-injury. Levels of hippocampal NGF mRNA expression increased by 1 hr. after injury and plateaued until 3 and 5 hrs. post-injury. These data are consistent with the possible regulatory role of endogenous *c-fos* on NGF expression following TBI.

Brain-derived neurotrophic factor (BDNF) and neurotrophic factor 3 (NT3) are neurotrophins present in rat brain (Hofer et al., 1990; Maisonpierre et al., 1990; Rocamora et al., 1992; Smith et al., 1995). Interestingly, the distributions of cells expressing BDNF and NT3 mRNA in the adult rat brain are unique for each factor. In the hippocampus, BDNF mRNA is expressed in the dentate gyrus and CA1-CA4 regions, whereas NT3 mRNA is expressed in a more restrictive pattern, being distributed only in the dentate gyrus, CA2, and medial CA1 regions (Rocamora et al, 1992; Smith et al., 1995). Outside of the hippocampus, higher levels of BDNF mRNA have been found in many regions of the brain, including the neocortex, piriform cortex, and amygdala, whereas NT3 mRNA is not markedly expressed in these areas (Lindvall et al., 1992; Rocamora et al., 1992; Hohn et al., 1990). Both neurotrophins, however, produce a similar neurotrophic effect on some neurons, while retaining distinct characteristics in other respects (Anderson et al., 1990; Hohn et al., 1990; Hyman et al., 1991; Knusel et al., 1992; Lindsay et al., 1985; Maisonpierre et al., 1990). Both BDNF and NT3 affect neurite outgrowth (Davies et al., 1986; Maisonpierre et al., 1990) and the survival of neural crest-derived sensory neurons (Barde et al., 1980; Davies et al., 1986; Hohn et al., 1990; Linday et al., 1985). Further studies indicate that BDNF may be trophic for a wide range of different types of neurons (DiStefano et al., 1992; Ip et al., 1993; Smith et al., 1995). BDNF, but not NT3, increases survival of cholinergic neurons (Anderson et al., 1990; Ballarin et al., 1991; Dixon et al., 1991) and dopaminergic neurons from the substantia nigra (Hyman et al., 1991; Knusel et al, 1991). In contrast, NT3 is considered to be particularly important in embryogenesis and development of the hippocampus (Collazo et al., 1992; Ernfors et al., 1990; Freidman et al., 1991).

Several studies have examined the effects of CNS injuries on the expression of BDNF and NT3. CNS insults associated with activation of glutamate transmission, increased intracellular calcium, and *c-fos* gene expression have demonstrated increased levels of BDNF gene expression. Increased BDNF expression has been reported following ischemia (Lindvall et al., 1992; Takeda et al., 1993), seizures (Gall & Lauterborn, 1992; Gall & Isackson, 1989; Isackson et al., 1991; Rocamora et al., 1992), hippocampal damage induced by kainic acid injection (Ballarin et al., 1991), insulin-induced hypoglycemic coma (Lindvall et al., 1992), glutamate-mediated spreading depression (Kokaia et al, 1993), and glucocorticoid-associated stress (Smith et al., 1995). Decreased NT3 mRNA expression has been reported following ischemia (Lindvall et al., 1992; Takeda et al., 1992), seizures (Ernfors et al., 1990; Gall & Lauterborn, 1992; Isackson et al., 1991; Rocamora et al., 1992), and insulin-induced hypoglycemic coma (Lindvall et al., 1992).

No studies have examined BDNF and NT3 mRNA expression following mechanical TBI. Thus, we employed a controlled cortical-impact rodent model of brain injury to investigate the co-expression of BDNF and NT3 in the rat brain. Levels of BDNF and NT3 mRNA expression were measured following unilateral injury to the cerebral cortex. To obtain reliable data on the co-expression of neurotrophin genes, adjacent coronal sections from the same rat brains were hybridized *in situ* with BDNF and NT3 cRNA probes. BDNF mRNA increased at 1 hr., 3 hrs., and 5 hrs. after unilateral cortical injury in the cortex ipsilateral to the injury site and bilaterally in the dorsal hippocampus. NT3 mRNA did not change significantly following injury. Our results suggest that TBI produces rapid increases in BDNF mRNA expression in rat brain without changes in NT3 mRNA expression, a finding which differs from studies of ischemia and seizures. It is possible that increased levels of BDNF mRNA rather than NT3 are important components of pathophysiological responses to TBI.

GENE TRANSFECTION OF NEUROTROPHINS AND EXOGENOUS ADMINISTRATION OF NEUROTROPHIN PROTEINS

The therapeutic potential of various neurotrophins for treatment of the injured CNS is widely recognized (Barinaga, 1994). Recent studies indicate that maintenance of hippocampal cultures in the presence of BDNF results in significant increases in NF protein (Ip et al., 1993). Although administration of exogenous proteins has generated important information about neurotrophins and has therapeutic potential, significant limitations imposed by protein degradation and by the blood brain barrier restrict the clinical utility of these approaches (Barinaga, 1994). Gene transfer is an alterative way to introduce BDNF into CNS cells and tissues. Although viral vectors have been widely studied to introduce genes into the CNS (Culver et al., 1992; Hefti, 1986; Horwitz, 1990; Johnson et al., 1992; Lagallasalle et al., 1993; Wolf et al., 1988), our laboratory is conducting systematic studies of the potential of cationic liposomes for gene transfection in the brain and spinal cord (Yang et al., 1994b, c). Recent studies report liposome-mediated b-galactosidase (b-gal) gene transfection and expression in adult mouse brain (Roessler & Davidson, 1994). Optimal concentrations of liposomes for transfection of the b-gal gene in primary septo-hippocampal cultures have been determined by our laboratory (Yang et al. 1994c). Furthermore, we have confirmed relatively long-lasting but not permanent expression of functional NGF in primary septo-hippocampal cell cultures by liposome-mediated gene transfer (Ibid.). The transient expression produced by liposome-mediated gene transfection may limit its application in diseases caused by genetic defects. However, liposomal transfection of trophic factors may prove useful for treatment of CNS injury by blunting transient pathological processes and/or facilitating recovery. Because of the simplicity, reproducibility, safety, and efficiency of cationic liposome-mediated gene transfection (Felgner et al., 1987; Hug & Sleight 1991; Nabel et al., 1992), we have examined liposome-mediated BDNF gene transfection *in vitro*. Importantly, this research also examined the therapeutic potential of BDNF transfection to restore NF loss following injury to CNS neurons.

Previous studies indicate that the cytomegalovirus (CMV) is a prudent initial choice of viral promoter (Fang et al., 1989; Giordano et al., 1991; Li et al., 1992; Thompson et al., 1993). We used a pUC19-based plasmid containing a CMV promoter as an expression vector for NGF transfection (MacGregor & Caskey, 1989; Yang et al., 1994c). Rat NGF DNA was subcloned into a unique Not1 site under the control of the CMV promoter. We used the commercially available DOTMA and DOPE (Gibco-BRL) liposome formulated from a 1:1 (w:w) mixture of the cationic lipid N-[1 -(2,3-dioleyloxy)propyl]-n,n,n-trimethylammoniumchloride (DOTMA) and dioleoyl phosphotidylethanolamine (DOPE) in membrane-filtered water.

Because of our laboratory's interest in injury mechanisms in the hippocampus and the preferential vulnerability of the hippocampus to traumatic or ischemic brain injury (Yang et al., 1994c; Yang et al., 1994a), we used mixed primary septo-hippocampal cell cultures for *in vitro* studies of liposome-mediated gene transfection of BDNF (Hayes et al., 1995). Cultures were incubated for 10 days prior to injury and/or transfection. By that time, astrocytes reached confluence and were no longer actively multiplying, while neurons were well differentiated and stable.

After BDNF gene transfection in uninjured cultures, RT-PCR and immunohistochemical staining confirmed increases in BDNF mRNA and protein in transfected cells (Figure 9.3A). Three days after depolarization injury, Western blot and immunohistochemical analyses detected significant loss of NF proteins in non-transfected cultures, while BDNF transfection produced marked increases in NF proteins following either transfection 48 hours prior to injury or transfection 24 hours following injury (Figure 9.3B). Immunohistochemical studies also detected enhanced immunolabelling of BDNF and total NF protein (phosphorylated and nonphosphorylated) in injured neurons following BDNF transfection or administration of exogenous BDNF protein, as compared to untransfected, injured controls.

To our knowledge, these results represent the first reported demonstration of liposome-mediated BDNF transfection in post-mitotic CNS cell cultures. In addition, there are no previously published reports that either exogenous BDNF protein or transfection of cDNA for BDNF can enhance recovery of NF loss produced by injury to CNS cells. Mechanisms mediating BDNF upregulation of NF proteins following injury are unknown, although previous *in vitro* studies have indicated that neurotrophins such as NGF can induce NF phosphorylation (see Clark & Lee, 1991). Although our data indicate that BDNF can increase total NF levels, future studies must analyze in more detail the potential effects of BDNF on phosphorylation state of NF proteins. Since the magnitude of depolarization injury employed in these studies does not produce cell death in septo-hippocampal cultures, our data suggest that BDNF protein or transfection of BDNF cDNA may be useful in restoring levels of NFs in injured but surviving neurons. Moreover, there may be a considerable therapeutic window of opportunity following injury, since transfection of BDNF cDNA even 24 hours following injury can substantially enhanced recovery of NF levels.

SUMMARY AND CONCLUSIONS

In summary, our laboratories have initiated systematic comparisons of the effects of injury on cytoskeletal derangements employing *in vivo* and *in vitro* models. Importantly, by employing an *in vitro* model that reproduces features of TBI *in vivo*, we have been able to demonstrate cytoskeletal derangements similar to those produced by TBI to the intact

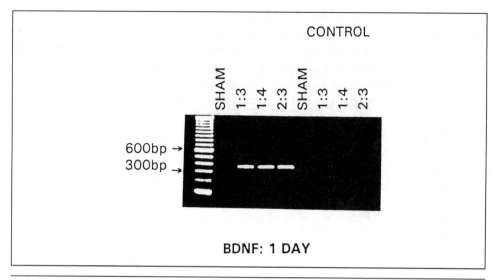

Figure 9.3A: RT-PCR analysis detected BDNF mRNA following liposome-mediated transfection. One day after liposome-mediated BDNF gene transfection (1:3; 1:4; 2:3mg DNA/ml liposomes/well), cells in culture were lysed by adding 0.2 ml of RNAzol B (Cinna/Biotec Laboratories, Inc.) per 10^6 cells. BDNF mRNA expression was increased in BDNF cDNA transfected cultures (lanes-1:3; 1:4; 2:3) compared to liposome-only treated cultures (Sham lane). To examine possible DNA contamination during RNA preparation, RNA samples were included without performing reverse transcription. These control studies confirm the absence of DNA contamination (Control lanes). Marker: 100 bp DNA ladder (Gibco BRL, Grand Island, NY). The RNA preparation was performed as previously described (Yang et al., 1994a). Total RNA from individual wells was used for DNA synthesis at 42°C for 2 hrs. using 200 units of M-MLV reverse transcriptase (Perkin-Elmer, Norwalk, CT), 40 nmole of dNTP, 200 nmole DTT and using oligo/dT as primers. For PCR, one pair of forward and backward primers of BDNF was used. The sequence of BDNF/5 primer was 5'-GCAAACATGTCTATGAGGGT-3', and of BDNF/3, was 5'- GGTCAGTGTACATACACAGG-3'⁵ (Yang et al., 1994b). Total DNA and 40 pmole of primer were used for PCR. PCR was carried out in a programmable heating block (Perkin-Elmer, Norwalk, CT) using cycles consisting of denaturation at 95°C for 1 min., followed by annealing at 55°C for 1 min., and DNA extension at 72°C for 2 min. After 25 cycles of PCR, samples were electrophoresed on 1.5% agarose gel. Gels were stained with ethidium bromide and photographed under UV light.

brain. Data from this *in vitro* system of CNS injury suggests that transfection of neurotrophins or administration of exogenous neurotrophin proteins can enhance recovery of lost cytoskeletal proteins in surviving neurons after brain injury. Equally important, these initial *in vitro* studies employed non-viral vector systems that may have considerable therapeutic potential for treatment of human head injury. However, experience with gene transfection suggests that it is considerably more difficult to develop effective transfection systems *in vivo* than *in vitro*. Thus, it will be important for future *in vivo* studies both to confirm that liposomes can produce efficient levels of gene transfection and to confirm that transfection and/or exogenous administration of neurotrophic proteins can enhance recovery of the injured neuronal cytoskeleton.

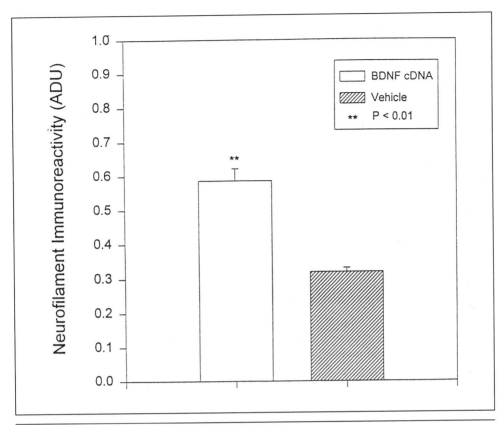

Figure 9.3B: Quantification of Western blot analyses in arbitrary densitometric units (ADU) indicated that BDNF transfection produced marked increases in intermediate NF proteins 3 days after injury, as compared to control cultures exposed only to liposomes, when BDNF cDNA was transfected 24 hrs. after injury (P<0.01 by Student's t-test).

REFERENCES

Adams, J., Graham, D., & Gennarelli, T. (1983). Head injury in man and experimental animals. *Acta. Neurochir, 32*, 15–30.

Anderson, R.F., Alterman, A.L., Barde, Y.A., & Lindsay, R.M. (1990). Brain-derived neurotrophic factor increases survival and differentiated functions of rat septal cholinergic neurons in culture. *Neuron, 5*, 297–306.

Arai, A., Kessler, M., Lee, K., & Lynch, G. (1990). Calpain inhibitors improve the recovery of synaptic transmission from hypoxia in hippocampal slices. *Brain Research, 532*, 63–68.

Arai, A., Vanderklish, P., Kessler, M., Lee, K., & Lynch, G. (1991). A brief period of hypoxia causes proteolysis of cytoskeletal proteins in hippocampal slices. *Brain Research, 555*, 276–280.

Ballarin, M., Ernfors, P., Lindefors, N., & Persson, H. (1991). Hippocampal damage and kainic acid injection induce a rapid increase in mRNA for BDNF and NGF in the rat brain. *Experimental Neurology, 114*, 35–43.

Barde, Y.A., Edgar, D., & Thoenen, H. (1980). Sensory neurons in culture: Changing requirement for survival factors during embryonic development. *Proceedings of the National Academy of Science USA, 77*, 1199–1230.

Barinaga, M. (1994). Solving the delivery puzzle. *Science, 264,* 772–774.

Beattie, M.S., Stokes, B.T., & Breshnahan, J.C. (1988). Experimental spinal cord injury: Strategies for acute and chronic intervention based on anatomic, physiological and behavioral studies. In D.G. Stein and B.S. Sabel (Eds.), *Pharmacological approaches to the treatment of brain and spinal cord injury* (pp. 43–74). New York: Plenum Press

Clark, E.A., & Lee, V.M.-Y. (1991). The differential role of protein kinase C isozymes in the rapid induction of neurofilament phosphorylation by nerve growth factor and phorbol esters in PC12 cells. *Journal of Neurochemistry, 57,* 802–810.

Collazo, D., Takahashi, H., & McKay, R.D.G. (1992). Cellular target and trophic functions of neurotrophin-3 in the developing rat hippocampus. *Neuron, 9,* 643–656.

Cork, L.A., Sternberger, N.H., Sternberger, L.A., Casanova, M.F., Struble, R.G., & Price, D.L. (1986). Phosphorylated neurofilament antigens in neurofibrillary tangles in Alzheimer's disease. *Journal of Neuropathology and Experimental Neurology, 45,* 56–64.

Culver, K.W., Ram, Z., Wallbridge, S., Ishii, H., Oldfield, E.H., & Blaese, R.M. (1992). *In vivo* gene transfer with retroviral vector-producer cells for treatment of experimental brain tumors. *Science, 256,* 1550–1552.

Curran, T., & Morgan, J. (1985). Superinduction of *c-fos* by nerve growth factor in the presence of peripherally active benzodiazepines. *Science, 229,* 1265–1268.

Dautingy, A., Pham-Dinh, D., Roussel, C., Felix, J.M., Nussbaum, J.L., & Jolles. (1988). The large neurofilament subunit (NF-H) of the rat: cDNA cloning and in situ detection. *Biochemistry and Biophysiology Research Communications, 154,* 1099–1106.

Davies, A.M., Thoenen, H., & Bard, Y.A. (1986). The response of chick sensory neurons to brain-derived neurotrophic factor. *Journal of Neuroscience, 6,* 1897–1904.

Dekosky, S.T., Gross, J.R., Miller, P.D., Styren, S.D., Kochanek, P.M., & Marion, D. (in press). Upregulation of nerve growth factor following cortical trauma. *Experimental Neurology.*

Dietzel, I., Lux, H.D., & Heinemann, U. (1986). Ionic changes and alterations in the size of the extracellular space during epileptic activity. *Advances in Neurology, 44,* 619–639.

DiStefano, P.S., Friedman, B., Radziejewski, C., Alexander, C., Boland, P., Schick, C.M., Lindsay, R.M., & Wiegand, S.J. (1992). The neurotrophins BDNF, NT-3, and NGF display distinct patterns of retrograde axonal transport in peripheral and central neurons. *Neuron, 8,* 983–993.

Dixon, C.E., Bao, J., & Hayes, R.L. (in review). Reduced evoked release of acetylcholine in the rodent hippocampus following traumatic brain injury.

Dixon, C.E., Clifton, G.L., Lighthall, J.W., Yaghmai, A.A., & Hayes, R.L. (1991). A controlled cortical impact model of traumatic brain injury in the rat. *Journal of Neuroscience Methods, 39,* 253–262.

Ernfors, P., Wetmore, C., Olson, & L., Persson, H. (1990). Identification of cells in rat brain and peripheral tissues expressing mRNA for members of the nerve growth factor family. *Neuron, 5,* 511–526.

Fang, X.J., Keating, A., Devillers, J., & Sherman, M. (1989). Tissue-specific activity of heterologous viral promoters in primary rat hepatocytes and Hep G2 cells. *Hepatology, 10(5),* 781–787.

Felgner, P.L., Gadek, T.R., Holm, M., Roman, R., Chan, H.W., Wenz, M., Northrop, J.P., Ringold, G.M., & Danielsen, M. (1987). Lipofection: A highly efficient, lipid-mediated DNA transfection procedure. *Proceedings of the National Academy of Science USA, 84,* 7413–7417.

Fineman, I., Hovda, D.A., Smith, M., Yoshino, A., & Becker, D.P. (1993). Concussive brain injury is associated with a prolonged accumulation of calcium: A ^{45}Ca autoradiographic study. *Brain Research, 624,* 94–102.

Forno, L.S., Sternberger, L.A., Sternberger, N.H., Strefling, A.M., Swanson, K., & Eng, L.F. (1986). Reaction of Lewy bodies with antibodies to phosphorylated and non-phosphorylated neurofilaments. *Neuroscience Letters, 64,* 253–258.

Franklin, J.L., & Johnson, E.M. (1992). Suppression of programmed neuronal death by sustained elevation of cytoplasmic calcium. *Trends in Neurosciences, 12,* 501–508.

Friedman, W.J., Ernfors, P., & Persson, H. (1991). Transient and persistent expression of NT-3/BDNF mRNA in the rat brain during postnatal development. *Journal of Neuroscience, 11,* 1577–1584.

Gall, C., & Isackson, P.J. (1989). Limbic seizures increase neuronal production of messenger RNA for nerve growth factor. *Science, 245,* 758–761.

Gall, C., & Lauterborn, J. (1992). The dentate gyrus: A model system for studies of neurotrophin regulation. *Epilepsy Research Suppl., 7,* 171–185.

Gall, C., Murray, K., & Isackson, P. (1991b). Kainic acid-induced seizures stimulate increased expression of nerve growth factor mRNA in rat hippocampus. *Molecular Brain Research, 9,* 113–123.

Gall, C., Lauterborn, J., Bundman, M., Murray, K., & Isackson, P. (1991a). Seizures and the regulation of neurotrophic factor and neuropeptide gene expression in brain. *Epilepsy Research Suppl., 4,* 225–245.

Gennarelli, T., Thibault, I., & Tipperman, R. (1989). Axonal injury in the optic nerve: A model stimulating diffuse axonal injury in the brain. *Journal of Neurosurgery, 67,* 24–53.

Ghosh, A., Carnahan, J., & Greenberg, M.E. (1994). Requirement for BDNF in activity-dependent survival of cortical neurons. *Science, 263,* 1618–1623.

Giordano, T., Howard, T.H., Coleman, J., Sakamoto, K., & Howard, B.H. (1991). Isolation of a population of transiently transfected quiscent and senescent cells by magnetic affinity cell sorting. *Experimental Cell Research, 992,* 993–997.

Gorman, L.K., Fu, K., Hovda, D.A., Becker, D.P., & Katayama, Y. (1989). Analysis of acetylcholine release following concussive brain injury in the rat. *Journal of Neurotrauma, 6,* 203–207.

Greenberg, M.E., Greene, L., & Ziff, E.B. (1985). Nerve growth factor and epidermal growth factor induces rapid transient changes in proto-oncogene transcription in PC 12 cells. *Journal of Biological Chemistry, 260,* 14101–14110.

Gwag, B.J., Sessler, F., Kimmerer, K., & Springer, J. (1994). Neurotrophic factor mRNA expression in dentate gyrus is increased following angular cundle transection. *Brain Research, 647,* 23–29.

Hamm, R.J., Dixon, C.E., Gbadebo, D.M., Singha, A.K., Jenkins, L.W., Lyeth, B.G., & Hayes, R.L. (1992). Cognitive deficits following traumatic brain injury produced by controlled cortical impact. *Journal of Neurotrauma, 9,* 11–20.

Hashimoto, Y., Kawatsura, H., Shiga, Y., Furukawa, S., & Shigeno, T. (1992). Significance of nerve growth factor content levels after transient forebrain ischemia in gerbils. *Neuroscience Letters, 139,* 45–46.

Hayes, R.L., Jenkins, L.W., & Lyeth, B.G. (1992). Neurotransmitter-mediated mechanisms of traumatic brain injury. *Journal of Neurotrauma, 9,* S173-S187.

Hayes, R.L., Yang, K., Whitson, J.S., Xue, J.J., Kampfl, A., Mu, X.S., Zhao, X., Faustinella, F., & Clifton, G.L. (1995). Rescue of injury-induced neurofilament loss by BDNF gene transfection in primary septo-hippocampal cell cultures. *Neuroscience Letters, 191,* 121–125.

Hefti, F. (1986). Nerve growth factor promotes survival of septal cholinergic neurons after fimbral transections. *Journal of Neuroscience, 8,* 2155–2162.

Hengerer, B., Lindholm, D., Heumann, R., Ruther, U., Wagner, E.F., & Thoenen, H. (1990). Lesion-induced increase in nerve growth factor mRNA is mediated by *c-fos. Proceedings of the National Academy of Science USA, 87,* 3899–3903.

Herrera, D.G., Maysinger, D., Gadient, R., Boeckh, C., Otten, U., & Cuello, A.C. (1993). Spreading depression induces *c-fos*-like immunoreactivity and NGF mRNA in the rat cerebral cortex. *Brain Research, 602,* 99–103.

Hofer, M., Pagliusi, S.R., Hohn, A., Leibrock, J., & Barde, Y.A. (1990). Regional distribution of brain-derived neurotrophic factor mRNA. *EMBO J, 19,* 2459–2464.

Hoffman, P.N., & Lasek, R.J. (1975). The slow component of axonal transport: Identification of major structural polypeptides of the axon and there generality among mammalian neurons. *Journal of Cellular Biology, 66,* 351–366.

Hohn, A., Leibrock, J., Bailey, K., & Bard, Y.A. (1990). Identification and characterization of a novel member of the nerve growth factor/brain-derived neurotrophic factor family. *Nature, 344,* 339–341.

Horwitz, M.S. (1990). Adenoviidade and their replication. In B.N. Fields and D.M. Knipe (Eds.), *Fields neurology* (2nd ed.) (pp. 1679–1721). New York: Raven Press.

Hug, P., & Sleight, R.G. (1991). Liposomes for the transformation of eukaryotic cells. *Biochem. et Biophys. Acta, 1097,* 1–17.

Hyman, C., Hofer, M., Barde, Y.A., Juhasz, M., Yancopoulos, G.D., Squinto, S.P., & Lindsay, R.M. (1991). BDNF is a neurotrophic factor for dopaminergic neurons of the substantia nigra. *Nature, 350,* 230–232.

Inuzuka, T., Tamura, A., Sato, S., Kirino, T., Toyoshima, I., & Miyatake, T. (1990a). Suppressive effect of E-64c on ischemic degradation of cerebral proteins following occlusion of the middle cerebral artery in rats. *Brain Research, 526,* 177–179.

Inuzuka, T., Tamura, A., Sato, S., Kirino, T., Yanagisawa, K., Toyoshima, I., & Miyatake, T. (1990b). Changes in the concentrations of cerebral proteins following occlusion of the middle cerebral artery in rats. *Stroke, 21,* 917–922.

Ip, N.Y., Li, Y., Yancopoulos, G.D., & Lindsay, R.M. (1993). Cultured hippocampal neurons show response to BDNF, NT-3, and NT-4, but not NGF. *Journal of Neuroscience, 13,* 3394–3405.

Isackson, P.J., Huntsman, M.M., Murray, M.D., & Gall, C.M. (1991). BDNF mRNA expression is increased in adult rat forebrain after limbic seizures: Temporal patterns of induction distinct from NGF. *Neuron, 6,* 937–948.

Jensen, A.M., & Chiu, S.W. (1990). Fluorescence measurement of changes in intracellular calcium induced by excitatory amino acids in cultured cortical astrocytes. *Journal of Neuroscience, 10,* 1165–1175.

Johnson, G.V.W., Litersky, J.M., & Jope, R.S. (1991). Degradation of microtubule-associated protein 2 (MAP2) and brain spectrin by calpain: a comparative study. *Journal of Neurochemistry, 56,* 1630–1638.

Johnson, P.A., Yoshida, K., Gage, F.H., & Friedmann, T. (1992). Effects of gene transfer into cultured CNS neurons with a replication-defective herpes simplex virus type 1 vector. *Molecular Brain Research, 12,* 95–102.

Julien, J.-P., & Mushynski, W.E. (1982). Multiple phosphorylation sites in mammalian neurofilament polypeptides. *Journal of Biological Chemistry, 257,* 10467–10470.

Kaku, Y., Yonekawa, Y., Tsukahara, T., Ogata, N., Kimura, T., & Taniguchi, T. (1993). Alterations of a 200 kDa neurofilament in the rat hippocampus after forebrain ischemia. *Journal of Cerebral Blood Flow and Metabolism, 13,* 402–408.

Kamakura, K., Ishiura, S., Susuki, K., Sugita, H., & Takaku, F. (1985). Calcium-activated neutral protease in the peripheral nerve, which requires uM order Ca^{2+}, and its effect on the neurofilament triplet. *Journal of Neuroscience Research, 13,* 391–403.

Katayama, Y., Becker, D.P., Tamura, T., & Hovda, D.A. (1990). Massive increases extracellular potassium and the indiscriminate release of glutamate following concussive brain injury. *Journal of Neurosurgery, 73,* 889–900.

Katayama, Y., Kawamata, T., Tamura, T., Hovda, D.A., Becker, D.P., & Tsubokawa, T. (1991). Calcium-dependent glutamate release concomitant with massive potassium flux during cerebral ischemia *in vivo. Brain Research, 558,* 136–140.

Knüsel, B., Winslow, J.W., Rosenthal, A., Burton, L.E., Seid, D.P., Nikolics, K., & Hefti, F. (1991). Promotion of central cholinergic and dopaminergic neuron differentiation by brain-derived neurotrophic factor but not neurotrophin-3. *Proceedings of the National Academy of Sciences USA, 88,* 961–965.

Knüsel, B., Winslow, J.W., Rosenthal, A., Burton, L.E., Beck, K.D., Rabin, S., Nikolics, K., & Hefti, F. (1992). K-252b selectively potentiates cellular actions and trk tyrosine phosphorylation mediated by neurotrophin-3. *Journal of Neurochemistry, 59,* 715–722.

Kokaia, Z., Gunilla, G., Ringstedt, T., Bengzon, J., Kokaia, M., Siesjo, B.K., Persson, H., & Lindvall, O. (1993). Rapid increase of BDNF mRNA levels in cortical neurons following spreading depression: regulation by glutamatergic mechanism independent of seizure activity. *Molecular Brain Research, 19,* 277–286.

Kruijer, W., Schubert, D., & Verma, I.M. (1985). Induction of the proto-oncogene fos by nerve growth factor. *Proceedings of the National Academy of Sciences USA, 82,* 7330–7334.

Kudo, T., Takeda, M., Tanimukai, S., & Nishimura, T. (1993). Neuropathological changes in the gerbil brain after chronic hypoperfusion. *Stroke, 24,* 259–265.

Ladenheim, R.G., Lacroix, I., Foignant, Chaverot, N., Strosberg, A.D., & Couraud, P.O. (1993). Endothelins stimulate *c-fos* and nerve growth factor expression in astrocytes and astrocytoma. *Journal of Neurochemistry, 60,* 260–266.

Lee, K.S., Frank, S., Vanderklish, Arai, A., & Lynch, G. (1991). Inhibition of proteolysis protects hippocampal neurons from ischemia. *Proceedings of the National Academy Science USA, 88,* 7233–7237.

Legallasalle, G., Robert, J.J., Berrard, S., Ridoux, V., Stratford-Perricaudet, L.D., Perricaudet, M., & Mallet, J. (1993). An adenovirus vector for gene transfer into neurons and glia in the brain. *Science, 259,* 988–990.

Liem, R.K.H. (1993). Molecular biology of neuronal intermediate filaments. *Cell Biology, 5,* 12–16.

Lindsay, R.M., Thoenen, H., & Barde, Y.A. (1985). Placode and neural crest-derived sensory neurons are responsive at early developmental stages to brain-derived neurotrophic factor. *Developmental Biology, 112,* 319–328.

Lindvall, O., Ernfors, P., Bengzon, J., Kokaia, Z., Smith, M.L., Siesjo, B.K., & Persson, H. (1992). Differential regulation of mRNAs for nerve growth factor, brain derived neurotrophic factor, and neurotrophin 3 in the adult rat brain following cerebral ischemia and hypoglycemic coma. *Proceedings of the National Academy of Sciences, 89,* 648–652.

Lyeth, B.G., Jenkins, L.W., Hamm, R.J., Dixon, C.E., Phillips, L.L., Clifton, G.L., Young, H.F., & Hayes, R.L. (1990). Prolonged memory impairment in the absence of hippocampal cell death following traumatic brain injury in the rat. *Brain Research, 526,* 249–258.

MacGregor, G.R., & Caskey, C.T. (1989). Construction of plasmids that express E. coli beta-galactosidase in mammalian cells. *Nucleic Acids Research, 17,* 2365.

Maisonpierre, P.C., Belluscio, L., Squinto, S., Ip, N.Y., Furth, M.E., Lindsay, R.M., & Yancopoulos, G.D. (1990). Neurotrophin-3: A neurotrophic factor related to NGF and BDNF. *Science, 247,* 1446–1451.

Mattson, M.P., Dou, P., & Kater, S.B. (1988). Outgrowth-regulating actions of glutamate in isolated hippocampal pyramidal neurons. *Journal of Neurosciences, 8,* 2087–2100.

Mocchetti, I., De Bernardi, M.A., Szekely, A.M., Alho, H., Brooker, G., & Costa, E. (1989). Regulation of nerve growth factor biosynthesis by b-adrenergic receptor activation in astrocytoma cells: A potential role of *c-fos* protein. *Proceedings of National Academy of Sciences USA, 86,* 3891–3895.

Morgan, J.I., & Curran, T. (1991). Proto-oncogene transcription factors and epilepsy. *Trends in Pharmacological Sciences, 12,* 343–349.

Nabel, E.G., Gordon, D., Yang, Z.Y., Xu, L., San, H., Plautz, G.E., Wu, B.Y., Gao, Huang, L., & Nabel, G.J. (1992). Gene transfer *in vivo* with DNA liposome complexes, lack of autoimmunity and gonadal localization. *Human Gene Therapy, 3,* 649–656.

Nakamura, M., Araki, M., Oguro, K. & Masuzawa, T. (1992). Differential distribution of 68 kD and 200 kD neurofilament proteins in the gerbil hippocampus and their early distributional changes following transient forebrain ischemia. *Experimental Brain Research, 89,* 31–39.

Nilsson, P., Hillered, L., Olsson, Y., Sheardown, M.J., & Hansen, A.J. (1993). Regional changes interstitial K+ and Ca2+ levels following cortical compression contusion trauma in rats. *Journal of Cerebral Blood Flow Metabolism, 13,* 183–192.

Nixon, A., & Marcotta, C.A. (1984). Degradation of neurofilament proteins by purified human brain cathespin D. *Journal of Neurochemistry, 43,* 507–516.

Nixon, A., & Shiag, R.K. (1991). Neurofilament phosphorylation: A new look at regulation and function. *TINS, 14,* 501–506.

Ogata, N., Yonekawa, Y., Taki, W., Kanngi, R., Murachi, T., Hamakubo, T., & Kikuchi, H. (1989). Degradation of neurofilament protein in cerebral ischemia. *Journal of Neurosurgery, 70,* 103–107.

Peng, Z.C., Chen, S., Fusco, M., Vantini, G., & Bentivoglio, M. (1993). Fos induction by nerve growth factor in the adult rat brain. *Brain Research, 632,* 57–67.

Perlmutter, L.S., Siman, R., Gall, C., Seubert, P., Baudry, M., & Lynch G. (1988). The ultrastructural localization of calcium activated protease "Calpain" in rat brain. *Synapse, 2,* 79–88.

Pietrini, V., Danielli D., Bevilacqua, P., & Lechi, A. (1993). Panencephalo-pathic type of Cruetzfeld-Jacob Disease with neuropathological features similar to Pick's Disease. *Clinical Neuropathology, 12,* 1–6.

Poltorak, M., Stevens, J.R., Freed, W.J., & Casanova, M.F. (1988). The expression of phosphorylated neurofilament epitopes in human brains. *Brain Research, 475,* 328–332.

Posmantur, R., Hayes, R.L., Dixon, C.E., & Taft, W.C. (1994). Neurofilament 68 and neurofilament 200 protein levels decrease after traumatic brain injury (TBI). *Journal of Neurotrauma, 11,* 533–545.

Posmantur, R., Taft, W.C., Dixon, C.E., Liu, S.J., & Hayes, R.L. (1994b). Acute structural derangements of cortical neurons in the rat following traumatic brain injury (TBI): An examination of neurofilament (NF) immunofluorescence. *Neurotrauma Society Abstracts.*

Posmantur, R., Kampfl, A., Liu, S.J., Heck, K., Taft, W.C., Clifton, G.L., & Hayes, R.L. (in press). Cytoskeletal derangements of cortical neuronal processes 3 hrs. after traumatic brain injury in rats: An immunofluorescence study. *Journal of Neuropathology and Experimental Neurology.*

Rocamora, N., Palacios, J.M., & Mengod, G. (1992). Limbic seizures induce a differential regulation of the expression of nerve growth factor, brain-derived neurotrophic factor and neurotrophin-3, in the rat hippocampus. *Molecular Brain Research, 13,* 27–33.

Roessler, B.J., & Davidson, B.L. (1994). Direct plasmid mediated transfection of adult murine brain cells *in vivo* using cationic liposomes. *Neuroscience Letters, 167,* 5–10.

Sambrook, J., Fritsch, E.F., & Maniatis, T. (1989). *Molecular Cloning* (2nd ed.) (pp. 18, 32). New York: Cold Spring Harbor Laboratory Press.

Sautter, J., Schwartz, M., Duvdevani, R., & Sabel, B.A. (1991). GM_1 ganglioside treatment reduces visual deficits after graded crush on the rat optic nerve. *Brain Research, 565,* 23–33.

Schalepfer, W.W., & Zimmerman, U.P. (1985b). Mechanisms underlying the neuronal response to ischemic injury. Calcium-activated proteolysis of neurofilaments. *Progress in Brain Research, 63,* 185–196.

Schalepfer, W.W., Lee, W., Lee, C., & Zimmerman, U.P. (1985a). An immunoblot study of neurofilament degradation *in situ* and during calcium-activated proteolysis. *Journal of Neurochemistry, 44,* 502–509.

Sharp, F.R., Gonzalez, M.F., Hisanage, K., Mobley, W.C., & Sagar, S.M. (1989). Induction of the *c-fos* gene product in the rat forebrain following cortical lesions and NGF injections. *Neuroscience Letters, 100,* 117–122.

Shaw, G. (1986). Neurofilaments: Abundant but mysterious structures. *Bioessays, 4,* 161–166.

Shozuhara, H., Onodera, H., Katoh-Semba, R., Kato, K., Yamasaki, Y., & Kogure, K. (1992). Temporal profiles of nerve growth factor beta-subunit level in rat brain regions after transient ischemia. *Journal of Neurochemistry, 59,* 175–180.

Siman, R., Baudry, M., & Lynch, G. (1984). Brain fodrin: Substrate for calpain 1, an endogenous calcium-activated protease. *Proceedings of the National Academy of Sciences USA, 81,* 3572–3576.

Smith, M.A., Makino, S., Kvetnansky, R., & Post, R.M. (1995). Stress and glucocorticoids affect the expression of brain-derived neurotrophic factor and neurotrophin-3 mRNAs in the hippocampus. *Journal of Neurosciences, 15,* 1768–1777.

Sternberger, L.A., & Sternberger, N.H. (1983). Monoclonal antibodies distinguish phosphorylated and nonphosphorylated forms of neurofilaments *in situ*. *Proceedings of the National Academy of Sciences USA, 80,* 6126–6130.

Sternberger, L.A., Sternberger, N.H., & Ulrich, J. (1985). Aberrant neurofilament phosphorylation in Alzheimer's disease. *Proceedings of the National Academy of Sciences USA, 82,* 4274–4276.

Szatkowski, M., & Attwell, D. (1994). Triggering and execution of neuronal death in brain ischemia: Two phases of glutamate release by different mechanisms. *Trends in Neurosciences, 17,* 359–365.

Taft, W.C., Yang, K., Dixon, C.E., & Hayes, R.L. (1992). Microtubule-associated protein 2 levels decrease in hippocampus following traumatic brain injury. *Journal of Neurotrauma, 9,* 281–290.

Taft, W.C., Yang, K., Dixon, C.E., Clifton, G.L., & Hayes, R.L. (1993). Hypothermia attenuates the loss of hippocampal microtubule-associated protein 2 (MAP2) levels following traumatic brain injury. *Journal of Cerebral Blood Flow and Metabolism, 13,* 796–802.

Takeda, A., Onodera, H., Sugimoto, A., Kogure, K., Obinata, M., & Shibahara, S. (1993). Coordinated expression of messenger RNAs for nerve growth factor, brain-derived neurotrophic factor and neurophin-3 in the rat hippocampus following transient forebrain ischemia. *Neurosciences, 55,* 23–31.

Thompson, T.A., Gould, M.N., Burkholder, J.K., & Yang, N.S. (1993). Transient promoter activity in primary rat mammary epithelial cells evaluated using particle bombardment gene transfer. *In Vitro Cell Development Biology, 29A,* 165–170.

Towbin, H., Staehelin, T., & Gordan, J. (1979). Electrophoretic transfer of proteins from polyacrylamide gels to nitrocellulose sheets: Procedure and some applications. *Proceedings of the National Academy of Sciences USA, 76,* 4340–4354.

Troost, D., Seilevis T., De-Johng J., & Swaab, D. (1992). Neurofilament and glial alterations in the cerebral cortex in ALS. *Acta Neuropathologica, 84,* 664–673.

Ulrich, J., Probst, A., Langui, D., Anderson, B., & Brion, J. (1987). Cytoskeletal immuno-histochemistry of Alzheimer's dementia and related diseases: A study with monoclonal antibodies. *Pathology Immunology Research, 6,* 273–283.

Varon, S., & Conner, J.M. (1994). Nerve growth factor in CNS repair. *Journal of Neurotrauma, 11,* 473–486

Wang, S., Hamberger, A., Yang, Q., & Haglid, K.G. (1994). Changes in neurofilament protein NF-L and NF-H immunoreactivity following kainic acid-induced seizures. *Journal of Neurochemistry, 62,* 739–748.

Weiss, J., Hartley, D.M., Koh, J.Y., & Choi, D.W. (1993). AMPA receptor activation potentiates zinc neurotoxicity. *Neuron, 10,* 43–49.

Whitson, J.S., Kampfl, A., Zhao, X., Dixon, C.E., & Hayes, R.L. (in press). Brief potassium depolarization decreases levels of neurofilament proteins in CNS culture. *Brain Research.*

Wolf, D., Richter-Landsberg, C., Short, M.P., Cepko, C., & Breakfield, X.O. (1988). Retrovirus mediated gene transfer of beta-nerve growth factor into mouse pituitary line AtT-20. *Molecular Brain Med, 5,* 43–49.

Yaghmai, A., & Povlishock, J. (1992). Traumatically induced reactive change as visualized through the use of monoclonal antibodies targeted to neurofilament subunits. *Journal of Neuropathology and Experimental Neurology, 51,* 158–176.

Yang, K., Mu, S., Xue, J.J., Liu, P.K., Whitson, J., Salminen, A., Dixon, C.E., & Hayes, R.L. (1994a). Increased expression of *c-fos* gene and AP-1 transcription factor after cortical impact injury in rodent model. *Brain Research, 664,* 141–147.

Yang, K., Faustinella, F., Xue, J.J., Whitson, J.S., Kampfl, A., Mu, S., Zhao, X., Taglialatela, G., Perez-Polo, J.R., Clifton, G.L., & Hayes, R.L. (1994b). Sustained expression of functional nerve growth factor in primary septo-hippocampal cell cultures by liposome-mediated gene transfer. *Neuroscience Letters, 182,* 291–294.

_____ (1994c). Optimizing liposome-mediated gene transfer in primary rat septo-hippocampal cell cultures. *Neuroscience Letters, 182,* 287–290.

Yang, K., Mu, X., Xue, J.J., Perez-Polo, J.R., & Hayes, R.L. (in press). Regional and temporal profiles of *c-fos* and NGF mRNA expression in rat brain after lateral cortical impact injury. *Journal of Neuroscience Research.*

Yang, K., Mu, X., Yan, H., Xue, J.J., Iwamoto, Y., Liu, S.J., Dixon, C.E., & Hayes, R.L. (in press). Increased expression of BDNF but not NT-3 mRNA in rat brain after cortical impact injury. *Journal of Neuroscience Research.*

Zheng, M., & Heinrich, G. (1988). Structural and functional analysis of the promoter region of the nerve growth factor gene. *Molecular Brain Research, 3,* 133–140.

10 Neural Transplants

Manuel Portavella

Laboratorio de Psicobiología, Facultad de Psicología
Universidad de Seville, Seville, Spain

INTRODUCTION

The history of neural grafting in the nervous system began with differential vitality studies in living animals (dogs, cats, and rabbits) using the transplant of adult cortical tissue as an experimental tool (Thompson, 1890). Dunn (1917) also managed to graft newborn brain tissue into the brain of newborn animals, although he was essentially interested in establishing the viability of grafting. Many studies have been carried out since the turn of the century using a variety of animals (fish, amphibians, and mammals) and several types of tissue, including neural (peripheral nerves, embryonic tissues, cerebral cortex, fetal cells) and nonneural tissues (epithelial, glandular, tumoral).

There were primarily two aims motivating these studies (Das, 1990): on the one hand, the need to understand the underlying embryonic mechanisms of neural development, and, on the other, the interest in achieving host brain regeneration. A review of past and present experimental results shows a clear differentiation both in the effectiveness of techniques used and in neural graft viability and host response in several vertebrate phyla. Results of regeneration and neural grafting studies in the central nervous system (CNS) of nonmammalian vertebrates (amphibians and fish) is noteworthy when compared to results obtained in mammalian studies. For example, experimental results of regeneration in cut optical nerves of frogs (Sperry, 1944) found recovery of vision, and retinal inputs showed neurospecificity with certain targets in the optical tectum. Mammals cannot recover visual capacities in these conditions. Thus, the CNS of cold-blooded vertebrates shows high regenerative capacities. Cajal's findings (1914) had led him to consider these capacities in mammalian CNSs to be virtually nonexistent. However, work by Liu and

Chambers (1958) showed some degree of regeneration in mammalian CNSs to be irrefutable. Nevertheless, this regeneration becomes less significant when compared with the regenerative capacities of poiquilothermal CNS and mammalian peripheral nervous system (PNS).

It was not until the early 1970s that research results began to establish the conditions necessary for grafting into the mammalian brain with the demonstration of connectivity formation between fetal cell graft and host tissue in newborn animals (Lund & Hauschka, 1976). Björklund et al. (1976) demonstrated that developing central neural tissue grafted into the brain established efferent and afferent connections with the host brain. Björklund and Stenevi (1979) demonstrated the effectiveness of neural transplants in the partial recovery of functions.

Therefore, there is an intimate relation between neural transplant viability and the underlying processes of regeneration, development, and differentiation in the nervous system. In fact, a successful graft integration may be due to regenerative effects on host axons, graft proliferation, and differentiation in the host brain or graft-derived trophic effects. In most cases, a combination of these processes is involved in graft viability.

Fetal tissue is presently considered to be the most suitable material for transplantation. This is because once it is grafted, it goes through phases of neuroepithelial differentiation, promoting host tissue regeneration and possibly having a trophic effect.

TECHNIQUES, MODELS, AND CONDITIONS FOR NEURAL GRAFTING

The introduction of this chapter indicates the aims that promoted research into neural transplants. Today, researchers are concerned with another objective—the development of grafting techniques that can be used as therapy to treat human neurodegenerative diseases (Alzheimer's, Huntington's, Parkinson's, and motor diseases). While recognizing that there are many neural grafting models and considering important data from nonmammalian vertebrate studies, this chapter focuses on grafting techniques developed in mammals and in animal models of human diseases. It also looks at the prospects for the therapeutic use of present-day techniques in human diseases.

Grafting Techniques Developed in Animals

Studies performed in nonmammal vertebrates (Harrison, 1935; Detwiler, 1964) demonstrate that the most successful material for *in vivo* transplantation is embryonic tissue, and they also show that grafting is much more successful when the host is also an embryo. This is because nondifferentiated tissues allow greater integration of both graft and host. These reports suggest several conditions for promoting embryonic graft viability in both mammal and nonmammal hosts: (1) growing embryonic tissue is most successful, (2) it is needed to make a cavity size sufficient for promoting growth of the grafted solid tissue, and (3) it also needs direct contact between graft and host (Das, 1990). Several types of tissue have been grafted in mammals: (1) homologous adult cortical tissue (Saltykow, 1905; Nissl, 1911; Altobelli, 1914); (2) sympathetic ganglia for determining its viability and integration (Ranson, 1909; Ramón y Cajal, 1914; Tidd, 1932; Le Gros Clarck, 1943); (3) peripheral nerves for determining both integration and axonal regeneration (Tello, 1911), regeneration level (Le Gros Clarck 1943), or for using it as a permissive environmental path in which CNS fibers regenerate and grow along the peripheral nerve (Aguayo et al., 1984); (4) intraventriculary endocrine tissue (Flerko & Szentagotay, 1957); (5) intraparenchymaly tissue from epiphysis and thymus (Green,

1967); (6) neural and nonneural tissues for determining neural grafting effects on endocrine tissue (Krieger & Gibson, 1984; Sladek & Gash, 1984)); (7) fetal neural tissue in newborn animals (LeGros Clark, 1940); (8) fetal cells in suspension (Björklund et al., 1980); and (9) genetically modified cells (Rosenberg et al. 1988).

A cavity is needed in the host brain to place a solid piece of tissue; this procedure produces host injuries such as axotomy and cellular death, isolation from the blood system, and, in cavity borders, proliferating astrocytes that build an isolating bar between necrotic and whole tissue (gliosis). This glia scar is a nonpermissive barrier for host growing regenerating axons.

These experiments provide important information giving rise to questions on several subjects:

- What is the most appropriate technique for each transplant?
- Which kind of tissue should be used?
- What is the critical age for grafting for both the donor and the host?
- When is it the right time to carry out grafting?
- What environmental conditions promote graft viability, regeneration, and integration of both tissues?
- Is there a CNS immunological response against grafting?

Early adult cortical transplant studies were performed by piece extraction from donors. This piece might be replaced into a donor cavity (homograft or autograft), or it might be inserted into another co-specific animal (allograft). These experiments showed little or no regeneration because in extracted pieces, there was a high cellular death rate since the loss of blood irrigation meant lower nutrients and gaseous exchange. In the host, some growing cells were observed, but only on the limits of the cavity. This research into mammal transplants indicates that CNS adult grafting is not viable.

However, from Cajal's reports (1914), it has been demonstrated that pieces of adult PNS remain in the mammal brain in several conditions. Grafting of sympathetic ganglia is partially successful. These ganglia are enveloped in a connective capsule so that there is no contact between donor and host cells. In addition, no axon has been seen to go through a connective capsule or glial scar; there is no real integration. In the case of grafting portions of peripheral nerve, it has been reported that regeneration is restricted to the region surrounding the point where the nerve is inserted; this is due to both axonal trauma and specially nonpermissive environmental characteristics of the CNS that are very restrictive. When using the peripheral nerve as a permissive environmental tool, CNS axonal regeneration is promoted. Davis and Aguayo (1981) managed to achieve partial regeneration between natural targets using the peripheral nerve as a bridge to allow axonal regeneration from the medulla oblongata to the spinal cord and vice-versa.

The grafting of fetal nervous tissue is considered to be the most successful. Grafting is said to be a success when the graft survives in the host brain, induces host regeneration, and improves physiological and behavioral deficits of a trauma or neurodegenerative illness (Stein, 1988). Neuroblasts are transplanted with success (the cells have not yet been fully differentiated), other differentiated elements are also anatomically integrated in the host brain, and grafted tissue keeps its structural characteristics. In other words, if we implant a portion of embryonic cerebellar cortex in an adult brain, it tends to conform to a cerebral cortex structure (Das, 1974). Fetal grafts survive in the animal for life. According to Das (1975), embryonic neocortical tissue undergoes stages typical of embryonic development, such as proliferation, migration, differentiation, and shaping of a rudimentary laminar cortex.

Another way to insert neural tissue is to inject a suspension of fetal cells into a specific region (Figure 10.1): (1) a piece is extracted from a desired region, (2) the cells of the piece are chemically (trypsin) and mechanically separated, and (3) from this mixture of fetal cells, a volume of fetal cells in suspension is extracted. These cells can then be injected into deeper forebrain regions (Björklund, 1983). This technique has several advantages over the insertion of a solid piece. In fact, before grafting a piece, it is necessary to make a cavity (traumatic lesion), and the deeper the region the piece is to be grafted into, the larger the lesion needed (Figure 10.1). In the case of the injection of fetal cells, the only damage caused is that of the syringe's needle.

Other techniques that have been developed recently involve the use of genetically modified cells (fibroblasts and immortalized cells from neuroblasts, gliomas, and nonneural tissues) to produce several substances that may induce tissue regeneration or enhance neurotransmission. These substance-secreting cells may be considered as biological "micropumps," which secrete substances more constantly than artificial secretory structures (intracerebral polymer capsules). By using various genetic manipulation techniques, certain cells can be programmed to produce, for example, the nerve growth factor (NGF) (Rosemberg et al., 1988). This factor can increase the survival rate of cholinergic neurons after a lesion; it might be fair to assume that it could have similar effects on cells threatened with the lethal effects of a neurodegenerative illness. These cells may also balance deficits in neurotransmitter levels. For example, genetically modified fibroblasts can produce the tyrosine-hydrolase enzyme; the activity of this enzyme produces L-dopa, and this substance improves the deficits of dopamine in Parkinson's disease (Fisher et al., 1991). Immortalized cells can also produce L-dopa and improve drug-induced behavioral deficits in animal models of Parkinson's disease (Wolff et al., 1989; Horellou et al., 1990). However, the drawback is that immortalized cells can give rise to tumors.

Neural Immunological Response and Grafting

From early studies into grafting, the CNS has been considered as an immunologically privileged system. Raju and Grogan (1977) even looked for immunologically privileged places to perform graft trials. This and other research demonstrated that neural and nonneural tissues (epithelial, endocrine, and muscular) were able to develop in host brains (Das 1990). Green (1943, 1967), using embryonic tissue from the kidney, pituitary gland, or thymus, reported that both isografts (tissue grafted between animals from the same strain) and xenografts (donor tissue grafted from a different species) survive and differentiate in the brain. The reason for this permissibility may be that these tissues are enveloped in a connective capsule, which impedes close contact with the host tissue and, as a result, this makes sensitization more difficult. Having said this, immunological rejection against xenografts that probably did not have this protection has been proven (Das, 1990).

Consideration of the CNS as an area with incomplete immunological protection may be based on (1) the brain having little or no relation with the lymphatic system, (2) the existence of a selective barrier between circulatory systems and the CNS (hematoencephalic barrier), (3) the presence of a connective capsule enveloping nonneural grafted tissues (documented in most research published on the subject), and (4) a poor expression of major histocompatibility complex (MHC), essentially expressed by the glias.

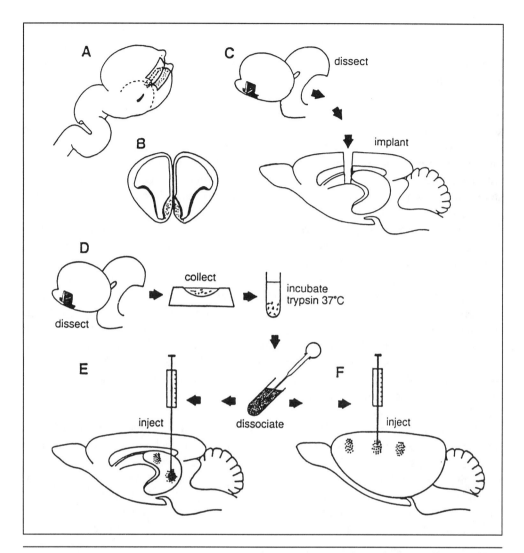

Figure 10.1: Septal transplantation techniques. (**A**) tissue rich in acetylcholine (ACh) (tinted area) is dissected from ventral forebrain area of the embryonic brain, taken 15–16 days of gestation age. (**B**) a coronal section through the rostral forebrain shows the ventromedial area containing the developing ACh neurons of septal and diagonal bands included in the dissection. (**C**) the transplants may be made by implanting "solid" pieces of tissue into an appropriate cavity in the host brain, such as through the fimbria-fornix where the graft tissue can be positioned immediately adjacent to the septal pole of the deafferented hippocampus. (**D**) alternatively, the graft tissue from many embryos can be pooled, digested in trypsin, washed, and mechanically dissociated to form a cell suspension. The tissue is injected stereotaxically in microliter aliquots into alternative target sites in the adult host brain, such as (**E**) the hippocampus or (**F**) neocortex. From Dunnett. Cholinergic grafts, memory and aging. *TINS, 14,* 311–376.

However, the CNS cannot be considered as a completely immunologically privileged place. In fact, immunological response may be a serious impediment to neural tissue being grafted from animals of the same (allograft) or different (xenograft) species. When the cavity allowing the graft insertion into the brain is made, blood vessels are broken that enable contact between host lymphocytes and donor tissue, and this contact may set off the immunological response. Moreover, several cellular components from the CNS (astrocytes, microglia, and endothelial cells) express certain substances involved in the immunological response (e.g., MHC). It has also been shown that when the host is in contact with donor antigens some days before grafting, the grafts are speedily rejected (Medawar, 1948). The more genetically different the donor tissue, the more speedily rejected the immunological response, something that happens within 20 days using xenografts (Sloan et al., 1991). The best evidence of the existence of this immune response is based on research carried out with animals that are immunodeficient or whose immune system is still developing. For example, grafts of neural tissue from rats survive without immune rejection in the brain of immunodeficient mice. The most revealing studies have been carried out grafting neural tissue from mice into the brain of newborn rats; they reported the survival of donor tissue. However, in the same animals, an immunological response could be provoked if tracts of the brain were injured, which, in turn, could activate glial-related immunological mechanisms and also disrupt the haematoencephalic barrier (Sloan et al., 1991).

In human grafting research, some partially developed techniques exist for protecting the graft against immune response, including immunosuppressor treatment, monoclonal antibodies treatment, and the selection of nonimmunogenic cells for grafting. Immunosuppressor treatment is the most widely used, but prolonged treatment can produce harmful effects. Monoclonal antibody techniques may be used to block certain molecules involved in the immunological response of T-lymphocytes. The last group of experiments would involve the preselection of embryonic neural cells as a result of their incapacity to produce MHC. This could give rise to the allografts and xenografts that were not rejected by the patient (Bartlett et al., 1990).

In summary, we could say (1) the CNS is immunogenic, (2) data indicating a poor immune response could well be related to the absence of contact between donor and host (connective capsule and glial scar), (3) in the CNS, there are several cells capable of producing MHC, (4) a lower level of immune response is related to the greater level of genetical identity of graft and host antigens, (5) extracting the glia, which produce MHCs, from the tissue to be grafted could minimize the risk of graft rejection (Sloan et al, 1991), and, finally, (6) the use of immunosuppressors is necessary, for the moment at least.

Conditions for Central Neural Grafting

The survival of a piece of neural tissue graft in the CNS depends on several conditions. The place where it is grafted must involve a fast vascularization (pia mater, ependymal canal, or ventricular choroid plexus) as the grafted piece needs rapid blood support for its survival. It must be exposed to the circulation of cerebrospinal liquid. This is why some graft trials are performed in the anterior eye chamber. Additionally, the natural or mechanically made graft insertion cavity must be large enough to allow the graft to grow. If the graft is made up of fetal cells in suspension, it may be placed in any region of the brain or spinal parenchyma. Graft size is also important, because if it is excessively large, blood support level and other variables may not be sufficient to allow the viability of most of the graft cells.

Graft age is also a very important factor. Grafting of tissue pieces carried out in rat and mice models showed a greater graft survival rate with fetal or newborn donor tissue. Generally, when the tissue is a week or more old, it is difficult for it to survive, and similarly adult tissue does not survive. Therefore, it is preferable to carry out grafts with fetal tissue. In embryonic development, not all tissues go through the same stages at the same time, so the time of extraction will depend on the type of material to be grafted (e.g., 19 days old for cortical cells and 16 days old for substantia nigra cells [Stein, 1988]). The right moment for extraction and grafting donor tissue is when the last cellular division and neuronal migration takes place, but this must happen before the axons have time to form extensive connections (Björklund, 1987).

The age of the host is also very important. It has been shown that in rats, the best moment is immediately after birth (newborn individuals). This is because a certain indifferentiation that facilitates reciprocal integration still exists in newborn individuals. It is clear that the older the host, the less effective the graft. Immature brains have fewer requirements than the adult brain, which is why they are more suited to grafting (placing, cavity space, and size).

With respect to techniques for graft insertion, it is necessary to make a cavity in the host brain to allow the insertion of a solid piece. In other words, a lesion is made resulting in axotomy, cellular death, glial scar shaping on the edges of the lesion, the release of substances into the environment (e.g., trophic factors and cell adhesion molecules), interactions between the oligodendrocyte surface, and growth cones and degenerative processes. All of these processes can interfere with graft viability. With so many things going on, it is vital to know just the right moment to graft after making the cavity (Stein, 1988). Nieto-Sampedro and Cotmant (1985) and Nieto-Sampedro et al. (1982) showed that if the graft is carried out 7–10 days after making the cavity, it is more viable than if the graft is done in under 7 days. A reason for this difference is that critical time is needed to produce a certain and necessary amount of trophic factors that create a permissive environment for graft viability, its growth, and, possibly, its integration (Nieto-Sampedro, 1988). This question has been tested by Stein et al. evaluating performance in a spatial discrimination task of rats (Labbe et al., 1983), which compared the performance of lesioned groups (frontal cortical lesion), sham operated groups, and others lesioned and grafted with 19-day-old (E19) fetal cortical cells. They were divided into 4 groups: grafting at 7 days, 14 days, 30 days, and 60 days after the lesion. Results showed clearly that performance was better in the 7- and 14-day groups than in the other two groups (30 and 60 days after), with the latter two producing no improvement at all (Figure 10.2). In the case of suspended fetal cell grafts, the same requirements exist in relation to the age of both host and donor tissues.

The cells used as "micropumps" need to meet certain conditions. Gage et al. (1987 and 1991) has set out ideal criteria:

1. they must be easy to get at and must be available in large quantities.
2. they must be viable *in vitro* cells and need to proliferate to allow the insertion of genetically-derived material.
3. they should survive indefinitely once grafted but should stop growing after the transplant (no tumoral processes).
4. they must be harmless "per se" and not interfere with host CNS functions.
5. if possible, they should not be immunogenic cells and, therefore, not require immunosuppression.

Cells from neuroblastoma (NS20 Y cell) capable of producing L-dopa have been tested successfully in Parkinsonian animal models with improvements in apomorphine-induced effects (turning behavior), which are provoked in nigral lesioned animals (6-hydroxydopamine is a neurotoxic against dopaminergic cells) (Horellou et al., 1990). Cells derived from tumors after grafting have a high probability of producing tumoral

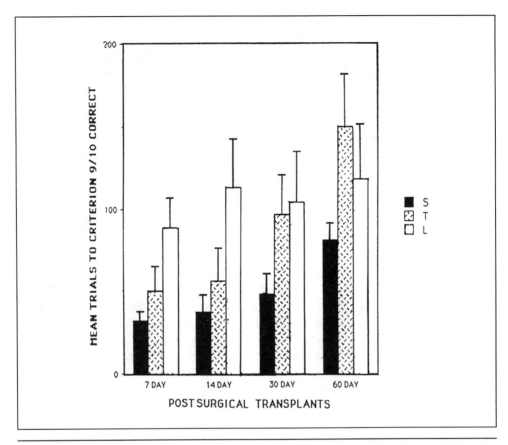

Figure 10.2: Trials to criteria on partial alternation task in rats with bilateral frontal cortex lesions give sham operations or transplants 7, 14, 30, or 60 days after the initial surgery. Black = sham-operated animals; hatched bars = the performance of rats with E19 frontal tissue transplants; gray bars = the rats with lesions only (modified from Stein, 1988).

processes. However, some studies demonstrate the effectiveness of antimitotic agents (mitomicin C), which produce amitotic cells from neuroblastoma used in grafting experiments (Gash et al., 1986). However, these cells continue to present many problems, apart from the continuous immunosuppression treatment.

Primary autologous fibroblasts seem to be the best material for transplantation. They can be obtained in large quantities from skin substrate from the same patient (the immunogenicity problem is reduced), they proliferate easily *in vitro*, and it seems that they stop growing following grafting. Essentially, two kinds of fibroblasts have been tested (Gage et al., 1991); one produces NFG, and the other carries the tyrosine-hydrolase (TH) gene that can produce L-dopa.

NEURAL GRAFT FUNCTIONS IN CNS

The clinical aim is to use the graft as a treatment that will improve symptoms without causing secondary effects. Neurodegenerative diseases involve cellular death and the loss of afferences and efferences.

It has been proven experimentally that the results of grafting can vary depending on the kind of neurotransmitter, neurotrophic factors, place, and graft conditions. In fact, the graft promotes regeneration of CNS neurites. Grafting studies of fetal tissue rich in both acetylcholine in the hippocampus and dopamine in the striatum of rats show a partial recovery of circuits. The degree of behavioral recovery depends on suitable graft placing and, therefore, reinnervation (Björklund & Stenevi, 1985, 1984).

Dunnet et al. (1982) showed that after the section of the septohippocampal connection, fetal grafts of septal cells (cholinergic cells) in the section point are integrated in the host hippocampus and recover the dentritic connection pattern of cholinergic cells. The animals can also perform a spatial discrimination task in a T-maze. The lesion of the septohippocampal connection impairs task performance.

To find out whether task performance improvements following grafting are mediated by graft-derived neurotrophic factors, Stein et al. (1988) carried out an experiment in which rats performed both a spatial navigation task in a water maze and a spatial alternation task in a T-maze. Animals lesioned in the frontal cortex and later grafted at 19 days learned to perform both tasks. Grafted animals which then had the graft extracted by aspiration after the original acquisition learning performed the task in the same time as the animals still with the graft (Figure 10.3). This study suggests that there is a graft-derived, restorative trophic effect on host tissue.

Grafts also show neurospecificity. Labbe et al. (1983) report that a rat with a fetal frontal cortical graft in a frontal cortical region (homotopic graft) showed behavioral recovery in a spatial discrimination task but did not show any learning improvement if the graft was from the cerebellar cortex (heterotopic graft) (Figure 10.4). Other experiments have been carried out recently (Escobar et al., 1994) in aversive conditioned taste tasks demonstrating different specificity between several cerebral cortical regions, with the only group showing any behavioral recovery being that of animals with a homotopic graft in combination with the NGF in the insular cortex.

Improvements after grafting may occur for several reasons: (1) grafted cells integrate (Sunde et al., 1984) and promote functional recovery (Dunnet et al., 1982), (2) the graft promotes the regeneration or support of host tissue (Fisher et al., 1991; Stein, 1988), and (3) a combination of the first and second reasons exists in most cases.

ANIMAL MODELS OF HUMAN DISEASES: THE EFFECTS OF GRAFTS ON PHYSIOLOGICAL AND BEHAVIORAL IMPROVEMENTS

Parkinson's Syndrome

Models are based on the selective lesion of dopaminergic neurons from the striatum, since part of the disease's impairments are related to the degeneration of the dopaminergic path from the substantia nigra to the striatum. Toxic substances that kill dopaminergic neurons are used; 6-hydroxydopamine (6-OHDA) is used in rat and nonhuman primate experiments, and 1-methyl-4-phenyl-1,2,3,6-tetrahydropyridine (MPTP) is used in non-human primate models. In rats, it is very difficult to distinguish the caudate nucleus of the putamen. This is not a problem in monkeys where it is easily distinguishable (Sinden et al., 1992).

From the grafting of both adrenal medullar cells, which have tyrosine-hydrolase activity (produce L-dopa), and fetal cells from the substantia nigra, which produce

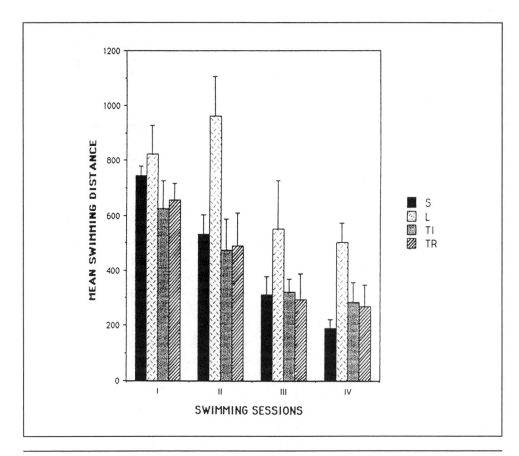

Figure 10.3: Spatial navigation performance in the water maze means swimming distance was recorded over sessions represented by roman numerals for animal with sham operations (black bars), lesions alone (hatched bars), transplants intact at the time of testing (gray bars), or transplants removed (diagonal lines) prior to testing. These data show that animals with lesions alone are impaired during training sessions, but those that had transplants for several months prior to testing were able to locate the submerged platform in the task of water. More importantly, even those animals with transplants intact at the time of testing from both groups were better than their lesions-alone counterparts (from Stein, 1988).

dopamine, diverse and stimulating results have been obtained. Grafting of substantia nigra pieces into the caudate nucleus improved motor deficits in monkeys previously treated with MPTP (Taylor et al., 1991). Likewise, grafts of fetal cells in dopamine-rich suspensions not only promote motor improvements but also improve the performance of motor skill tasks like grasping and reaching (Annett et al., 1991). Also, in the Parkinson's model using Rhesus monkeys, after autologous grafting from the adrenal medulla, the pot-sprouting of dopaminergic fibers has been correlated with improvements in drug-induced responses (turning behavior). After 10 months, several sham-operated control and operated monkeys lost grafted cells, and the postmortem study revealed an axonal sprouting of dopaminergic cells from the accumbens nucleus to the cavity or grafting site. In later experiments, anatomical analyses after six months with both fetal dopaminergic grafts (Bamkiewicz et al., 1990) and nondopaminergic grafts from cerebellar or spinal tissue (Ibid., 1991) showed similar results. These results may indicate a graft-derived

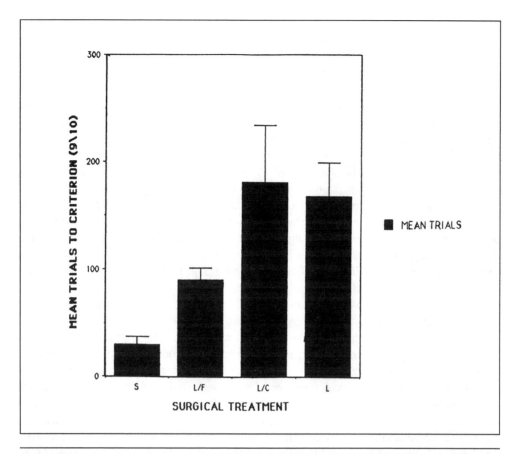

Figure 10.4: Average trials to criteria and standard errors on spatial alternation learning. Adult rats received operations (S) or bilateral frontal cortex lesions followed/days later by transplants of E19 frontal cortex (L/F9) or E19 cerebellar tissue (L/C). The L/F group performed the learned alternation significantly better than the L/C group or those with lesions alone. (Modified from Stein, 1988).

trophic effect promoting the sprouting of dopaminergic fibers. *In vitro* studies have demonstrated the effects of several trophic factors in dopaminergic cells survival. Brain-derived neurotrophic factor (BNDF) enhanced cell survival and protected it against the toxic effects of MPTP's metabolites (Hyman et al., 1991). Another experiment showed that BNDF and b-FGF (basic Fibroblast Growth Factor) enhanced neurotransmitter storing activity (Knusel et al., 1991). These data support the trophic effect theory. In fact, in rat experiments, it was shown that adrenal medulla grafting, together with NGF infusion, promoted survival and aided the functional effects of the graft (Strömberg et al., 1985).

Nikkhah et al. (1994), in an experimental Parkinsonian rat model, achieved an increase in the survival of grafted fetal nigral cells and the promotion of a fuller striatal reinervation using a micrografting technique, reaching the point of grafting 450,000 cells in many places of the striatum. Enhancing the graft's number may enhance graft effectiveness. Experimental results demonstrate that the graft promotes physiological and behavioral improvements if it is placed near the denervated site. This does not happen in more distant zones (e.g., ventral mesencephalum), where it would be desirable in order to recompose the original neural system because the distance within the CNS is too great.

It should also be said that grafted dopaminergic cells integrate poorly in host brain tissue (Lindvall, 1991; Gage et al., 1992).

Alzheimer's Disease or Senile Dementia

Degeneration of the cholinergic system and memory impairments are two characteristic of Alzheimer's. The disease is also related to the aging process and the loss of learning capacity. However, there are also many symptoms not related to cholinergic degeneration, so research has catered to this multiplicity. The majority of studies carried out involve lesions in the septo-hippocampal system, which is involved in memory and learning processes and is also very rich in cholinergic activity. This area of research uses animal models with old rats, cognitive impairment rats, and rats with excitotoxic lesions (Lindvall, 1991). The experiments with old rat models have been carried out using learning paradigms such as spatial learning (T-maze and Morris water maze), avoidance, and motor coordination tasks showing that animal task performance was related to the grafting of one or several neurotransmitters (Dunnett, 1991). Nigral grafts rich in dopamine improved motor coordination deficits in old rats (Gage et al., 1983). Septal grafts rich in cholinergic cells inserted into the hippocampus improved task performance in the water maze (Gage et al., 1984). Grafts from the locus coeruleus, rich in nor-adrenergic cells, improved learning deficits in a passive avoidance task (Collier et al., 1988).

Experiments with the transection of the rat fimbria-fornix make the animal incapable of performing a spatial learning task, along with producing other cognitive disturbances. In the case of the spatial task, septal grafts restore task performance deficits (Dunnet et al., 1982). However, it is not a full recovery; in fact, the fimbria-fornix section produces total denervation of subcortical afferences from the hippocampus (cholinergic, nor-adrenergic, and serotonergic afferences), and it may be necessary to recompose different kinds of afferences to compensate for deficit amounts. Research by Nilsson et al. (1990) and Ritcher-Levin and Segal (1989) shows that the combined grafting of septal and raphe tissues (colinergic and serotonergic enriched cells, respectively) induces greater improvements in water maze performance than septal tissue grafting alone. Nucleus basalis magnocellularis (NBM) is involved in the degeneration of basal forebrain cholinergic fibers reaching the hippocampus and neocortex. Excitoxic lesions in NBM is a dementia model, and a great many deficits have been shown here. Cholinergic grafts in the neocortex improved several deficits of avoidance and spatial learning and also improved others with no apparent cognitive function (sensory-motor neglect). It has been suggested that cholinergic deficits may be related to a metabolic failure. Bearing this in mind, intraventricular injections of NGF have been used in old rats, and they have been shown to reduce atrophy of septal cholinergic cells and improve learning retention of spatial navigation between sessions blocks (Fischer et al., 1987). Nonhuman primate experiments (marmosets) have tested fetal cholinergic cell grafting following fimbria fornix sectioning or chemical lesioning; the results showed learning deficit improvements in visuospatial tasks (Ridley & Baker, 1991). There are many more experiments in this field, but we can conclude that (1) cholinergic grafting improves deficits of hippocampal and neocortical lesions (Dunnett, 1991), (2) grafting two different tissues (cholinergic and serotonergic) in the hippocampus produces a remarkable recovery, (3) many memory deficits in aging are related to cholinergic disturbances, (4) underlying dementia are deep processes of atrophy of both intrinsical cortical neurons and subcortical inputs, (5) underlying dementia is also a broad range of degenerative phenomena from which cholinergic degeneration may be a secondary effect, and (6) at present, neural grafting is not considered a treatment for Alzheimer's disease (Dunnett, 1990).

Huntington's Disease

Degeneration of striatal GABAergic fibers is considered a symptom of this illness. Animal models are based on excitotoxic lesions produced by kainic and ibotenic acid injections into both caudate nucleus and putamen in nonhuman primate models (Hantraye et al., 1990) and into striatum in rat models (Dunnett & Iversen, 1981). This disease involves motor disorders (e.g., chorea) and dementia. Animal models involve motor disorders and cognitive deficiencies. Isacson et al. (1986) reported that in striatal ibotenic lesioned rats and monkeys that underwent grafts of fetal striatal tissue, this tissue is anatomically and functionally integrated and, to a certain extent, improves motor (less locomotor activity) and cognitive (delayed alternation task and T-maze) deficits. Eight- to ten-week-old human fetal cells have been grafted in striatal lesioned rats with the same procedure as above, showing growth and development of the cells and reinervation of the globus pallidus and substantia nigra. However, it is not known whether any functional improvement occurs (Wictorin et al., 1990).

Heredity Ataxia

This illness involves the degeneration of the cerebellar cortex. The animal model uses a mutant mouse suffering from a degeneration of Purkinje's cells (Lindvall, 1991). Sotelo and Alvarado-Mallart (1991) have reported that after grafting 12-day-old pieces or suspension cells from a pcd mouse, embryonary Purkinje cells invade the host cortex, migrating to corresponding domains, and induce axonal and dentritic outgrowth of host cells until integrating synaptically in the cerebellar cortex. However, these axons do not establish connections with deep nuclei. Although the results are very persuasive, it is not known whether any functional recovery takes place. In fact, the nonestablishment of deep nuclei connections already makes its functioning much more difficult.

Amyotrophic Lateral Sclerosis

This is a motor system disease involving muscular paralysis. Animal models involve the breaking of spinal ventral roots in newborn rats or spinal cord excitotoxic lesions with kainic acid (Lindvall, 1991). Studies carried out have used embryonic tissue from spinal medulla. They showed survival and anatomical integration of the graft in host medulla, receiving host connections and projecting to peripheral nerves. Recent studies into chicken sciatic nerve lesions have shown that local application of neural cell adhesion molecule (NCAM) helps to improve graft connectivity recovery and functioning (Daniloff et al., 1995).

HUMAN GRAFTING: BEHAVIORAL AND MOTOR EFFECTS

There are, at present, still no grafting techniques for general use in neurodegenerative illnesses; there are too few clinical studies and too many controversial interpretations. There are also many unanswered questions about the causes of disease. However, one case where some limited advances have been made has led to the development of techniques for the treatment of Parkinson's disease. These basically consist of obtaining fetal tissue from noncontaminated abortions and grafting this tissue to patients with immunosuppression, and the fetal tissue is able to survive in the human brain. The surgical techniques used are limited to two kinds. First, there is the esterotaxic grafting of fetal cell suspensions that involves a less traumatic effect due to the injection's needle. The second technique involves the grafting of a solid piece from fetal nigral tissue, which involves a microsurgical operation and requires opening a cavity in the caudatus nucleus.

Parkinson's Disease Treatment

In Parkinson's disease, the most widely used treatment consists of grafting from the adrenal medulla. Madrazo et al. (1987) showed an improvement in results that has not been achieved by others since then. Allen (1989) reports modest improvements related to an increase in the response to L-dopa. Ahlskog et al. (1990) and Olanow et al. (1990) suggested that graft effects do not persist. The studies of Petersen et al. (1989) determined that virtually all the adrenal cells died and that there was an absence of tyrosine-hydrolase activity.

However, Madrazo et al. (1990) published a subsequent study that lasted three years and covered 34 post-operatory cases after adrenal grafting in the caudate head. They reported that 60% showed good improvements, 20% moderate improvements, and 20% poor improvements. The effects of improvement were bilateral, involving both a decrease in rigidity, bradykinesis and postural instability, and improvements in walking performance. It also managed to reduce the L-dopa treatment dose to 60%. In another subsequent study of 200 patients, Lindvall reported less spectacular results than Madrazo, showing only modest improvements in 30–50 patients, with the motor fluctuations characteristic of the syndrome remaining along with the L-dopa dose level. We have learned from animal studies that adrenal grafts do not seem to integrate with the host, so their action in improvements might involve a neurotrophic effect, and they could stimulate the sprouting of the host's intact dopaminergic neurons. Another possibility may be that the adrenal medulla increases dopamine and other catecholamine levels. This has been tested in humans with adrenal grafts by injecting intraventricular NGF for a four-week period, inducing a larger dopaminergic cell survival and increasing catecholaminergic neurotransmitter levels. Motor improvements have also been described (Olson et al., 1991).

Embryonic fetal cells have also been used in human treatment. This grafting has been performed in the caudate nucleus and in the putamen, and in both of them simultaneously with grafting in 1–10 different locations (Lindvall, 1991). Most of the patients undergoing this treatment received immunosuppression. Lindvall has summarized the results; improvements were partial or moderate, except with one patient where the improvements were complete. The L-dopa response was enhanced (the same dose was more effective), and there was an increase in the duration of the "on" phase accompanied by reduced hypokinesis and rigidity ("off" phase). The appearance of positive effects varied from the time immediately following grafting in some patients to 3–4 months later in others. Some other improvements took up to eight months to appear. No undesirable side effects were observed following grafting, and postmortem studies showed graft survival in some patients (Lindvall, 1991). The study of positron emission tomography (PET) in one patient showed fluor-dopa captation (i.e., it showed a dopamine synthesis increase in both graft and surrounding host tissue). There were many differences among patient responses and initial conditions: on the one hand, immunosuppression treatment, and on the other, the level of degeneration of each patient and their age. Several researchers suggest that patient improvements are related to a dopaminergic sprouting in the patient's CNS (Freed, 1990). This has been demonstrated in animals but not in humans.

The development of an effective therapy for Parkinson's disease runs up against many obstacles, as clinical data do not yet recommend a universal treatment. In most cases, the graft does not survive or survives unsatisfactorily, and the reinervation is short and restricted to the striatum. However, in experiments where human mesencephalical tissue has been grafted to immunosuppressed rats, 20 thousand grafted human cells survived in the rat brain. Fetal grafting restored 30–40% of total cell amount. PET experiments following fluor-dopa uptake demonstrated a low fetal graft survival rate and poor levels of improvement.

To say these diseases have no single cause, that dopaminergic grafting acts only on one level, does not decrease deficits related, for example, to locus coeruleus nor-adrenergic paths, which have been related to intellectual deficits and depressions in Parkinson's disease. Dopaminergic grafted cells may die for several reasons: (1) there may be environmental or endogenous neurotoxins in the process of the illness itself, or there may be a neurotrophical shortcoming; (2) there might also be noxious effects from the L-dopa treatment (however, this has not been shown to interfere in graft viability in rats); and (3) immunological rejection could take place, as happened with a patient who deteriorated after 10 months. For this reason, it is necessary to extend an immunosuppressive treatment that may produce noxious effects in graft viability, although in the vast majority of cases, graft failure seems to be the result of other causes (space and growth ability). This immunological problem may be minimized by extracting the cells that can trigger immunological responses, such as glial and endothelial cells (Lindvall, 1991).

Huntington's Disease

The development of neural grafting treatment for this disease will most probably follow the path laid by the treatment of Parkinson's. Huntington's disease has a short life expectancy, and this is obviously a critical factor when contemplating a medical approach to applying grafting techniques. Some of the symptoms (chorea) may be treated with dopaminergic antagonists, but the associated dementia cannot.

Although animal experimentation results suggest that neural grafting may be a useful therapy for Huntington's disease, the existence of some unanswered questions prevents its application:

1. What age must the donor be?
2. What is the most suitable surgical procedure?
3. How much striatal tissue is needed for grafting?
4. Is there a need for developing clinical, neurophysiological, and neuropsychological procedures to follow graft functions?
5. Is it necessary to demonstrate the graft survival, which it can be monitored by means of the PET and magnetic resonance imaging (MRI)?

Something that is critical in this illness is the time grafting takes place. This is because the illness involves the temporal progress of some structural abnormalities, such as striatal atrophy, dilation of the lateral ventricle, and moderate cerebral cortex atrophy. There are no guarantees without previous clinical experience that the neural graft will not degenerate or that it will have no use in the advanced stages of the disease. In most of the rodent and nonhuman primate studies of striatal fetal tissue, the grafting involved does not form a good model for looking at long-term degeneration because it has been carried out soon after the excitotoxic lesion. We need to know more about chronically lesioned animals, which could be more closely compared to advanced pathological stages of the disease in humans (Lindvall, 1991).

Another important question to do with the time that the graft is performed concerns the possibility that if the graft is carried out in the early stages, it might counteract degenerative changes in other regions of the brain. If striatal neurons are replaced by neural grafts when the first dysfunctional disease symptoms appear, this may preserve the brain's afferent neural systems against degenerative processes.

Dementia

Given the complexity of the disease's degenerative effects and the results of research into dementia, the development of an effective grafting technique is still a long way off. We still do not know where, what, or when to graft (Dunnet, 1990).

CONCLUDING REMARKS

Transplant techniques, as a clinical therapy, are still in their initial stages with many unanswered questions of a scientific, clinical, economic, and ethical nature still to be resolved.

The results of scientific research using animal experimentation have and will continue to provide valuable data for the application of techniques. However, we still have insufficient data regarding something that is fundamental to treating a neurodegenerative illness (Alzheimer's, Parkinson's, Huntington's, etc.)—the delimitation of the causes and the process of the illness. Does degeneration occur first in one system which then affects others, or does it occur simultaneously in several systems? Is degeneration the work of a toxic endogene or is it a metabolic problem that reduces the number and effectiveness of neurotrophic factors? Are any other factors, such as adhesion proteins, involved?

Present-day research and techniques of genetic manipulation are producing very significant data about the genetic markers of these and many other diseases and hereditary mental disorders. But as yet, they do not allow us to describe and delimit the causes and processes of these illnesses. It is logical to suppose that if the causes and subsequent development of these syndromes are discovered, it will be easier to find and use adequate therapy, whether this occurs in the form of prevention or treatment with grafts, trophic factors, pharmacological medication, or an appropriate combination of all of these.

It is undoubtedly in the area of Parkinson's disease where the most progress has been made both in animal research and in clinical testing. It has been shown that the use of trophic factors in the dopaminergic system assists graft viability, its functioning, and the survival of host cells. Animal research has shown that neurotrophic factors have the same beneficial effects in models of Alzheimer's and Huntington's syndromes. The same could be said of illnesses affecting the spinal medulla. It has also been shown that the application of cellular NCAM adhesion proteins at the site of a lesion (sciatic nerve) increases regeneration, neuron-evoked response capacity is recuperated, and motor response recuperation occurs (Daniloff et al., 1995).

As far as the material to be used in grafts is concerned, candidates include various types of cells. First, there are fetal cells that have a high survival rate, and it has been shown that they do, in some cases, integrate themselves into the host tissue. Their grafting is correlated with the "de novo" formation of connections (in the case of septal grafts, in the hippocampus) and motor and behavioral functional recuperation, including tasks that involve a cognitive process. The main drawback with them is that they require treatment with immunodepressors with the corresponding problems that this represents, combined with the danger of becoming affected by the degenerative processes affecting the host neurons (a toxin that kills host dopaminergic cells will probably do the same to grafted ones).

The grafting of heterotopic allogenic material, such as adrenal chromafin cells, is the most widely used technique, but there is no consensus as to the effectiveness of its grafting. There are results from studies that, if not entirely contradictory, take very different views of the effectiveness of the graft. Findings suggest that as the extent of the illness and the age of the patient increases, the effectiveness of the treatment might be reduced. There is no uniform pattern to the type of patient or his/her age, and there is normally no previous knowledge of the extent of degeneration existing in the neurotransmitter systems.

Cells modified by genetic engineering are capable of synthesizing and expelling neurotransmitter metabolic precursors (L-dopa) or neurotrophic factors (NFG or BDNF) into the surrounding environment. This ability makes them a possible preventive instrument against degeneration. These cells also seem to be less affected by degenerative processes than fetal cells.

Neuroepitelial fetal cells are the first to develop in the individual; they are multipotential, and, with advances in the understanding of neural development, they could become a very useful material for grafting, given the advantages they possess. We know that in the first stages of embryonal development of the nervous system, a series of morphogenetic mechanisms exist—via interaction with the surrounding environment—that induce the formation of a certain neuronal type from these multipotential cells. Understanding of these mechanisms would allow us to induce and create the material to be transplanted (Cattaneo & McKay, 1991). However, its applicability is still at a very preliminary stage.

Neural transplants have been shown to be effective in many animal models; they have promoted regeneration, have avoided degeneration, and have produced motor and behavioral improvements. Interesting conclusions have been drawn for the application of these techniques in humans. But for maximum effectiveness, it will be necessary to meet the following requirements:

1. Possess a more thorough understanding of the process, if not of the cause or causes, of neurodegenerative illnesses.
2. Know when is the most suitable moment for grafting, with respect to the process of the illness and the patient's age, as the latter could indicate the type of therapy to be used.
3. Find the simplest and most economic material for use in the graft. This may mean taking it from an aborted fetus or selecting a more plastic material from which a certain type of cell could be obtained (neuroepitelial cells from the crest and neural tube). This involves ethical and economic factors.
4. Select the type of material depending on how far the damage has spread. For example, fetal cells that act as micropumps secrete a specific neurotrophic factor that would prevent the degeneration of a certain system of neurotransmitters that, in turn, would safeguard the survival of others (preventive therapy).
5. Restore the functionality of the patient's neural system not only by an external replacement of neurons but also by stimulating the regeneration of those that are still alive.

6. Find out how a treatment with immunosuppressors or one with medications (L-dopa) interferes with the viability and effectiveness of the graft. It needs to be established whether this is because of what the medication provides *in situ* (genetically modified fibroblasts that secrete the substance), because a material is introduced with a greater genetic similarity to the host (fibroblast autograft), or because a material is selected to make the immune response less intense (grafts from which the glia have been extracted).

In light of present experimental results, the effectiveness of the technique seems to result from a combination of factors. On the one hand, there is the grafting of tissue—on the other, the inoculation of substances (neurotrophic factors) that favor regeneration and protect against degeneration, the grafting of secretory capsules, or the grafting of cells that produce them. Although it should be said that at the moment, given the complex set of factors involved in neurodegenerative diseases such as senile dementia, the use of grafting is so far minimal. As O. Lindvall (1991) states, "The future of cell transplantation as a treatment for human neurodegenerative disorders will depend on the application of systematic scientific approaches to solve both basic and clinical problems."

There is also an important ethical angle to the use of these techniques. This centers mainly on where the material that is to be grafted comes from. Today, it comes from aborted fetal tissue. Apart from the problem this represents with respect to the limited availability of supply, it raises a serious ethical problem. In some countries legislation has been tightened regarding the use of this type of material; the only alternative would be to use material coming from the actual patient (e.g., fibroblasts). In other countries (mainly the United States, Canada, and the EU) legislation has been introduced to protect on the one hand, the rights of patients and relatives (if, for example, they do not want to receive treatment for moral or religious reasons), and, on the other, to prevent profit-making and other abuses which, depending on the level of control in a country, are more or less inevitable. There are definitely no easy solutions to this question, and it is bound to produce much debate during the coming years. Let us not forget that when organ transplants began, there was also a great deal of similar argument (Hoffer & Olson, 1991).

REFERENCES

Aguayo, A.J., Björklund, A., Stenevi, U., & Carlstedt, T. (1984). Fetal mesencephalic neurons survive and extend long axons across PNS grafts inserted into the adult striatum. *Neurosci. Letts*, *45*, 53–58.

Ahlskog, J.E, Kelly, P.J., van Heerden, J.A., Stoddard, S.L., Tyce, G.M, Windbebank, A.J., Bailey, P.A., Bell, G.N., Blexrud, M.D., & Carmichael, S.W. (1990). Adrenal medullary transplantation into the brain for treatment of Parkinson's disease: Clinical outcome and neurochemical studies. *Mayo Clin. Proc.*, *65*, 305–328.

Allen, G.S., Burns, R.S., Tulipan, N.B., & Parker, R.A. (1989) Adrenal medullary transplantation to the caudate nucleus in Parkinson's disease. *Arch. Neurol.*, *316*, 487–491.

Altobelli, R. (1914). Inesti cerebrali. *Gazz. Int. Med. Chir.*, *17*, 25–34.

Annett, L.E., Dunnett, S.B., Torres, E.M., Ridley, R.M., Baker, H.F., & Marsden, C.D. (1991). Behavioural assessment of embryonic nigral graft placed in the caudate nucleus and/or putamen of 6-OHDA lesioned marmoset. *Eur. J. Neurosci.*, *4*, 248.

Bamkiewicz, K.S., Plunkett, R.J., Jacobowitz, D.M., Kopin, I.J., & Olfield, E.H. (1991). Fetal nondopaminergic neural implants in Parkinsonian primates. *J. Neurosurg.*, *74*, 97–104.

Bamkiewicz, K.S., Plunkett, R.J., Jacobowitz, D.M., Porrino, L., Di Porzio, U., London W.T., Kopin, I.J., & Olfield, E.H. (1990). The effect of fetal mesencephalon implants on primate MPTP-induced Parkinsonism: Histochemical and behavioral studies. *J. Neurosurg.*, *72*, 231–144.

Björklund, A. (1987). Brain implants, transplants. In G. Adelman (Ed.), *Encyclopedia of neuroscience* (Vol. 1) (pp. 165–167). Boston: Birkhäuser Edt.

Björklund, A., & Stenevi, U. (1979). Regeneration of monoaminergic and cholinergic neurons in the mammalian central nervous system. *Physiol. Rev., 59,* 62–100.

————. (1984). Intracerebral neural implants: Neuronal replacement and reconstruction of damaged circuitries. *Ann. Rev. Neurosci., 7,* 279–308.

———— (Eds.). (1985). *Neural grafting in the mammalian CNS.* Amsterdam: Elsevier.

Björklund, A., Schmidt, R.H., & Stenevi, U. (1980). Functional reinervation of the neostriatum in the adult rat by use of intraparenchymal grafting of dissociated cell suspensions from the substantia nigra. *Cell. Tiss. Res., 212,* 39, 45.

Björklund, A., Stenevi, U., & Svendgaard, N.-Aa. (1976). Growth of transplanted monoaminergic neurones into adult hippocampus along the perforant path. *Nature, 262,* 787–790.

Björklund, A., Stenevi, U., Schmidt, R.H., Dunnett, S.B., & Gage, F.H. (1983). Intracerebral grafting of neuronal cell suspensions. *Acta Physiol. Scand., 522* (Suppl.), 1–75.

Cattaneo, E., & McKay, R. (1991). Identifying and manipulating neuronal stem cells. *TINS., 14,* 338–340.

Collier, T.J., Gash, D.M., & Sladek, J.R. (1988). Transplantation of norepinephrine into aged rats improves performance of learned task. *Brain Res., 448,* 77–87.

Daniloff, J.K., Shoemaker, R.S., Lee, A.F., Strain, G.M., & Remsen, L.G. (1995). N-CAM promotes recovery in injured nerves. *Restor. Neurol. Neurosci., 7,* 137–144.

Das, G.D. (1974). Transplantation of embryonic neural tissue in the mammalian brain. I. Growth and differentiation of neuroblast from various regions of the embryonic brain in the cerebellum of neonate rats. *J. Life Sci., 4,* 93–124.

————. (1975). Differentiation of dentrites in the transplanted neuroblast in the mammalian brain. In G.W. Kreuztberg (Ed.), *Advances in neurology: Physiology and pathology of dendrites* (Vol. 12). New York: Raven Press.

————. (1990). Neural transplantation: an historical perspective. *Neurosci. Biobehav. Rev., 14,* 389–401.

David, S., & Aguayo, A.J. (1981). Spinal motoneuron requirement in man: Rank deordering with direction but not speed of voluntary movement. *Science, 214,* 931–933.

Detwiler, S.R. (1964). *Neuroembryology: An experimental study.* New York: Hafner Publishing Co.

Dund, E.H. (1917). Primary and secondary findings in a series attempts to transplant cortex in the albino rat. *J. Comp. Neurol., 27,* 565–582.

Dunnett, S.B. (1990). Neural transplantation in animals models of dementia. *Eur. J. Neurosci., 2,* 567–587.

————. (1991). Cholinergic grafts, memory and ageing. *TINS., 14,* 11–76.

Dunnett, S.B., & Iversen, S.D. (1981). *Behav. Brain Res., 2,* 189–209.

Dunnet, S.B., Low, W.C., Iversen, S.D., Stenevi, U., & Björklund, A. (1982). Septal transplants restore maze learning in rats with fombria-fornix lesions. *Brain Res., 251,* 335–348.

Escobar, M.L., Russell, R.W., Booth, R.A., & Bermúdez-Rattoni, F. (1994). Accelerating behavioral recovery after cortical lesions. I. Homotopic implants plus NGF. *Behav. Neural Biol., 61,* 73–80.

Fischer W., Wictorin, K., Björklund, A., Williams, L.R., Varon, S., & Gage, F.H. (1987). Amelioration of cholinergic neurons atrophy and spatial memory impairment in aged rats by nerve growth factor. *Nature, 329,* 65–68. Fisher, L.J., Jinnah, H.A., Kale, L.C., Higginns G.A., & Gage F.H. (1991). Survival and function of intrastriatally grafted primary fibroblast genetically modified to produce L-dopa. *Neuron, 6,* 371–380.

Freed, W.J. (1990). Fetal brain grafts and Parkinson's disease. *Science, 250,* 1434.

Gage F.H.., Kang, U.J., & Fisher, L.J. (1992). Intracerebral grafting in the dopaminergic system: Issues and controversy. *Cur. Opinion Neurobiol., 1,* 414–419.

Gage, F.H., Kawaja, M.D., & L.J. Fisher. (1991). Genetically modified cells: Applications for intracerebral grafting. *TINS., 14,* 328–333.

Gage, F.H., Björklund, A., Stenevi, U., & Dunnet, S.B. (1983). Aged rats: Recovery of motor impairments by striatal nigral grafts. *Science, 221,* 966–969.

Gage, F.H., Björklund, A., Stenevi, U., Dunnet, S.B., & Kelley, P.A.T. (1984). Intrahippocampal septal grafts ameliorate deficits in aged rats. *J. Neurosci., 4,* 2856–2865.

Gash, D.M., Notter, M.F.D., Okawara, S.H., Kraus, A.L., & Joynt, R.J. (1986). Amitotic neuroblastoma cells used for neural implants in monkeys. *Science, 223,* 1420–1422.

Green, H.S.N. (1967). The use of transplanted tissues in biology and histology. In G.H. Bourne (Ed.), *In vivo techniques in histology* (pp. 80–102). Baltimore: Williams & Wilkins.

Hantraye, P., Riche, D., Maziere, M., & Isacson, O. (1990). A primate model of Huntington's disease: Behavioral and anatomical studies of unilateral excitotoxic lesions of the caudate-putamen in the baboon. *Exp. Neurol., 108,* 91–104.

Harrison, R.G. (1935). On the origin and development of the nervous system studied by methods of experimental embryology. *Proc. R. Soc. Lond. (B), 118,* 155–196.

Hoffer, B.J., & Olson, L. (1991). Ethical issues in brain cell transplantation. *TINS., 14,* 384–388.

Horellou, P., Marlier, L. Privat, A., & Mallet, J. (1990). Behavioral effects of engineered cells that synthesize L-dopa or dopamine after grafting into the rat neostriatum. *Eur. J. Neurosci., 2,* 116–119.

Hyman, C., Hofer, M., Barde, Y.-A., Juhasz, M. Yancopoulos, G.D., Squinto, S.P., & Lindsay, R.M. (1991). BDNF is a neurotrophic factor for dopaminergic neurons of the substantia nigra. *Nature, 350,* 230–232.

Isacson O., Dunnett, S.B., & Björklund, A. (1986). Graft-induced behavioral recovery in an animal model of Huntington's disease. *Proc. Natl. Acad. Sci. U.S.A., 83,* 2728–2732.

Knusel B. Winslow, J.W., Rosenthal, A., Barton, L.E., Seid, D.P., Nikolics, K., & Hepti. F. (1991). Promotion of central cholinergic and dopaminergic neuron differentiation by brain-derived neurotrophic factor but not neurotrophin-3. *Proc. Natl. Acad. Sci. USA, 88,* 961–965.

Krieger, D.T., & Gibson, M.J. (1984). Correction of genetic gonadotropic hormone-releasing hormone deficiency by preoptic area transplants. In J.R. Sladek Jr. and D.M. Gash (Eds.), *Neural transplants: Development and functions* (pp. 187–204). New York: Plenum Press.

Labbe, R., Firl, A.C., Mufson, E.J., & Stein D.G. (1983). Fetal brain transplants: Reduction deficits in rat with frontal cortex lesions. *Science, 217,* 470–472.

Le Gros Clark, W.E. (1940). Neural differentiation in implanted fetal cortical tissue. *J. Neurol. Psychiatry, 3,* 263–272.

———. (1943). The problem of neural regeneration in the central nervous system. II. The insertion of peripheral nerve stumps into the brain. *J. Anat., 77,* 251–259.

Lindvall, O. (1991). Prospects of transplantation in human neurodegenerative diseases. *TINS, 14,* 376–384.

Lindvall, O., Björklund, A., & Widner, H. (Eds.). (1991). *Proceedings of E.K. Fernstrom Symposium on intracerebral transplantation in movement disorders: Experimental and clinical experiences.* Amsterdam: Elsevier.

Liu C.N., & Chambers W.W. (1958). Intraspinal sprouting of dorsal root axons. *AMA. Archiv. Neurol. Psych., 79,* 46–61.

Lund, R.D., & Hauschka, S.D. (1976). Transplanted neural tissues develops connections with host rat brain. *Science, 193,* 582–584.

Madrazo, I., Drucker-Colin, R., Diaz, V., Martinez-Mata, J., Torres, C., & Becerril, J.J. (1987). Open microsurgical autograft of adrenal medulla to the right caudate nucleus in two patients with intractable Parkinson's disease. *N. Eng. J. Med., 216,* 831–834.

Madrazo, I., Franco-Bourland, R., Ostrosky-Solis, P., Aguilera, M., Cuevas, C., Zamorano, C., Morelos, A., Megallon, E., & Guizar-Sahagun, G. (1990). Fetal homotransplants (ventral mesencephalon and adrenal tissue) to striatum of Parkisonian subjects. *Arch. Neurol., 47,* 1281–1285.

Medawar, P.B. (1948). Immunity to homologous grafted skin. III. The fate of skin homografts transplanted to the brain, to subcutaneus tissue, and anterior chamber of the eye. *Br. J. Exp. Pathol., 29,* 58–69.

Nieto-Sampedro, M. (1988). Growth factor induction and order of events in CNS repair. In D.G. Stein and B. Sabel (Eds.), *Pharmacological approaches to the treatment of brain and spinal cord injuries.* New York: Plenum Press.

Nieto-Sampedro, M., & Cotmant, C.W. (1985). Growth factor induction and order of events in CNS repair. In C.W. Cotman (Ed.), *Synaptic plasticity* (pp. 407–456). New York: Guilford Press.

Nieto-Sampedro, M. Lewis, E.R., Cotman, C.W., Manthorpe, M. Skaper S.D., Barbin, G., Longo F.M., & Varon, S. (1982). Brain injury causes a time-dependent increase in neurotrophic activity at the lesion site. *Science, 221*, 860–861.

Nikkhah, G., Cunningham, M.G., Jodicke, A. Knappe, U., & Björklund, A. (1994). Improved graft survival and striatal reinnervation by microtransplantation of fetal nigral cell suspensions in the Parkinsonian model. *Brain Res., 633*, 133–143.

Nilsson O.G., Brundin P., & Björklund, A. (1990). Amelioration of spatial memory impairment by intrahippocampal grafts of mixed septal and raphe tissue in rats with combined cholinergic and serotonergic denervation of the forebrain. *Brain Res., 515*, 193–206.

Nissl, F. (1911). Experimentell anatomische Untersuchungen über die Hirnrinde. *Vehr. Ges. Deut. Natur. Arzte., 83*, 353–355.

Olanow, C.W., Koller, W., Goetz, C.G., Stebbins, G.T., Cahill, D.W., Gauger, L.L., Morantz, R. Penn, R.D., Tanner, C.M., & Klawans, H.L. (1990). Autologous transplantation of adrenal medulla in Parkinson's disease. *Arch. Neurol., 47*, 1286–1289.

Olson, I., Backlund, E.O., Ebendal, T., Freedman, R., Hamberger, B., Hansson, P., Hoffer, B., Lindblom, U., et al. (1991). Intraputamental infusion of nerve growth factor to support adrenal medullary autografts in Parkinson's disease: One-year follow-up of first clinical trial. *Arch. Neurol., 48*, 373–381.

Petersen, D.I., Price, M.L., & Small, C.S. (1989). Autopsy findings in a patient who had adrenal-to-brain transplant for Parkinson's disease. *Neurology, 39*, 235–238.

Plunkett, R.J., Bankiewicz, K.S., Cummins A.C., Miletich, R.S., Schwartz, J.P., & Oldfield E.H. (1990). Long-term evaluation of hemiparkisonian monkeys after adrenal autografting or cavitation alone. *J. Neurosurg., 73*, 918–926.

Raju, S., & Grogan, J.B. (1977). Immunologic study of the brain as a privileged site. *Transplant Proc., 9*, 1187–1191.

Ramón y Cajal, S. (1914). *Estudios sobre la degeneración y regeneración del sistema nervioso*. Madrid: N. Moya.

Ranson, W. (1909). Transplantation of the spinal ganglion into the brain. *Q. Bull. Northwest Univ. Med. School, 11*, 176–178.

Ridley R.M., & Baker, H.F. (1991). Can fetal neural transplants restore function in monkeys with lesion-induced behavioral deficits? *TINS., 14*, 365–370.

Ritcher-Levin G., & Segal M. (1989). Raphe cells grafted into hippocampus can ameliorate spatial memory deficits in rats with combined serotonergic/cholinergic deficiencies. *Brain Res., 477*, 404–407.

Rosemberg, M.B., Friedman, T., Robertson, R.C., Tuszinsky, M., Wolff, J.A., Breakefield, X.O., and Gage, F.H. (1988). Grafting genetically modified cells to damaged brain: Restorative effects of NGF expression. *Science, 242*, 1575–1578.

Saltykow, S. (1905). Versuche über Genhirnreplantation, zugleich ein Beintrag zur Kenntniss der Vorgänge an den zelligen Gehirnelementen. *Arch. Psychiatry, 40*, 329–390.

Sinden, J.D., Patel, S.N., & Hodges, H. (1992). Neural transplantation: Problems and prospects for therapeutic application. *Cur. Opinion Neurol. Neurosur., 5*, 902–908.

Sladek, J.R., & Gash, D.M. (1984). Morphological and functional properties of transplanted vasopressin neurons. In J.R. Sladek, Jr. and D.M. Gash (Eds.), *Neural transplants:Development and functions* (pp. 243–282). New York: Plenum Press.

Sloan, D.J., Wood, M.J., & Charlton, H.M. (1991). The immune response to intracerebral neural grafts. *TINS., 14*, 341–346.

Sotelo, C., & Alvarado-Mallart, R.M. (1991). The reconstruction of cerebellar circuits. *TINS., 14*, 350–355.

Sperry, R.W. (1944). Optic nerve regeneration with return of visions in anurans. *J. Neurophysiol., 7*, 57–69.

Stein, D.G. (1988). Practical and theoretical issues in the uses of fetal brain tissue transplants to promote recovery from brain injury. In T.E. LeVere, C.R. Almli, & D.G. Stein (Eds.), *Brain injury and recovery: Theoretical and controversial issues* (pp. 249–272). New York: Plenum Press.

Strömberg, I., Herrera-Marschitz, M., Ungerstedt, U., Ebendal, T., & Olson, L. (1985). Chronic implants of chromaffin tissue into the dopamine-denervated striatum. Effects of NGF on graft survival, fiber growth and rotational behavior. *Exp. Brain Res., 60,* 335–349.

Sunde, N., Laurberg, S., & Zimmer. (1984). Brain grafts can restore damaged connections in newborn rats. *Nature, 310,* 51–53.

Taylor, J.R., Elsworth, J.D., Roth, R.H., Sladek J.R., Collier T.J., & Redmond, D.E. (1991). Grafting of fetal substantia nigra to striatum reverses behavioral deficits induced by MPTP in primates: A comparison with other types of grafts as controls. *Exp. Brain Res., 85,* 335–348.

Tello, F. (1911). La influencia del neurotropismo en la regeneración de los centros nerviosos. *Trab. Lab. Invest. Biol., 9,* 123–160.

Thompson, W.G. (1890). Successful brain grafting. *NY Med. J., 51,* 701–702.

Tidd, C.W. (1932). The transplantation of spinal ganglia in the white rat: A study of the morphological changes in surviving cells. *J. Comp. Neurol., 55,* 531–543.

Wictorin, K., Clarke, D.J. Bolam, J.P, & Björklund, A. (1990). Fetal striatal neurons grafted into the ibotenate lesioned adult striatum: Efferent projections and synaptic contacts in the host globus pallidus. *Neuroscience, 37,* 301–315.

Wolff, J.A., Fisher, L.J. Jinnah, H.A., Langlais, P.J., Iuvone, P.M., O'Malley, K.I., Rosemberg, M.B., Shimohama, S. Friedmann, T., & Gage F.H. (1989). Grafting fibroblast genetically modified to produce L-dopa in a rat model of Parkinson's disease. *Proc. Natl. Acad. Sci. USA, 86,* 9011–9014.

11 Neuropharmacological Treatment Following Traumatic Brain Injury: Problems and Perspectives

Claudio Perino and Roberto Rago

Centro di Medicina Riabilitativa "AUSILIATRICE"
Via Peyron 42, 10143 Torino, Italy

> At the molecular level, an explanation of the action of a drug is often possible, at the cellular level it is sometimes possible, but at the behavioral level, our ignorance is abysmal.
> —Cooper, Bloom, Roth. *The Biochemical Basis of Neuropharmacology,* 1986

INTRODUCTION

Traditionally, most physicians in the field of rehabilitation have relied on nonpharmacological modalities for the treatment of long-term traumatic brain injury (TBI) consequences. More recently, physiatrists and neurologists alike started to realize that many TBI sequelae, particularly in the subacute and chronic stages, may be lessened, alleviated, and sometimes cured through an appropriate use of a number of neuropharmacological and psychopharmacological compounds (Zasler, 1992; Cope, 1994; Stein et al., 1994). However, in spite of increased knowledge and experience, practical pharmacology in this realm remains somewhat between *the art of probability and the science of uncertainty*; the following condensed review is a summary of general considerations on TBI neuropathology, sporadic studies published in specialized books and journals, and a number of personal experiences and observations (Perino, 1990).

At first, we should consider a few related and interconnected problems.

1. There is an extreme complexity and a remarkable individual variability in the human central nervous system (CNS). Every person is *unique* for multiple genetic, prenatal, environmental, developmental, and social factors. A casual combination of a great number of parameters, within the limits and potentiality of the species, accounts for the wide variety of personal differences (Gardner, 1985; Geschwind & Galaburda, 1987). This has no equal in other organs or

functions and explains the primary difficulties that are found by neuropharmaco-logical research. Consequently, results in this area may be inconclusive, conflict-ing, and nonreplicable.

2. Subjects who suffer TBI are also very heterogeneous in terms of modality, site and extension of lesions, secondary damage, neurological and cognitive deficits, functional capacity for compensation, etc. In practice, every patient should be considered a "unicum" and thus treated (Cope, 1990). Moreover, even consider-ing some interesting proposals for classification (Zappala, 1988), we still lack a clear nosographic interpretation of post-traumatic neurological syndromes.

3. The selection of drugs to be employed in this field is derived from acquired knowledge in other areas of neurology and psychiatry (e.g., dementia, cere-brovascular disease, developmental retardation, and various psychiatric syn-dromes), and often their use is conducted through trial and error, as we lack standardized protocols for TBI sequelae (Wilsher et al., 1979; Giurgea et al., 1983; Saletu et al., 1985; McLean et al., 1991).

4. Many pharmacological substances that are active on the human CNS have varying effects on different individuals. Sometimes this can be dose-dependent; in other cases, it seems that there may be groups of "non-responders" or "hyper-responders" within the general population for reasons not yet fully understood (Whyte, 1988). Many active compounds have also numerous "side effects." This may be an improper term, as it encourages the notion that they are casual or incidental. In reality, they should be called "undesired effects," as they are always a direct part of the pharmacological properties of the drug and cannot, therefore, be eliminated without simultaneously dismissing its actual clinical therapeutic efficacy (Eames, 1989).

5. Many proposed treatments have only an empirical basis (i.e., we cannot be sure about their mechanisms of action, if not in terms of general unverified hypoth-esis). Some drugs have also various activities on pathological conditions very far from one another (e.g., amantadine, which was introduced as an antiviral agent, has subsequently also been attributed anti-Parkinsonian effects [Gualtieri et al., 1989]).

6. We still have great difficulty in measuring neurological and neuropsychological change due to a lack of international standards, especially when group studies are involved. Also, psychometric batteries may often be inadequate for this type of pathology (Cope, 1990). Should we, therefore, measure impairment, disability, handicap, a combination of these, or something else?

7. Neuropharmacological intervention cannot be isolated from other complex treat-ment procedures for TBI patients such as appropriate nutrition, environment modification, and motor, cognitive, behavioral, and social rehabilitation. In fact, benefits from a given substance often cannot be shown if we are unable to simultaneously control many other variables (Trexler, 1991).

RESEARCH ISSUES

Usually the clinical efficacy of a new drug is tested with a group trial, where a given number of patients are administered the substance and then compared with another group, as similar as possible, which assumes a placebo or another well-established compound. Of course, these studies have to meet all ethical requirements and be scientifically unbiased (randomized and double-blind). Effective products, thus certified, will be predictably active on most of the subjects treated (e.g., most diabetics will have a blood-sugar reduction proportional to the quantity of injected insulin).

On the other hand, with neuropsychopharmacological drugs, the results may be extensively complicated by the more individualized response to the given substance and by the numerous difficulties of correct clinical and instrumental measurement. Group trials may thus become extremely complex and expensive; the large numbers of subjects involved, needed to statistically minimize individual variables and to match two homogeneous samples, may most of the time hinder any research at all. Sometimes this may be overcome by the use of simplified measuring instruments with the drawback of obtaining unspecific or useless results.

For these economic and scientific considerations, it has therefore been proposed to use a single-case study model or a collection of similar single-study cases, as suggested by Whyte (1988) and well exemplified by Seliger (1992). Following this model, an individual clinical situation is carefully analyzed and matched with the theoretical knowledge about the drug to be tested. Variable clinical signs or behavior should then be transferred into some kind of reference measure as accurately as possible (e.g., impairment or disability scales, neuropsychological testing, instrumental measures such as EEG, SPECT, rCBF, EP, etc.), and a "baseline" starting point should be established (Barlow & Hersen, 1984). Areas of measurement might be neurophysiological, neurological, or neuropsychological depending on the theoretical activity of the drug, on the problem to be treated, and on the consensus reached by the neurorehabilitation team.

In general, however, we should remember that:

1. In the context of neurological rehabilitation, "measurement" in the pure scientific sense is rarely possible; there are few aspects that can be easily quantified, and standard units are generally absent.
2. The term "assessment," referring to the process of recognizing and determining the cause and extent of a patient's problems, is becoming more frequent and accurate in describing the researcher's work.
3. In practice, assessment and measurement are closely related. Many, but not all, measures generate numbers, which often do not carry the significance of ordinary numbers.
4. The most important consideration, when choosing any measure, is to know *why* the information is being sought.
5. All tests can have varying numbers of false-positives and/or false-negatives.
6. The final crucial consideration is that measures should be *reliable* (how much is any difference due to a real change and how much is random or biased error), *sensible* (can they detect the change expected), *valid* (can they measure whatever they are supposed to), as *simple* as possible (without losing sensitivity), and easily *communicable* to others.

At this point, after meeting as many of these requirements and considerations as feasible, the given substance may be tested in the individual subject, either with an open trial or in a double-blind modality, following, for example, an A-B-A-B model alternating drug and placebo.

Subsequent assessment or measures should be taken at given intervals that follow the predetermined study protocol. At the end of the trial, data should be analyzed and related to all clinical observations that have been collected in the meantime. Some final considerations should be written in a formalized report, and results should be discussed, explained, and commented upon.

From a collection of analogous clinical trials and situations, hopefully, it will then be possible to draw larger generalizations on a subpopulation of clinically similar patients (Sloan et al., 1992). Implementing such methods may at least enable clinicians to acquire simultaneously more scientific experience and more practical knowledge in their every-day activity.

Formal scientific validity is probably limited to the work of professional researchers who can more easily control experimental conditions, variability, and factor analysis, but at least these procedures may teach everyone a better pragmatic use of some substances and the elimination of less useful or potentially harmful compounds (Guyett et al., 1986).

MAIN NEUROCHEMICAL SYSTEMS

Although numerous neurotransmitters (close to 100) have been currently identified in the human CNS, most can be grouped into four categories: acetylcholine, monoamines, amino-acids, and proteins (small peptides). Their interaction is overwhelmingly complex; moreover, besides a well-known synaptic mechanism of "neurotransmission," some poorly understood "neuroregulation-neuromodulation" functions may exist. The latter can be partially compared to hormonal activities (extracellular diffusion of transmitters—far- and long-acting—and nonsynaptic information transmission). As a prerequisite to further pharmacological considerations, present knowledge is here very briefly summarized.

Cholinergic Systems

There are two major classes of receptors: nicotinic and muscarinic. Functionally, cholinergic neurons in the CNS (at the levels of upper brainstem, ventral forebrain, hippocampus, striatum, mesial cortex, etc.) have been theorized to play a role in arousal, attention, memory, learning processes, motor control, and affective disorders (Bradley, 1989; Woolf, 1991).

Dopaminergic Systems

Their projections are usually divided into categories based on length: long, short, and ultrashort. The first originate from the ventral tegmentum (mesolimbic/mesocortical tracts) and the substantia nigra (nigrostriatal tract) and are more easily damaged in case of diffuse axonal injury (DAI) linked to cerebral trauma. It has also been shown that there are several subtypes of dopaminergic receptors and systems (Koller et al., 1989). Functionally, they are mainly connected to motor activity but are also involved in arousal, hypothalamic activities, and motivational drives.

Nor-adrenergic Systems

Adrenergic cells are identified in many CNS structures including the locus ceruleus, forebrain, lateral tegmental nuclei, pons, and spinal cord. Receptors are divided into alpha 1, alpha 2, beta 1, and beta 2. Central nor-adrenergic pathways are involved in many functions (e.g., vigilance, nociception, learning behavior, sleep/wake cycle, mood, and motivational drives [Snyder, 1986]).

Serotonergic Systems

Cell bodies are prevalent in the brainstem and raphe nuclei, projecting mainly into the frontal lobes, the cerebellum, and the limbic system. Multiple subtypes of central receptors (at least seven) have been identified and functionally linked to mood and emotion regulation, aggression, sexual behavior, feeding, and thermoregulation.

Amino-Acids

They are the most common of all neurotransmitters, usually divided into two broad categories: excitatory (i.e., aspartate and glutamate) and inhibitory (i.e., glycine and gamma-aminobutyric acid). GABA is involved both in the regulation of movement (cerebellum, striatum, spinal cord) through a modulation of reflexes and in the control of complex states (e.g., anxiety and epilepsy).

Neuropeptides

They have been studied extensively in recent years, as they are thought to be responsible for nonsynaptic neuromodulation. The opioid systems (beta-endorphines, enkephalines, dynorphines) have a role in pain and stress perception, while hormone-like peptides (substance P, ACTH, vasopressin, oxytocin, somatostatin, and protireline, to name just a few) have been investigated for their potential clinical use in many instances (Stein et al., 1994; Chujo et al., 1980). Their mechanisms of action in the human CNS, however, remain obscure and open to different speculations.

Finally, we should remember that the notion that one neuron secretes one neurotransmitter at all its terminals no longer holds true; there are several examples of neurocells that produce multiple biologically active substances both in the form of monoamines and short-chain peptides. The significance of this phenomenon is still unclear and opens the way to new paths of research and future treatment implications.

PHARMACOLOGICAL INSTANCES

At the clinical level, it is not easy to transfer the little theoretical knowledge that we possess.

In the area of traumatic brain injury (TBI) sequelae, there are few specific indications, and the use of different drugs is often linked to pragmatic considerations following analogies with other similar neurological syndromes, past experience in individual cases, and laboratory studies on animal models. A review of the international literature does not supply uniform guidelines to follow in treating these patients for a number of reasons which we have in part already examined.

We believe that, at the conceptual level, neurodrugs to be used with TBI patients should be divided into two categories:

1. **structural drugs**, whose action should be to protect "neuronal hardware" from secondary insults through different trophic restorative mechanisms, and
2. **neurochemical drugs,** whose activity, following neurotransmitter mechanisms, should enhance the "software," directly and indirectly, at the synaptic level.

Some compounds may be theoretically active at both levels, but this first differentiation may allow us to identify which substances should be used in the acute, subacute, and chronic phases following the primary insult. In fact, initially, the goal may be to save neurons and glial cells from secondary damage (hypoxic, metabolic, cytotoxic, etc.), while at a later stage, the goal may become optimal functional performance, at the software level, of all intact remaining neuronal networks (reorganization and potentiation of existing functioning neuropathways).

The third theoretical aspect of neuropharmacological intervention is contained in the Latin maxim *primum non nocere*; every effort should be made to eliminate or reduce the use of all substances that may have a negative effect on the recovery of a traumatically lesioned CNS (Perino, 1993). Among these, we should at least mention *benzodiazepines*, which may interfere with memory and learning (Sharf et al., 1988); *ethanol,* which produces cholinergic deficits (Parson, 1977); and *antidepressants* and *neuroleptics,* which may be neurotoxic, anticholinergic, antidopaminergic, and produce sedation, memory and attentional deficits and also interfere with movement recovery (Feeney et al., 1982; Judd et al., 1987). *Baclofen* (antispastic), *phenytoin,* and *phenobarbital* (antiseizure) can all have multiple negative effects on neurological and cognitive recovery (Sandy & Gillman, 1985; Andrewes et al., 1986; Prichard, 1980; Dikmen et al., 1991; Trimble, 1991) and should be employed carefully.

Politherapy, or overdosage, may greatly increase risks of unwanted negative consequences. It is thus mandatory to remember that the use of the above substances should be frequently verified in terms of advantage/disadvantage ratio and that their use should be reduced to a minimum or completely abandoned in patients who have suffered TBI

STRUCTURAL COMPOUNDS

Theoretically, they include all substances that may prevent the secondary extension of primary neurological insult through mechanisms of neuroprotection (from Ca^{++} influx and free radicals) of partially damaged neurons and glia, restoration of the blood/brain barrier and cell function, and resolution of "diaschisis." They should be used within hours (4–12) from the event or, at most, within a few days.

For example, *nimodipine*, among the calcium channel antagonists, has been shown to improve the neurological outcome of patients with subarachnoid hemorrhage (SAH) due to a traumatic cause (European Study Group, 1994).

A glycolipid, *monosialoganglioside GM1,* has been investigated for its active mechanism of neuroprotection through glutamate inhibition and membrane stabilization. It seems to improve, in animal models of neurotrauma, the recovery of movement and general functional outcome (Stein et al., 1994).

CDP-choline, as a constituent of cell membranes, has been theoretically indicated to facilitate structural restoration of damaged neurons and has been put to clinical trials with somewhat favorable results (Cohadon & Richer, 1984).

More recently, clinical research has been directed towards investigations of *lazaroids*, which are scavengers of free radicals largely implicated in the extension of secondary neuronal damage after a traumatic event. *Tirilazad mesilate*, the most important of these compounds, is under scrutiny for registration as a neuroprotective substance for the acute phase following TBI (Pasqualin, 1994).

Another investigated free radical scavenger, with the same rationale and indication, is the protein *PEG superoxide dismutase* (PEG-SOD).

Finally, one should briefly mention the possible role of other natural products (*vitamin E, gingko biloba extracts, magnesium*) and of *progesterone*, which have significantly influenced the recovery of traumatically brain-damaged rats (Stein et al., 1994). We should, at this point, also emphasize that there are grounds for caution before treatments in animal models can be applied to humans; incidentally, the latter substances are easily available and sufficiently safe to use but too inexpensive to be of particular interest for drug companies' research priorities.

DOPAMINERGIC AGONISTS

The main drug in this class has historically been *L-dopa* (levodopa), frequently combined with *carbidopa,* to increase CNS effects and to minimize peripheral side effects (Lal et al., 1988; Sohn et al., 1987). Typical Parkinsonism is an infrequent consequence of TBI; however, one well-recognized syndrome occurs after repeated boxing insults (dementia pugilistica or punch-drunk syndrome) (Katz, 1990).

Amantadine, initially used as an antiviral agent, has shown some anti-Parkinsonian activity, through pre- and post-synaptic dopaminergic mechanisms and as a glutamate antagonist. It has also been experimented with in post-traumatic agitation and aggressive behavior (Gualtieri et al., 1989). *Bromocriptine, pergolide,* and *lisuride* have been considered possible dopaminergic alternatives, especially in regard to treatment of akinetic mutism (Crismon et al., 1988). One has to remember, however, that post-traumatic Parkinsonism may be resistant or minimally responsive to therapy.

NOR-ADRENERGIC AGONISTS

The classic "psychostimulant" drugs have been theorized to have mixed nor-adrenergic, dopaminergic, and indoleaminergic (5-HT) activities.

Dextroamphetamine, methylphenidate, and *pemoline* have all positive effects on vigilance and cognition (Kupietz et al., 1985; Lipper et al., 1976; Stern, 1978) but numerous possible adverse consequences (agitation, psychiatric disturbances, irritability, anxiety, insomnia, anorexia, etc.) (Angrist, 1978), and, therefore, their use with TBI patients poses problems and risks (Chiarello et al., 1987). Some authors, however, feel that stimulant therapies may be safe, in most cases, at low doses and in the hands of responsible practitioners (Gualtieri, 1988; Gualtieri & Evans, 1988).

CHOLINERGIC AGONISTS

Most of these substances cannot be used clinically due to lack of CNS specificity, a short half-life, and a negative peripheral side-effects profile. Direct administration of *choline* or *lecitine,* for example, does not improve memory in elderly subjects (Blusztain & Wurtman, 1983; McEntee & Crook, 1990).

A precursor, *alpha-glyceryl-phosphoryl-choline,* seems, on the contrary, to have some positive effects on the aging brain (Amenta, 1992). Also, *nicotine* (given transdermally) has been shown to improve some cognitive parameters, but its clinical use is not established at the moment (Peeke et al., 1984).

In the field of post-traumatic brain injury syndrome, the use of some indirect cholinergic drugs, called *nootropic,* could yield some interesting results. One should at least mention *L-acetyl-carnitine,* under investigation for the treatment of dementia and cerebrovascular diseases (McEntee & Crook, 1990; Patti et al., 1988), *codergocrine* (Weil, 1988; Imperato et al., 1994), *oxiracetam* (Moglia et al., 1984; Itil et al., 1986), and *piracetam,* which has been tested for the treatment of acute TBI sequelae (Carrington Da Costa et al., 1978). However, the lack of more clinical trials with these compounds cannot justify undue optimism, even if they may appear theoretically sound and safe to employ in the cure of cognitive related problems.

SEROTONERGIC AGONISTS

Their use is indicated for the treatment of aggressive behavior, emotional incontinence, and post-traumatic organic depression. They include *trazodone, buspirone, fluoxetine* and *citalopram* (Sloan et al., 1992; Eison & Temple, 1986; Cassidy, 1989; Mendels, 1987) and are still experimental in patients who have suffered TBI. *Carbamazepine* and *lithium*, which are partially serotonergic, may be included in this category. They should always be administered by specialists with direct competence of their effects to individualize dosage, to monitor clinical consequences, and to reduce unwanted problems (Glenn et al., 1986; Mc Allister, 1985).

GABAMINERGIC AGONISTS

They should be mentioned here again for the risk of undesired negative cognitive effects; their use during rehabilitation, if really necessary, should be closely monitored. In particular *ethanol, diazepam,* and *baclofen* should be avoided. Benzodiazepines, in fact, can reduce learning through interference with memory mechanisms or may cause state-dependent learning (study-drunk/test-drunk effect) (Healey et al., 1983; O'Shanick & Parmelee, 1989).

Phenobarbital, used to prevent or to control post-traumatic epilepsy, should be substituted whenever possible (Pellock, 1989; Wroblewski et al., 1989).

NEUROPEPTIDES

They are endogenous ubiquitary proteins that are present at different CNS levels and are responsible for complex and mostly unknown hormone-like neuromodulatory mechanisms (Drago, 1988). Many of them (i.e., ACTH, VIP, vasopressin, substance P, somatostatin, oxytocin, etc.) do not present a possibility of practical clinical use at the moment (Stein et al., 1994). Only *protireline* (TRH-T) has been studied and can be employed to treat the post-traumatic comatose syndrome (Hatanaka et al., 1980; Agnoli et al., 1988). From personal experience, it seems to be, if correctly used, the best solution to improve vigilance in subjects already emerging from coma. Its activity is probably linked to modulation and enhancement of hypothalamic, mesolimbic, and brainstem reticular formation structures (Sano et al., 1979).

SPECIFIC CLINICAL ISSUES

From a practical point of view, the most common clinical situations can be grouped into six main categories: (1) emergence from coma and recovery of basic neurological functions; (2) prevention or control of post-traumatic seizures; (3) recovery of movements and prevention of limb contractures; (4) correction of unbalanced homeostatic and neuroendocrine mechanisms; (5) control and correction of post-traumatic neuropsychiatric disturbances; and (6) compensation of cognitive deficits and enhancement of residual abilities.

1. This section incorporates acute care, therapies to minimize secondary neurological damage, treatment of all early complications (i.e., infective, metabolic, etc.), and the possible use of substances to enhance arousal and recovery of consciousness. Some of these issues have already been examined in the previous paragraphs, and some go beyond the frame of this review. We should, however,

emphasize that from a strictly formal scientific standpoint and in accordance with the lack of a specific therapy for cerebrovascular diseases, there are no drugs directly registered for the treatment of acute TBI sequelae.

2. It also goes beyond the scope of this work to deal with post-traumatic epilepsy. However, we would like to stress again, in agreement with other authors (Pellock, 1989; Wroblewski et al., 1989; Yablon, 1993), that the use of phenytoin and phenobarbital should be abandoned whenever possible in favor of the use of carbamazepine, valproic acid, or lamotrigine. For an extensive review, please refer to the chapter in this book by F. Monaco.

3. Movement disturbances (i.e., dystonia, spasticity, tremors, Parkinsonism, myoclonus, dyskinesias, etc.) can be treated with some degree of success following brain injury. On this matter, please refer to a study by Katz (1990). We also suggest, in cases of severe spasticity, the employment of dantrolene sodium (Davidoff, 1985; O'Shanick & Zasler, 1990). For Parkinsonian-like disturbances, various different personalized therapies have been suggested (Eames, 1989; Sohn et al., 1987 Santosh et al., 1988). Tremors and myoclonus need careful investigation, some guesswork, and sound clinical judgment to choose between beta-blockers, piracetam, and benzodiazepines (Biary et al., 1989; Jankovic et al., 1986). For the prevention of heterotopic ossification, the use of etidronate disodium and nonsteroidal anti-inflammatory agents has been proposed, remembering, however, that most recommendations are based on spinal cord injury literature (Boutke, 1988).

4. DAI can produce hypothalamic and neurohypophysial damage in a certain proportion of the most severe TBI cases (10–20%). Consequences may include hypertension, hyperthermia, disregulation of fluid and nutrient metabolisms, and disruption of sleep-wake and circadian cycles; hormonal malfunctioning may also ensue. These medical complications should be dealt with by all appropriate specialists, always remembering the importance, in the acute stage, of nutrient and fluid intake, of thermic regulation, and of a well-functioning immune system in avoiding secondary complications and damage. Hypertension should be treated only if persistent or premorbid, and a preference should be for beta-blockers (e.g., atenolol) and for calcium channel antagonists (Wroblewski et al., 1987). Most commonly, hormonal disregulations include hypothyroidism, hypogonadism, and hypocorticalism. Therapies should be conducted only after endocrinological consultations (Klingbeil & Cline, 1985; Norman et al., 1980).

5. The treatment of aggressive, disruptive, or maladaptive behavior is among the problems usually encountered in the late postacute or chronic phase of recovery. The first task is to analyze premorbid personality and life-style, residual cognitive disturbances, environmental conditions, physical pain, and stress and fatigue reactions, as all these factors may play a role in the direction of generating unacceptable behavior. The correction and elimination of these concurrent causes, whenever possible, should be one of the priorities. The use and choice of an appropriate drug should be considered only as a secondary instance, also, in relation to the uncertainty of neuropharmacological action to control behavior. Theoretically, it is supposed that aggressive behavior may be suppressed through a modulation of fronto-temporo-limbic structures, with potentiation of the serotoninergic systems and inhibition of the nor-adrenergic. The substance of first choice in this direction may be carbamazepine, which is relatively free from

adverse cognitive effects and is also effective as a protective agent against undiagnosed temporal lobe epilepsy (Evans & Gualtieri, 1985). As alternatives, other compounds may be indicated: fluoxetine (Sloan et al., 1992), amantadine (Gualtieri et al., 1989), lithium (Glenn et al., 1986), and trazodone or amitriptyline (Mysiw et al., 1988). If clear signs of hyperadrenergic activity are present (hypertension, tachycardia, profuse sweating, etc.), beta-blockers or clonidine may be considered (Greendyke & Kukol, 1987; Greendyke et al., 1989; Bond, 1986). Medication effects will only be evident after at least two weeks of treatment, and pharmacological intervention alone is unable, most of the time, to control disruptive behavior completely. Thus, other measures should be used simultaneously, if necessary (i.e., neurobehavioral techniques, environment modification, pain relief, and cognitive and psychological interventions).

6. The last issue, already briefly mentioned elsewhere, deals with the theoretical possibility of enhancing cognitive capacities through pharmacological treatment (Gualtieri & Evans, 1988). The use of nootropic substances (i.e., L-acetylcarnitine, oxiracetam, etc.) or of psychostimulants (nicotine, caffeine, amphetamine, etc.) has not yet proven to be effective on a large statistically significant scale, and the whole matter is still open to speculation.

CONCLUSIONS

Finally, we would like to draw, in accordance with other authors, some final considerations and general guidelines (Zasler, 1992; Cope, 1994; Gualtieri, 1991).

We would suggest the following practical clinical notes:

1. Conduct a careful differential analysis of the problems to be treated.
2. Consider all nonpharmacological alternatives.
3. Evaluate if the pharmacological choice is still the most appropriate.
4. Prepare a list of all known pharmacological possibilities containing indications, drawbacks, and interactions of employable drugs.
5. Choose the substance with the best risk/benefit ratio.
6. Individualize posology, with a preference for a daily monodose, if possible.
7. Consider every therapy a trial, always amenable to change or suspension.
8. Control as objectively as possible the individual clinical results and be well aware of undesired effects.
9. Verify compliance and patient's subjective tolerability.
10. Use other specialists' competence whenever necessary.

On the research side, on the other hand, there is documented preliminary evidence that a number of drugs may prove beneficial in the treatment of human TBI, and thus a special effort should be made in this direction. Too many subjects are at present denied opportunities for a better recovery by lack of therapy or by misuse of available resources.

We also have to remember that the question of validating treatment methods is related to the issue of developing meaningful measures of functional recovery, which is yet to be resolved by rehabilitation specialists.

The search for new treatment protocols seems to proceed following two parallel pathways: on the one hand, to reduce undesired effects of "hard" drugs and to make them more selective; on the other hand, to improve efficacy of biologically "soft" compounds (Stein et al., 1994). At present, a correct clinical methodology and a multidisciplinary approach are the only means of taking up this great challenge before the end of the century.

REFERENCES

Agnoli, A., et al. (1988). *TRH-T: Pharmacological and clinical studies. Recent advances and perspectives.* London: John Libbey.

Amenta, F. (1992). Colina alfoscerato e terapia dell'invecchiamento cerebrale (Choline alphoscerate and brain aging therapy). *Brit. Med. J.* (Italian ed.), *17,* 51–58.

Andrewes, D., et al. (1986). A comparative study of the cognitive effects of phenytoin and carbamazepine in new referrals with epilepsy. *Epilepsia, 27,* 128–134.

Angrist, B.M. (1978). Toxic manifestations of amphetamine. *Psych. Ann., 8,* 13–18.

Barlow, D., & Hersen, M. (1984). *Single-case experimental designs* (2nd ed.). New York: Pergamon Press.

Biary, N., et al. (1989). Post-traumatic tremor. *Dept. Neurol., 1,* 103–106.

Blusztain, J. K., & Wurtman, R.J. (1983). Choline and cholinergic neurons. *Science, 221,* 614–616.

Bond, V.S. (1986). Psychiatric indications for clonidine: The neuropharmacological and clinical basis. *J. Clin. Psycopharm., 6,* 81–87.

Boutke, C. F. (1988). Pharmacologic treatment of heterotopic ossification. *J. Head Tr. Rehabil., 3,* 86–89.

Bradley, P.B. (1989). *Introduction to neuropharmacology.* Boston, MA: Wright.

Carrington Da Costa, R.B., et al. (1978). Studio controllato di piracetam verso placebo nei disturbi della coscienza dovuti a traumi cranici (Controlled study of piracetam versus placebo for TBI consciousness disturbances). *Acta Therapeutica, 4,* 109–118.

Cassidy, J.W. (1989). Fluoxetine: A new serotonergically active antidepressant. *J. Head Trauma Rehabil., 2,* 67–69.

Chiarello, R.J., et al. (1987). The use of psychostimulants in general psychiatry. *Arch. Gen. Psych., 44,* 286–295.

Chujo, T., et al. (1980). Experimental and clinical studies on TRH-T for treatment of disturbances of consciousness. *Neurol. Medico-Chirurgica, 20,* 289–301.

Cohadon, F., & Richer, E. (1984). CDP-choline in severe traumatic coma: A double-blind study. In *International meeting on CDP-choline* (pp. 299–303). New York: Elsevier.

Cope, D.N. (1990). Pharmacology for behavioral deficits: Disorders of cognition and affect. In R. Wood (Ed.), *Neurobehavioural sequelae of TBI* (pp. 250–273). London: Taylor and Francis Ltd.

Cope, D.N. (1994). Head trauma destiny: Interactions of neuropharmacology and personality. In A.L. Christensen & B. Uzzell (Eds.), *Brain injury and neuropsychological rehabilitation: An international perspective* (pp. 41–56). Hillsdale, NJ: Lawrence Erlbaum Associates.

Crismon, M.L., et al. (1988). The effect of bromocriptine on speech dysfunction in patients with diffuse brain injury and akinetic mutism. *Clin. Neuropharm., 11,* 462–466.

Davidoff, R. (1985). Antispasticity drugs: Mechanisms of action. *Ann. Neurol., 17,* 106–166.

Dikmen, S., et al. (1991). Neurobehavioral effects of phenytoin prophylaxis of post-traumatic seizures. *J.A.M.A., 265,* 1271–1277.

Drago, F. (1988). Neuropeptides in human therapy: Pharmacology and clinical perspectives of TRH-T. *TB-Today, 15* (Suppl. 4), Catania, Italy.

Eames P. (1989). Risk-benefit considerations in drug treatment. In R. Wood & P. Eames (Eds.), *Models of brain injury rehabilitation* (pp. 164–179). London: Chapman and Hall.

Eison, A.S., & Temple, D.L. (1986). Buspirone: review of its pharmacology and current perspectives of action. *Ann. J. Med., 80,* 1–9.

European Study Group. (1994). A multicenter trial of the efficacy of nimodipine on outcome after severe head injury. *J. Neurosurg., 80,* 797–804.

Evans, R.W., & Gualtieri, C.T. (1985). Carbamazepine: A neuropsychological and psychiatric profile. *Clin. Neuropharmacol., 8,* 221–241.

Feeney, D.M., et al. (1982). Amphetamine, haloperidol and experience interact to affect rate of recovery after motor cortex injury. *Science, 217,* 855–857.

Gardner, H. (1985). *Frames of mind: The theory of multiple intelligences.* New York: Basic Book Inc.

Geschwind, N., & Galaburda. (1987). A.M. *Cerebral lateralization: Biochemical mechanism, associations and pathology.* Cambridge, MA: M.I.T. Press.

Giurgea, C., et al. (1983). Nootropic drugs and ageing. *Acta Psych. Belgica, 83,* 349–358.

Glenn, M.B., et al. (1986). Lithium carbonate for aggressive behavior or emotional lability in nine brain-injured patients. *Arch. Phys. Med. Rehabil., 67,* 634.

Greendyke, R.M., et al. (1989). Treatment of behavioral problems with pindolol. *Acad. Psychosom. Med., 30,* 161–165.

Greendyke, R.M., & Kukol, R.J. (1987, April). Intermittent explosive disorder: successive treatment with propanolol and pindolol. *V.A. Practitioner,* 47–55.

Gualtieri, C. T. (1991). The psychopharmacology of TBI. In *Neuropsychiatry and behavioral pharmacology* (pp. 37–88). New York: Springer-Verlag.

Gualtieri, C.T. (1988). Pharmacotherapy and the neurobehavioral sequelae of TBI. *Brain Injury, 2,* 101–129.

Gualtieri, C.T., & Evans, R.W. (1988). Stimulant treatment for the neurobehavioral sequelae of TBI. *Brain Injury, 2,* 273–290.

Gualtieri, T., et al. (1989). Amantadine: A new clinical profile for TBI. *Clin. Neuropharm., 12,* 258–270.

Guyett, G., et al. (1986). Determining optimal therapy-randomized trials in individual patients. *N. Engl. J. Med, 314,* 899–902.

Hatanaka, M., et al. (1980). Clinical effect of TRH-T on consciousness disturbances. *J. N. Rem. Clin., 29,* 57–60.

Healey, M., et al. (1983). Effects of chlorazepate, diazepam, lorazepam and placebo on human memory. *J. Clin. Psych., 44,* 436–439.

Imperato, A., et al. (1994). Codergocrine (hydergine) regulates striatal and hippocampal acetylcholine release through D receptors. *Neuro Report, 5,* 674–676.

Itil, T.M., et al. (1986). CNS pharmacology and clinical therapeutic effects of oxiracetam. *Clin. Neuropharm., 9,* 570.

Jankovic, J., et al. (1986). Segmental myoclonus: Clinical and pharmacologic study. *Arch. Neurol., 43,* 1025–1031.

Judd, L., et al. (1987). Effects of psychotropic drugs on cognition and memory in normal humans and animals. In H. Melzer (Ed.), *Psychopharmacology: The third generation of progress* (p. 146). New York: Raven Press.

Katz, D. (1990). Movement disorders following traumatic head injury. *J. Head. Trauma Rehabil., 5,* 86–90.

Klingbeil, G., & Cline, P. (1985). Anterior hypopituitarism: A consequence of head injury. *Arch. Phys. Med. Rehabil., 66,* 44–46.

Koller, W.C., et al. (1989). D1 and D2 dopamine receptor mechanisms in dopaminergic behaviours. *Clin. Neuropharm., 11,* 221–231.

Kupietz, S.S., et al. (1985). Psychostimulants: Plasma concentration and learning performance. *J. Clin. Psychopharm., 5,* 293–295.

Lal, S., et al. (1988). Modification of function in head-injured patients with Sinemet. *Brain Injury, 2,* 225–233.

Lipper, S., et al. (1976). Treatment of chronic post-traumatic organic brain syndrome with dextro-amphetamine: First reported case. *J. Nerv. Ment. Dis., 162,* 366–371.

McAllister, T.W. (1985). Carbamazepine in mixed frontal lobe and psychiatric disorders. *J. Clin. Psych., 46,* 393–394.

McEntee, W.J., & Crook, T.H. (1990). Age-associated memory impairments. *Neurology, 10,* 526–530.

McLean, A., et al. (1991). Placebo-controlled study of pramiracetam in young males with memory and cognitive problems resulting from head injury and anoxia. *Brain Injury, 5,* 375–380.

Mendels, J. (1987). Clinical experience with serotonin reuptake-inhibiting antidepressants. *J. Clin. Psych., 48,* 26–30.

Moglia, A., et al. (1984). Activity of oxiracetam in patients with organic brain syndrome: A neuropsychological study. *Clin. Neuropharm., 7,* 784.

Mysiw, W.J., et al. (1988). Amitriptyline for post-traumatic agitation. *Am. J. Phys. Med. Rehab., 88,* 29–33.

Norman, D., et al. (1980). Permanent diabetes insipidus following head trauma: Observation on 10 patients. *J. Trauma, 20,* 599–602.

O'Shanick, G.J., & Parmelee, D.X. (1989). Psychopharmacologic agents in the treatment of brain injury. In D. Ellis & A.L. Christensen (Eds.), *Neuropsychological treatment after brain injury* (pp. 91–104). Boston: Martinus Nijhoff.

O'Shanick, G.J., & Zasler, N.D. (1990). Neuropsychopharmacological approaches to TBI. In J. Kreutzer & P. Wehman (Eds.), *Community integration following TBI* (pp. 15–27). Baltimore: P.H. Brooks.

Parson, O.A. (1977). Neuropsychological deficits in alcoholics: Facts and fancies. *Alcoholism, 1,* 51.

Pasqualin, A. (1994). Tirilazad mesylate in subaracnoid haemorrage: Results of the European-Australian study. Atti del Congresso Internazionale sul Trauma Cranico grave. Parma, Italy, October 1994.

Patti, F., et al. (1988). Effects of L-acetylcarnitine on functional recovery of hemiplegic patients. *Clin. Trials J., 25* (Suppl. 1), 87–101.

Peeke, S.C., et al. (1984). Attention, memory and cigarette smoking. *Psychopharmacology, 84,* 205–216.

Pellock, J. M. (1989). Editorial: Who should receive prophylactic antiepileptic drug following head injury? *Brain Injury, 3,* 107–108.

Perino, C. (1993). Il trattamento neuropsicofarmacologico del danno celebrale post-traumatico (Neuropharmacological treatment of TBI). In R. Rago & C. Perino (Eds.), *La riabilitazione dei T.C.E. nell'adulto* (pp. 209–220). Milano, Italy: Ed. Ghedini.

Perino. C. (1990). Neurofarmaci e memoria: Quale interazione? (Neurodrugs and memory: Which interaction?). In L. Caldana (Ed.), *La riabilitazione della memoria dopo danno cerebrale* (pp. 177–184). Rome, Italy: Editore Marrapese.

Prichard, J. (1980). Antiepileptic drugs: Phenobarbital. In G. Glaser et al. (Eds.), *Antiepileptic drugs and mechanisms of action* (p. 473). New York: Raven Press.

Saletu, B., et al. (1985). Double-blind placebo-controlled clinical psychometric and neuropsychological investigations with oxiracetam in the organic brain syndrome of late life. *Neuropsychobiology, 13,* 44–52.

Sandy, K., & Gillman M. (1985). Baclofene-induced memory impairment. *Clin. Neuroph., 8,* 294–295.

Sano, K., et al. (1979). Clinical studies on TRH-T for the treatment of disturbances of consciousness (Part 1). *Jap. J. Clin. Exp. Med., 56,* 248-258: (Part 2) *Neurol. Sc., 23,* 184-210.

Santosh, L., et al. (1988). Modification of function in head-injured patients with Sinemet. *Brain Injury, 2,* 225–233.

Seliger, G., et al. (1992). Fluoxetine improves emotional incontinence. *Brain Injury, 6,* 267–270.

Sharf, M.B., et al. (1988). Comparative amnestic effects of benzodiazepine hypnotic agents. *J. Clin. Psych., 49,* 134.

Sloan, R., et al. (1992). Fluoxetine as a treatment for emotional lability after brain injury. *Brain Injury, 6,* 315–319.

Snyder, S.H. (1986). *Drugs and the brain.* New York: Scientific American Books, Inc.

Sohn, D.G., et al. (1987). Levodopa-carbidopa therapy for movement disorders. *Arch. Phys. Med. Rehabil., 68,* 745–746.

Stein, D., et al. (1994). Pharmacological treatments for brain injury repair: Progress and prognosis. *Neuropsychol. Rehabil., 4,* 337–357.

Stern, J.M. (1978). Cranio-cerebral injured patients: A psychiatric clinical description. *Scand. J. Rehabil. Med., 10,* 7–10.

Trexler, L.E. (1991). Neuropsychological assessment and rehabilitation of TBI in the USA. *Giorn. Ital. Med. Riabil., I,* 41–52.

Trimble, M. (1991). Cognitive effects of anti-convulsants. *Neurology, 41,* 1326.

Weil, C. (1988). *Hydergine: Pharmacologic and clinical facts.* Berlin: Springer-Verlag.

Whyte, J. (1988). Clinical drug evaluation. *J. Head Trauma Rehab., 3,* 95–99.

Wilsher, C., et al. (1979). Piracetam as an aid to learning in dislexia. *Psychopharmacology, 65,* 107–109.

Woolf, N.J. (1991). Cholinergic systems in the mammalian brain and spinal cord. *Progr. Neurobiol., 37,* 475–524.

Wroblewski, B.A., et al. (1987). Chronic hypertension after TBI: Pharmacologic options. *J. Head Tr. Rehabil.*, 2, 87–89.

Wroblewski, B.A., et al. (1989). Carbamazepine replacement of phenytoin, phenobarbital and primidone in a rehabilitation setting: Effect on seizure control. *Brain Injury*, 3, 149–156.

Yablon, S.A. (1993). Review article: Post-traumatic seizures. *Arch. Phys. Med. Rehabil.*, 74, 983–1001.

Zappalà, G. (1988). Traumatismi cerebrali da incidenti: Approccio multidisciplinare e riabilitazione neuropsicologica. (TBI: Multidisciplinary approach and neuropsychological rehabilitation). *Riabilit. e Apprend.*, 8, 337–346.

Zasler, N.D. (1992). Review: Advances in neuropharmacological rehabilitation for brain dysfunction. *Brain Injury*, 6, 1–14.

12 Acquired Brain Injury Physical Rehabilitation

Paolo Pietrapiana, Maria Pia Bronzino, Claudio Perino, and Roberto Rago

Centro di Medicina Riabilitativa "AUSILIATRICE"
Via Peyron 42, 10143 Torino, Italy

INTRODUCTION

The description and classification of sensory-motor damage caused by traumatic brain injury (TBI) is extremely helpful in understanding rehabilitative problems (Cope, 1990).

In this complex and varied field, the best approach should be holistic, integrated, and interdisciplinary, helping individuals to recover their motor abilities as an expression of their interaction with the outside world (Trexler & Zappalà, 1988). Formulating a global treatment and rehabilitation plan related to presenting clinical features means, therefore, finding appropriate compenation in the organization of function and behavior. It is the aim of therapy to employ dynamic and balanced strategies and to promote the patient's progress following realistic objectives with appropriate techniques along a continuum of care (Table 12.1).

NEUROPATHOLOGY AND CLINICAL FEATURES

Three main types of neuropathological lesions are usually found following TBI (Jaggi, Obrist, Gennarelli, & Langfitt, 1990): (1) focal damage, (2) diffuse axonal injury (DAI), and (3) secondary ischemic damage. A combination of these, although not always evident at neuroimaging, can be responsible for coma if brainstem structures are involved (Zappalà, 1988). There can also be focal lesions in various areas (e.g., frontal lobes, temporal lobes, occipital lobes) sometimes associated with vascular or meningeal lesions (Jennett, Teasdale, Braakman, Minderhoud, Heiden, & Kurze, 1979). These pathological combinations may give some idea of the variability of motor disturbances in different patients.

	STRUCTURES	OBJECTIVES
First Phase	MOBILE UNIT	First aid, maintenance of vital functions Safe transportation of patient
	INTENSIVE CARE, NEUROSURGICAL AND TRAUMA UNITS	Maintainance of vital functions Specific treatment of lesions
Second Phase	SPECIAL TBI REHABILITATION UNIT	Assessment of damage Integrated rehabilitative projects Sensory regulation Prevention of secondary and tertiary damage Rehabilitative treatment Training for staff and the patient's family Quality control
Third Phase	COMMUNITY REHABILITATION SERVICE OR SHELTERED ACCOMODATION FAMILY SOCIAL STRUCTURES	Rehabilitative maintainance treatment Preparation for social reintegration Return to family, social life and work/school activities Reduction of handicap Quality of life improvement

In order to obtain a clear picture and to set therapeutic goals, it is useful to differentiate the neurological aspects of TBI. Taxonomic studies have identified three main syndromes: orbito-frontal, dorso-lateral, and cerebellar-brainstem (Zappalà, 1988). Other authors prefer to describe all the "pure" possible neurological forms that can be present, often simultaneously, in the same patient (Griffith & Mayer, 1990). For rehabilitation purposes, it is useful to refer to some neurological features that represent more classically the evolution of motor deficits associated with head injury (Table 12.2).

Table 12.2: Predominant Motor Deficits

Absent or minimal motor impairment
Motor neglect and/or apraxia
Hemiparesis or hemiplegia
Central asymmetrical tetraparesis (or double hemiparesis)
Ataxic cerebellar syndrome
Extrapyramidal syndrome

Absent or Minimal Motor Impairment

Regaining correct functional movements can depend on there being no lasting damage to motor areas, spontaneous recovery, and plasticity of the central nervous system (CNS). In this case, rehabilitation is directed towards training the patient to improve execution of movements at various levels of performance (speed, strength, variations in trajectory, coordination, etc.).

Motor Neglect and/or Apraxia

The subject shows few single motor deficits, but there is serious impairment at the executive level. Rehabilitation is based on integrating neuropsychological components with the production of motor functions of increasing complexity.

Hemiparesis or Hemiplegia

The patient presents with a focal lesion that is generally evident from neuroradiological examination. The severity of the sensory-motor deficit varies according to the site and extension (cortical, subcortical, or both) of the cerebral lesion. In all cases, signs of injury to the pyramidal system can be found: alterations in muscle tone, abnormal reactions to stimuli, and loss of mobility. In less serious cases, the deficits become evident only during activities of daily life, and rehabilitation is directed to these areas.

Central Asymmetrical Tetraparesis (or Double Hemiparesis)

In these cases, damage is bilaterally pyramidal, with a stronger tendency to one side. The evolution toward spasticity is frequent but not the rule; most often, the motor deficit is primarily distal. Sometimes cortico-bulbar deficits are associated, causing a reduction in ability to speak and swallow. If this occurs, together with a defect in postural control of the head and trunk, it can interfere with nutrition and cleanliness. Rehabilitation is, therefore, directed initially towards postural control, then to training movements for daily activities.

Ataxic Cerebellar Syndrome

In these patients, cerebellar damage is predominant even if there may be associated pyramidal damage. The greatest difficulties are seen in functional activities, in transfers, and in walking. Some of these subjects can improve significantly after specific neuromotor rehabilitation (postural control, balance, and coordination exercises).

Extrapyramidal Syndrome

Lesions of the various extrapyramidal components interfere with autonomous walking and self-care. Subjects, therefore, need assistance with transfers, personal hygiene, and activities of daily life. Although pharmacological treatment is probably the primary intervention, it is nonetheless useful to undertake early neuromotor rehabilitation.

In tracing the rehabilitative path for brain-injured patients, it is also possible to subdivide its evolution into three distinct phases according to the presenting symptoms: acute, post-acute, and late. Each of these is identified on the basis of specific clinical data, type of healthcare structure, time from injury, professional figures involved, means of intervention, and therapeutic objectives.

FIRST PHASE

It begins at the moment of trauma and lasts until the vital cardiovascular and respiratory functions are reestablished (from a few days to several weeks) (Jennett, 1990). Primary level healthcare structures are usually involved at this stage: the accident and emergency unit, intensive care, trauma care, and neurosurgery. Their task is to guarantee the patient's survival, with surgical intervention to the lesions if necessary.

With a favorable prognosis "quoad vitam," rehabilitative treatment is then begun soon after hospitalization. The severity of the patient's condition does not exempt the rehabilitation team from a thorough assessment and a treatment plan. In fact, early rehabilitation allows the patient's potential for recovery to be exploited to the maximum and limits secondary and tertiary damage (Cope & Hall, 1982; Hackler & Tobis, 1990; Namerow, 1987; Rusk, Block, & Lowman, 1969). In this phase, treatment objectives can be summarized as follows:

1. Forming an early prognosis, circumstances permitting. This is reached by an accurate assessment of injury, of the level of consciousness, and of associated lesions.

2. Preventing secondary and tertiary complications at the following levels: cutaneous (pressure sores), respiratory (reduction in pulmonary ventilation and efficiency), osteoarticular (calcification of soft tissues, muscle-tendon shortening, joint rigidity).

3. Controlling pathological movements and eliciting correct postures and movements.

4. Enabling the patient to regain contact with the environment.

5. Monitoring neurological progress.

Physiatrist's Assessment

The physiatrist's assessment of TBI in the acute phase consists of

- **Medical history** and interviews with relatives to obtain information about the patient's premorbid personality, social and family environment, and his/her studies or work.
- **Patient observation**, noting expression of body movements, vital functions and various support systems, presence of peripheral nerve lesions, conditions of muscles and joints, damage to sensory organs, medical complications, etc.
- **Kinesiologic assessment.**
- **Assessment of level of consciousness and neurological damage.** The Glasgow Coma Scale will have been used already at the beginning of the patient's hospitalization. It defines scores for neurological indices of severity of coma by analyzing verbal, ocular, and motor responses. The rehabilitation specialist adds to this findings from an assessment of reflex responses (Table 12.3). This information completes and defines the level of cerebral damage.

Neuroradiological and neurophysiological assessments (CT scan, MRI, SPECT, EEG, EMG, EP, etc.) complete the monitoring of the evolution of post-traumatic lesions.

Table 12.3: Assessment of Reflex Responses

PHASIC REFLEXES	TONIC REFLEXES
Pupillary	Postural in decortication
Vestibular-ocular	Postural in decerebration
Corneal	Tonic-labyrinthine
Extrinsic oculomotor	Tonic-asymmetrical of the neck
Pharyngeal	Tonic-symmetrical of the neck
Tendon and cutaneous	

Rehabilitation Plan

The rehabilitation plan is made on the basis of the data obtained in the above examinations and consists of

1. *Integrated rehabilitative nursing.* The nursing staff is trained by the rehabilitation therapists to avoid the potential damage of prolonged immobility. Two types of intervention are necessary:

    - **Postural control in bed.** This prevents pressure sores, maintains the joints in correct positioning, and encourages better pulmonary ventilation.
    - **Range of motion exercises.** The aim of this practice is to prevent articular rigidity and muscle-tendon contractures (Goldspink & Williams, 1990). The patient's general condition often requires that these treatments must be brief and spread out during the day. In some cases, casting is useful to maintain positions obtained during mobilization.

2. *Respiratory assistance and/or training.* This is fundamental for preventing secondary hypoxic damage to the CNS and for limiting respiratory complications. Respiratory training, if possible, must be practiced several times a day to maintain ventilation in the lower airways and to enable bronchial secretions to be eliminated. When autonomous respiratory function has been reestablished, the patient must be "weaned" from the respiratory pump. Close collaboration between the anesthesiologist and the therapist is essential at this point. The tracheal tube is often left in place to protect the airways from the risk of aspiration and to enable the removal of bronchial secretions. It must be remembered, however, that this can be a significant pathway for serious infection and can impede early recovery of swallowing and speech.

3. *Sensory regulation.* This consists of a dual intervention:

    - **Controlled sensory stimulation.** Different channels can be periodically stimulated (acoustic, visual, gustatory, olfactory, tactile, and osteoarticular receptors), although there is no proof of efficacy (Rinehart et al., 1990). Nursing maneuvers, postural regulation and selective mobilization, all of which involve direct contact between staff and patient, must be performed with caution to avoid painful stimuli and increase of intracranial pressure.
    - **Environmental regulation.** A quiet and reassuring environment should be created where voices, sounds, and lights are modulated. The presence of family members at the bedside needs to be organized and supervised.

4. *Help and information for the patient's family.* The role of the patient's family is fundamental from the very first hours in intensive care, and relatives can be gradually involved in the patient's early rehabilitation. The neuropsychologist and the rehabilitation specialist need to establish early contact with the family to provide support in three principal ways:

    - **Informative.** The "quoad vitam" prognosis, made in the intensive care unit, must be integrated with a clear explanation of the possible lasting consequences for the patient's motor, cognitive, and behavioral conditions. The importance of the family's help must be strongly encouraged. It needs to be emphasized, however, that they are not substitutes for the nursing staff, nor must they initiate therapy from their own ideas.

- **Educational**. The relatives need to be trained to assist the patient and to monitor his/her evolving level of consciousness.
- **Preventive**. The aim is to prevent burnout in the family members who accompany the patient.

SECOND PHASE

This begins when vital functions become stabilized or there is an improvement in the state of consciousness. The discriminating parameter for beginning a more structured and assiduous rehabilitation therapy is the subject's responsiveness to the environment. This cannot be carried out in intensive care or neurosurgical departments because of the difference in clinical aims and resources required. The patient needs, at this point, to be transferred to a rehabilitation department; it is always a delicate moment, and it is difficult to establish fail-safe criteria for clinical conduct.

It is useful here to refer to the Ranch Los Amigos Assessment Scale, which distinguishes eight levels of cognitive performance on the basis of ability to respond to environmental stimuli (Table 12.4).

In our experience, level III is the minimum necessary for a transfer to a rehabilitation unit. In some cases, an improvement in the state of consciousness is not accompanied by sufficient stability of vital functions. Subjects in this category may need an intermediate structure, defined as "post-intensive operative unit with rehabilitative value," where more assiduous and specific therapy is guaranteed.

Mobilization, integrated nursing, respiratory assistance, and sensory regulation, already proposed during the acute phase, can here be carried out with more suitable aids and equipment such as a tilting bed, objects to increase awareness, and video and sound equipment to attract the subject's attention and stimulate an emotional response.

The presence of the patient's family should be permitted, and their involvement, correctly guided, is an indispensable part of this phase.

When the patient no longer needs clinical monitoring, he/she should be transferred to a special rehabilitation unit. The treatment of TBI patients in a general rehabilitation department is not usually practicable, as they need particular therapies that require a specific environment.

Special units (Figure 12.1) are structured to meet the global needs of these patients and to guarantee (1) the best logistical environment; (2) the continuation of rehabilitative integrated nursing; (3) integrated, interdisciplinary diagnosis and therapy; and (4) planning and implementation of specific rehabilitative treatment.

1. *The best logistical environment.* This should be a treatment area structured and equipped like a small apartment, where personalized living conditions can be created with some comfort. Furnishings can include a table and chairs, an armchair, a television and VCR, a radio-cassette player and tapes, pictures, posters, a clock, and a calendar. There should be an individual bathroom with wheelchair access. Next to the living-room, there should be a room for individual treatment such as motor rehabilitation, occupational therapy, and ergonomic therapy. Isolated rooms are also needed for treating communication disorders, swallowing problems, and neuropsychological impairments. Lastly, one or two larger common rooms on the floor are required for group therapy or training.

Table 12.4: Rancho Los Amigos Scale (from the Professional Staff Association of R.L.A. Hospital, Inc., Downey, CA, 1980)

RANCHO LOS AMIGOS SCALE
Levels of cognitive functioning

I—No response
Patient appears to be in a deep sleep and is completely unresponsive to any stimuli presented to him/her.

II—Generalized response
Patient reacts inconsistently and non-purposefully to stimuli in a nonspecific manner. Responses are limited in nature and are often the same regardless of stimulus presented. Responses may be physiological changes, gross body movements, and vocalization. Responses are likely to be delayed. The earliest response is to deep pain.

III—Localized response
Patient reacts specifically but inconsistently to stimuli. Responses are directly related to the type of stimulus presented, as turning head toward a sound or focusing on an object presented. The patient may withdraw an extremity and vocalize when presented with a painful stimulus. S/he may follow simple commands in an inconsistent, delayed manner, such as closing his/her eyes, or squeezing or extending an extremity. Once external stimuli are removed, s/he may lie quietly. S/he may also show a vague awareness of self and body by responding to discomfort by pulling at the nasogastric tube or catheter or by resisting restraints. S/he may show a bias toward responding to some persons, especially family and friends, but not to others.

IV—Confused/agitated
Patient is in a heightened state of activity with severely decreased ability to process information. S/he is detached from the present and responds primarily to his/her own internal confusion. Behavior is frequently bizarre and nonpurposeful relative to his/her immediate environment. S/he may cry out or scream out of proportion to stimuli even after removal, may show aggressive behavior, attempt to remove restraints or a tube, or crawl out of bed in a purposeful manner. S/he does not discriminate between persons or objects and is unable to cooperate directly with treatment efforts. Verbalization is frequently incoherent or inappropriate to the enviroment. Confabulation may be present; s/he may be hostile. Gross attention to environment is very brief, and selective attention is often nonexistent. Being unaware of present events, patient lacks short-term recall and may be reacting to past events. S/he is unable to perform self-care activities without maximum assistance. If not disabled physically, s/he may perform automatic motor activities such as sitting, reaching, and ambulating, as part of his/her agitated state but not as a purposeful act or necessarily on request.

V—Confused/inappropriate
Patient appears alert and able to respond to simple command fairly consistently. However, with increased complexity of commands or lack of any external structure, responses are nonpurposeful, random, or at best, fragmented away from any desired goal. S/he may show agitated behavior, but not on an internal basis as in level IV, but rather as a result of exernal stimuli and usually out of proportion to the stimulus. S/he has gross attention for the enviroment, is highly distractible, and lacks ability to focus attention to a specific task without frequent redirection. With structure, s/he may able to converse on a social-automatic level for short periods of time. Verbalization is often inappropriate; confabulation may be triggered by present events. Memory is severely impaired, with confusion of past and present in reaction to ongoing activity. Patient lacks initiation of functional tasks and often shows inappropriate use of objects without external direction. S/he may be able to perform previously learned tasks when structured for him/her, but is unable to learn new information. S/he responds best to self, body, comfort and, often, family members. The patient can usually perform self-care activities with assistance and may accomplish feeding with supervision. Management on the unit is often a problem if the patient is physically mobile, as s/he may wander off either randomly or with vague intention of "going home."

VI—Confused/appropriate
Patient shows goal-directed behavior, but is dependent on external input for direction. Response to discomfort is appropriate, and s/he is able to tolerate unpleasant stimuli, e.g., NG tube, when need is explained. S/he follows simple directions consistently and shows carryover for tasks s/he has relearned, e.g., self-care. S/he is at least supervised with old learning and is unable to be maximally assisted for new learning, with little or no carryover. Responses may be incorrect due to memory problems but are appropriate to the situation. They may be delayed to immediate, and s/he shows decreased ability to process information with little or no anticipation or prediction of events. Past memories show more depth and detail than recent memory. The patient may show beginning awareness of his/her situation by realizing s/he doesn't know an answer. S/he no longer wanders and is inconsistently oriented to time and place. Selective attention to tasks may be impaired, especially with difficult tasks and in unstructured settings, but s/he is now functional for common daily activities. S/he may show vague recognition of some staff and has increased awareness of self, family, and basic needs.

VII—Automatic/appropriate
Patient appears appropriate and oriented within hospital and home settings, goes through daily routine automatically but robot-like, with minimal to absent confusion, and has shallow recall of what s/he has been doing. S/he shows increased awareness of self, body, family, food, people, and interaction in the environment. S/he has superficial awareness of, but lacks insight into, his/her condition, decreased judgment, and problem solving, and lacks realistic planning for his/her future. S/he shows carryover for new learning. S/he requires at least minimal supervision for learning at a decreased rate. S/he is independent in self-care activities and supervised in home and community skills for safety. With structure, s/he is able to initiate tasks or social and recreational activities in which s/he now has interest. His/her judgment remains impaired. Prevocational evaluation and counseling may be indicated.

Table 12.4: Rancho Los Amigos Scale cont.

RANCHO LOS AMIGOS SCALE Levels of cognitive functioning
VIII—Purposeful/appropriate Patient is alert and oriented, is able to recall and integrate past and recent events, and is aware of and responsive to his/her culture. S/he shows carryover for new learning if acceptable to him/her and his/her life role, and needs no supervision once activities are learned. Within his /her physical capabilities, s/he is independent in home and community skills. Vocational rehabilitation, to determine ability to return as a contributor to society, perhaps in a new capability, is indicated. S/he may continue to show decreases relative to premorbid abilities in quality and rate of processing, abstract reasoning, tolerance for stress, and judgment in emergencies or unusual circumstances. His/her social, emotional, and intellectual capacities may continue to be at a decreased level for him/her, but functional within society.

2. *Rehabilitative integrated nursing.* This is carried out by the nursing staff and the patient's relatives. Nursing assistance is of particular relevance here, because, of all the treatment team members, the ones who are in most continuous contact with the patient are the nurses. They must be completely integrated in the rehabilitation program in order to be able to carry out their duties of assistance, given the patient's communicative and behavioral disturbances. The relatives are kept informed about the patient's changing physical and mental state. They supervise and observe the patient while in the room, and they reassure the patient emotionally. The relatives and nursing staff meet with the therapists at regular intervals to exchange information and pass on advice and suggestions.

3. *Integrated, interdisciplinary diagnosis and therapy.* In most cases, the brain-injured patient presents with a multiple pathology, directly caused by the polytrauma, to different organs and structures. The compromising of vital functions

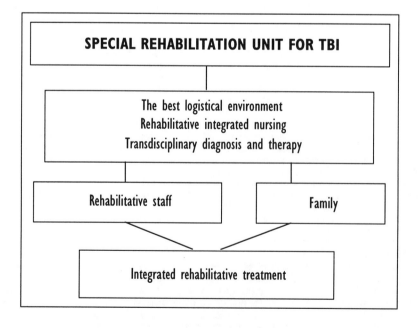

Figure 12.1: Special rehabilitation for TBI.

means that various medical specialists are jointly involved; indeed, often in the acute phase, their work has been essential to guarantee the patient's survival. When general conditions become stable and the patient is transferred to the special rehabilitation unit, the collaboration of various specialists to assess and plan treatment is essential to maximize recovery. The priority in this phase is to lead the patient towards the greatest possible autonomy in activities of daily life. The presence of dysphagia justifies an early assessment by an ORL specialist, followed by a specific treatment plan. For example, the need to regain the standing position as soon as possible, with correct postural alignment, requires the attention of the orthopedic specialist to study the patient's osteoarticular condition and to suggest the most suitable treatment according to level of progress. Visual disorders (defined as "post-trauma vision syndrome"), which can cause loss of binocular vision, headache, inability to read or write, staring, and related disturbances (proprioceptive and postural), need the attention of an opthalmologist. Other professionals are introduced according to need: the plastic surgeon, the urologist, the gastroenterologist, etc. Their advice can solve specific problems and allow the continuation of the patient's rehabilitative journey.

4. ***Planning and practice of specific rehabilitative treatment.*** When taken on for treatment in the special unit, the patient has a treatment plan formulated for him/her according to his/her sensory-motor and cognitive conditions (Figure 12.2). Realistic objectives and strategies are established on the basis of priority of injury, improvement in state of consciousness, and with consideration of the patient's level of collaboration. It is useful to divide rehabilitative treatment in terms of short-, medium-, and long-term goals. Failure or delay in reaching established objectives should induce modification of the treatment plan, not only in the qualitative aspect (type of treatment), but also in the quantitative aspect

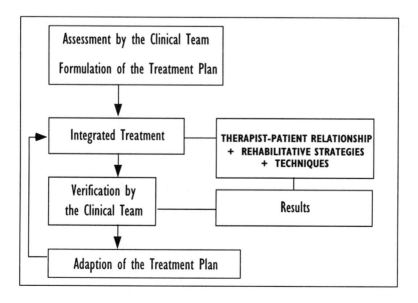

Figure 12.2: Rehabilitative process.

(frequency and duration of treatment). Rapid neuromotor or behavioral progress requires accurate and frequent checking of results in order to adapt and modify treatment, even on a daily basis. It is important that these checks be carried out by all members of the rehabilitation team—physiatrist, dietitian, ORL specialist, neuropsychologist, physiotherapist, speech therapist, occupational therapist, social worker, and nurse (Cope, 1990). Coming, as they do, from different cultural and professional backgrounds, the team members need a certain amount of homogenization and common training to ensure coherence in diagnosis and treatment. Treatment planning requires the precise division of the day's timetable between the various therapeutic activities (Figure 12.3) and careful use of the rooms available. This division of activities helps the patient to gradually adapt to a more organized scheme of time and space, even if this adaptation is difficult due to fatigue and attention problems.

The coordinating or primary therapist in the rehabilitation team is important as a liaison between the staff, for treatment planning, and for relatives' training and thus becomes the point of reference for the patient and his/her family.

Physiatrist's Assessment

An initial sensory-motor assessment is essential for a correct and efficient therapeutic approach; here, the physiatrist is joined by the neuropsychologist, the orthopedic specialist, the neurologist, and the therapists for respiratory and swallowing problems.

The motor behavior assessment needs to focus on signs of interaction and adaptability to the environment, rather than evoking nonspecific reflexes. These are not directly connected to the severity of cognitive disorders and have a prevalently prognostic value.

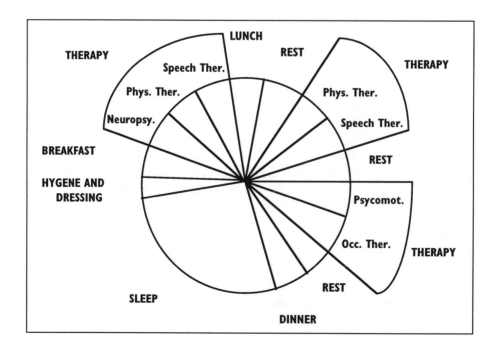

Figure 12.3: Therapy timetable.

Table 12.5 summarizes the useful elements of TBI assessment.

The sensory assessment is carried out by stimulating the patient's vision, hearing, touch, proprioception, and taste. Initially, the stimuli must be weak, in order to avoid a neurovegetative crisis and an increase in intracranial pressure or abnormal reflex responses, but they must be of sufficient strength to be able to evoke reactions according to the level of consciousness and, if possible, to stimulate an interaction between the patient and his/her environment.

Table 12.5: Sensory-Motor Assessment

- Pathological and clinical medical history
- Observation of posture and spontaneous movements
- Sensory assessment
  - sight-visual ability
  - hearing
  - touch-localization
  - proprioception
  - taste
- Selective evaluation of joint movements
- Muscle tone assessment
- Response to verbal commands
- Oral/facial mobility
- Postural evaluation (sitting, standing, balance and righting reactions)
- Walking
- Manipulation, stereognosis
- Activities of daily life

To record the reactions to visual stimuli, the patient must be able to stare at an object. In fact, eye opening, which often occurs quite precociously after post-traumatic coma, does not always mean that the patient is in contact with the environment. The chosen object for visual assessment must be familiar to the patient and have some emotional significance. Asymmetry of visual field, persistence of glance, ability to follow a moving object, and exploration of the visual field are all assessed.

For the hearing assessment, stimuli already familiar to the patient are used, spoken or musical, always at a low volume. In this way, attention and reactions may be tested, noting attempts by the patient to trace the source of the sounds with his/her eyes or by turning the head.

The tactile assessment carries notable emotional value, even in healthy subjects. For brain-injured patients, touch is often the first and most simple method of communication. At first, the reactions are of a global type; later, they are associated with eye-opening and staring at the therapist. From initial stimulation of medium intensity, other stimuli with more emotional meaning may be used, requiring identification and discrimination of place if attention improves and responses become progressively more oriented.

Finally, reactions to taste stimuli can be assessed at an early stage, even before feeding is restored, because their emotional significance is notable and provides important connections with the environment.

Speech assessment, if possible, is always important and should be directed towards finding out possible limitations in articulation and their causes and characteristics. If done early, it is of great value in preventing later problems.

Similarly, the checks on muscle tone and on limb mobility have prognostic value following the evolution of the pathology, and these findings are used to set therapeutic goals. Initially, the primitive and instinctive movements that the patient presents are assessed, and later a comparison is made with the quality of spontaneous and voluntary movements, analyzing postural control and balance. Then, the patient's ability to perform complex motor tasks is examined. The oral/facial assessment, essential for feeding and speech, can be inserted here. Finally, perceptive motor activity is assessed, as well as the ability to control and regulate complex, purposeful behavior.

Together with assessments of personal autonomy, mobility, and transfers, these checks give useful indications for the patient's family reintegration.

Even though it is not the therapist's sole responsibility, the swallowing assessment is fundamental for the patient's therapeutic program. In fact, as it is vital for the patient's survival, this function also has significant physical and psychological repercussions on recovery, in addition to having great emotional and social value. A correct assessment (Table 12.6) should consist of

- **Medical history and clinical data** (possible respiratory complications, aspiration, position of nasogastric tube or abdominal feeding tube, vocal cord paralysis from intubation, etc.).
- **Observation** of the patient and examination of functions.
- **Instrumental semiotics**—indirect laryngoscopy, rinopharingolaryngoscopy with optic fibers, and dynamic video-fluorographic examination (Cancialosi, Gonella, & Rago, 1993; Cot & Desharnais, 1989).

Table 12.6: Swallowing Assessment

Aspecific

Observations:
- consciousness level
- trunk control in sitting
- saliva control
- sensitivity of face, lips, tongue, palate (response, temperature, pressure)
- taste (sweet, savory, acid, bitter)

Functions and reflexes:
- breathing (apnea, co-ordination between apnea and swallowing)
- cough (reflex, voluntary)
- throat-clearing (reflex, voluntary)

Associated deficits:
- dysphonia (aphonia, hoarseness, gurgling voice)
- oral/facial apraxia (mouth opening, extending the tongue, blowing out the cheeks, blowing, smiling)
- dysartria
- aphasia

Specific

Oral preparation phase
- difficulty with introducing the food
- difficulty with keeping the food in the mouth
- difficulty with chewing
- food pocketing in cheeks
- difficulty with positioning and moving the bolus

Oral phase
- alteration of propulsion of bolus towards the pharynx in repeated attempts
- extended time of oral transit
- fall of bolus in hypopharynx before the start of the swallowing reflex
- pre-swallowing aspiration

Pharyngeal phase
- alteration in swallowing reflex
- insufficient closure of soft palate
- laryngeal elevation compromised
- pharyngeal peristalsis compromised
- glottical closure and horizontalisation of epiglottis compromised
- mid-swallowing aspiration
- food pocketing in glosso-epiglottal vallecula
- pocketing in pyriform sinus

Oesophagal phase
- pharyngeal-oesophagal peristalsis compromised
- alteration in the crico-pharyngeal opening
- post-swallowing aspiration
- oesophagal reflux

In our work, two functional scales are used to quantify and summarize the gathered data, establish short- and mid-term objectives, and verify over time the progress made during rehabilitation: the Functional Independence Measure (FIM),[1] and the Functional Assessment Measure (FAM).[2] The FIM, already used to measure disability through a number of activities essential for independence in daily living, is integrated with the appropriate FAM for cognitive and behavioral deficits following brain injury (Tables 12.6 and 12.7).

Rehabilitation

1. *Treatment of basic vital functions.* During the first stage of treatment of a brain-injured patient, the aim is to reestablish the independent functioning of respiration, feeding, and sphincter control, which are generally maintained artificially during the acute phase. One of the priorities is, therefore, to wean the patient from mechanical support systems: the drip, the urinary catheter, the endotracheal tube, the nasogastric feeding, and/or percutaneous endoscopic gastrostomy (PEG), all of which have significant repercussions for rehabilitation.

   - **Sphincter control training.** Bladder and bowel incontinence is often a feature of brain injury in the acute and post-acute phases, while urinary retention is rather rare. Loss of sphincter control may ensue from disturbances in the level of consciousness and attention, which prevent effective voluntary control over excretory functions; this is often worsened by prolonged use of a catheter. Even if an improvement in consciousness and in collaboration on the patient's part enables renewed sphincter control, return to normality requires rigorous training by the nursing staff and the patient's relatives (Figure 12.4).

   - **Respiratory training.** The patient is often transferred to the special rehabilitation unit with the endotracheal tube still in place. The endotracheal tube guarantees the possibility of broncho-aspiration, in case food or gastric matter enters the airways. The tube is, however, a potential carrier of infections that can endanger the patient's ventilation, already precarious because of prolonged mechanical assistance. Respiratory therapy consists of

     1. Daily drainage of secretions, mobilization of the thoracic cage, and, level of consciousness permitting, active participation on the patient's part (deep breathing, coughing, breath-holding, forced breathing out).
     2. Weaning from the tracheal tube.
     3. Possible surgical closure of the stoma.

   - **Swallowing training.** Most patients with severe TBI present with swallowing problems that require for some time the use of the nasogastric tube or PEG (D'Amelio, Hammond, Spain, & Sutyak, 1994; Kirby et al., 1991). In these cases, recovery of function depends not so much on the patient's level of consciousness as on the concomitant neurological damage. Treatment of dysphagia is carried out by the speech therapist, who collaborates with the nursing staff and the patient's relatives (Cancialosi, Gonella, & Rago, 1993; Field & Weiss, 1989). According to the patient's abilities, this can consist of:

     ◎ **Aspecific treatment.** The aim is to increase the patient's attention span and motivation by passively stimulating movements that are

Table 12.7: Functional Assessment Worksheet

FUNCTIONAL ASSESSMENT WORKSHEET (FIM + FAM)				
SELF-CARE ITEMS	Adm	Goal	D/C	F/U
1 Eating	___	___	___	___
2 Grooming	___	___	___	___
3 Bathing	___	___	___	___
4 Dressing upper body	___	___	___	___
5 Dressing lower body	___	___	___	___
6 Toileting	___	___	___	___
7 Swallowing	___	___	___	___
SPHINTERIC ITEMS				
8 Bladder management	___	___	___	___
9 Bowel management	___	___	___	___
MOBILITY ITEMS				
Transfer technique				
10 Bed, chair, wheelchair	___	___	___	___
11 Toilet	___	___	___	___
12 Tub or shower	___	___	___	___
13 Car transfer	___	___	___	___
Locomotion				
14 Walking/wheelchair (circle one)	___	___	___	___
15 Stairs	___	___	___	___
16 Community access	___	___	___	___
COMMUNITY ITEMS				
17 Comprehension—Aud/Vis	___	___	___	___
18 Expression verbal/non-verbal	___	___	___	___
19 Reading	___	___	___	___
20 Writing	___	___	___	___
21 Speech intelligibility	___	___	___	___
PSYCHOSOCIAL ADJUSTMENT ITEMS				
22 Social interaction	___	___	___	___
23 Emotional status	___	___	___	___
24 Adjustment to limitations—Psych	___	___	___	___
25 Employability	___	___	___	___
COGNITIVE FUNCTION ITEMS				
26 Problem solving	___	___	___	___
27 Memory	___	___	___	___
28 Orientation	___	___	___	___
29 Attention	___	___	___	___
30 Safety judgement	___	___	___	___

Scale 7   Complete indipendence (timely, safely)   3   Moderate assist (50–74% of task)
       6   Modified indipendence (extra time, device)   2   Maximal assist (25–49% of task)
       5   Supervision (cueing)   1   Total assist (subiect performs < 25% of task)
       4   Minimal assist (75% or more of task)

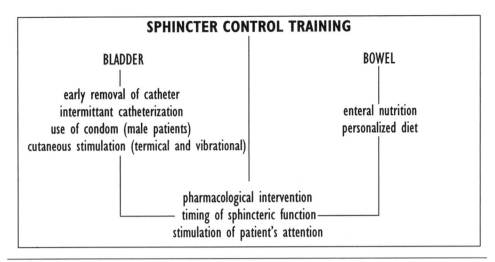

Figure 12.4: Procedure for sphincter control.

generally active in order to obtain the reflex action of swallowing. This can already be started while the patient is in intensive care and, in all cases, when the patient is not compliant.

◎ **Specific treatment.** What is required is a minimum of attention span, not necessarily constant throughout the day, and the ability to understand and carry out simple commands. The aim is to achieve conscious and effective swallowing in a short time with a low risk of aspiration (Table 12.8).

2. *Sensory-motor treatment.* It is fundamentally important in treating subjects with TBI to always consider the unity of the mind and body in which the physical and the psychological, the fruits of personality, experience, and environment, are indissolubly fused. Since brain injury brings destruction to the organization of self, this is very hard to recover. Evoking the semiautomatic mechanisms still present (e.g., standing, walking) may reinforce cortical motor systems in order to

Table 12.8: Swallowing Training

Sensory stimulation of the oral cavity	General treatment of attention, sensitivity (localized), posture, respiration, protective reflexes (coughing, throat-cleaning)
Breathing training	Treatment to improve movement, strength, speed of the swallowing muscles
Stimulation of oro-facial movement	Special rehabilitative techniques: • posture
Inhibition of pathological reflexes (biting and sucking)	• type and consistency of food • compensatory strategies
Treatment of muscle spasticity	(stimulation of pharyngeal swallowing, head and neck postures, Mendhelson manoeuvers, swallowing break-down)
Stimulation of automatic swallowing reflex	

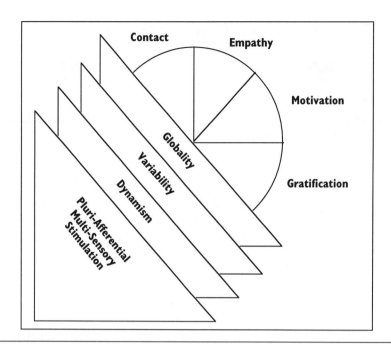

Figure 12.5: Therapeutic exercise.

reacquire successfully complex and flexible voluntary movement strategies. For these reasons, the reorganization of all the functional systems that allow maximum motor and cognitive interaction is considered a priority (Figure 12.5).

In the early stages, therefore, the aim of treatment is to reintegrate the physical and cognitive parts of the person, using global movement with its strong potential to reactivate the unity of the individual. Early standing, for example, may be justified, despite the severity of the patient's neuromotor deficits and low level of consciousness, because of the awakening action it may bring. The amount of difficulty the rehabilitation specialist meets in selecting treatment strategies and in applying them effectively also depends on the presence of behavioral problems such as aggression, akinesis, apathy, mutism, disinhibition, and attention lapses (Brooks, 1988; Lezak, 1987). For this reason, it is essential that the therapist establish a solid interpersonal relationship with the patient, with reciprocal trust. The therapist should be able to empathize with the patient's problems, focusing on the most pressing aspects and becoming, in a certain respect, a confidant. This is made possible by careful and accurate assessment of the most effective means of communication available (verbal, gestural, behavioral), on the basis of which is built, day by day, the most suitable treatment plan. This relationship, while difficult to establish, is far from easy to maintain over time. The patient will oscillate between acceptance and refusal, imposing demands on the relationship; the therapist must maintain it using knowledge of behavioral strategies (gratification, reinforcement, favor, reassurance, valuing, ignoring, etc.), choosing those which prove to be the most efficient for maximizing rehabilitation and overcoming negative phases and for increasing self-awareness (Attanasio, Careddu, & Malvicino, 1995).

These preliminary considerations are essential and now allow us to describe in more detail therapeutic work as it is carried out.

In sensory-motor rehabilitation for brain-injured patients, it can be very difficult and often frustrating to apply the classical rehabilitative methods, because they do not always prove to be decisive in modifying the natural evolution of the pathology. In our view, techniques (such as Bobath's) have more significance as formative influences on the therapist than as determining instruments for treatment form.

For explanatory purposes, therapeutic treatment can be divided into *early* and *late*. In the early phase, as soon as voluntary movements begin, active mobilization is carried out, first in bed and then in the gym. Early standing is very important, first using the plinth, and then, when the patient regains head control, using the standing-frame. This also assists cardio-circulatory and respiratory recovery, stimulates tonic-postural reflexes and spatial orientation, prevents muscle contractions, and improves the patient's contact with the environment (Table 12.9).

Activation of complex, semiautomatic motor sequences is then sought, including movement changes (supine, prone, sitting, standing) that require voluntary control of pathological components. The progressive recovery of control over axial movement is, in

Table 12.9: Rehabilitative Treatment in the Second Phase

(A) EARLY

    Bed/Wheelchair
- correct posture
- cautious passive mobilization
- progressive introduction of active movement
- indication for passive use of splints
- early weight-bearing
- physiotherapy in therapeutic pool

(B) LATE

  Physical therapy
    Floor work
- work towards bodily symmetry and symmetrical points of support in various positions
- global, assisted active mobilization, which must not be reduced to just segmental treatment
- neuro-muscular techniques that allow the voluntary recovery of movement (e.g., Bobath)
- prone-lying with trunk extension; active control of the cervical-cephalic axis
- attaining and maintaining a balanced position on all fours and also the "sphinx" position
- active movement assisted by indipendent movement of pelvic and scapular girdles

    Sitting work
- independent movement of pelvic and scapular girdles working towards complete movements with trunk symmetry
- trunk flexion and transfer of weight onto the lower limbs, helped by the therapist; working towards active extension at hip and knee, with maintained correct posture and lateral transfers
- attainement of standing

    Standing work
- correction of pathological movements
- homogeneous static trunk control that counteracts axial dystonia
- lateral and antero-posterior transfers of weight with visual and electromyographic feedback
- walking practice: break-down of walking pattern, forwards, backwards, sideways, and going downstairs/upstairs

  Ergotherapy and occupational therapy
  Psycho-motor therapy
  Treatment of peripheral nerve lesions
  Home visits for aids and adaptations

fact, a prerequisite for the functional use of the limbs in transfers, personal care, independent feeding, communication, and in other complex tasks of daily life. In our view, the various techniques are valuable insofar as they contribute to the reorganization of the connections between movement, consciousness, and external reality (Table 12.9).

In this phase, psychomotor therapy is an integral part of the treatment plan. The psychomotor approach uses movement as a means of expression and communication and acts on the subject's psychosomatic integrity. Psychomotor therapy aims to improve the patient's relationship with his/her own body and to focus on emotional and behavioral experience (Lapierre et al., 1991). Through play, conditions can be created to facilitate the emergence of the patient's motor and cognitive abilities without necessarily focusing on his/her difficulties. The aim is to recover the notions of body scheme, spatial and temporal relations, gestures, and eye-body coordination (Table 12.10).

Table 12.10: A Sequence of Motor Activity in Psychomotor Therapy

| (1) Throw the ball forward, near, behind, in front |
| (2) Pass the ball through the legs or over the head |
| (3) Touch in sequence objects spread out on the floor, walking diagonally |
| (4) Perform the previous task moving in the opposite direction |
| (5) Correctly put back the objects on the floor after having done the above task |
| (6) Draw the arrangement of the objects in the correct order on a piece of paper |
| (7) Invert a numerical sequence in correct temporal succession |
| (8) Find the shortest or the longest way to reach a point in the room |
| (9) Trace the source of a sound, blindfold |

Ergotherapy and occupational therapy complete the rehabilitation program and focus on perfecting the motor ability necessary for autonomy in daily activity and for a possible return to work (Belio, Conte, & Coste, 1987). In this usually lengthy phase of hospitalization, the rehabilitative team periodically plans weekend home visits for the patient. These are considered therapeutic in themselves. They should have well-defined prerequisites, objectives, and strategies. (Table 12.11).

In our experience, home visits, even for brief periods, help the patient to control early behavioral problems such as attention lapses, aggression, and depression and have a positive effect on the time taken for recovery. Furthermore, the family becomes aware of the patient's real condition; this should also help relatives to overcome problems of refusal or misunderstanding, which are often difficult to deal with successfully in the hospital setting.

Table 12.11: Framework for Therapeutic Home Visits

PREREQUISITES	**OBJECTIVES**
• stable medical condition	• early return to the family environment
• postural control (sitting and/or standing)	• verifying behavioral problems
• absence of feeding problems	• improving awareness of deficits
• absence of urinary retention	• increasing motivation to recovery
• suitable family environment	• training the family in handling the patient
	• adaptation of rehabilitative strategies

THIRD PHASE

This is better defined as the phase of social integration or as "community rehabilitation" (Hackler & Tobis, 1990; Ben-Yishay & Gold, 1990). Many consider that it begins most often at about six months after the trauma (Jennett, 1990). In our opinion, however, temporal criteria are not always valid because much depends on the severity of the injury. Discharge from the special rehabilitation unit depends on (1) stabilization of neurological condition and (2) the possibility of care at home or in a day hospital. In fact, although the patient still needs integrated rehabilitative treatments, he/she can already spend the main part of the day at home or in his/her environment.

In order to reach community reintegration, it is useful for the patient to participate in a day treatment program in which activity is organized at least four days a week (Table 12.12). The day hospital provides the key link between the complete return to social life and hospital rehabilitation, where traditionally the patient is protected and therapy is, inevitably, practiced in an artificial setting, rather separate from ordinary life. The aims of the day hospital are not only to maintain the functional abilities already gained by the patient but, above all, to work towards re-entry into family and school or work (Jennett, 1990; Hackler & Tobis, 1990; Namerow, 1987; Rao, Sulton, Young, & Harvey, 1986). An outline of the patient's personal needs and a functional profile is prepared in order to

- establish a maximum autonomy goal,
- raise awareness of personal strengths and limits,
- encourage compensatory techniques and strategies,
- encourage the highest standard possible in ordinary life (quality of life),
- rebuild important interpersonal relationships, and
- prepare return to school or work.

Because a person's disability has complex consequences at individual, family, and social levels (Table 12.13), it is imperative, at this stage, to plan the treatment program with a team consisting of physiatrist, neuropsychologist, physiotherapist, occupational therapist,

Table 12.12: Example of a Weekly Timetable of Day Hospital Structured Activities for Brain-Injured Patients

Time	Mon	Tues	Wed	Thur	Fri
9	STAFF ORGANIZATION	NEURO-PSYCHOLOGY GROUP			
9:30		NEURO-PSYCHOLOGY, EDUCATIONAL PSYCHOLOGY , SPEECH THERAPY, PHYSIOTHERAPY (INDIVIDUAL OR GROUP)			
11	STAFF MEETING	BREAK			
11:20		PHYSIOTHERAPY GROUP	SWIMMING	OCCUPATIONAL THERAPY	DRAMA GROUP
13		LUNCH			
13:45	MEETINGS WITH PATIENT'S RELATIVES	PSYCHOMOTOR THERAPY	OCCUPATIONAL THERAPY	MUSIC GROUP	ART GROUP
15—16	STAFF WORK	VARIOUS ACTIVITIES AND RETURN HOME			

Table 12.13: Consequences of Disability in TBI

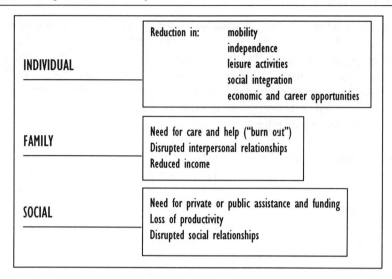

INDIVIDUAL	Reduction in:	mobility independence leisure activities social integration economic and career opportunities
FAMILY	Need for care and help ("burn out") Disrupted interpersonal relationships Reduced income	
SOCIAL	Need for private or public assistance and funding Loss of productivity Disrupted social relationships	

psychomotor therapist, speech therapist, social worker, and, in our experience, a teacher of the arts. The employment of teachers of the expressive arts along with traditional therapists and the inclusion of artistic sessions in which gesture, speech, and movement are integrated assist the recovery of movement as affective, intellectual, and behavioral expression (Montagna, Gentina, Bricco, Frus, Venturino, & Rago, 1995).

In this phase, the goals of physiotherapy are to improve walking and transfers, coordination, and dexterity in bi-manual activity and to regain, where possible, the ability to practice sports (swimming, riding, etc.). To stimulate and consolidate the highest integration of motor abilities (as well as communication, relationships, and behavior), the patient also participates in group therapy (Prigatano & Fordyce, 1986). Group therapy brings the following benefits:

- It helps the subject to overcome the dualistic therapist-patient relationship.
- It reduces isolation and the sense of being abandoned.
- It stimulates the ability to interact with others and with the environment.
- It heightens awareness of limits and of personal resources.
- It improves motivation and initiative for general mobility.

Along with traditional techniques, other methods more recently introduced into physical rehabilitation may be included (such as the Feldenkrais Method, T'ai Chi Chu'an, etc.). The aim of these techniques is to globally rationalize posture and movement by increasing coordination, flexibility, and scope of action.

Occupational therapy, individually or in groups, should be done daily, as it completes and maximizes the work done in physiotherapy. The goals of occupational therapy, including creative manual work, are:

- To improve practical abilities and thus increase strength, coordination, and mobility.
- To maintain correct posture in sitting and standing.
- To develop fitness and stamina (e.g., standing tolerance, work pacing).
- To help the patient coexist with his/her remaining physical and cognitive problems by developing compensatory techniques.

- Where appropriate, to teach the use of aids and adaptations that can enable the patient to complete tasks otherwise impossible.
- To normalize the patient's habits of daily self-care.
- To assess the patient's vocational potential with the social worker for a possible return to work or retraining program (Willard & Spackman, 1988).

VEGETATIVE STATE AND REHABILITATION

Jennet and Plum (1972) first used the term "persistent vegetative state" to describe the condition of a patient emerging from coma after a severe brain injury who is without communicative verbal contact or appreciable evidence of cognitive activity. The condition can be clinically defined by the summary in Table 12.14.

This condition is clinically distinguished from brain death (absence of brainstem functions, corneal and pupillary reflexes, postural reaction, motor response to pain, presence of convulsions, very severe EEG abnormalities), from coma (eyes always closed, lack of response to verbal commands, lack of communication, presence of automatic defensive movements to painful stimuli), and also from the "locked-in syndrome" (absence of voluntary movement, partial or total maintenance of cognitive ability, communication possible only by eye or head movements) (Young, Blume, & Lynch, 1989; Plum & Posner, 1982). Many authors agree that the diagnosis of permanent vegetative state must only be given after a long period of clinical monitoring: one year for patients coming out of post-traumatic coma, 3–6 months for post-anoxic coma (Bricolo, Turazzi, & Feriotti, 1987). During this period, while the prognosis is still uncertain, rehabilitative treatment, along with intensive nursing care and medical care, is justified with the aims of preventing secondary and tertiary damage and of stimulating, where possible, the recovery of consciousness and contact with the environment.

Rehabilitation for these patients takes the following forms:

1. *Clinical supervision.* This requires continuous attention in order to note if a response appears to environmental stimuli. The patient needs to be clinically monitored to avoid general complications that would cause his/her neurological state to worsen.
2. *Rehabilitative nursing.* This is the principal and most demanding treatment for patients in the vegetative state. It integrates the movements required for personal hygiene, posture, and mobilization with controlled multi-modal stimuli. Nursing care also ensures that ulcers and pressure sores are avoided.

Table 12.14: Clinical Definition of Vegetative State

• Spontaneous eye-opening
• Regaining of the sleep/wake cycle
• Spontaneous maintenance of vital functions
• Absence of purposeful motor responses
• Absence of understandable speech and/or inconsistent emission of incomprehensible vocal sounds
• Failure to carry out simple commands
• Absence of sustained, completed ocular movements
• Presence of oral and bucco-facial automatisms

Table 12.15: Framework for Prevention and Treatment of Orthopedic Problems in TBI

CAUSE	TYPE OF TREATMENT
C N S PARALYSIS	PREVENTION • static and dynamic splints TREATMENT • dynamic and static splints • corrective surgery for soft tissues and bones
P N S PARALYSIS	PREVENTION • correct orthopedic treatment in the acute phase • appropriate nursing • control of EO and spasticity TREATMENT • peripheral neurosurgery • splints and physiotherapy • symptomatic functional surgery
POST-TRAMATIC DEFORMITY DELAYED AND INCORRECT FRACTURE CONSOLIDATION	PREVENTION • correct orthopaedic treatment • control of spasticity TREATMENT • functional surgery
HETEROTOPIC CALCIFICATION (periarticular, miofascial, etc.)	PREVENTION • pharmacological • control of inflammatory processes and of joint traumatisms TREATMENT • surgical removal • physical therapy

3. *Prevention of thrombi and emboli.* The high risk of thrombus and embolus, brought about by immobility, can be countered by regular and frequent mobilization in bed and by appropriate pharmacological treatment.

4. *Prevention of neuro-orthopedic complications.* Correct posture with sufficient maintenance of articularity and muscle functions will avoid articular blocks, muscle tendon contractures, and the calcification of peri-articular tissues (heterotopic ossification).

5. *Prevention of respiratory complications.* Prolonged intubation and artificial ventilation often cause vocal cord lesions, tracheal stenosis and malacia, changes in pulmonary function, and infections of the airways. For this reason, chest physiotherapy and bronchial drainage should be included, along with nursing and medical care, to encourage secretion elimination and clearing of air passages.

6. *Nutritional control.* With patients in the vegetative state in which nutritional needs are increased, enteral feeding is the rule. It allows a complete and balanced caloric intake, and it avoids the possibility of food being aspirated into the air passages with consequent "ab ingestis" pneumonia. In the initial phases, however, gentle tactile, thermic, and gustatory stimuli in the patient's mouth and oropharynge remain a part of daily therapy.

7. *Support for the patient's family.* The complex ways in which a family adapts to the situation imposed by the traumatic event depend on many factors: the patient's premorbid condition and role, the relatives' psychological resources and economic position, and the progress of the clinical situation (Rosin, 1977). The role of the rehabilitation team is to support and empathize with the relatives as they adapt to the changed situation. Since family members are involved with helping and

supervising the patient, they must be trained in handling their relative to prepare for a return home, if and when possible. Once the vegetative state is considered irreversible, though, they may assist with feeding, hygiene, and mobilization.

ORTHOPEDIC PROBLEMS IN TBI REHABILITATION

Traumatic lesions of the musculoskeletal frame are often found concomitant with brain injury. Surgical stabilization of fracture sites must be a priority, even when basic vital functions are severely compromised and when the "quoad vitam" prognosis has not been established yet. Fundamentally, treatment of traumatic lesions consists of (1) reducing the factors that aggravate the state of shock, (2) avoiding the development of post-traumatic deformities, (3) enabling suitable and adequate nursing for the patient, and (4) allowing early rehabilitation.

Successively, in the post-acute and chronic phases, orthopedic treatment may be necessary to complement the sensory-motor therapy undergone by the patient. Certain pathological conditions, in fact, occur with some frequency during the recovery process and have a negative effect on it. The causes are generally (1) primitive lesions misunderstood in the acute phase; (2) insufficient, unsuitable, or mis-timed traumatological treatment; and (3) neurochemical and circulatory changes.

The most frequent neuro-orthopedic injuries can be classified as follows:

1. **Injury secondary to paralysis.** Spasticity and imbalance between muscle groups are often caused by the lesion in the CNS. They can cause limb postural changes that progress slowly towards structural deformity.

2. **Peripheral nerve lesions.** They can be divided into early and late. The first can be caused directly by the traumatic agent through contusion, crushing, or tearing. Late lesions are often consequences of structural deformities, heterotopic ossification, or inadequate nursing during a period in which a compression or traction mechanism is used.

3. **Incorrect consolidation and post-traumatic deformity.** Fractures that unite in malalignment and the consequent deformities are not rare events in the post-comatose patient. The most frequent causes are misdiagnosis in the acute phase or loss of reduction of the fracture because of insufficient fixation. Only when the correction of the deformity is essential to the patient's functional recovery is surgical correction carried out.

4. **Heterotopic calcification and heterotopic ossification.** This consists of deposits of calcium salts in the extra-skeletal tissues without the structural organization of bony matter. They tend to be found in areas where soft tissues have been sites of inflammatory processes or have received traumatic damage. Their presence can lead to articular complications, such as ankylosis or subluxation, or trophic complications such as pressure sores and trapped peripheral nerves. Early surgical removal of heterotopic ossification, although posing an increased risk of relapse, is now considered essential for accelerating functional recovery (Debelleix, 1987).

In all these cases, the best results are obtained through correct prevention, requiring early attention and assessment of need by the orthopedic surgeon and the rehabilitation specialist working together. In the most serious cases in which preventive techniques have been insufficient, physiotherapy and splinting are used to reinforce surgical treatment and to maintain the benefits it has conferred (Table 12.15).

ENDNOTES

1. Developed by the Uniform Data System for Medical Rehabilitation, State University of New York at Buffalo, 232 Parker Hall, SUNY South Campus, 3435 Main St., Buffalo, New York.
2. Developed at Santa Clara Valley Medical Center, 751 So. Bascom Ave., Box A421, San José, California.

REFERENCES

Attanasio, C., Careddu, L., & Malvicino, A. (1995). Riorganizzazione globale del movimento (Global movement reorganization). In R. Rago & C. Perino (Eds.), *Riabilitazione e reinserimento sociale negli esiti di trauma encefalico* (Rehabilitation and social reintegration after TBI). Rome, Italy: Ed. Marrapese.

Belio, C., Conte, B., & Coste, B. (1987). Ergothèrapie et traumatisés craniens. In *Rééducation et réadaptation des traumatisés craniens*. Paris, France: Ed. Masson.

Ben-Yishay, Y., & Gold, J. (1990). Therapeutic milieu approach to neuropsychological rehabilitation. In R. Wood (Ed.), *Neurobehavioral sequelae of traumatic brain injury*. London, UK: Taylor and Francis.

Bricolo, A., Turazzi, S., & Feriotti, G. (1980). Prolonged post-traumatic unconsciousness: Therapeutic assets and liabilities. *Journal of Neurosurgery, 52,* 625–634.

Brooks, N. (1988). Personality change after severe head injury. *Acta Neurochirurgica (Suppl.), 44,* 59–64.

Cancialosi, P., Gonella, M.L., & Rago, R. (1993). La rieducazione della deglutizione (Swallowing rehabilitation). In R. Rago & C. Perino (Eds.), *La riabilitazione dei traumi cranio encefalici nell'adulto* (Rehabilitation of TBI in the adult). Milano, Italy: Ghedini Editore.

Cope, D.N. (1990). Physiatric assessment for rehabilitation. In M. Rosenthal et al. (Eds.), *Rehabilitation of the adult and child with traumatic brain injury*. Philadelphia: F.A. Davis Company.

Cope, D.N., & Hall, K. (1982). Head injury rehabilitation: Benefit of early intervention. *Arch. Phys. Med. Rehabil., 63,* 433–437.

Cot, F., & Desharnais, G. (1989). *La dysphagie chez l'adulte: Évaluation et traitement*. Paris, France: Edisem.

D'Amelio, L.F., Hammond, J.S., Spain, D.A., & Sutyak, J.P. (1994). Tracheostomy and percutaneous endoscopic gastrostomy in the management of the head-injured trauma patient. *Am. Surg., 60,* 180–185.

Debelleix, X. (1987). Complications neuroorthopédiques des traumatisés craniens. In *Rééducation et réadaptation des traumatisés craniens*. Paris, France: Ed. Masson.

Field, L.H., & Weiss, C.J. (1989). Dysphagia with head injury. *Brain Injury, 3,* 19–26.

Goldspink, G., & Williams, P. (1990). Muscle fibre and connective tissue changes associated with use and disuse. In L. Ada & C. Canning (Eds.), *Key issues in neurological physiotherapy*. Oxford, UK: Butterworth Heinemann.

Griffith, E.R., & Mayer, N.H. (1990). Hypertonicity and movement disorders. In M. Rosenthal et al. (Eds.), *Rehabilitation of the adult and child with traumatic brain injury*. Philadelphia: F.A. Davis Company.

Hackler, E., & Tobis, J.S. (1990). Reintegration into the community. In M. Rosenthal et al. (Eds.), *Rehabilitation of the adult and child with traumatic brain injury*. Philadelphia: F.A. Davis Company.

Jaggi, J., Obrist, W., Gennarelli, T.A., & Langfitt, T. (1990). Relationship of early cerebral blood flow and metabolism to outcome in acute head injury. *Journal of Neurosurgery, 72,* 176–182.

Jennett, B. (1990). Scale and scope of the problem. In M. Rosenthal et al. (Eds.), *Rehabilitation of the adult and child with traumatic brain injury*. Philadelphia: F.A. Davis Company.

Jennett, B., & Plum, F. (1972). Persistent vegetative state after brain damage. *Lancet, 4,* 734–737.

Jennett, B., Teasdale, G., Braakman, R., Minderhoud, J., Heiden, J., & Kurze, T. (1979). Prognosis of patients with severe head injury. *Neurosurgery, 4,* 283–289.

Kirby, D.F., Clifton, G.L., Turner, H., et al. (1991). Early enteral nutrition after brain injury by percutaneous endoscopic gastrojejunostomy. *J.P.E.N., 15,* 298–302.

Lapierre, A., et al. (1991). *Il corpo nella relazione* (Body and relationship). Rome, Italy: Ed Armando.

Lezak, M.D. (1987). Relationships between personality disorder, social disturbances, and physical disability following traumatic brain injury. *J. Head Trauma Rehabil., 2,* 57–69.

Montagna, C., Gentina, E., Bricco, M., Frus, L., Venturino, A., & Rago, R. (1995). L'espressione artistica in riabilitazione (Artistical expression in rehabilitation). In R. Rago & C. Perino (Eds.), *Riabilitazione e reinserimento sociale negli esiti di trauma encefalico* (Rehabilitation and social reintegration after TBI). Rome, Italy: Ed. Marrapese.

Namerow, N.S. (1987). Current concepts and advances in brain injury rehabilitation. *J. Neuro. Rehab., 1,* 101–114.

Plum, F., & Posner, J.B. (1982). *Diagnosis of stupor and coma.* (3rd ed.) Philadelphia: F.A. Davis Company.

Prigatano, G.P., & Fordyce, D.J. (1986). *Neuropsychological rehabilitation after brain injury.* Baltimore, MD: Johns Hopkins University.

Rao, N., Sulton, L., Young, C.L., & Harvey, R.F. (1986). Rehabilitation team and family assessment of initial home pass. *Arch. Phys. Med. Rehabil., 67,* 759–761.

Rinehart, M.A. et al. (1990). Strategies for improving motor performance. In M. Rosenthal et al. (Eds.), *Rehabilitation of the adult and child with traumatic brain injury.* Philadelphia: F.A. Davis Company.

Rosin, J. (1977). Reactions of families of brain-injured patients who remain in a vegetative state. *Scand. J. Rehab. Med., 9,* 1–5.

Rusk, H.A., Block, J.E., & Lowman, E.W. (1969). Rehabilitation following traumatic brain damage: Immediate and long-term follow-up results in 127 cases. *Med. Clin. North Am., 53,* 677–684.

Trexler, L.E. & Zappalà, G. (1988). Neuropathological determinants of acquired attention disorders in traumatic brain injury. *Brain and Cognition, 8,* 291–302.

Willard, H.S., & Spackman, C.S. (1988). *Terapia occupazionale* (Occupational therapy). Cosenza, Italy: Ed. Brenner.

Young, B., Blume, W., & Lynch, T.N. (1989). Brain death and persistent vegetative state: Similarities and contrasts. *Can. J. Neurol. Sci., 16,* 388–393.

Zappalà, G. (1988). Multidisciplinary approach in head injury rehabilitation. *Functional Neurology, 4* (Suppl. 3), 143–145.

13 Post-Traumatic Seizures and Post-Traumatic Epilepsy: Pharmacological Prophylaxis and Treatment

Francesco Monaco

Professor of Neurology
University of Sassari, Italy

INTRODUCTION

The study of epileptic phenomena following brain injury is particularly related to the area of epileptogenesis, as a traumatic event causing a series of biochemical effects which, in the end, lead to neuronal damage and critical activity. It is, therefore, necessary to report briefly some basic neurophysiological and neurochemical data, as they represent the essential premises for understanding the subsequent therapeutic implications.

MECHANISMS OF EPILEPTOGENESIS

Post-traumatic epilepsy is the best way to investigate the natural course of epileptogenesis, as the time of focal insult can be more easily documented. The studies of Jennett (1979) on epilepsy secondary to head trauma have furnished the proof of the pathophysiological distinction between early post-traumatic seizures (during the first weeks following the event) and late post-traumatic seizures. Risk factors, and hence basic mechanisms, of seizure types are, therefore, different (Table 13.1).

Those studies also confirmed that the silent period between trauma and the first unprovoked epileptic seizure may vary from a few days to more than ten years. It is likely that genetic factors may influence the development of late epilepsy (Eaves, 1982), but, undoubtedly, the most interesting data are gathered from experiments concerning models of "iron epilepsy" (Willmore, Sypert, Munson, & Hurd, 1978). These studies show that intra-cortical injection of blood, or blood components (haemoglobin, ferritin, or iron chloride), in cats, rats, and guinea pigs causes a chronic epileptogenic focus. The histological aspect is characterized by cavitary necrosis, neuronal loss, neuronal iron stockades, and astroglial reactions similar to human post-traumatic foci.

Table 13.1: Risk Factors after Non-Missile Traumatic Brain Injury

<u>Early post-traumatic seizures</u>

> Intra-cranial hematoma
> Focal neurological signs
> Post-traumatic amnesia >24 hrs.
> Depressed skull fracture
> Subarachnoid hemorrhage
> Age below 5 yrs.
> Linear skull fracture

<u>Late post-traumatic seizures</u>

> Intra-cranial hematoma
> Early post-traumatic seizures
> Depressed skull fracture
> Post-traumatic amnesia >24 hrs.
> Age above 16 yrs.

These experiments may provide a suitable model for events following trauma (i.e., iron may further worsen brain damage, in part catalyzing chemical reactions that yield free toxic radicals [Aust, Morehouse, & Thomas, 1985]). Other implicated mechanisms are connected to the inhibition of ATPase and the peroxidation of lipoproteins of microsomal membranes (Victoria & Barber, 1969). Iron, or iron components in an added aqueous solution or a suspension of polyunsaturated fatty acids, cause the formation of free oxygen radicals, hydroxylic radicals, peroxides, singlet oxygen, and peripheral ions (Aust & Svingen, 1982).

These highly reactive oxidizing agents that are believed to be formed by iron-catalyzed Haber-Weiss reactions (Koppenol, Buttler, & Van Leeuwen, 1978) start and propagate the polyunsaturated fatty acids peroxidation through the extraction of hydrogen from the carbonyl bonds (Koppenol, Buttler, & Van Leeuwen, 1978), thus causing the breakdown of the lipid membranes of microsomes, mitochondria, lysosomes, and erithrocytes (Wills, 1969).

The products of non-enzymatic peroxidation catalyzed by iron also cause a degradation of deoxyribose (Halliwell & Gutteridge, 1981) and amino acids (Gutteridge, 1981) and a release of arachidonic acid (Niehaus & Samuelson, 1968) with the formation of prostaglandins that yields some dienic conjugates, the malonylaldehyde chromogene (MDA-reactive of 2-thiobarbituric acid [TBA]), fluorescent Schiff bases, and gas (Chio & Tappel, 1969).

Though several volatile and nonvolatile products are formed during the lipidic peroxidation, the reaction with TBA creates a complex with the volatile reactants and provides the appropriate means for an estimate of peroxidation that has occurred (Dirks, Faiman, & Huyser, 1982). Figure 13.1 shows that biochemical cascade of events described above.

NEUROPROTECTIVE AGENTS

Alpha-tocopherol (natural vitamin E) prevents peroxidative sulphydryl damage of groups of glycolipids and glycoproteins by the reaction of phenolic hydroxylic groups with radicals propagated by oxidative carbonyl-hydrogen abstraction (Witting, 1980). In

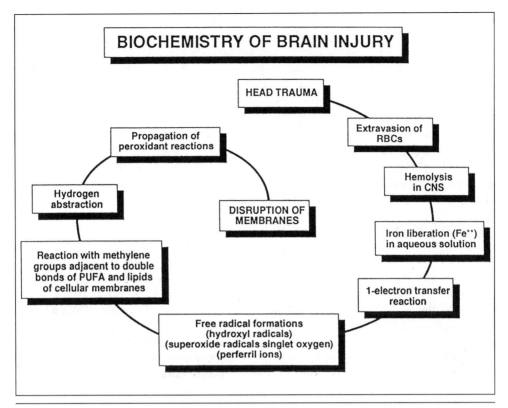

Figure 13.1: The biochemical cascade of events following brain injury, from head trauma to the disruption of cell membranes.

addition, the phytyl side chain tocopherol may intercalate within the acyl chains of polyunsaturated phospholipids, causing lipid membrane stabilization and reduction in membrane permeability (Diplock & Lucy, 1973; Lucy, 1972). Tocopherol may also act as a free radical scavenger and singlet oxygen quenching agent (Witting, 1980).

The sulphydryl group of glutathione also prevents cellular membranes from peroxidation (Singh & Nath Patak, 1990). Intracellular formation of hydrogen peroxide and free radicals are reduced by glutathione peroxidase, with selenium as a metallic cofactor and glutathione as a co-substrate (Smith, Tappel, & Chow, 1974). Thus, administration of selenium and tocopherol results in synergistic protection of cellular membranes against lipid peroxidation (Hafeman, Sunde, & Hoekstra, 1974; Willmore & Rubin, 1981). In fact, it has been shown that these two neuroprotective agents, when administered five days before the epileptogenic lesion and for six weeks afterwards to rats with experimental iron epilepsy, cause a marked reduction of epileptic activity (Willmore & Rubin, 1981).

Theoretically, iron chelating agents and/or calcium channel antagonists also might be able to block the iron cellular injury (Halliwell & Gutteridge, 1986).

The 21-aminosteroid tirilazad is a steroid-like molecule without glucorticoid activity; it is an antioxidant agent capable of scavenging lipid peroxyl radicals and decreasing the formation of hydroxyl radicals (Hall, 1993). It has been shown to reduce Vitamin E following reperfusion to an occluded area of the brain (Marmarou, 1994) and to stabilize membranes, slowing the rate of lipid peroxidation (Hall, Yonkers, McCall, & Braughler, 1988).

One of the body's natural neuroprotective agents against free radicals is superoxide dismutase, an enzyme that specifically scavenges superoxide anions. It acts extracellularly to protect against peroxidation of brain phospholipids (Gutteridge, 1981) and, therefore, can be used in the prevention of the cellular damage by free radicals. However, the clinical value of natural, unmodified superoxide dismutase is limited because its half-life is six minutes. If superoxide dismutase is linked with strands of polyethlyene glycol (pegorgotein, polyethlyene glyco-superoxide dismutase), its half-life is extended to about five days, and it also improves the drug's access to endothelial cells, the probable sites of superoxide production (Marmarou, 1994).

Finally, nerve growth factors, glutamate inhibitors, and opiod receptor antagonists might prove helpful in preventing the degenerative processes caused by brain injury, but to date, their use remains experimental (Bullock, 1993).

HUMAN POST-TRAUMATIC EPILEPSY

Of all cases with brain injury, about 5% develop early post-traumatic seizures, and another 5% develop late post-traumatic seizures. In most subjects, late post-traumatic seizures occur during the first year after head trauma (70–75%), with a decreasing risk over the passage of time in the following 10 years (Annegers et al., 1980). The wide epdemiological studies performed on the U.S. Vietnam veteran population have indicated an overall risk percentage for post-traumatic epilepsy by missile wounds of about 50% (Salazar et al., 1985).

It is likely that the range of epileptogenic risk may vary from a minimum of 5% in the civilian population to a maximum of 35% in the military population, as, in this case, the trauma is more often a penetrating one (Caveness et al., 1979; Willmore, 1992).

PROPHYLAXIS AND TREATMENT

Prophylaxis

Before facing the problem of prophylaxis and treatment of human post-traumatic epilepsy, we must refer once more to experimental data (Mutani et al., 1991).

In rats, phenobarbital administered prophylactically (i.e., before the onset of epilepsy) prevents the occurrence of audiogenic seizures (Servit, 1960), and in guinea pigs with alumina gel epilepsy, "mirror" foci are prevented in a similar manner (Morrell & Baker, 1961). Rapport and Ojemann (1975) suggested that the prophylactic administration of phenytoin might prevent the maturation of the epileptogenic focus in cobalt-induced epilepsy. Animal studies regarding kindling mechanisms have also suggested that there may be experimental evidence to support a preventive rationale for anticonvulsant prophylaxis (McNamara et al, 1989; Wada et al, 1976).

So, encouraged by animal experimentation, retrospective and non-randomized open trials in humans were conducted during the past 30 years with somewhat favorable results (Yablon, 1993), but decidedly less impressive results were observed among randomized controlled perspective investigation. Table 13.2 summarizes the three main double-blind, placebo-controlled perspective studies on the efficacy of anti-epileptic drugs as prophylaxis of post-traumatic epilepsy. They fail to substantiate evidence of efficacy for anti-epileptic drugs prophylaxis in late post-traumatic seizures (Penry, White, & Brackett, 1979; Temkin et al., 1990). Most studies used phenytoin as prophylaxis, though similar results were also observed in one trial primarily administering carbamazepine (Glozner et al., 1983).

Table 13.2: Summary of Double-Blind, Placebo-Controlled Prospective Studies of the Efficacy of Anti-Epileptic Drugs as Prophylaxis of Post-Traumatic Epilepsy

| Authors | Drugs | Percent Developing Epilepsy | |
		Control (%)	Treated (%)
Penry et al., 1979	Phenytoin	13.0	23.0
	Phenobarbital		
Young et al., 1983	Phenytoin	10.8	12.9
Temkin et al., 1990	Phenyton	21.1	27.5

Other anti-epileptic drugs, such as valproic acid (VPA), vigabatrin (GVG), or lamotrigine (LTG) might prove prophylactically useful in the future (Anderson et al., 1991).

Therefore, it seems necessary to perform a preliminary evaluation of the realistic risk of post-traumatic epilepsy development in relation to a severity scale suggested by selective studies (Table 13.3).

Table 13.3: Risk Factors for Late Post-Traumatic Seizures

Factor(s)	Incidence of late seizures (%)
Penetrating injury caused by missile-parietal lobe	74
Depressed fracture, post-traumatic amnesia >24 hr. and early seizures	60
Penetrating injury caused by missile	42
Intracranial hematoma	35
Depressed fracture, post-traumatic amnesia >24 hr.	32
Focal signs, early seizure	32
Focal cerebral damage on CT	32
Depressed fracture, early seizure	26
Depressed fracture, focal signs	26
Centroparietal damage (including contusion, hemorrhage or abscess)	25
Early-onset seizure(s)	25
Depressed fracture, dura torn	24
Extradural or subdural hemorrhage	20
Hemiplegia, hemiparesis, or aphasia	20
Depressed skull fracture	15
Brain contusion	14
Loss of consciousness >24 hr.	5
Post-traumatic amnesia >1 hr.	5
Linear skull fracture	5
Mild concussion	1

Threshold risk is usually estimated to be equal or above 15% (Dugan & Howell, 1944), and a tentative treatment protocol is shown in Table 13.4, where it results that phenobarbital or phenytoin may be administered indifferently in selected patients immediately after head trauma (Oles & Penry, 1985). It may also be that a period of six months, as indicated, is not sufficient in the most severe cases, and that prophylaxis may be prolonged up to two years.

Table 13.4: Prophylactic Dosing Protocol

	Phenytoin	Phenobarbital
IV Loading Dose*		
Dose	18 mg/kg	1 mg/kg each hr. x 4
Concentration	15–20 µg/ in normal saline	
Rate	25–50 mg/min	≤60 mg/min
Total time	≤1 hr.	4 hrs.
Serum Concentration Monitoring		
To achieve	15–20 µg/ml	15–40 µg/ml**
Monitor	1 hr following loading dose	
Readjust dose	1 mg/kg for each µg/ml	1 mg/kg for each µg/ml
Monitor	24 hrs.	24 hrs.
	As needed on oral maintenance at 1–2 weeks, 1 month	As needed on oral maintenance at 1–2 weeks, 1 month
Duration of Treatment		
Time at full dosage	6 months	6 months
Tapering	25%/wk t	25%/wk t

*	Assuming no prior phenytoin or phenobarbital
**	May take 1 week to achieve
t	Taper drugs one at a time

Treatment

The term "treatment" can be used, in this case, as a synonym for "symptomatic management" (Yablon, 1993) as a therapeutic approach to post-traumatic seizures and post-traumatic epilepsy, since they are similar to epileptic seizures in the general population. Obviously, it is far beyond the scope of this chapter to examine the enormous amount of literature on this matter, and it is recommended that the reader refer to excellent textbooks for exhaustive information on the choice of drugs, duration of treatment, and other related problems (Levy, Mattson, & Meldrum, 1995; Willie, 1993). Table 13.5 shows the main anti-epileptic drugs and their clinical use.

People working in a rehabilitation setting need to be aware of the effects of anti-epileptic drugs, as both post-traumatic epilepsy and anti-epileptic drugs may strongly influence patients' treatment results. From this point of view, the main concern is the potential for possible cognitive and behavioral adverse effects of anti-epileptic drugs (Dodrill, 1988), and therefore, some information must be presented on this topic.

COGNITIVE EFFECTS OF ANTI-EPILEPTIC DRUGS

It is known that the sedative action of some anti-epileptic drugs, such as phenobarbital, primidone, and benzodiazepines, is similar in terms of impairment of cognitive function (Meador, Loring, & Huh, 1990), though their effect is not permanent and the discontinuation of these medications is associated with return to normal function. Phenobarbital and primidone induce memory impairment (especially in short-term memory and attention), though some studies have demonstrated a lack of influence of intellectual development in children (Camfield & Camfield, 1981). Phenytoin has also been investigated, and Dilantin dementia was described by Rosen in 1966, but a relationship seems to

Table 13.5: Main Anti-Epileptic Drugs

Drug	Clinical use	Plasma therapeutic level (μg/ml)	Days to reach steady-state
Phenobarbital	GCS	15–40	15
Dyphenyl-Hydantoin	GCS	10–20	7–9
	CPS		
Primidone	GCS	8–12	4–7
	GNCS		
	CPS		
Carbamazepine	GCS	4–12	4–5
	CPS		
Valproid Acid	GNCS	40–100	2–4
	GCS		
	CPS		
Vigabatrin	GCS	n.n.	1–2
	CPS		
Lamotrigine	GCS	1–3	6–7
	CPS		

GCS = Generalized convulsive seizures
GNCS = Generalized nonconvulsive seizures
CPS = Complex partial seizures
n.n. = not necessary

exist only with high drug plasma concentrations (Reynolds, 1983). The neuropsychological side effects seem to be less relevant using some other agents, such as ethosuximide, clobazam, or carbamazepine (Willie, 1993).

Among anti-epileptic drugs, vigabatrin (gamma-vinyl-GABA) is the compound on which researchers have focused the greatest attention. Several studies, including the ones performed by our group, have confirmed that it has no detrimental effect on cognition (Dodrill et al., 1995; Monaco et al., 1996). Similarly, lamotrigine does not worsen cognition; it may show a positive effect on a depressed mood (Leach & Brodie, 1995a). Gabapentin, another GABAergic drug, does not differ from carbamazepine as far as cognitive effects are concerned (Dodrill et al., 1992). Finally, there are no significant differential cognitive effects from oxcarbazepine, the 10-keto analogue of carbamazepine and phenytoin (Aikia & Kalvainen, 1992).

In accordance with our previous experience (Monaco et al., 1976) and other reports (Katz, 1988), carbamazepine should be strongly considered as an alternative drug treatment to phenbarbital or phenytoin whenever cognitive or behavioral side effects appear. In any case and with any drug, careful therapeutic plasma drug monitoring must always be performed to insure proper blood levels (Kutt, 1992).

As oxcarbazepine has shown comparable efficacy to the mother drug with a lower incidence of side effects (Leach & Brodie, 1995b), it might represent a good substitute for carbamazepine in the future.

REFERENCES

Äikiä, M., Kalvainen, R., & Sivenius, J. (1992). Cognitive effects of oxcarbazepine and phenytoin monotherapy in newly diagnosed epilepsy: One year follow-up. *Epilepsy Res, 11*, 199–203.

Anderson, G.D., Chabal, S., Gidal, B.E., Hendryx, R.J., Wilensky, A.J., & Temkin, N.R. (1991). Effect of valproate on coagulation parameters in a post-traumatic head injury population. *Epilepsia* (Suppl. 3), *32*, 10.

Annegers, J.F., Grabow, J.D., Broover, R.V., Laws, E.R., Elveback, L.R., & Kurland, L.T. (1980). Seizures after head trauma: A population study. *Neurology, 30*, 683–689.

Aust, S.D., & Svingen, B.A. (1982). The role of iron in enzymatic lipid peroxidation. In W.A. Prior (Ed.), *Free radicals in biology* (Vol. 5) (pp. 1–28). New York: Academic Press.

Aust, S.D., Morehause, L.A., & Tomas, C.E. (1985). Role of metals in oxygen radical reactions. *Free Radical Biol. Med., 1*, 3–25.

Bullock, R. (1993). Opportunities for neuroprotective drugs in clinical management of head injury. *J. Emerg. Med., 11*, 23–30.

Camfield, C.S., & Camfield, P.R. (1981). Behavioral and cognitive effects of phenobarbital in toddlers. In K.B. Nelson & J.H. Ellenberg (Eds.), *Febrile seizures* (pp. 203–210). New York: Raven Press.

Caveness, W.F., Mejrowsky, A.M., Rish, B.L., Kistler, J.P., Dillon, J.D., Weiss, & J.H. (1979). The nature of post-traumatic epilepsy. *Neurosurg., 50*, 545–553.

Chio, K.S., & Tappel, A.L. (1969). Synthesis and characterization of the fluorescent products derived from malonaldehyde and amino acids. *Biochemistry, 8*, 2821–2827.

Diplock, A.T., & Lucy J.A. (1973). The biochemical modes of action of vitamin E and selenium: A hypothesis. *FEBS Lett., 29*, 205–210.

Dirks, R.C., Faiman, M.D., & Huyser, E.S. (1982). The role of lipid, free radical initiator, and oxygen on the kinetics of lipid peroxidation. *Toxicol. Appl. Pharmacol., 63*, 21–28.

Dodrill, C.B. (1988). Cognitive effects of anti-epileptic drugs. *J. Clin. Psychiatry* (Suppl. 3), *49*, 31–34.

Dodrill, C.B., Arnett, J.L., Sommerville, K.W., & Sussman, N.M. (1995). Effects of different dosages of Vigabatrin (Sabril) on cognitive abilities and quality of life in epilepsy. *Epilepsia, 36*, 164–173.

Dodrill, C.B., Wilensky, A.J., Ojeman, L., Temkin, N., & Shellenberger, K. (1992). Neuropsychological, mood and psychosocial effects of gabapentin. *Epilepsia, 33* (Suppl. 3), 117.

Dugan, M., & Howell, J.M. (1994). Post-traumatic seizures. *Emerg. Med. Clin. North America, 12*, 1081–1087.

Eaves, L.J. (1982). The utility of twins. In V.R. Anderson, J.K., Penry, & C.F. Sing (Eds.), *Genetic basis of the epilepsies* (pp. 249–276). New York: Raven Press.

Glozner, F.L., Haubitz, I., Miltner, F., Kapp, G., & Pflughaupt, K.W. (1983). Epilepsy prophylaxis with carbamazepine in severe brain injuries. *Neurochirurgia, 26*, 66–79.

Gutteridge, J.M.C. (1981). Thiobarbituric acid reactivity following iron-dependent free radical damage to aminoacid and carbohydrates. *FEBS Lett., 128*, 343–345.

———. (1982). The protective action of superoxide dismutase on metal ion catalyzed peroxidation of phospholipids. *Biochem. Biophys. Res. Comm., 77*, 379–386.

Hafeman, D.J., Sunde, R.A., & Hoekstra, W.G. (1974). Effects of dietary selenium on erithrocyte and liver glutathione peroxidase in the rat. *J. Nutr., 104*, 580–587.

Hall, E.D. (1993). The role of oxygen radicals in traumatic injury: Clinical implications. *J. Emerg. Med., 11*, 31–36.

Hall, E.D., Yonkers, P.A., McCall, J.M., & Braughler, J.M. (1988). Effects of the 21-aminosteroid U74006F on experimental head injury in mice. *J. Neurosurg., 68*, 456–461.

Halliwell, B., & Gutteridge, J.M.C. (1981). Formation of a thiobarbituric acid reactive substance from deoxyribose in the presence of iron salts. *FEBS Lett., 128*, 347–352.

———. (1986). Iron and free radical reaction: two aspects of antioxidant protection. *TIBS, 11*, 372–375.

Jennett, B. (1975). *Epilepsy after non-missile head injury* (2nd ed.). Chicago: Williams Heinemann.

Katz, R.T. (1988). Seizure disorder in the rehabilitation setting. *Concepts Rehabil. Med., 4*, 15–20.

Koppenol, W.H., Butler, J., & van Leeuwen, W. (1978). The Haber-Weiss cycle. *Photochem. Photobiol., 28*, 650–660.

Kutt, H. (1992). Pharmacologic principles. In S.R. Resor& H. Kutt (Eds.), *The medical treatment of epilepsy* (pp. 27–42). New York: Marcel Dekker.

Leach, J.P., & Brodie, M.J. (1995a). Lamotrigine: Clinical use. In R.H. Levy, R.H., Mattson, & B.S. Meldrum (Eds.), *Anti-epileptics drugs,* (4th ed.) (pp. 889–895). Cedar Knolls: Lippincott-Raven Healthcare.

———. (1995b). New anti-epileptic drugs—an explosion of activity. *Seizure, 4,* 5–17.

Levy, R.H., Mattson, R.H., & Meldrum, B.S. (1995). *Anti-epileptic Drugs* (4th ed.). Cedar Knolls: Lippincott-Raven Healthcare.

Lucy, J.A. (1972). Functional and structural aspects of biological membranes: a suggested structural role of vitamin E in the control of membrane permeability and stability. *Ann. N.Y. Acad. Sci. 203,* 4–11.

Marmarou, A. (1994). Traumatic brain injury: Understanding the pathway to recovery. *Neurol. News Update, 2,* 1–2.

McNamara, J.O., Rigsbee, L.C., Butler, L.S., & Shin, C. (1989). Intravenous pheytoin is an effective anti-convulsant in the kindling model. *Ann. Neurol., 26,* 675-678.

Meador, K.J., Loring, D.W., & Huh, K. (1990). Comparative cognitive effects of anti-convulsant. *Neurology, 40,* 391–394.

Monaco, F., Riccio, A., Covacic, A., Durelli, L., Mutani, R., & Morselli P.L. (1976). Further observations on carbamazepine plasma levels in epileptic patients: Relationships with therapeutic and side effects. *Neurology, 26,* 936–943.

Monaco, F., et al. (in press). Cognitive effects of vigabatrin: A review. *Neurology.*

Morrell, F., & Baker, L. (1961). Effects of drugs on secondary epiloptogenic lesions. *Neurology, 11,* 651–664.

Mutani, R., Monaco, F., Cantello, R., Gianelli, M., Civardi, C., & Naldi P. (1991). Pharmacological prophylaxis of post-traumatic epileptogenesis: An update on the experimental models. In L. Murri, G. Parienti, & J.F. Annegers (Eds.), *Pharmacological prophylaxis for post-traumatic epilepsy* (pp. 17–21). Pisa: Pacini.

Niehaus, W.G., & Samuelsson. (1968). Formation of malonaldehyde from lipid arachinodate during microsomal lipid peroxidation. *Eur. J. Biochem., 6,* 126–130.

Oles, K.S., & Penry, J.K. (1985). Pharmacological prophylaxis of post-traumatic seizures. In R.T. Johnson (Ed.), *Current therapy in neurologic disease* (pp. 46–51). Philadelphia: Decker & Mosby.

Penty, J.K., White, B.G., & Brackett, C.E. (1979). A controlled prospective study of the pharmacologic prophylaxis of post-traumatic epilepsy. *Neurology, 29,* 600–601.

Rapport, R.L., & Ojeman, G.A. (1975). Prophylactically administered phenytoin: Effects on the development of chronic cobalt induced epilepsy in the cat. *Neurology, 32,* 532–548.

Reynolds, E.H. (1983). Mental effects of anti-epileptic medication: A review. *Epilepsia* (Suppl. 2), *24,* S85–S95.

Rosen, J.A. (1966). Dilantin dementia. *Trans. Am. Neurol. Ass., 93,* 276.

Salazar, A.M., Jabbar, B., Vance, S.C., Graffmann, J., Amin, D., & Dillon, J.D. (1985). Epilepsy after penetrating head injury. I. Clinical correlates: A report of the Vietnam Head Injury Study. *Neurology, 35,* 1406–1414.

Schmutz, M., Klebs, K., & Baltzer, V. (1988). Inhibition of enhancement of kindling evolution by anti-epileptics. *Neural. Transm., 72,* 245–257.

Servit, Z. (1960). Prophylactic treatment of post-traumatic epilepsy. *Nature* (London), *188,* 669.

Singh, R., & Nath Patak, D. (1990). Lipid peroxidation, and glutathione peroxidase, glutathione reductase, superoxide dismutase, catalase, and glucose-6-phosphate dehydrogenase activities in $FeCl_3$-induced epileptogenic foci in the rat brain. *Epilepsia, 31,* 15–26.

Smith, P.J., Tappel, A. L., & Chow, C.K. (1974). Glutathione peroxidase activity as a function of dietary selenomethionine. *Nature* (London), *247,* 392–393.

Temkin, N.R., Dikmen, S.S., Wilensky, A.J., Keihm, J., Chabal, S., & Winn, H.R. (1990). A randomized, double-blind study of phenytoin for the prevention of post-traumatic seizures. *N. Engl. J. Med., 323,* 497–502.

Victoria, E.J., & Barber, A.A. (1969). Peroxydation of microsomal membranes protein-lipid complexes. *Lipids, 4,* 582–588.

Wada, J.A., Sato, M., Waka, A., Green, J.F., & Troupin, A.S. (1976). Prophylactic effects of phenytoin phenobarbital and carbamazepine examined in kindling cat preparations. *Arch Neurol., 33,* 426–434.

Willie, E. (1993). *The treatment of epilepsy: Principles and practice.* Philadelphia: Lea and Phebiger.

Willmore, L.J. (1992). Post-traumatic epilepsy. *Neurol. Clin., 10,* 869–878.

Willmore, L.J., & Rubin, J.J. (1981). Antiperoxidant pre-treatment and iron-induced epileptiform discharge in the rat: EEG and histopathology study. *Neurology, 31,* 63–69.

Willmore, L.J., Sypert, G.W, Munson, J.B., & Hurd, R.W. (1978). Chronic focal epileptiform discharges induced by injection of iron into rat and cat cortex. *Science, 200,* 1501–1503.

Wills, E.D. (1969). Lipid peroxide formation in microsomes: The role of non-haeme iron. *Biochem. J., 113,* 325–332.

Witting, L.A. (1980). Vitamin E and lipid antioxidants in free-radical-initiated reactions. In W.A. Pryor (Ed.), *Free radicals in biology* (Vol. 4) (pp. 295–319). New York: Academic Press.

Yablon, S.A. (1993). Post-traumatic seizures. *Arch. Phys. Med. Rehabil., 74,* 983–1001.

Young, B., Rapp, R., Brooks, W.H., Norton, J.A., Haack, D., & Walsh J.W. (1983). Failure of prophylactically, administered phenytoin to prevent late post-traumatic seizures. *J. Neurosurg., 58,* 236–241.

14 Treatment and Rehabilitation of Sleep Disorders in Patients with Brain Damage

Javier Espinar-Sierra

Sleep Unit, Hospital Universitario San Carlos
Madrid, Spain

INTRODUCTION

Sleep disorders are frequent in patients with neurological impairment. They do not always originate from brain damage but can also be caused by other concurrent factors, such as those related to the deterioration of the sleep-wake rhythm, psychological disturbances, drugs, etc. In many cases, these factors have a greater influence on the abnormality of sleep than the brain damage itself. This should be considered when evaluating, treating, and rehabilitating the patient with brain damage and complaints of sleep disorders.

NEUROPHYSIOLOGY AND NEUROANATOMY OF SLEEP AND WAKE

The neuronal systems that control sleep and wakefulness are located in the brainstem, hypothalamus, and basal portion of the forebrain, with relay nuclei located in the thalamus and target organs in the cortex. Thus, affectation of these systems can cause abnormalities of sleep and wakefulness.

In the regulation of wakefulness, several interrelated and redundant systems intervene, mainly the reticular formation of the mesencephalon, pons, and medulla that provokes the activation and desynchronization of the cortex through three routes: that which relays in the nonspecific nuclei of the thalamus, that of Meynert's nucleus (via ponto-basal-cortical), and that which passes through the posterior hypothalamus. The locus coeruleus (nor-adrenergic), which diffusely projects into the cortex and receives afferents from the posterior hypothalamus and the medulla and intervenes in the selective attention and discrimination of information, participates in wakefulness as well. The adrenergic system of the medulla sends afferents to the locus coeruleus and is the main relay of the excitatory sympathetic system and, therefore, regulates the vegetative response of wakefulness. The nigrostraital dopaminergic system maintains behavioral wakefulness, and the mesolimbic and mesocortical systems of the ventromedial tegmentum are necessary for cognitive processes and focalized attention. The ventrolateral posterior hypothalamus (histaminogen) guarantees the regulation of wakefulness and sends projections to the anterior hypothalamus, to the basal nuclei of Meynert, and to the cortex. Finally, the raphe systems (serotoninergic) have a complex or paradoxical function, since the serotoninergic neurons are active during wakefulness; however, if they are inactivated, insomnia occurs. It seems that the axonal release of serotonin during wakefulness would prepare sleep by favoring the synthesis of hypnogenic substances in unknown structures. This would facilitate drowsiness and, during all of the sleep, would control the serotoninergic permissive systems so that it would have a direct and differed influence in the regulation of the wakefulness states (Adrien, 1994).

In the regulation of slow wave sleep (SWS), the preoptic region of the anterior hypothalamus plays a principal role. Besides promoting sleep, it inhibits the posterior hypothalamus that promotes wakefulness. The anterior hypothalamus provokes the drowsiness necessary to initiate the remaining regulatory structures of slow sleep. In the control of the SWS, GABAergic cells of the Meynert nucleus also intervene. In turn, these inhibit the cholinergic cells of the same nucleus and those of the posterior hypothalamus and facilitate the appearance of the spindles (generated by the reticular nucleus of the thalamus by the interaction between the GABAergic neurons of the Meynert nucleus and the thalamocortical neurons) and the slow sleep waves. These are produced by the hyperpolarization of the thalamocortical neurons that result from the decrease of cholinergic influences from the brainstem.

The SWS is regulated by three processes: a circadian process, an ultradian process that regulates its periodic appearance during the night, and an accumulative or homeostatic (process S) process that charges during wakefulness and discharges during sleep (Borbeley, 1982).

REM sleep is preferentially generated in medullar and pons structures through several superimposed and overlapping mechanisms in which we can distinguish direct control, hypothalamus-hypophysial influences, and several humoral influences. In the direct control of sleep (initiation, maintenance, and interruption), the executive and permissive mechanisms are distinguished. The executive structures are those that are active during the entire length of REM sleep (REM-On neurons) and the permissive ones that discontinue their activity during REM sleep (REM-Off neurons) (Steriade & McCarley, 1990). The executive mechanisms depend on the cholinergic cholinoceptive neurons of the medulla (n. magnocellular) and pons (pontopeduncular tegmentum, laterodorsal tegmentum, alpha locus coeruleus). The permissive mechanisms of REM sleep depend on monoaminergic cells (REM off) more diffusely arranged in the brainstem, principally in the locus coeruleus and in the serotoninergic neurons of the raphe.

Production of REM sleep depends on the activation of all of the executive structures and the discontinuation of the activity of the monoaminergic permissive structures. The substances involved in the neurohumoral regulation of REM sleep are not known, but the preoptic region of the anterior hypothalamus seems to be essential for the inhibition of the posterior hypothalamus, which has a tonic inhibition on REM production. On the other hand, there is a series of substances that facilitate REM sleep such as the vasoactive intestinal peptide (facilitating NREM and REM), the corticotropin-like intermediary peptide, the growth hormone, and somatostatin. Temperature and metabolism can also modify the balance between regulator neurons of REM sleep.

ENCEPHALIC LESIONS THAT ALTER SLEEP AND WAKEFULNESS

From the above discussion, it is well understood that for normal sleep to be produced, the integrity of the mentioned encephalic structures would be necessary and also that the lesions produced in them would provoke different disorders of sleep and wakefulness (Figure 14.1).

Lesions of the brain hemispheres alter the expression of the different stages of sleep. In one case of laminar necrosis of the entire brain cortex, the disappearance of SWS and of the spindles and the alteration of the ultradian organization of sleep were observed (Autret et al., 1975). However, the brain hemispheres do not seem to be necessary for the generation of sleep itself, since alternation of sleep and wake has been described in a child with anencephalia (Nielsen & Sedgwick, 1949). Certain modulating influences arise from the basal portion of the brain and reach the mesencephalon from the basal part of the forebrain, making up the so-called Nauta and Haymaker circuit (Culebras, 1992).

For some time, the influence of the thalamus in the regulation of the sleep-wake cycle was denied, but experiments in diencephalic and athalamic cats which had chronic insomnia (Villablanca, 1974) and the recent description by Lugaresi et al. (1986) of the

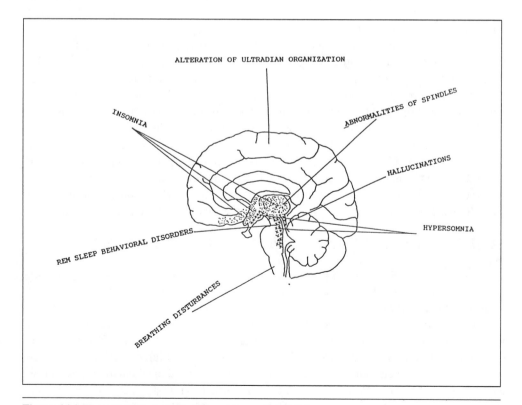

Figure 14.1: Encephalic lesions that alter sleep and wakefulness.

"Fatal Familial Insomnia Syndrome" have made it necessary to reconsider this presumption. Fatal Familial Insomnia is characterized by incapacity to sleep associated with vegetative hyperactivity and the later appearance of motor and endocrine disorders. This disease is inherited in a dominant autosomic fashion and exists in a selective or prevalent degeneration of the dorsomedian or anterior nuclei of the thalamus by the exclusion of the hypothalamus from the cortical inhibitory control (Lugaresi, 1992).

Lesions of the posterior hypothalamus provoke coma, lethargy, and hypersomnia, since both the cellular bodies and the fibers that pass through it form a part of the ascendent activating reticular system. Lesions of the anterior hypothalamus cause insomnia because of its inhibiting effect on the posterior hypothalamus. Cases of narcolepsy-cataplexy that are symptomatic of a craniopharyngioma and lesions of the hypothalamic and of the third ventricle have been described (Aldrich & Naylor, 1989).

The lesions of the medial portion of the mesencephalon provoke a decrease in wakefulness, paralysis of the vertical gaze, and pupillary abnormalities, since, in this zone, the rostral portion of the activating reticular system and the nucleus of the third cranial nerve are found. Some patients have the so-called "peduncular hallucinations," which are intense visual hallucinations having great color related to the content of the consciousness, and that are probably related to REM sleep, since the peduncular hallucinations appear in patients with sleep disorders (Culebras, 1992).

In patients with tumors located in the rostral portion of the brainstem that invade the floor of the third ventricle, sleep attacks, episodes of cataplexy, and sleep paralysis have been described (Stahl et al., 1980). The lesions of the inferior mesencephalon and the superior tegmentum of the pons that affect the area surrounding the locus coeruleus are causes of the "REM Sleep Behavior Disorder" (RSBD), which is a syndrome that exists with an REM sleep without atonia (Schenck et al., 1986).

The dorsal lesions of the tegmentum of the pons that affect the reticular formation produce unconsciousness, while the pontine ventral lesions that do not affect the reticular do not affect the consciousness. Extensive lesions of the pontine tegmentum provoke insomnia, abnormalities, and even the abolition of the NREM and REM sleep, and paralysis of the horizontal gaze is associated. In lesions of the medium raphe of the pons and the mesencephalon, there can be loss of NREM sleep (Culebras, 1992).

The lesions of the medulla affect respiration during sleep and can produce a complete failure of the automatic control of respiration, resulting in a clinical picture similar to that of Ondine's syndrome or congenital alveolar hypoventilation. The medulla centers of respiration are also affected in the Arnold-Chiari syndrome in which apneas appear during sleep (Noya et al., 1993) and in poliomyelitis if the medulla or the pons are affected.

SLEEP-WAKE RHYTHM IN PATIENTS WITH BRAIN DAMAGE

The sleep-wake cycle is a circadian biological rhythm that permits a better adaptation of the organism to the environment. It is regulated by the interaction of internal "biological clocks," environmental influences, and different processes that promote sleep and wakefulness. Humans have at least two internal synchronizers with different periods (Folkard, Minors, & Waterhouse, 1984). One of the oscillators is located in the suprachiasmatic nucleus, and the other would be a biochemical mechanism of production and use of a substance (Factor S). The most important external synchronizers, the so-called "Zeitgebers" or time markers, are the light-darkness or day-night alternation, eating schedule, and social schedule (family, work, TV, etc.). To a lesser degree, temperature, relative humidity, and other environmental changes have an influence. Maladjustment or nonperception of these time markers would also provoke sleep-wake disorders in patients with brain damage, mainly in those with cognitive deterioration, sensorial deprivation, and handicaps, and who are confined to bed.

PSYCHOLOGICAL FACTORS

Psychological factors have a great significance in the pathophysiology of sleep disorders. In many patients with brain damage, different psychological disorders can be observed. These are mainly anxiety and depression that are, in most cases, a consequence of the clinical condition of the patient more than of the specific lesions.

DRUGS

The neurological patients often receive drugs that affect the central nervous system (CNS) and that can provoke sleep disorders (Corruble et al., 1994; Warot, Corruble, & Puech, 1994). Some drugs do so by exaggerating their effect (i.e., insomnia with the use of CNS stimulants), and others by an unexpected effect (night terrors and use of levodopa). The effect can appear during the administration of the drug or when it is discontinued. Neurological patients may also receive drugs whose primary effect is not on the CNS (theophylline, antihypertensives) but that have secondary effects on sleep. Table 14.1 shows the drugs that alter sleep. The possible use of these drugs should be considered when evaluating patients with brain damage.

REHABILITATION OF SLEEP DISORDERS

The objective of sleep rehabilitation is to obtain healthy sleep habits by using different procedures that will depend on the abnormality of the sleep and the baseline

Table 14.1: Drug-Related Sleep Disorders

INSOMNIA:
Antibiotics, Anti-convulsants, Antidepressants, Antiinflammatory, Antirheumatics, Bronchodilators, Cardiovascular Agents, CNS-Stimulants, Diuretics, Hypnotics and Sedatives—Tolerance and Rebound, Levodopa, Methysergide, Neuroleptics, Steroids, Thyroid Hormone

DAYTIME SLEEPINESS:
Analgesics, Anorectic Agents, Anti-convulsants, Anticholinergics, Antidepressants, Antihistamines, Antihypertensive Agents, Benzodiazepinics, Chemotherapics, Griseofulvine, Methysergide, Non-Steroid Antiinflammatory, Progesterone

SLEEP APNEA SYNDROME:
Anesthesia, Antidepressants, Barbiturates, Benzodiazepinics, Betablockers, Narcotics, Sedatives, Steroids, Testosterone

PARASOMNIAS:
Nightmares (Amantadine, Antidepressants, Baclofen, Betablockers, Dapsone, Digitalis, Fenfluramine, Levodopa, Pentazocine)
Nocturnal Terrors and Somnambulism
(Anti-convulsants, Anticholinergics, Antidepressants, Antihistamines, Hypnotics, Levodopa, Lithium, Neuroleptics, Sedatives)
Enuresis (Anti-convulsants)
Bruxism (Amphetamines, Fenfluramine)
Sleep Paralysis (MOA-Inhibitors)
Nocturnal Myoclonus (Anticholinergics, L-dopa, MAO-Inhibitors)

disease of the patient. Principally, sleep hygiene regimes, behavioral techniques, and modification of the synchronizers of the sleep-wake cycle are used.

Sleep Hygiene

Sleep hygiene is fundamental for the prevention and rehabilitation of sleep disorders, and in some of them, generally the mildest ones, it may be the only treatment. Sleep hygiene is supported by a series of practices (Table 14.2); time spent in bed should be strictly limited to sleep needs and sexual activities, and other activities such as reading, TV, radio, etc. should be avoided in bed. A schedule for going to bed and getting up should be established and should be independent of whether it is a work day or holiday and whether the person has slept well or badly. Moderate exercise is recommended but should not be performed close to bedtime, since exercise changes the body temperature and produces fatigue, two mechanisms that cause arousal. As far as possible, a pleasant environment should be created in the bedroom. It should not be too cold or too warm, and there should be acceptable relative humidity. Clearly, noise and anything else that can cause the person to wake up should be avoided. Mealtimes contribute to shape the circadian cycle, and, therefore, a regular schedule is recommended. Furthermore, dinners should neither be heavy nor should the subject go to bed fasting, since both situations make sleep difficult. Hypnotics should only be used when necessary, and the patient should be warned about the risks of self-medicating. The use of drugs and stimulants, including spirits, should be avoided, above all, close to bedtime. The patient should be advised not to think about the day's problems while in bed since this increases anxiety and makes it difficult to sleep. Naps are only permitted in patients who have no sleep conciliation difficulties; insomnia patients should avoid them (Hauri, 1977; De Koninck, 1994; Zarcone, 1994).

Table 14.2: Sleep Hygiene

1.	Limit time in bed.
2.	Establish bed time and getting up time.
3.	Perform moderate exercise.
4.	Create a pleasant environment in temperature and humidity.
5.	Avoid noises.
6.	Have regular meal times and avoid heavy dinners or going to bed hungry.
7.	Take hypnotic drugs only when prescribed by the doctor.
8.	Avoid medications and stimulants (including caffeine and spirits).
9.	Do not take problems to bed.
10.	Naps should be short and only if there is no difficulty with nocturnal sleep.

"Resynchronization" of the Sleep-Wake Rhythm

There are two basic mechanisms in sleep-wake rhythm disorders that can be easily evaluated and "rehabilitated." On the one hand, it is known that the longer the wakefulness before going to bed, the easier it is for sleep to appear and that this will be better (longer and deeper) if one goes to sleep at the right moment. The two moments in the day in which the biological clock favors sleep is during the nighttime and towards noon (siesta). On the other hand, exposure to bright light in the final hours of the afternoon tends to delay the sleep phase, while intense light during the first hours of the morning tends to advance it (Czeisler et al., 1989). In latitudes in which there is sunlight at these times, a one-hour walk outside is enough. In winter and in the northern countries, intense artificial light will be necessary (Hauri & Esther, 1990). Social customs that function as external synchronizers should also be reinforced. Taking cold showers in the morning and hot showers in the afternoon has been recommended (Saletu, 1986).

Behavioral Treatment

Behavioral treatment is based on learning and conditioning of good sleep habits. Stimulus control and restricting the time in bed are the most used methods.

Stimulus Control

Stimulus control (SC) is based on the fact that some insomnia patients associate the bedroom with feelings of frustration and arousal, which should be modified by conditioning the sensation of sleep with the fact of going to bed. For this, the patient should be instructed to go to bed only when he is sleepy. He should only go to bed to sleep (not to read, watch TV, etc.), and if he cannot sleep, he should go to another room and return to the bedroom only when he is sleepy again. If he does not sleep then, he should get up. This should be repeated as often as necessary during the night. It is important that, regardless of how the subject sleeps, he should get out of bed at the same time every day and should not take any naps (Bootzin & Nicassio, 1978).

Restriction of Time in Bed

Restriction of time in bed (RTB) is based on the observation that when the time in bed is prolonged, sleep is fragmented by long periods of awakenings and becomes superficial. In the RTB, the patient is asked to drastically decrease the time spent in bed. After this, he is progressively permitted to increase it in order to produce continuity and deepness of sleep. Other behavioral techniques have not been verified in the treatment of sleep disorders (Hauri & Esther, 1990; Saletu, 1986).

SLEEP DISORDERS IN PATIENTS WITH BRAIN DAMAGE

Head Trauma

After a head trauma, there can be excessive daytime sleepiness, difficulty in initiating and maintaining sleep, and more rarely, parasomnias. After coma, there is generally a slow recovery of the state of consciousness, with the patient remaining somnolent during the day and falling asleep during monotonous situations or even while being cured. Normal wakefulness generally takes a long time to appear, and sleep patterns can remain abnormal long after the head trauma (Parkes, 1985)).

In general, somnolence that appears after a head trauma usually forms a part of the post-traumatic subjective syndrome (PSS). In the PSS or post-concussional syndrome, daytime sleepiness or nonrestorative sleep is associated with cognitive and neurovegetative disorders that include complaints such as migraines, cervicalgias, eating disorders (anorexia or bulimia), and loss of libido, as well as psychiatric disorders, mainly depression (Carlander, 1994: Culebras, 1992). In the PSS, sleepiness is not always verified by studies of naps, but nighttime sleep is generally fragmented (Prigatano et al., 1982). At times, somnolence occurs in an isolated way, and no psychiatric disorder is seen so that no diagnosis of PSS can be made (Carlander, 1994). It is in these cases when it is best to speak of post-traumatic sleepiness or hypersomnia (PTH), which is defined as excessive somnolence that occurs as a consequence of a trauma that affects the CNS (ASDA, 1990). This disorder means a clear change in the sleep pattern regarding the moment before the trauma. Excessive daytime sleepiness may or may not be resistible and followed by a period of sleep. It is generally clearer immediately after the head trauma and can disappear in weeks or months, but a residual somnolence may continue and even worsen during the following 6–18 months. The somnolence that appears in some patients after a head trauma may be due also to a sleep apnea syndrome (SAS). Guilleminault et al. (1980) described the presence of an SAS in eight of the 20 patients who presented daytime somnolence after a head trauma. This SAS can be explained by a direct lesion of the medullar respiratory centers or of the fibers of the motoneurons of the cervical spinal cord that go to the diaphragm (Bonekat, Andersen, & Squires, 1990) and also by simple snoring existing before the trauma, decompensated by weight gain or the administration of psychotropic drugs (Carlander, 1994) and, sometimes, by lesions of the facial structure or the upper respiratory tract.

Cognitive deterioration and psychopathology are frequent in the SAS and should be differentiated from the post-traumatic subjective syndrome. In the SAS, improvement of sleepiness and psychopathology do not occur simultaneously, because while improvement in sleepiness is immediate, that of the psychopathological disorders associated with SAS is only obtained after several months of treatment (Ramos-Platon & Espinar-Sierra, 1992).

Exceptionally, the appearance of narcolepsy during a head trauma has been described. However, most of the authors believe that the trauma can provoke coma, stupor, hypersomnolence, and drowsiness but cannot provoke a real narcoleptic syndrome (Parkes, 1985). In any event, when it is verified that the patient has an HLA-DR15-DQ6 haplotype, it should be questioned if the trauma only had a precipitating role in the appearance of the symptoms (Carlander, 1994).

In the evaluation of the somnolent patient after the trauma, the possibility that the somnolence existed before and is even the cause of the head trauma should not be overlooked since pathological somnolence is a frequent cause of work and traffic accidents. Patients with SAS more often have traffic accidents that are more severe than those suffered by the normal population (Findley, Unverzagt, & Suratt, 1988).

Treatment of post-traumatic hypersomnia is preferentially symptomatic with CNS stimulants such as methylphenidate or pemoline. Regarding the post-traumatic subjective syndrome dependent symptomatology, the patient can generally benefit from energizing tricyclic antidepressants (clomipramine) or fluoxetine. In any event, the patient would benefit from good sleep hygiene and the regulation of the sleep-wake cycle, fixing the bedtime and getting up time, and he/she should be encouraged to exercise regularly far from the bedtime, avoiding that which could alter nighttime sleep and abstaining from the use of alcohol. Severe sleep apnea syndrome would be treated by the home administration of nasal continuous positive airway pressure (nasal-CPAP) (Sullivan et al., 1981). In mild cases, general hygienic measures such as weight loss, suppression of spirits and sedatives, and respiratory depressors would be sufficient. In some cases, when these have been previously malformed or damaged by the trauma, corrective surgery of the airways or maxillofacial structures (Powell, Guilleminault, & Riley, 1994) could be applied. Reconstruction of the upper airways by uvulopalatopharyngoplasty generally offers good results in patients who are not heavy and have a moderate or mild SAS.

As a part of the post-traumatic subjective syndrome, insomnia can also appear and is seen a few hours or days after consciousness is recovered. It generally disappears after some days, although in some patients, it lasts for a long time. In post-traumatic insomnia, the lost of sleep-wake rhythm because of the hospital stay should also be considered, and hygienic and behavior measures are best indicated here, above all, in patients with no neurological sequelae. In those patients in which PSS is identified or in which social or work problems consequent to the trauma overlap, the use of drugs is generally necessary. When the mood is affected, antidepressants having sedative effects (amitriptyline), which are generally efficacious with moderate doses before going to bed, should be used.

Tumors

Tumors can provoke sleep disorders directly or through endocranial hypertension, hydrocephalus, or both. Sleep abnormalities will depend on the site of the lesion. Several patients have been described with a narcolepsy syndrome secondary to tumors located in different parts of the brain (Aldrich & Naylor, 1989; Stahl et al., 1980): glioblastoma of the mesencephalon, craniopharyngioma, glioma of the third ventricle, hypophysial adenoma, and in colloid cyst of third ventricle. In tumors located in the rostral portion of the brainstem that invade the floor of the third ventricle, episodes of cataplexy, attacks of sleep, and sleep paralysis have been described (Stahl et al., 1980). Most of these patients have attacks of sleep and cataplexy and generally present the HLA-DR2 antigen of histocompatibility, but there are descriptions of HLA DR2- and DQ1-negative patients who have developed symptomatic narcolepsy because of a diencephalic lesion. Thus, belonging to type HLA DR2 seems to be a favoring but not essential factor (Aldrich & Naylor, 1989). Occasionally, the appearance of recurrent hypersomnias similar to the Kleine-Levin syndrome (Roth, 1980) and to recurrent hypersomnia linked to the menstrual cycle (L'Hermitte & Kiriaco, 1929) have been described in the context of brain tumors.

Vascular Diseases

As in the tumors, the abnormalities of sleep that appear in the vascular diseases of the brain will depend on the site of the lesion. In general, in the days following the stroke, an inversion of the sleep-wake rhythm is produced, and there is lethargy during the day and agitated wakefulness during the night. Daytime lethargy can sometimes be misinterpreted as a sign of deterioration of the neurological situation (Culebras, 1992). In the acute stage, there can also be apneas and hypopneas with significant oxygen desaturations (Askenasy & Goldhammer, 1988). In the chronic stages, both ischemic and hemorrhagic accidents can damage the regulatory structures of sleep and leave sequelae on it. In lacunar infarcts that affect the mesencephalon and the pons, REM Sleep Behavior Disorders (RSBD) can appear. This can be due to the disconnection of the tegmentoreticular tract and of the centers that surround the locus coeruleus that are responsible for the muscular atonia of the REM sleep (Culebras & Moore, 1989).

Multiple Sclerosis

Complaints of sleep in multiple sclerosis (MS) are three times more frequent than in the normal population. In a sample of 143 patients with a definite diagnosis of MS, one fourth have some difficulty with sleep, principally with its onset or maintenance (Clark et al., 1992). These difficulties are related to the presence of depression and to the lesions that provoke motor symptomatology. Thus, treating the depression to relieve the sleep symptoms in patients with definite MS would take priority. The narcolepsy-cataplexy syndrome associated with MS has also been described. Some of the cases appeared after a long evolution of MS, which suggests that the MS would provoke or favor the appearance of narcolepsy. However, as is generally observed in HLA DR2-positive patients, this would indicate a common genetic susceptibility (Autret, 1994).

Degenerative Diseases of the CNS

In Parkinson's disease, sleep disorders are frequent. The most common abnormalities are fragmentation and lengthening of the sleep latency, which condition an important decrease in sleep efficiency. This would lessen with greater daytime symptomatology. The SWS is generally reduced, and the REM sleep can also be reduced but to a lesser degree, while there is an increase in the stages of light sleep (stages 1 and 2). Patients who have hypertonia and rigidity usually present less REM sleep than those who have normal muscle tone during sleep (Monret, 1975). REM sleep and total sleep time are even more decreased in patients with nocturnal hallucinations (Comella, Tanner, & Ristanovic, 1991).

Aldrich (1994) distinguishes several factors in the origin of sleep disorders of Parkinsonians: (1) neurochemical changes in the regulatory systems of sleep-wake would provoke interruption of sleep and decrease in REM and NREM sleep, (2) lesser mobility in bed due to bradykinesia and rigidity would condition discomfort and more waking up, (3) abnormal movements during sleep (periodic movements of sleep, tremors, myoclonias induced by medication) would provoke waking-up, (4) the respiratory disorders during sleep, and (5) circadian and sleep-wake pattern disorders affected by the disease or medication would mean insomnia, fatigue, and/or daytime sleepiness. To establish the origin of the sleep disorder in each case, a detailed clinical history must be obtained. The course of the disease and sleep disorder and information from the bed-mate on movements, rigidity, tremors, respiratory disorders, and waking up during the night are very important to know. Regarding medication, the administration schedule must be known since if the dopaminergic medication is not given near bedtime, rigidity will alter the sleep. If it is too close, it will provoke insomnia at the beginning. Furthermore, it should be considered that low-dose dopaminergic medication induces sleep, while high doses make it difficult. Anticholinergic medication, on the other hand, can affect the amount of REM sleep and worsen the respiratory problem (Aldrich, 1994.). If the effect of the medication can be ruled out, a disorder of the circadian rhythm must be considered (advance or delay of the phase or inversion of the sleep-wake rhythm). Behavioral, psychiatric, and social factors that can condition the sleep disorder must also be considered.

Once the causes are identified, the best treatment for each case should be started. In any event, good sleep hygiene should commence, and the bedroom conditions should be improved; sometimes a simple portable commode can improve the sleep disorder (Ibid.). In the advanced stages of the disease, a suggestion may be made to the spouse to sleep in another bed or room, since the sleep disorder may make cohabitation with the patient unacceptable and cause institutionalization.

The dosage and time in which the drug is administered should be adapted to the sleep disorder in question. However, and more importantly, how a change in the dosage will affect the control of the daytime symptomatology must be considered. In insomnia patients without hallucinations or vocalization, Aldrich (1994) recommends adding 100 mg of levodopa and 25 of carbidopa at bedtime and a similar amount at 2:00 A.M. or 3:00 A.M. in the morning if the patient wakes up. Improvement of insomnia would be obtained by the decrease in rigidity and bradykinesia. Variability of response depends on the causes involved in the sleep treatment. As has been said, dopaminergic medication can provoke sleep disorders (vivid dreams, nightmares, and night terrors), above all, in patients with dementia; thus, if this occurs, the mid-day and night dosage should be reduced. If insomnia continues, benzodiazepinic hypnotic agents can be used for short periods of time. Amitriptyline-type tricyclic antidepressants can be useful in the treatment of difficulty of sleep onset because of their sedative effects, and they can also be beneficial for daytime symptomatology due to their anticholinergic effects. However, they can potentially induce deliriums in patients with cognitive deterioration.

When insomnia is due to dyskinetic movements during sleep, it generally responds to low doses of dopaminergics, to clonacepan, and to other benzodiazepines. Respiratory disorders of the Parkinson's disease during sleep should be treated in the usual way (nasal-CPAP, weight reduction, surgery, etc.).

Shy-Drager syndrome is a multisystemic degeneration that is generally associated to a Parkinsonian syndrome, to orthostatic hypotension, and to other signs of autonomic nervous system failure. In this context, central and obstructive type apneas and the appearance of REM Sleep Behavior Disorders (Sforza et al., 1988) that can precede other signs of neurological deficit (Culebras, 1992) are frequent during sleep. In progressive supranuclear paralysis (PSP), there is subcortical dementia, paralysis of the vertical gaze and axial rigidity, and insomnia with a decrease in the amount of sleep and fragmentation of it, bad organization of the NREM sleep, few spindles, and decrease of REM sleep. Insomnia of the progressive supranuclear paralysis is mild at the onset of the disease and is characterized by difficulty in getting to sleep. As the disease advances, fragmentation of sleep is produced, and insomnia becomes worse, but there is no difficulty at the onset or early morning waking. This insomnia would be due to the neuronal loss of the brain structures that regulate sleep due to the degeneration of the tegmental structures of the rostral portion of the brainstem, the subthalamus, and the medial thalamus (Aldrich et al., 1989). Factors associated with the severity of the disease such as discomfort, affectation of mobility or nocturnal disorientation, and possibly diurnal naps, would also be involved. However, the insomnia of these patients is much greater than that seen in other patients with dementia and affectation of mobility (Ibid.). In patients with olivopontocerebellar atrophy (OPCA), phenomena of REM sleep without atonia (RSBD) have also been described (Schenck et al., 1986; Sforza et al., 1988; Quera-Salva & Guilleminault, 1986) since the neurons of the pons that generate REM sleep and motor inhibition are affected. In the OPCA, there is a reduction of the density of rapid eye movements and the amount of REM and NREM sleep. The growing increase of the amount of REM sleep has been associated with a progressive affectation of the sleep generators of the pontine tegmental structures (Culebras, 1992). Central- and obstructive-type sleep apneas that are probably related to autonomic dysfunction have also been described (Chokroverty, Sachdeo, & Masdeu). In spinocerebellar degeneration, there is absence of REM sleep and decrease in NREM sleep and undetermined sleep, as well as sleep apneas that can condition the prognosis of these patients due to the associated autonomic dysfunction and cardiac arrhythmias. Bedridden patients with snoring, respiratory arrhythmias, and medullar symptoms have a high risk of sudden death during sleep (Katayama, Hirano, & Yoyama, 1987).

Sleep Disorders in Dementia

Patients with dementia frequently present insomnia and inversion of the sleep-wake rhythm that is generally associated with nocturnal agitation. In the beginning, when the subject has a problem getting to sleep, he/she is not generally worried by it and does not consult the doctor, but little by little, this becomes worse, and the impact on diurnal wakefulness increases due to the loss of autonomy and familial relationship of the patient. When the insomnia becomes worse, it is more difficult for the patient to stay awake or sleep for long periods. In this stage, the so-called *sundown syndrome* can appear. This disorder is the one that most commonly alters the sleep of the demented. Some authors call it nocturnal delirium, but while delirium is a diagnosis, sundowning is a behavior (Vitiello, Bliwise, & Prinz, 1992). Sundowning can appear in the evening or later at night and is defined as the nocturnal exacerbation of abnormal behavior and agitation (Ibid.). It is generally the most frequent cause of institutionalization, since the family generally tolerates other signs of cognitive deterioration (confusion, memory loss, incontinency) better but does not feel capable of living with an agitated patient who shouts and has nocturnal wandering (Bliwise, 1993). Patients with sundowning frequently, although not always, are demented, have recently changed rooms, have incontinency, and present less medical diagnosis than those who do not present sundowning (Evans, 1987).

The sleep-wake rhythm disorder in dementias is due to the following factors: (1) sensorial privation and absence of sensorial stimuli during the day, (2) absence of physical and mental exercise during the day, and (3) organic factors such as the abnormalities of respiration during sleep (Okawa et al., 1991).

Infectious, toxic, pharmacological, and metabolic causes should be disregarded (Lipowski, 1989). In the absence of these, nocturnal agitation should be treated with neuroleptic medication, since benzodiazepines are not very efficacious and even can be the cause of confusional behavior. Haloperidol (0.5–1 mg) and thioridazine (25 mg) are effective. They can present side effects in the long term (Bliwise, 1993), and the drug should be periodically discontinued to verify its need and prevent side effects (Bliwise, 1993; Devanand, Sackeim, & Mayeux, 1988).

To rehabilitate the sleep of the demented, action should be taken on the different factors that condition it.

1. The environment surrounding the patient should be improved, maintaining an appropriate sensorial atmosphere, with a visible clock, calendar, and family photos in a calm and well-lighted room (Lipowski, 1989).

2. In institutionalized patients, moderate exercise and a schedule of regulated nocturnal activities should be established and directed by an occupational therapist, and this will serve to minimize the lack of comfort to other patients and to the personnel of the institution (Bliwise, 1993).

3. Nurses are essential in reinforcing the social interaction with the patient (speaking, walking), since this seems to improve the disorders of the sleep-wake rhythm and the nocturnal behavior in some patients (Okawa et all., 1991)

4. Naps should be eliminated to decrease the fragmentation of sleep and nocturnal waking the following night. For this same reason, unnecessary visits by the nursing staff should be avoided.

5. Exposure to light generally improves sleep in the demented, but effects of activation and restlessness appear immediately, probably due to the effect of the light on macular degeneration (Bliwise, 1993).

6. The association of SAS and dementia is frequent (Figure 14.2), even more so in multi-infarct than in Alzheimer's disease (Erkinjuntti et al., 1987), and the severity of the dementia is related to the number and hypoxia consequent to the apneas (Ibid.). The treatment of the SAS would be similar to other types of

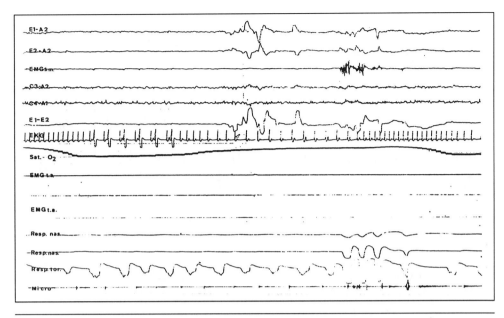

Figure 14.2: Polysomnogram of a 62-year-old female with Alzheimer's disease and severe sleep apnea syndrome that demonstrates obstructive apnea, oxygen desaturation, and cardiac arrhythmia.

patients. However, many times, the cooperation of the patient with the use of nasal-CPAP is not possible.

Sleep Disorders in Early Brain Damage

Children with an important mental retardation usually have sleep disorders. Institutionalized patients generally have irregular and fragmented sleep during the entire day and spend most of the day asleep or with a low activity level (Landesman-Dwyer & Sackett, 1978). Half of the patients who live at home also have sleep disorders, and two-thirds wake up frequently at night (Quine, 1991). In most of the cases, the sleep abnormalities are not due to brain lesions but to loss of the "zeitgebers" or external synchronizers. The newborn with brain lesions sometimes has a maturation delay and/or delay in perception of the visual stimuli that can affect the development of the circadian rhythms, and the same occurs due to the loss of or difficulty in social contact that these children have. Thus, action taken on the sleep-wake cycle should be that which makes it possible to better regulate sleep. Although there are few controlled studies that evaluate the effectiveness of these procedures, there are some descriptions that support them (Summers, Lynch, & Harris, 1992). In the rehabilitation of the disorders of the sleep of the retarded child, it is important to eliminate the diurnal naps and to accumulate all the sleep in the nighttime hours. To reduce the nocturnal wake-ups, the intake of fluids in the afternoons should be reduced so that nighttime miction does not cause awakening, and the bedtime and getting up time should be strictly established. In some cases, it is necessary to add medication, and the best results are obtained with the combination of behavioral treatment and pharmacological treatment with chloral hydrate or diphenhydramine-type antihistamines, although after some time, diphenhydramine can be substituted by a placebo without modifying the results (Ibid.).

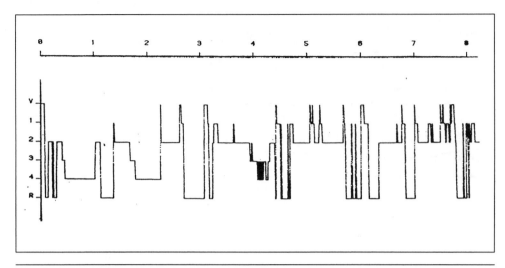

Figure 14.3: Hypnogram of a 9-year-old girl with the Prader Willi syndrome that demonstrates sleep onset in REM sleep (SOREM) and numerous REM cycles.

Prader-Willi syndrome (PWS) is due to the deletion or disomy of the long arm of chromosome 15 and is clinically characterized by neonatal hypotonia, dysmorphic facies, short stature, eating and behavior disorders, hypogonadism, and mild mental retardation. Most of the patients with Prader-Willi Syndrome suffer excessive daytime sleepiness and other abnormalities of sleep and respiration during it. Vela-Bueno et al. (1980, 1984) described the sleep onset REM stage (SOREM) for the first time (Figure 14.3). Other abnormalities of REM sleep observed are the appearance of REM sleep during the day, fragmentation and decrease in REM sleep time (Helbing-Zwanenburg, Kamphuisen, & Mourtazaev, 1980), greater number of sleep cycles, and variable REM latency (Hertz, Cataletto, Feinsilver, & Angulo, 1993). These abnormalities, similar to those found in narcolepsy, have led some authors to think about the possibility of a secondary narcolepsy, but as it is not associated with HLA DR2, this explanation is not very plausible. In the PWS, there are generally breathing abnormalities during sleep, mainly nocturnal hypoventilation (Vela-Bueno et al., 1984), but patients who develop SAS are rare. Both the sleep and respiration disorder are related to the hypothalamic dysfunction (Vela-Bueno et al., 1984; Hertz et al. 1993) that is responsible for the rest of the symptomatology (obesity, hypogenitalism, etc.).

CNS-stimulants similar to those used in narcolepsy (caffeine methylphenidate or amphetamines) have been recommended in the treatment of diurnal sleepiness. However, these medications can provoke important side effects, above all, in those patients whose state of mood is altered. Consequently, an attempt should be made to treat this sleepiness with programmed naps during the day (Helbing-Zwanenburg, Kamphuisen, & Mourtazaev, 1993). Two to three naps of at least 20 minutes during the day when the patient is usually sleepy should be recommended. Weight control in these patients is fundamental for their good evolution. When severe nocturnal hypoventilation is associated, nasal-CPAP (bi-level positive airway pressure [BIPAP]) should be used, and weight control should be intensified since there is some relation between severity of oxygen desaturation and obesity (Hertz et al., 1993).

Rett's syndrome (RS) affects girls without a family history or birth problems in whom, after a period of normal psychomotor development, there is a regression of the previously acquired skills, detention of cephalic growth, walking difficulties, very characteristic stereotypes of the hands, and pseudoautistic behavior. Three-fourths of the girls with RS have sleep disorders (Coleman et al., 1988). The parents report that their daughters wake up in the middle of the night laughing. These episodes that appear periodically are sometimes long and disturb the continuity of sleep. Some girls in stage III of the disorder present violent shouting during sleep that can be associated with the nighttime laughing mentioned. It is also of interest to record sleep in the RS because the only objective finding of the syndrome is sometimes the presence of paroxystic discharges (Figure 14.4) that are more persistent during sleep even in patients who do not have epileptic seizures (Hagberg et al., 1983; Espinar-Sierra et al., 1990). Attention is also brought to the scarce development of the normal electrophysiologic phenomena of sleep, particularly of the spindles (Espinar-Sierra et al., 1990).

In the Down Syndrome (DS), sleep is characterized by an increase in waking up during sleep, decrease in REM sleep and, above all, in the density of eye movements, frequent body movements, and a decrease in the transition periods between NREM and REM sleep and vice versa. In adolescents with Down Syndrome, sleep is generally somewhat longer than normal (Okawa & Sasaki, 1987). The scarcity of REM sleep and spindles has been related to mental retardation (Castaldo, 1969). Down Syndrome is frequently observed in association with a sleep apnea syndrome (Loughlin, Wynne, &

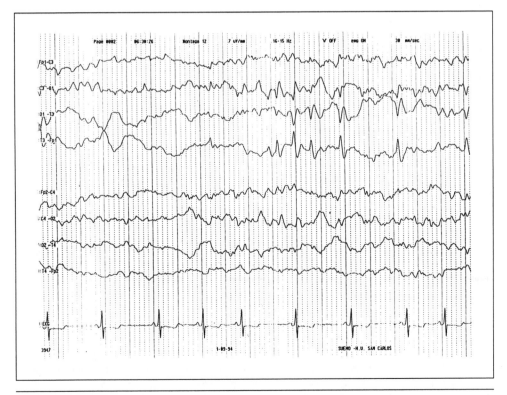

Figure 14.4: Polygraphic recording of a 6-year-old girl with Rett's syndrome that demonstrates paroxystic discharges in left temporal area.

Victorica, 1981), which does not always have a favorable response to adenoidectomy or tonsillectomy as does SAS in other children (Marcus, Keens, & Bautista, 1991), because other factors such as macroglossia or hypotonia are generally more important in the DS (Strome, 1986). In these cases, nasal-CPAP is administered.

Epilepsy (see also Chapter 13)

There are multiple relationships between epilepsy and sleep. Both deprivation of sleep, arousal of sleep, and sleep itself are activators of epileptic seizures and some epileptic seizures that only occur in certain stages of sleep (Shouse, 1987). Seizures by themselves can alter the continuity and quality of nocturnal sleep, while anti-convulsants can provoke sleepiness, insomnia, and even parasomnias (Table 14.1). Epileptic patients should take great pains with sleep hygiene, avoiding acute or chronic sleep deprivation and irregular sleep habits.

CONCLUSIONS

Sleep disorders presented by brain-damaged patients are not only due to the neurological affectation but also to the alteration of the sleep-wake rhythm, to concurrent psychological factors, to drugs administered, and to other factors. This should be taken into account when evaluating these patients. Sleep rehabilitation endeavors focus on the patients' learning to sleep again, which is obtained by behavioral techniques, sleep hygiene regimes, and modification of the external and internal synchronizers of the sleep-wake rhythm.

REFERENCES

Adrien, J. (1994). Neurobiologie du cycle veille-sommeil. In M. Billiard (Ed.), *Le sommeil normal et pathologique. Troubles du sommeil et de eveil* (pp. 27–38). Paris: Masson.

Aldrich, M.S. (1994). Parkinsonism. In M.S. Kryger, T. Roth, & W.C. Dement (Eds.), *Principles and practice of sleep medicine* (pp. 783–789). Philadelphia: WB Sanders Company.

Aldrich, M.S., & Naylor, M.W. (1989). Narcolepsy associated with lesion of the diencephalon. *Neurology, 39,* 1505–1508.

Aldrich, M.S., Foster, N.L., White, R.F., Bluemlein, I., & Prokopowicz, G. (1988). Sleep abnormalities in progressive supranuclear palsy. *Ann. Neurol., 25,* 557–581.

American Sleep Disorders Association (ASDA). (1990). *The international classification of sleep disorders.* Rochester: ASDA.

Askenasy, J.J., & Goldhammer, I. (1988). Sleep apnea as a feature of bulbar stroke. *Stroke, 19,* 637–639.

Autret, A. (1994). Sommeil et affections neurologiques (a l'exclusion des épilepsies). In M. Billiard (Ed.), *Le sommeil normal et pathologique: Troubles du sommeil et de eveil* (pp. 496–506). Paris: Masson.

Autret. A., Carrier, H., Thommasin, M., Jouvet, M., & Schott, B. (1975). Etude physiopathologique et neuro-pathologique d'un syndrome de décortication cérébrale. *Rev. Neurol., 131,* 491–504.

Bliwise, D.L. (1993). Sleep in normal aging and dementia. *Sleep, 16,* 40–41.

Bonekat, H.W., Andersen, G., & Squires, J. (1990). Obstructive disordered breathing during sleep in patients with spinal cord injury. *Paraplegia, 28,* 292–298

Bootzin, R.R., & Nicassio, P. (1978). Behavioral treatment of insomnia. In M. Hersen, R. Eisler, & P. Miller (Eds.), *Progress in behavior modification* (Vol. 6) (pp. 1–45). New York: Academic Press.

Borbeley, A.A. (1982). A two-process model of sleep regulation. *Human Neurobiology, 1,* 195–204.

Carlander, B. Les autres causes de somnolence pathologique. In M. Billiard (Ed.), *Le sommeil normal et pathologique: Troubles du sommeil et de eveil* (pp. 288–295). Paris: Masson.

Castaldo, V. (1969). Down's syndrome: A study of sleep patterns related to level of mental retardation. *Am. J. Ment. Defic., 74,* 187–190.

Chokroverty, S., Sachdeo, R., & Masdeu, J. (1984). Autonomic dysfunction and sleep apnea in olivopontocerebellar degeneration. *Arch. Neurol., 41,* 926–931.

Clark, C.M., Fleming, J.A., Li, D., Oger, J., Klonoff, H., & Paty, D. (1992). Sleep disturbance, depression, and lesion site in patients with multiple sclerosis. *Arch. Neurol., 49,* 641–643.

Coleman, M., Brubaker, J., Hunter, K., & Smith, G. (1988). Rett syndrome: A survey of North American patients. *J. Ment. Def. Res., 11,* 102–109.

Comella, C.L., Tanner, C.M., & Ristanovic, R.K. (1991). Sleep disturbances and hallucinations in Parkinson's disease: Results of quantitative sleep studies. *Ann. Neurol., 30,* 295.

Corruble, E., Warot, D., Solibrie, C.L., & Puech, A. (1994). Les insomnies liées aux medicaments. In M. Billiard (Ed.), *Le sommeil normal et pathologique: Troubles du sommeil et de eveil* (pp. 187–193). Paris: Masson.

Culebras, A. (1992). Neuroanatomic and neurologic correlates of sleep disturbances. *Neurology, 42* (Suppl. 6), 19–27.

Culebras, A., & Moore, J.T. (1989). Magnetic resonance finding in REM sleep behavioral disorder. *Neurology, 39,* 1519–1523.

Czeisler, C.A., Kronauer, R.E., Alla, J.S., Duffy, J.F., Jewett, M.E., Brown, E.N., & Ronda, J.M. (1989). Bright light induction of strong (type 0) resetting of the human circadian pacemaker. *Science, 244,* 566–568.

De Koninck, J. (1994). Hygieène du sommeil et traitements comportementaux de l'insomnie. In M. Billiard (Ed.), *Le sommeil normal et pathologique: Troubles du sommeil et de eveil* (pp. 208–215). Paris: Masson.

Devanand, D.P., Sackeim, H.A., & Mayeux, R. (1988). Psychosis, behavioral disturbance and the use of neuroleptic in dementia. *Comp. Psychiatry, 29,* 387–401.

Erkinjuntti, T., Partinen, M., Sulkava, R., Telakivi, T., Salmi, T., & Tilvis, R. (1987). Sleep apnea in multiinfarct dementia and Alzheimer's disease. *Sleep, 10,* 419–425.

Espinar-Sierra, J., Toledano, M.A., Franco, C., Campos-Castello J., Gonzalez-Hidalgo, M., Oliete, F., Garcia-Nart, M. (1990). Rett's Syndrome: A neurophysiological study. *Neurophysiol. Clin., 20,* 35–42.

Evans, L.K. (1987). Sundown syndrome in institutionalized elderly. *J. Am. Geriat. Soc., 35,* 101–108.

Findley, L.J., Unverzagt, M.E., & Suratt, P.M. (1988). Automobile accidents involving patients with obstructive sleep apnea. *Am. Rev. Respir. Dis., 138,* 337–340.

Folkard, S., Minors, D.S., & Waterhouse, J.M. (1984) Is there more than one circadian clock in humans? Evidence from fractional desyncronization studies. *J. Physiol., 357,* 341–356.

Guilleminault, C., Faull, K.M., Miles, L., & van den Hoed, J. (1980). Post-traumatic excessive daytime sleepiness: A review of 20 patients. *Neurology, 33,* 1584–1589

Hagberg, B., Aicardi, J., Dias, K., & Ramos, O. (1983). A progressive syndrome of autism, dementia, ataxia, and loss of purposeful hand use in girls. Rett's syndrome: Report of 35 cases. *Ann. Neurol., 14,* 471–479.

Hauri, P. (1977). *The sleep disorders.* Kalamazoo: The Upjohn Company.

Hauri, P., & Esther, M.S. (1990). Insomnia. *Mayo Clin. Proc., 65,* 869–882.

Helbing-Zwanenburg, B., Kamphuisen, H.A.C., & Mourtazaev, M.S. (1993). The origin of excessive daytime sleepiness in the Prader-Willi syndrome. *J. Intelect. Disab. Res., 37,* 533–541.

Hertz, G., Cataletto, M., Feinsilver, S.H., & Angulo, M. (1993). Sleep and breathing patterns in patients with Prader Willi Syndrome (PWS): Effects of age and gender. *Sleep, 16,* 366–341.

Katayama, S., Hirano, Y., & Yoyama, S. (1987). Nocturnal sudden death in cases with spinocerebellar degeneration. *Sleep Res., 16,* 483.

L'Hermitte, J., & Kiriaco, N. (1929). Hypersomnie périodique reguliérement rhytmée par les régles dans un cas de tumeur basilaire du cerveau. *Rev. Neuro., 36,* 715–719.

Landesman-Dwyer, S., & Sackett, G.P. (1978). Behavioral changes in nonambulatory, profoundly mentally retarded individuals. *Monogr. Am. J. Ment. Defic., 3,* 44.

Lipowski, Z.J. (1989). Delirium in the elderly patient. *N. Engl. J. Med., 320,* 578–582.

Loughlin, G.M., Wynne, J.V., & Victorica, B.E. (1981). Sleep apnea as a possible cause of pulmonary hypertension in Down Syndrome. *J. Pediatr., 98,* 435.

Lugaresi, E. (1992). The thalamus and insomnia. *Neurology, 42* (Suppl. 6), 28–33.

Lugaresi, E., Medori, R., Montagna, P., Baruzzi, A., Cortelli, P., Lugaresi, A. Tinuper, P., Zucconi, M., & Gambetti, P. (1986). Fatal familial insomnia and dysautonomia with selective degeneration of thalamic nuclei. *N. Engl. J. Med., 315,* 997–1003.

Marcus, C.L., Keens, T.L.,& Bautista, D.B. (1991). Obstructive sleep apnea in children with Down Syndrome. *Pediatrics, 88,* 132

Monret, J. (1975). Differences in sleep in patients with Parkinson's disease. *Electroenceph. Clin. Neurophysiol., 38,* 653–657

Nielsen, J.M., & Sedgwick, R.P. (1949). Instincts an emotions in an anencephalic monster. *J. Nerv. Ment. Dis., 110,* 387–394.

Noya, E., Lasheras, M., Sanchez-Algaba, A., Bueno, G., Balboa, F., Campos J., & Espinar, J. (1993). Malformacion de Arnold Chiari tipo II y apneas. *An. Esp. Pediatr., 39,* 248–250

Okawa, M., & Sasaki, H. (1987). Sleep disorders in mentally retarded and brain-impaired children. In C. Guilleminault (Ed.), *Sleep and its disorders in children* (pp. 269–289). New York: Raven Press.

Okawa, M., Mishima, K., Hishikawa, Y., Hozumi, S., Hori, H., & Takahashi, K. (1991). Circadian rhythm disorders in sleep-waking and body temperature in elderly patients with dementia and their treatment. *Sleep, 14,* 478–85.

Parkes, J.D. (1985). *Sleep and its disorders.* London: WB Saunders Company.

Powell, N.B., Guilleminault, C., & Riley, R.W. (1994). Surgical therapy for obstructive sleep apnea. In M.S. Kryger, T. Roth, & W.C. Dement (Eds.), *Principles and practice of sleep medicine* (pp. 706-721). Philadelphia: WB Sanders Company.

Prigatano, G.P., Stahl, M.L., Orr, W.C., & Zeiner, H.K. (1982). Sleep and dreaming disturbance in closed head injury patients. *J. Neurol. Neurosurg. Neuropsychiatry, 45,* 78–80.

Quera-Salva, M.A., & Guilleminault, C. (1986). Olivopontocerebellar degeneration, abnormal sleep and REM sleep without atonia. *Neurology, 36,* 576–577.

Quine, L. (1991). Sleep problems in children with mental handicap. *J. Ment. Def. Res., 33,* 269

Ramos-Platon, M.J., & Espinar-Sierra, J. (1992). Changes in psychopathological symptoms in sleep apnea patients after treatment with nasal continuous positive airway pressure. *Intern. J. Neuroscience, 62,* 173–195.

Roth, B. (1980). Narcolepsy and hypersomnia. Basel: Karger.

Saletu, B. (1986). Therapy for sleep disorders in depressives. *Psychopathology, 19,* (Suppl. 2), 239–262.

Schenck, C.H., Bundlie, S.R., Ettinger, M.G., Mahowald, M.W. (1986). Chronic behavioral disorders of human REM sleep: A new category of parasomnia. *Sleep, 9,* 293–308.

Sforza, E., Zucconi, M., Petronelli, R., Lugaresi, E., & Cirignotta, F. (1988). REM sleep behavioral disorders. *Eur. Neurol., 28,* 295–300.

Shouse, M.N. (1987). Sleep, sleep disorders, and epilepsy in children. In C. Guilleminault (Ed.), *Sleep and its disorders in children* (pp. 291–307). New York: Raven Press.

Spielman, A.J., Saskin, P., & Thorpy, M.J. (1987). Treatment of chronic insomnia by restriction of time in bed. *Sleep, 10,* 45–56.

Stahl, S.M., Layezer, R.B., Aminoff, M.J., Townsend, J.J., & Feldon, S. (1980). Continuous cataplexy in a patient with a midbrain tumor: The limp-man syndrome. *Neurology, 30,* 1115–1118, 1980.

Steriade, M., & McCarley, R. (Eds.). (1990). *Brainstem control of wakefulness and sleep.* New York: Plenum Press.

Strome, M. (1986). Obstructive sleep apnea in Down's Syndrome children: A surgical approach. *Laryngoscope, 96,* 1340.

Sullivan, C.E., Issa, F.G., Berthon-Jones, M., & Eves, I. (1981). Reversal of obstructive sleep apnea by continuous positive airway pressure applied through the nares. *Lancet, 1,* 862–865.

Summers, J.A., Lynch, P.S., & Harris, J.C. (1992). A combined behavioral/pharmacological treatment of sleep-wake schedule disorder in Angelman Syndrome. *J. Dev. Behav. Pediatr., 13,* 284.

Vela-Bueno, A., Campos-Castello, J., & Cabranes, J.A. (1980). Hipersomnia en el síndrome de Prader-Willi con comienzo del sueño en fase REM: Presentación de un caso. *Psiquis, 1,* 45–50.

Vela-Bueno, A., Kales, A., Soldatos, C.R., Dobladez, B., Espino, P., & Olivan, J. (1984). Sleep in the Prader Willi Syndrome: Clinical and polygraphic findings. *Arch. Neurol, 41,* 294–29.

Villablanca, J. (1974). Role of the thalamus in sleep control: Sleep-wakefulness studies in chronic diencephalic and athalamic cats. In O. Petre-Quadens & J.D. Schalg (Eds.), *Basic sleep mechanism* (pp. 166–307). New York: Academic Press.

Vitiello, M.V., Bliwise, D.L., & Prinz, P.N. (1992). Sleep in Alzheimer's disease and the sundown syndrome. *Neurology, 42* (Suppl. 6), 83–94.

Warot, D., Corruble, E., & Puech, A. (1994). Somnolence liée aux medicaments. In M. Billiard (Ed.), *Le sommeil normal et pathologique: Troubles du sommeil et de eveil* (pp. 253–261). Paris: Masson.

Yesagave, J., Bliwise, D., Guilleminault, C., Carskadon, M., & Dement, W.C. (1985). Preliminary communication: Intellectual deficit and sleep-related respiratory disturbances in the elderly. *Sleep, 8,* 30–33.

Zarcone, V.P. (1994). Sleep hygiene. In M.S. Kryger, T. Roth, & W.C. Dement (Eds.), *Principles and practice of sleep medicine* (pp. 542–546). Philadelphia: WB Sanders Company.

PART III:

REHABILITATION OF NEUROCOGNITIVE PROCESSES

15 Rehabilitation of Individuals with Frontal Lobe Impairment

Catherine A. Mateer

University of Victoria
Victoria, B.C., Canada

INTRODUCTION

Individuals with frontal lobe damage and associated executive function compromise can be among the most baffling and challenging patients that rehabilitation specialists work with. These patients may demonstrate average or even above-average intellectual abilities, seemingly adequate recall of information, and apparent knowledge when a verbal response is asked for. Yet they may demonstrate organizational, self-regulatory, and behavioral problems such that they fail to accomplish goals or complete even the simplest of tasks in the absence of cuing or structure.

This chapter discusses various approaches to treating and working with patients who have sustained frontal system compromise. The first step involves an assessment of frontal and executive system functions. This is often a challenging task, particularly when the goal is to identify goals for rehabilitation. Typically, the process of rehabilitation itself is viewed as a combination of *restorative* and *compensatory approaches. Restorative* approaches are those that may improve or restore executive function or control. *Compensatory* approaches involve the training of procedures or techniques that allow the individual to function more effectively despite their impairments. This category of approaches may also use environmental modifications to help reduce the demand on impaired cognitive functioning.

FUNCTIONS OF THE FRONTAL LOBE

The functions of the frontal lobe have been somewhat elusive despite the fact that frontal lobe dysfunction can seriously impair many aspects of cognitive ability and independent functioning. The frontal lobes do not have a unitary function; rather, different regions of the frontal system are important in different aspects of cognition and behavior (Di Pellegrino & Wise, 1991; Luria, 1980; Stuss & Benson, 1986). Portions of the frontal lobes play an important role in the initiation of action and behavior. Disruption of this system can result in spontaneity or behavioral inertia (Fuster, 1990). Individuals with such disorders are often capable of speaking or behaving quite normally but, without substantial external cuing, fail to do so. The frontal lobes are also important in identifying goals, in planning and organizing behavior to accomplish relevant goals, and in monitoring goal-directed activity (Shallice, 1982; Shallice & Burgess, 1991a). Disruption in this system may result in behavior that seems random, disorganized, or without purpose.

The frontal lobes are also important in many aspects of attention (see Van Zomeren & Brouwer, 1994). Working memory, the capacity to hold information in a mental store during active information processing, appears dependent on frontal systems. The ability to switch attention between tasks and the capacity for divided attention also appears to be, at least in part, dependent on frontal systems. In novel situations, when overlearned skills, knowledge, or responses cannot be used successfully, the frontal lobes are important in monitoring the effectiveness of behavior (Shallice & Burgess, 1991b). As a situation becomes more familiar or a pattern of response more routine, there is a decreased need for frontal involvement.

Although recall of specific declarative or semantic information does not seem to be dependent on the frontal regions, there are an increasing number of mnemonic functions, such as memory for temporal order, which have been ascribed to the frontal regions (Baddeley & Wilson, 1988; Janowsky, Shimamura, Kritchevsky, & Squire, 1989; Milner, Petrides, & Smith, 1985; Schacter, 1987). Although memory for content per se may not be frontally dependent, memory for contextual information (e.g., source memory and recent memory) have been found to be disrupted in patients with frontal involvement. Certain aspects of metamemory, such as "feelings of knowing," appear to be frontally mediated (Janowsky, Shimamura, & Squire, 1989). Finally, the capacity for "remembering to remember" or prospective memory has also been related to frontal system functioning.

Another major function of the frontal system appears to involve the regulation of mood and emotion. Patients with frontal lobe dysfunction have been described as more labile in their mood, more quick to respond emotionally with anger or frustration, and less sensitive to the feelings or needs of others. Family members often describe patients with frontal lobe injuries as quite different in terms of personality and behavior (Lezak, 1978, 1987; Prigatano, 1992).

EVALUATION OF FRONTAL LOBE FUNCTIONING

Before a treatment program can be implemented, it is important to conduct a thorough evaluation to determine the nature and degree of cognitive and behavioral impairment. It is widely acknowledged that functions associated with the frontal lobe are difficult to evaluate (Lezak, 1982, 1993). Most cognitive abilities are assessed through the use of psychometric measures. In such testing, there are usually very explicit instructions identifying what is expected, and there are strong cues to initiate and maintain responses. Given such inherent cues and support, many patients with frontal lesions often perform quite well, while in more naturalistic situations, they may fail to use the abilities that they possess. It is also hard to design tests of problem solving, planning, and organizing which capture the same underlying abilities that are needed for the myriad of activities required for adaptive functioning in everyday life.

For these reasons, there are substantial limits to conventional psychometric testing that form the base of most neuropsychological evaluations. There are, however, a number of measures that appear to have some utility in demonstrating frontal impairments, although none of them can be considered a litmus test for frontal dysfunction or for lack of frontal involvement. The Wisconsin Card Sorting Test (WCST) (Heaton, 1981) may reveal some of the difficulties some frontal patients demonstrate in identifying relevant information for processing, establishing behavioral sets, using environmental feedback, and shifting from one response set to another (Anderson, Damasio, Jones et al., 1991). The Brown Peterson Technique—Consonant Trigrams Format was found to be useful in identifying problems with working memory and mental control in frontally impaired patients (Stuss, Ely, & Hugenholtz, 1985). Various versions of the Stroop Test are often used to identify the difficulty frontally impaired patients have in shifting from a more automatic to a more controlled or focused response. Various measures of *fluency,* both verbal and nonverbal, have been used successfully in some patients to demonstrate problems with generation of material according to new or unusual categories. This generative fluency seems to correspond to behavioral spontaneity, mental flexibility, and sustained mental effort. Although using one or more of these measures might well suggest the likelihood of frontal involvement, poor performance on any of these measures does not necessarily inform the examiner as to how or under what circumstances such frontal deficits might be manifest in everyday life. They should not be an endpoint in the evaluation but a cue to further explore the possible manifestation of frontal impairment in natural contexts.

In the last few years, several new tests have been designed to more closely simulate the demands of everyday life. Wilson and her colleagues developed the Rivermead Everyday Memory Test (Wilson, Cockburn, & Halligan, 1985). The test uses naturalistic tasks to evaluate the integrity of various memory functions, some potentially dependent on frontal systems. Included in the measure are several prospective memory tasks that evaluate the patient's ability to remember to do certain actions at some point in the future. These items are described as having a better predictive capacity for level of independence in the community than do more traditional retrospective memory tests that are normally undertaken in psychometric examination. Sohlberg and Mateer (1989a) published the Prospective Memory Screening Test (PROMS), which is designed to sample prospective memory tasks that are either externally cued or which must be initiated based on internally generated prompts. They describe significant problems in prospective memory ability in a group of brain-injured patients, many of whom had frontal involvement. The use of measures such as these may capture aspects of frontal memory impairment that might not be seen on more traditional memory measures. In a similar attempt to capture everyday aspects of attentional ability, Robertson, Ward, Ridgeway, and Ninno-Smith (1994) developed the Test of Everyday Attention, which samples both basic attentional skills such as sustained attention, and higher level attention skills, including alternating and divided attention, in tasks that are realistic and similar in demand to everyday situations.

Tests such as the Tower of London (Shallice, 1982) and Tower of Hanoi (Glosser & Goodglass, 1990) have been used to examine various aspects of problem solving such as thinking ahead and planning future actions, and they have been shown to have some use in the assessment of frontal dysfunction. There have also been some innovative attempts to look at planning, organizing, and problem-solving abilities by constructing tasks that are more open-ended and allow more room for variation in performance than most psychometric tasks. The Tinkertoy Test (Lezak, 1982), which involves a fairly open-ended construction using multiple parts, allows the patient to undertake initiation, planning, and structuring of a potentially complex activity and to carry it out independently. The Route Finding Task (Boyd & Sautter, in press), requires that the patient find a specified location (e.g., a gift shop in a hospital). The measure allows for scoring of such dimensions as remembering the target location, the discovery and use of information or cues to find the location, and the use of a systematic approach for seeking the target location.

In a similar vein, Shallice and Burgess (1991b) reported on use of the Six Elements Test, a measure in which six different activities (two each of three types) must be started in a specified time period. The only additional restriction is that no two tasks of the same type may be done in sequence. Successful completion of this task requires the ability to think ahead, recall what has been done and what must yet be done, adhere to the rules set forth, and monitor the passage of time. The authors reported that patients with frontal involvement were often severely impaired on this task, despite average or even above-average intellectual and cognitive ability. Shallice and Burgess (1991b) described another task involving completion of multiple actions within in a particular time frame and according to a particular set of rules. The Multiple Errands Test differed in that it took place in a natural context, a shopping area, in which many natural distractors, cues, constraints, and other situational features were present. Again, patients with frontal involvement were described to have significant difficulty with completion of the errands. Problems emerged with breaking of rules, failing to complete individual tasks correctly, and losing track of time and of task demands.

The use of one or more open-ended or multi-tasking measures such as those described above are highly recommended in the evaluation of functioning that will be used in the development of a rehabilitation plan. Both formal results and informal observations made during such measures can yield valuable information about the practical impact of executive function impairments.

Another approach to evaluation of the practical impact of frontal lobe dysfunction involves the use of rating scales designed to identify everyday cognitive failures. These approaches do not rely on direct observation of a patient's performance on specific tests or tasks. Rather, they are designed to structure the observations of others who are in a position to observe the patients in a variety of situations or settings. Ratings of behavior in different domains by therapists, nurses, and family members can yield valuable information about the patient's level of independent and organized functioning in natural contexts.

Sohlberg and her colleagues (1992) developed the Profile of the Executive Control System (PRO-EX). The PRO-EX has rating scales for six different domains of cognitive/behavioral functioning that are, at least in part, dependent on the frontal system. The domains include *Goal Selection, Planning/Sequencing, Initiation, Execution, Timesense, Awareness of Deficits,* and *Self-Monitoring.* The level of functioning in each domain is listed on a 7-point scale. The scale can be used by clinicians after they have had the opportunity to observe the patient/client in various settings on a variety of tasks. The scale can also be used as a basis for discussion with families, to gain additional information about the patient's functioning in the home environment, and to assist in providing information and education to the family about the effects of frontal lobe injury.

Dywan, Roden, and Murphy (1995) have developed another measure designed to evaluate higher level integrative functions and adaptive behaviors in everyday life. The Brock Adaptive Functioning Questionnaire (BAFQ) asks for ratings of functioning on different tasks and abilities that sample five functional domains which have been theoretically associated with frontal lobe processes. These include *Planning, Initiation, Attention/ Memory, Arousal/Inhibition,* and *Social Monitoring.* In a preliminary study, the BAFQ has been shown to correlate with both psychometric measures of frontal lobe functioning and to ERP measures known to be sensitive to frontal activity in a group of individuals who had sustained traumatic brain injury (TBI) (Dywan & Segalowitz, in press). The scale has forms to allow both rating by caregivers and by patients themselves. It might also be used to assess effects of treatment on cognitive and behavioral activities related to frontal lobe functioning.

In summary, it must be recognized that the evaluation of frontal lobe functioning is a complex and challenging process. Although there are some psychometric measures that may suggest the probability of frontal involvement, it is the impact of this involvement on functional capacities that is most critical for rehabilitation planning. Frontal lobe impairments are not played out in isolation but in real world contexts. The level of demand for problem solving, mental flexibility, and complex information management interacts with the level of cuing and support provided in the environment to determine the functional impact of the impairment. Use of not only psychometrics but observations and rating of performance on open-ended tasks is an important part of the evolution of executive functions.

Finally, many individuals with frontal involvement display little insight into or awareness about the nature or degree of problems they demonstrate (Prigatano, 1991) and may tend to underestimate behavioral limitations (Prigatano, Altman, & O'Brien, 1990). For this reason, it is important to use information from others (e.g., family members, other therapists, etc.) who have had the opportunity to observe the individual in other contexts to gain information about initiation, flexibility of behavior, capacity to set and reach goals, and regulation of mood and emotion. Although information from the injured patients themselves about their functioning may not be reliable, it is important to ascertain the degree of insight a person demonstrates. Lack of awareness is not only an indicator of possible frontal involvement but an important factor in the person's rehabilitation plan. A formal plan to increase awareness is often appropriate, since commitment to and involvement in the therapeutic process and the recognition of the need to use strategies to compensate for deficits are often dependent on a degree of awareness of those same deficits.

THE PROCESS OF REHABILITATION

The goal of rehabilitation should be to improve the adaptive functioning of the individual in the setting in which they will be living and working. Following an evaluation of the cognitive/behavioral profile and the probable real world impact of the deficits, it is necessary to establish specific goals given current and future circumstances. An approach to intervention is then selected. The intervention plan or program is delivered, and data is kept on performance or behavior as appropriate. Once gains are made, a generalization plan should be developed and implemented. Finally, there should be an evaluation of the efficacy of the intervention, and the impact of functioning in the natural context should be determined (Sohlberg & Mateer, 1989b).

As indicated in the introduction, intervention for cognitive/behavioral impairments can take the form of process-oriented training designed to improve underlying skills or of compensatory training designed to assist the person in implementing strategies to compensate for underlying impairments. When dealing with frontal lobe impairments, another distinction between approaches is often useful. This distinction is between altering factors that are external to the patient and altering capacities of the patient himself.

Altering Factors External to the Client

One set of approaches to rehabilitation focuses on making manipulations to or of the environment. Such "external manipulations" would alter factors external to the client with minimal or no expectation of underlying change in the individual's capacities. Included under this rubric are such manipulations as altering the demands on the patient. This might be accomplished by simplifying tasks, eliminating the need to do certain tasks, or allowing longer time frames to complete activities. Such a manipulation can be made at a very basic level (e.g., dressing) or at a very high level (e.g., in a work setting). Other manipulations consistent with this approach would include the provision of external support in the form of oral or written cue systems, checklists to follow, or the training of task-specific routines. Yet another manipulation in this vein is the altering of environmental parameters, including the reduction of noise, clutter, or other potential distractions. There is an inherent assumption that such external manipulations would need to remain in place if the change in functioning or behavior is to continue, although it is possible that behaviors might become routine.

The use of behavioral interventions might also be considered an external manipulation, at least at the start. Behavioral interventions have as their goal increases or decreases in the frequency of certain behaviors or a change in their quality through the use of response contingencies (positive or negative reinforcement). In some instances, implementation of such programs may result in a change in behavior that stabilizes to the extent that the contingency can be withdrawn. In other cases, however, it is necessary to maintain the behavioral programming indefinitely or to move into another phase of training to effect behavior change in a different context.

Altering Factors Internal to the Individual

In contrast to approaches that focus on environmental manipulations or modification of factors external to the patient, there are approaches that have as a goal a change within the patient. This would include a myriad of approaches for improving underlying cognitive skills such as attention, memory, or problem solving. It would also include the training of compensatory behaviors or skills such as the ability to record in and refer to a memory system or organizer. Approaches that attempt to increase self-awareness or that teach self-instructional or metacognitive strategies could also be considered here.

In general, patients who demonstrate little behavioral initiative or flexibility, who are environmentally dependent with apparently minimal response to internal cues and/or who are minimally aware of their deficits, tend to respond better and more consistently to external manipulations. For these patients, environmental manipulations, behavioral strategies, and external cuing systems are often effective in increasing function. Patients who demonstrate greater behavioral initiative and flexibility, who initiate and direct their own behavior to some degree, and who are somewhat aware of the change in their abilities resulting from their injury are more likely to demonstrate improvements with specific cognitive training, training in the use of compensatory devices, and training in the use of self-instructional and metacognitive strategies. It is important, therefore, in working with frontally impaired patients to match the profile of the patient with the intervention approach (Sohlberg, Mateer, & Stuss, 1993). In the following sections, rehabilitation in several cognitive and behavioral domains commonly disrupted following frontal injury will be discussed.

THE REHABILITATION OF ATTENTIONAL IMPAIRMENTS

Many patients with frontal lobe impairments retain their basic premorbid knowledge and demonstrate essentially intact language processing capabilities. They are unlikely to have primary auditory, visual, or somatosensory impairments. They are very likely, however, to demonstrate problems with attention and concentration. If brainstem and mid-brain systems are essentially intact, it is likely that basic arousal mechanisms and focused attention will be spared. However, patients with frontal lobe impairment may demonstrate problems with sustained vigilance to task and are likely to have difficulty with distractibility and with smooth and effective allocation of attentional resources on more complex tasks (Van Zomeren & Brouwer, 1987, 1994). They are also likely to have difficulty shifting attention and performing efficiently on tasks that require divided attention capabilities (Stablum, Leonardi, Mazzoldi, Umilta, & Morra, 1994; Stuss, Stethem, Hugenholtz, Picton, Pivik, & Richard, 1989).

Many individuals with TBI, including those with significant frontal lobe impairment, have been shown to benefit substantially from exercise and training of attentional skills. Indeed, some of the earliest work in cognitive rehabilitation demonstrating positive findings involved systematic intervention with the attentional system (Ben-Yishay, Piasetsky, & Rattock, 1987; Kewman, Seigerman, Kinter, Chu, Henson, & Reeder, 1985; Gray, Robertson, Pentland, & Anderson, 1992). Sohlberg and Mateer (1987) developed a package of attention-training materials (Attention Process Training) that was based on a hierarchical model with five levels of attention including focused, sustained, selective, alternating, and divided attention. A large set of both auditory and visual tasks designed to exercise and challenge different aspects of attention were used in treatment sessions over periods of 6–8 weeks in length. The efficacy of this training in improving attentional capacities has been supported in a series of single-case designs and in group pre- and post-treatment comparisons (Mateer, Sohlberg, & Youngman, 1990). It was also demonstrated that improved attentional function was associated with improved anterograde memory function in individuals who received attention but not memory training (Mateer & Sohlberg, 1988; Mateer, 1992). Positive findings were also reported in a controlled group study that used attention training (Niemann, Ruff, & Baser, 1990). There is reason to believe that improved attentional control, with increased vigilance, decreased susceptibility to distraction, and improved capacity to deal with more than one task at a time would positively influence problem-solving, organizational, and communication skills. A first line of intervention, then, in the treatment of an individual with frontal lobe impairment, might profitably include the maximization of attentional capacity through formal attention training (see Mateer & Mapou, in press, for a review of assessment and management of attentional impairments following TBI).

BEHAVIOR MODIFICATION TO IMPROVE INITIATION AND DRIVE

The frontal lobes are essential for the effective initiation and sequencing of action programs. Clinically, action programs can be disrupted by problems with initiation or lack of drive. This might manifest in apparent disinterest or inactivity; there may also be a significant disassociation between verbal output (i.e., what someone says they will do) and their corresponding actions. Generally, it is not the case that the patient with frontal lobe deficits cannot perform an action; rather, it may not occur to them to perform the action at the appropriate time or place, or they may begin an activity but fail to maintain it. Generally, such patients respond quite well to external cues or prompts to initiate activity, and their behavior can be modified through traditional behavior modification techniques, although cuing and reinforcement may need to be maintained. Stuss, Delgado, and Guzman (1987) described the use of a verbal self-regulation approach in an individual with motor impersistence. The patient altered his behavior, but he continued to need to be cued to maintain the self-regulation strategy.

Some individuals with frontal system impairment may demonstrate adequate knowledge of what is going on in the environment but show little apparent interest or involvement. Sohlberg, Sprunk, and Metzelaar (1988) demonstrated that an individual with severe frontal lobe impairment and marked initiation problems did respond differentially with different types of cuing. During a group activity, the patient was provided with a cue at which time he was to ask himself whether or not he was initiating conversation. His verbal interactions during the group sessions clearly increased over a baseline period during and following a treatment phase in which such prompts were provided. Experimental control of the behavior was demonstrated by means of comparison to another measured behavior—response acknowledgments; these responses did not increase during the baseline or initial intervention stage but did when response acknowledgments were specifically trained and then cued by a similar prompted self-evaluation system.

Although differential reinforcement may be useful in some individual patients, loss of executive skills can impair the ability of the individual to initiate use of specific preserved abilities, monitor performance, and use feedback effectively to regulate behavior. Alderman and his colleagues (Alderman & Burgess, 1990; Alderman & Ward, 1991) have demonstrated effective use of another behavior modification technique—response cost—in assisting individuals who have not responded to reinforcement or extinction techniques to gain greater inhibitory control over their behavior. In this technique, the patient is given a number of tokens that are subsequently exchanged for tangible rewards at a later time. However, in the interim, the individual is prompted to give the therapist one token and state the reason for its loss whenever a target behavior (negative) is observed. The advantages of this procedure are that it (1) facilitates directing the patient's attention to aspects of his/her behavior that are not being monitored, (2) enables salient feedback to be extracted from the environment, (3) places minimal load on memory, (4) facilitates procedural learning, and (5) increases awareness. Alderman and his colleagues (Alderman, Fry, & Youngson, 1995) described the use of a response cost program to reduce verbalizations in a brain-injured woman who demonstrated a constant stream of verbal output. Although inhibition of speech was obtained in the institutional training environment, results did not automatically transfer to a second environment. A new program of self-monitoring training was successfully implemented to teach inhibitory control in the new environment. These results suggested that a number of even severe disorders of behavior could come under specific control in patients with frontal mise through the use of traditional behavioral management techniques.

TRAINING PROSPECTIVE MEMORY

At the action program level, functional difficulties may be manifested in failures of what has been termed *prospective memory*. Individuals with frontal lobe impairment frequently fail to act on future intended actions. They may have formed an intent to do something, but at the time that the action is required, they may fail to remember to act. Prospective memory requires that the person carry out a particular action at a specified time in the future based on a self-initiated and internally generated plan of action. Prospective memory can involve such practical and useful activities as remembering to take medications, remembering to make a phone call, or remembering to bring home items when shopping. This capacity may differ sharply from performance on more traditional measures of anterograde, semantic, or episodic memory that are traditionally tested by providing a cue or prompt for recall.

Performance on specific prospective memory tasks are included on the Rivermead Everyday Memory Test (Wilson, Cockburn, & Baddeley, 1985), which has been shown to be more closely correlated with functional independence in the community than has performance on more traditional measures of cued recall. Sohlberg, White, Evans, and Mateer (1992a, b) demonstrated the capacity to improve prospective memory functioning in patients with problems in this area. The goal of prospective memory training is to increase the amount of time between the instruction and the carrying out of a specific action with gradual introduction of distractors during the prospective memory interval. Using this procedure, it was demonstrated that even amnestic patients, initially unable to hold an instruction for even a minute or two, were able to improve and respond to 15-minute prospective tasks. Though still severely impaired, such patients are often capable of a higher level of independence after such training; with improved prospective memory, their capacity to use other memory and organizational systems and to move from room to room or task to task while maintaining an intention appears to be enhanced. Prospective memory can sometimes be compensated for by systematic training in the use of memory books or daily planners/organizers (Sohlberg & Mateer, 1989) and/or by use of cuing devices such as watch alarms or paging systems.

REHABILITATION OF EXECUTIVE FUNCTIONS

Executive functions, in this context, involve the capacity to organize sequences of behavior and to carry out both familiar and novel activities. Since most activities have to be done within somewhat specified time frames, it is important to look at time management strategies as well. At this level, a variety of management and treatment activities might be used, including restorative as well as compensatory strategies. Principals of delivery, regardless of the underlying intent, would be the same. It is important to keep data on the tasks presented and to build skills in a hierarchical fashion going from more structured to less structured tasks and vice versa.

Compensatory Strategies

If the patient is very acute in the rehabilitation process and/or is demonstrating very severe executive function disturbance, it may be profitable to initially focus on *teaching task-specific routines*. The assumption here is that the patient will not be capable of a wide variety of different action plans in different settings because of stimulus boundedness, perseveration, severe related cognitive disorders of attention or memory, or extremely limited insight and awareness. In such individuals, it may not be reasonable to facilitate flexible individually determined sequences, but training of particular sequences for standard highly repetitive functional activities may be possible (Craine, 1982). Included here would be a variety of grooming and dressing procedures such as showering, taking care of one's toilet, or dressing. Another common task-specific routine that might be taught is preparation of a very simple meal (e.g., preparing a simple breakfast). If executive functions are severely impaired, there should probably be a limited number of food items used and an avoidance of potential dangers such as use of the stove or waste disposers, with more emphasis, instead, on safer appliances. The patient might, however, be taught a simple sequence for preparing juice, coffee, and cereal, which could be done the same way each day. Geyer and colleagues (1987) prepared a handbook for teaching such task-specific routines for just this purpose. Behavioral techniques involving shaping of behavior and reinforcement are commonly a complementary adjunct to functional skills-training approaches (Giles & Clarke-Wilson, 1988). Burke and his colleagues described systematic use of checklists to guide behavior, combined with a self-instructional technique (Burke, Zenicus, Wesolowski, & Doubleday, 1991).

Another compensatory approach would include *environmental restructuring*. This would involve organizing the environment to reduce distractions or potentially dangerous situations, providing specific labels in the environment such as on kitchen cupboards or bathroom drawers, and/or setting up a variety of cuing systems. Cuing systems might involve training to use a watch with an alarm, a calendar system, or a card-cuing system to prompt activities throughout the day. It might also involve more complex computer-based or interactive systems that might provide greater flexibility but also might prove more costly and difficult to manage. Unfortunately, there is often a tendency for clinicians to spend less time actively training when compensatory strategies or devices are introduced, perhaps because it seems that the use of such devices should be obvious. Experience in rehabilitation clearly reveals, however, that active and systematic training is required for effective use of compensatory strategies and devices. An example of this type of systematic approach can be found in Sohlberg and Mateer (1989c) in their description of a comprehensive three-stage behavior approach to the training of compensatory strategies in an individual with severe amnestic as well as executive function disorders.

Restorative Approaches

Restorative approaches include a wide variety of structured exercises that would provide multiple opportunities for the initiation, planning, and carrying out of goal-directed activities. For each activity, there may be a variety of ways to complete it. The goal of treatment is for the patient to successfully take on increasing responsibility for carrying out multi-step plans and activities. In the following sections, several specific approaches to working with patients with executive function impairments will be discussed.

Therapy Planning Exercises

In most formal therapy sessions in rehabilitation settings, the actual planning and scheduling of the treatment period is under the control of the therapist. The therapist usually decides what activities will be done, over what duration of time, and in what order, thereby, in some sense, obviating the need for the patient's management of that period of time. When working with an individual with executive function compromise, it is often useful to turn the requirement for the treatment session planning over to the patient. The patient can be given general parameters such as that a certain number of tasks should be used and that a particular time frame is available. The patient, however, decides in what sequence and for what duration each activity is undertaken. One could look, for example, at the capacity to plan a period of 30 or 60 minutes and then look at the capability of the patient to stay within that scheduled plan. Once a patient is able to plan and maintain the time schedule, it would be useful to introduce something that would require the patient to alter or modify the plan. The therapist could indicate that a certain treatment area cannot be used, or that certain materials need to be used by someone else and are not available, or that the entire session needs to be shortened but that the same number of tasks must be incorporated. This allows for observations as to whether or not the patient can modify the plan in accordance with new information or new requirements. The author, in clinical practice, has found that independent scheduling of activity on the part of the patient is often quite revealing with regard to their capacity for scheduling and time management in everyday life.

Planning and Repair Activities

These tasks also address both initiation and organizational skills. The patient is given an errand either within the hospital or within the community. The patient is then scored on his/her ability to complete the errand. Training in strategies such as recording the errand in a memory book or organizational system may be necessary to complete such tasks. The clinician can organize errands hierarchically from easiest to hardest and can introduce the need for a variety of repair strategies. In many settings, it will be possible to move from hypothetical planning to actually carrying out the planning for a real life activity (e.g., patients could initially write or dictate the steps and tasks involved in planning a party, a recreational activity, or a trip; once they have mastered the written plan, they could be provided with opportunities and resources to actually carry out the plan).

Clinicians need to be creative in providing opportunities that meet the constraints of a particular work setting. If a clinician is working one-on-one in a private practice, he/she might suggest that the patients plan to arrange for refreshments. In a group setting, the clinician might ask the patient to plan an activity for the group (e.g., a breakfast, a birthday party, or a community outing). Again, opportunities for modifying plans are a necessity. In real life, for example, if one were organizing refreshments, it is certainly possible someone could be allergic to a particular food that had been planned; such contingencies should be included in patient exercises to increase the patient's flexibility and divergent thinking. For all these types of clinical exercises, it is imperative that data collection pertaining to the ability to plan hypothetical and/or real activities be scored. This can be done using any of a variety of charts or checklists.

In the author's experience, it is useful to evaluate patients' performance on complex, multiple-step tasks on the following parameters: (1) task understanding, (2) incorporation of information seeking, (3) direction retaining, (4) error detection, (5) error correction, and (6) on-task behavior. The second, fourth, fifth, and sixth parameters directly relate to the executive functions of planning, self-monitoring, and use of feedback. It is also useful to pay attention to the types and level of cuing a patient requires to complete activities. Specific cues provide information relevant to how to actually execute the task (e.g., "Have you turned on the stove?") Non-specific cues are used to remind the patient to self-monitor (e.g., "Is there something you should be doing now?"). Systematic manipulation of these two levels of cuing can figure prominently in a hierarchy for training executive functions. Over the course of training, one targets a decreased need for specific cues and greater ability to use non-specific cues. The eventual goal is for a reduction in the need for cues in general.

The foregoing tasks are included under the executive function component, as they all require the organization of output and the integration of complex patterns, relationships, and associations. Many patients with severe frontal lobe compromise may demonstrate only partial recovery of function at this level and may need to rely on compensatory approaches.

METACOGNITIVE TRAINING APPROACHES

Insight, self-awareness, and self-regulatory capacity are felt to reflect the highest level of frontal lobe activity (Stuss, 1991). As many persons with frontal lobe damage demonstrate limited insight into their problems and require explicit behavioral objectives in order to understand and progress in therapy, treatment in this area presents a tremendous challenge for the rehabilitation professional.

Awareness training can take a variety of forms. Usually, patients are given didactic information about the nature of their injury, the way in which it affects their behavior, and the reasons why a particular behavior is or is not appropriate or acceptable. Although sometimes helpful and often necessary, such didactic training is usually not sufficient to bring about the desirable change in behavior (Crossen, Barco & Velozo, 1989).

One approach to measuring self-awareness is to inform the patient that they tend to exhibit a particular behavior, be it desirable or undesirable (e.g., escalating to a loud voice, limited eye contact). The patient is then told to mark a piece of paper every time he/she believes he/she has exhibited the behavior during a designated time period. This recording can be done during a spontaneous conversation, in a one-on-one session, or during a group session. The clinician simultaneously keeps track of the behavior; video tapes may be made as an additional source of information. The patient's awareness may be increased by comparing his/her observations to those of the clinician or those observed on a tape.

Another kind of intervention at this level involves teaching self-instructional procedures before and during the execution of a training task. Cicerone and Wood (1987) reported successful treatment of a patient who exhibited impaired planning ability and poor self-control four years after closed head injury using such a procedure. They used, as a training task, a modified version of the Tower of London. Training in the self-instructional technique involved three distinct phases: overt verbalization, overt self-guidance, and covert internalized self-monitoring. To promote generalization following the program, the client was presented with a structured interpersonal problem and asked to solve it by applying principles learned in the self-instructional training. The results supported the clinical efficacy of verbal mediation training in treating executive functions. The authors noted, however, that generalization of training occurred only after direct, extended training using real life situations. Additional work in the use of self-instructional strategies has been carried out by Cicerone and Giacino (1992).

Von Cramon and Matthes-von Cramon (1990) described positive results in a series of patients with frontal lobe dysfunction using a training procedure that involved enabling patients to help reduce the complexity of a multi-stage problem by breaking it down into more manageable proportions. Problem-solving training incorporated four modules. The first involved the generation of goal-directed ideas, a kind of "brainstorming" designed to produce a variety of alternatives to a given problem. The second module involved training in systematic and careful comparison of information provided about a problem to be solved. The third, consisted of tasks requiring simultaneous analysis of information from multiple sources (such as having the patient compare catalogues from several tourist offices in order to find the most favorable trip to England for a family of four). The fourth module focused on improving the patient's abilities to draw inferences. The authors used short detective stories and had subjects uncover discrepancies and detect "clues" about how crimes could have been committed. The authors reported significant psychometric as well as functional gains in a group receiving this training when compared to a group receiving more generic memory training.

As with several of the other treatment approaches discussed, the use of metacognitive strategies and self-instructional programs for patients with acquired frontal injuries is just beginning to be formally evaluated. It is encouraging, however, that there have been positive outcomes reported and that there are numerous reports of success with such approaches in a variety of clinical populations.

GENERAL TREATMENT PRINCIPLES

A variety of approaches have been discussed with reference to the treatment of individuals with frontal lobe impairment. In general, they involve moving from simple structured activities with significant external cuing and support to more complex, multi-step activities in which external support is gradually reduced and internal support or self-direction is required. Although a variety of articles have suggested success in using these techniques, there are as yet a very small number of cases and a limited number of studies in which such techniques have been experimentally evaluated. Clearly, more work in this area is needed. In addition to the more formal intervention procedures already described, some generic interventions should not be forgotten. Certainly, education of the family and significant others in how to respond to a person with frontal lobe injury is important. Often, an appreciation for the organic or non-volitional nature of the behavior is helpful in alleviating the fears and misconceptions of family members and caregivers. As many different terms can be used to describe these behaviors and capacities, it is important to use consistent language and understandable terminology.

Repetition will be a key factor, and no matter what kind of intervention is used, whether it be restorative or compensatory, multiple opportunities for practice must be incorporated into the treatment program. Behavioral programs need to be well planned and consistently carried out. Finally, it is vital that clinicians actively train for generalization. One should not expect generalization but rather provide systematic opportunities during which skills and behaviors can be trained and stabilized.

Individuals with executive function compromise pose one of the greatest challenges to clinicians and the rehabilitation system. In the last decade, we have made great strides in understanding at least some of the many multi-faceted functions of the frontal lobes. With greater knowledge and understanding, we should be able to identify, develop, apply, and test specific interventions to mediate the effect of frontal system impairments. Executive function compromise, more so than physical limitations, or even many other cognitive impairments, has the potential to disrupt and limit an individual's capacity for independent, meaningful, and socially integrated functioning. Strides that we make in understanding and treating these impairments will be invaluable to our patients, their families, and society.

REFERENCES

Alderman, N., & Burgess, P.W. (1990). Integrating cognition and behaviour: A pragmatic approach to brain injury rehabilitation. In R.L. Wood & I. Fussey (Eds.), *Cognitive rehabilitation in perspective*. Basingstoke: Taylor Francis Ltd.

Alderman, N., & Ward, A. (1991). Behavioural treatment of the dysexecutive syndrome: reduction of repetitive speech using response cost and cognitive overlearning. *Neuropsychological Rehabilitation, 1*, 65–80.

Alderman, N., Fry, R.K., & Youngson, H.A. (1995). Improvement of self-monitoring skills, reduction of behaviour disturbance and the dysexecutive syndrome: Comparison of response cost and a new programme of self-monitoring training. *Neuropsychological Rehabilitation, 5*, 193–221.

Anderson, S.W., Damasio, H., & Jones, R.D. (1991). Wisconsin Card Sorting Test performance as a measure of frontal lobe pathology. *Journal of Clinical and Experimental Neuropsychology, 13*, 909–922.

Baddeley, A., & Wilson, B. (1988). Frontal amnesia and the dysexecutive syndrome. *Brain and Cognition, 7*, 23–30.

Ben-Yishay, Y., Piasetsky, E.B., & Rattock, J. (1987). A systematic method for ameliorating disorders in basic attention. In M.J. Meyer, A.L. Benton, & L. Diller (Eds.), *Neuropsychological rehabilitation*. Edinburgh: Churchill Livingstone.

Boyd, T., & Sautter, S.W. (in press). Route finding: A measure of everyday executive function in the head-injured adult. *Applied Cognitive Psychology*.

Burke, W.H., Zenicus, A.H., Wesolowski, M.D., & Doubleday, F. (1991). Improving executive function disorders in brain-injured clients. *Brain Injury, 5*, 25–28.

Cicerone, K.D., & Giacino, J.T. (1992). Remediation of executive function deficits after traumatic brain injury. *Neuropsychological Rehabilitation, 2*, 12–22.

Cicerone, K.D., & Wood, J.C. (1987). Planning disorder after closed head injury: A case study. *Archives of Physical Medicine and Rehabilitation, 68*, 111–115.

Craine, S.F. (1982). The retraining of frontal lobe dysfunction. In L.E. Trexler (Ed.), *Cognitive rehabilitation: Conceptualization and intervention*. New York: Plenum.

Crossen, B., Barco, P.P., & Velozo, C.A. (1989). Awareness and compensation in post-acute head injury rehabilitation. *Journal of Head Trauma Rehabilitation, 23*, 46–54.

Di Pelligrino, G., & Wise, S.P. (1991). A neurophysiological comparison of three distinct regions of the primate frontal-lobe. *Brain, 114*, 951–978.

Dywan, J., & Segalowitz, J. (1996). Self and family ratings of adaptive behavior after traumatic brain injury: Psychometric scores and frontally generated ERPs. *Journal of Head Trauma Rehabilitation, 11*, 79–95.

Dywan, J., Roden, R., & Murphy, T. (1995). Orbiotofrontal symptoms are predicted by mild head injury among normal adolescents. Paper presented at the International Neuropsychological Society, Seattle, Washington.

Fuster, J.M. (1990). Prefrontal cortex and the bridging of temporal gaps in the perception-action cycle. *Annals of the New York Academy of Sciences, 608*, 318–336.

Geyer, S. (1989). *Training executive function skills*. Puyallup, WA: Good Samaritan Hospital.

Giles, G.G., & Clarke-Wilson, J. (1988). The use of behavioral techniques in functional skills training after severe brain injury. *American Journal of Occupational Therapy, 42*, 658–665.

Glosser, G., & Goodglass, H. (1990). Disorders in executive control functions among aphasic and other brain-damaged patients. *Journal of Clinical and Experimental Neuropsychology, 12*, 485–501.

Gray, J.M., Robertson, I., Pentland, B., & Anderson, S. (1992). Microcomputer-based attentional retraining after brain damage: A randomised group controlled trial. *Neuropsychological Rehabilitation, 2*, 97–115.

Heaton, R.K. (1981). *Wisconsin Card Sorting Test Manual*. Odessa, FL: Psychological Assessment Resources.

Janowsky, J.S., Shimamura, A.P., & Squire, L.R. (1989). Memory and metamemory: Comparisons between patients with frontal lobe lesions and amnesic patients. *Psychobiology, 17*, 3–11.

Janowsky, J.S., Shimamura, A.P., Kritchevsky, M., & Squire, L.R. (1989). Cognitive impairment following frontal lobe damage and its relevance to human amnesia. *Behavioral Neuroscience, 103,* 548–560.

Kewman, D.G., Seigerman, C., Kinter, H., Chu, S., Henson, D., & Reeder, C. (1985). Stimulation and training of psychomotor skills: teaching the brain-injured to drive. *Rehabilitation Psychology, 30,* 11–27.

Lezak, M. (1978). Living with the characterilogically altered brain damaged patient. *Journal of Clinical Psychology, 39,* 592–598.

———. (1982). The problem of assessing executive functions. *International Journal of Psychology, 17,* 281–297.

———. (1987). Relationships between personality disorders, social disturbances, and physical disability following traumatic brain injury. *Journal of Head Trauma Rehabilitation, 2,* 57–69.

———. (1993). Newer contributions to the neuropsychological assessment of executive functions. *Journal of Head Trauma Rehabilitation, 8,* 24–31.

Luria, A.R. (1980). *Higher cortical functions in man.* New York: Basic Books.

Mateer, C.A. (1992). Systems of care for post-concussive syndrome. In L. J. Horn & N. D. Zasler (Eds.), *Rehabilitation of post-concussive disorders.* Philadelphia: Henley & Belfus.

Mateer, C.A., & Mapou, R. (1996). Understanding, evaluating and managing attentional disorders following traumatic brain injury. *Journal of Head Trauma Rehabilitation, 11,* 1–16.

Mateer, C.A., & Sohlberg, M.M. (1988). A paradigm shift in memory rehabilitation. In H. Whitaker (Ed.), *Neuropsychological studies of nonfocal brain injury: Dementia and closed head injury.* New York: Springer-Verlag.

Mateer, C.A., Sohlberg, M.M., & Youngman, P. (1990). The management of acquired attentional and memory disorders following mild closed head injury. In R. Wood (Ed.), *Cognitive rehabilitation in perspective.* London: Taylor and Francis.

Milner, B., Petrides, M., & Smith, M. (1985). Frontal lobes and the temporal organization of memory. *Human Neurobiology, 4,* 137–142.

Niemann, H., Ruff, R.M., & Baser, C.A. (1990). Computer assisted attention training in head injured individuals: A controlled efficacy study of an outpatient program. *Journal of Clinical and Consulting Psychology, 58,* 811–817.

Prigatano, G.P. (1991). Disturbances of self-awareness of deficit after traumatic brain injury. In G.P. Prigatano & D.L. Schacter (Eds.), *Awareness of deficit after brain injury: Clinical and theoretical perspectives.* New York: Oxford University Press.

———. (1992). Personality disturbances associated with traumatic brain injury. *Journal of Consulting and Clinical Psychology, 60,* 360–368.

Prigatano, G.P., Altman, I.M., & O'Brien, K.P. (1990). Behavioral limitations traumatic brain injured patients tend to underestimate. *Clinical Neuropsychologist, 4,* 163–176.

Robertson, I.H., Ward, T., Ridgeway, V., & Nimmo-Smith, I. (1994). *The Test of Everyday Attention.* Flempton, Bury St. Edmunds, Suffolk: Thames Valley Test Company.

Schacter, D.L. (1987). Memory, amnesia and frontal lobe dysfunction. *Psychobiology, 15,* 2–36.

Shallice, T. (1982). Specific impairments of planning. *Philosophical Trans Royal Society of London, 298,* 199–209.

Shallice, T., & Burgess, P.W. (1991a). Higher-order cognitive impairments and frontal-lobe lesions in man. In H. Levin, H.M. Eisenberg, & A.L. Benton (Eds.), *Frontal lobe function and injury.* Oxford: Oxford University Press.

———. (1991b). Deficits in strategy application following frontal lobe damage in man. *Brain, 114,* 727–741.

Sohlberg, M.M. (1992). *Manual for the profile of executive control system.* Puyallup, WA: AFNRD.

Sohlberg, M.M., & Mateer, C.A. (1987). Effectiveness of an attention training program. *Journal of Clinical and Experimental Neuropsychology, 19,* 117–130.

———. (1989a). *Prospective memory screening.* Puyallup, WA: AFNRD.

———. (1989b). *Introduction to cognitive rehabilitation: Theory and practice.* New York: Guilford Press.

————. (1989c). Training use of compensatory memory books: A three stage behavioral approach. *Journal of Clinical and Experimental Neuropsychology, 11*, 871–891.

Sohlberg, M.M., Mateer, C.A., & Stuss, D.T. (1993). Contemporary approaches to the management of executive control dysfunction. *Journal of Head Trauma Rehabilitation, 8*, 45–58.

Sohlberg, M.M., Sprunk, H., & Metzelaar, K. (1988). Efficacy of an external cuing system in an individual with severe frontal lobe damage. *Cognitive Rehabilitation, 4*, 36–40.

Sohlberg, M.M., White, O., Evans, E., & Mateer, C.A. (1992a). Background and initial case studies into the effects of prospective memory training. *Brain Injury, 5*, 129–138.

————. (1992b). An investigation of the effects of prospective memory training. *Brain Injury, 5*, 139–154.

Stablum, F., Leonardi, G., Mazzoldi, M., Unilta, C., & Morra, S. (1994). Attention and control deficits following closed head injury. *Cortex, 30*, 603–618.

Stuss, D.T. (1991). Self, awareness and the frontal lobes: A neuropsychological perspective. In G.R. Goethals & J. Struss (Eds.), *The self: An interdisciplinary approach*. New York: Springer-Verlag.

Stuss, D.T., & Benson, D.F. (1986). *The frontal lobes*. New York: Raven Press.

Stuss, D.T., Delgado, M., & Guzman, D.A. (1987). Verbal regulation in the control of motor impersistence. *Journal of Neurological Rehabilitation, 1*, 19–24.

Stuss, D.T., Ely, P., & Hugenholtz, H. (1985). Subtle neuropsychological deficits in patients with good recovery after closed head injury. *Neurosurgery, 17*, 41–47.

Stuss, D.T., Stethem, L.L., Hugenholtz, H., Picton, T., Pivik, J., & Richard, M.T. (1989). Reaction time after head injury: Fatigue, divided and focused attention, and consistency of performance. *Journal of Neurology, Neurosurgery, and Psychiatry, 52*, 742–748.

van Zomeren, A.H., & Brauwer, W.H. (1987). Head injury and concepts of attention. In H. J. Levin, J. Grafman, & H.M. Eisenberg (Eds.), *Neurobehavioral recovery from head injury*. New York: Oxford University Press.

————. (1994). *Clinical neuropsychology of attention*. New York: Oxford University Press.

von Cramon, D.Y., Matthes-von Cramon, G., & Mai, N. (1991). Problem solving deficits in brain injured patients: A therapeutic approach. *Neuropsychological Rehabilitation, 1*, 45–64.

Wilson, B.A., Cockburn, J., & Halligan, P. (1985). *The Rivermead Everyday Memory Test*. Flempton, Bury St. Edmunds, Suffolk: Thames Valley Test Company.

16 The Problem of Impaired Self-Awareness in Neuropsychological Rehabilitation

George P. Prigatano

Barrow Neurological Institute
St. Joseph's Hospital and Medical Center
Phoenix, AZ

INTRODUCTION

The highest of all integrative brain functions may be our ability to consciously process information about ourselves in a manner that reflects a relatively objective view while maintaining our unique phenomenological or subjective sense of self. Damage to the heteromodal regions of the human brain seems to negatively influence the capacity for self-awareness, albeit in different ways (Prigatano, 1991a). After severe traumatic brain injury (TBI) in which there often is bilateral but asymmetrical injuries to frontal/temporal structures in the presence of diffuse axonal injury (DAI) (Zimmerman & Bilaniuk, 1989), disturbances of self-awareness are common (Prigatano, Altman, & O'Brien, 1990; Prigatano & Altman, 1990; Prigatano, 1991b; Crossen, Barco, Velozo, Bolesta, Cooper, Werts, & Brobeck, 1989; Godfrey, Partridge, Knight, & Bishara, 1993; Prigatano & Leathem, 1993; Prigatano, in press). Attempts to rehabilitate these individuals suggest that this particular impairment represents a major barrier to successful rehabilitation (Prigatano et al., 1984, 1994; Prigatano et al., 1986; Ben-Yishay & Prigatano, 1990; Rattok et al., 1992). This chapter reviews research on the problem of impaired self-awareness after brain injury and discusses an approach to dealing with this problem within the context of neuropsychological rehabilitation.

IMPAIRED SELF-AWARENESS AFTER BRAIN INJURY: A NEGATIVE SYMPTOM

In 1955, Weinstein and Kahn summarized the earlier literature on anosognosia after brain injury and in so doing, attempted to distinguish it from what might broadly be called

---

denial of illness. Weinstein and Kahn's (1955) conception has often been misunderstood. Researchers have tended to interpret Weinstein's statement that premorbid personality factors contribute to denial phenomenon as a statement that disturbed self-awareness after brain injury primarily is motivated by some form of psychological defense. Weinstein (see Prigatano & Weinstein, in press) has been explicit in stating that a patient's behavior after brain injury is related to a number of factors, including the following: (1) the type, severity, rate of onset, location, and extent of brain injury pathology; (2) the nature of the disability; (3) the meaning of the incapacity as determined by the patient's premorbid experience and values; and (4) the milieu in which the behavior is elicited and observed.

Within the context of this model, brain injury can affect behavior in a direct and indirect manner. Injuries to the brain produce what John Hughlings Jackson called a *negative symptom* and what Goldstein later called a *direct symptom* (Goldstein, 1942). A negative symptom represents a true loss of function and an absence of information about the nature of that lost function.

Thus, patients may have a complete left-sided hemiplegia and report no disturbance whatsoever in motor functioning. They also can be cortically blind and state that their vision is "fine" but that the room is dark (see Bisiach & Geminiani, 1991). In these dramatic cases, the damage to the brain seems to deprive the individual of true knowledge that they have been affected. As time progresses, the patient's knowledge of their impairment may improve but not always. In the latter case, the term *anosognosia* or impaired self-awareness is appropriate.

Prigatano and Schacter (1991) have summarized historical and contemporary concepts concerning impaired self-awareness or anosognosia. They suggest that different levels or forms of impaired awareness can exist depending on the brain regions (systems) that have been rendered dysfunctional. When there is bilateral and extensive frontal lobe damage, it is not uncommon for the individual to demonstrate impaired insight about their socially inappropriate behaviors, as well as changes in their ability to plan, initiate, or execute a series of higher-order cognitive tasks. In contrast, lesions in the parietal area may adversely affect an individual's ability to consciously perceive disturbances in spatial perception or in visuomotor impairments. They may be unaware, for example, of a dressing dyspraxia. Case reports of patients who have focal lesions in the right frontal area versus those with lesions in the right parietal occipital areas tend to support this view (Prigatano & O'Brien, 1991).

Literature also suggests that lesions in the left temporal area may disturb not only language function but the patient's capacity to consciously perceive a disturbance in language function when it is present. Lebrun (1987), for example, has reported an aphasic patient who, once recovered from his TBI, was totally surprised to find that he had been paraphasic during the early phases of recovery. This type of phenomenon is seen repeatedly in the context of neuropsychological rehabilitation. These are classic neurobehavioral disturbances that reflect patients' lack of insight into their disability. This lack of insight seems directly related to destroyed brain tissue and can be considered a "negative symptom."

DENIAL OF DISABILITY AFTER BRAIN INJURY: A POSITIVE SYMPTOM

Associated with this former class of neurobehavioral disorders are disturbances in which individuals have *partial* knowledge of their disabilities or impairments. Here, the individual may report, for example, having a memory impairment but be unable to describe adequately the extent of the memory impairment or its psychosocial impact. For example, Logue, Durward, Pratt, Piercy, and Nixon (1968), in studying the quality of life of patients who had a ruptured anterior cerebral or anterior communicating artery aneurysm, asked patients and their relatives about changes in memory and intellectual functioning. While reports of memory impairments were common, the patients often had "poor insight" about the degree of memory impairment. This observation has been reported several times with TBI patients with frontal lobe pathology (Oddy et al., 1985; Prigatano et al., 1986; Prigatano, 1991a).

In this case, the individual appears to attempt to cope with this partial information and to "make sense" of his/her environment or social situation. Premorbid methods of coping may well influence a patient's "denial" of a difficult situation. In such instances, one would expect that cultural factors could indeed influence denial phenomenon. For example, northern Italians show less "denial of illness" than Swiss brain dysfunctional patients (Gainotti, 1975), and TBI patients of Maori ancestry report more disability than New Zealanders of English ancestry (Prigatano & Leathem, 1993). In both cases, there was clear evidence of brain dysfunction. However, how patients describe their dysfunction can and should be considered apart from the dysfunction itself. With this distinction in mind, it may be helpful to reexamine the problem of impaired self-awareness from the perspective of it representing either a positive or negative symptom. True impaired self-awareness is a negative symptom, and denial of disability is a positive symptom. In both cases, there is brain injury underlying the impaired awareness, but, in one case, there is a complete or almost complete lack of information, and, in the latter case, there is partial information.

If this dichotomy is useful, methods potentially can be developed to separate patients who show primarily impaired self-awareness versus those exhibiting denial of disability. Patients showing behavioral signs of greater bilateral and diffuse brain dysfunction affecting particularly the heteromodal cortex should show greater impaired self-awareness compared to individuals showing denial of disability phenomenon. One behavioral marker of this type of cerebral dysfunction is the speed of finger tapping. Weiller, Ramsay, Wise, Friston, and Frackowiak (1993) have shown that after an infarction in the internal capsule, patients who are able to normally tap their fingers to the pace of a metronome show bilateral activation of the two cerebral hemispheres during execution of the task. Areas that show notably increased metabolic activity typically include the frontal and parietal regions bilaterally. Based on this information, it was predicated that patients with impaired self-awareness versus denial of disability will exhibit slower finger tapping. In fact, patients with impaired self-awareness after brain injury more often tap with one or both hands at ≤ 35 taps/10 sec. using the Halstead Finger Tapping Test. Patients who were judged as free of any brain dysfunction but who tended to overestimate possible neuropsychological impairment (i.e., underestimating neuropsychological abilities) did not show this pattern (Prigatano & Klonoff, 1995). Although the data are tentative, they suggest that there are testable hypotheses concerning the potential separation of impaired self-awareness from denial of disability after brain injury.

THE PROBLEM OF RESISTANCE IN NEUROPSYCHOLOGICAL REHABILITATION

In his article on the effects of brain damage on personality, Goldstein (1952) clearly documented that impairment in the abstract attitude could compromise patients' ability to understand how they have been affected as well as their ability to function in the real world. He also pointed out that when patients emerge from coma, they often display an irritability, at least in the early stages. When one attempts to help a patient become more consciously aware of disturbances after brain injury, even in the post-acute phase, some form of resistance often is encountered.

Therapists should not view this resistance as reflecting an uncooperative attitude on the part of the patient. Rather, this resistance is often a normal consequence of disturbed higher cerebral functioning in which there is incomplete awareness of such disturbances. If the therapist can enter the patient's phenomenological field and experience some of what the patient is experiencing, this resistance can diminish (Prigatano et al., 1986; Prigatano, 1992, 1994, 1995). The importance of entering the patient's phenomenological field as a way of reducing the natural frustration/confusion the patient experiences has been described elsewhere (Prigatano, 1995). Often when the therapist understands what is frustrating the patient and can take steps to reduce the cognitive "confusion" of the patient, a therapeutic alliance is established. The quality of the "therapeutic alliance" directly relates to the outcome (Prigatano et al., 1994). Patients who establish a good therapeutic or working alliance with the therapist during rehabilitation tend to become productive. The same finding also applies to the quality of the therapeutic alliance with the patient's family. Having a good working alliance with the patient's family is associated with the productivity of brain dysfunctional patients after rehabilitation.

It is beyond the scope of this chapter to discuss psychotherapeutic efforts aimed at reducing resistance, but this issue is a very important part of neuropsychologically oriented rehabilitation (Prigatano, 1991, 1994). A brief discussion of the components of neuropsychologically oriented rehabilitation and how the establishment of a therapeutic milieu helps foster greater insight or awareness during the rehabilitation process is presented below.

COMPONENTS OF NEUROPSYCHOLOGICAL REHABILITATION

Table 16.1 illustrates a typical weekly program for patients in neuropsychological rehabilitation. The goal is to return patients to work or at least to a productive lifestyle after brain injury.

Table 16.1: Typical Weekly Work Re-entry Program*

	Monday	Tuesday	Wednesday	Thursday	Friday
8:15–8:55	Cognitive retraining	Cognitive retraining	Cognitive retraining	Cognitive retraining	Work trial
9:00–9:40	Individual therapies	Individual therapies	Individual therapies	Individual therapies	
9:40–9:50	Break	Break	Break	Break	
9:50–10:25	Individual/group	Individual/group	Individual/group	Individual/group	
10:30–11:10	Cognitive group	Cognitive group	Cognitive group	Cognitive group	
11:15–11:45	Group psychotherapy	Group psychotherapy	Group psychotherapy	Group psychotherapy	
11:45–12:00	Milieu	Milieu	Milieu	Milieu	
12:00–1:00	Lunch	Lunch	Lunch	Lunch	
1:00–5:00	Work trial	Work trial	Work trial	Work trial	Work trial (opt)
1:45–2:45		Relatives' group			
3:30–4:30	Staff meeting	Staff meeting	Staff meeting	Staff meeting	
5:00–6:00		Relatives' group			

*From Prigatano (1988). Reprinted with permission of the Barrow Neurological Institute.

Although this program has been modified over the years, Table 16.1 depicts the basic treatment activities and when they are incorporated during a rehabilitation day. During the first week of the work trial, patients will work 2 hrs./day, then move to 3–4 hrs. in the second week, if they can handle it. By the third week, the goal is to have the patients working 3–4 hrs., 4 days/wk., depending on the needs of the work supervisor and patient. Generally, months 3–6 are designated for less supervised activities.

Neuropsychological rehabilitation consists of five basic ingredients: cognitive remediation, psychotherapy, the establishment of a therapeutic milieu, the placement of patients in a productive work-trial, and the active involvement of the patient's family in the rehabilitative process (Prigatano et al., 1986, 1994; Prigatano, 1995).

In the context of this model, patients' cognitive deficits, as well as their emotional and motivational disturbances, are addressed in both individual and small-group therapies. Most importantly, however, these activities occur in the context of a therapeutic milieu. A therapeutic milieu is an environment specifically designed to anticipate patients' cognitive problems and to help them learn how brain injury has influenced their abilities. This goal is accomplished, of course, in the context of a supportive environment but one that is based on reality. The establishment of a therapeutic milieu is not easy and requires both administrative support from a hospital as well as a sophisticated and frankly psychologically mature rehabilitation staff (see Prigatano, 1989a, 1990).

The first component of a neuropsychological oriented rehabilitation is the establishment of a therapeutic milieu. The purpose of this milieu is to provide a treatment environment that, by its very nature, fosters a therapeutic impact on patients. After brain injury, patients are often frustrated and confused. The cognitively oriented therapies must attempt to reduce this confusion and help patients with their frustrations. Therapists should literally ask patients what most frustrates them after their brain injury and try to develop cognitive retraining activities (as well as other therapeutic activities) that reduce the confusion. Working on simple cognitive tasks that help patients begin to monitor their performance aids in developing this awareness (Klonoff, O'Brien, Prigatano, Chiapello, Cunningham, & Shepherd, 1989). Patients are asked to record their responses to the various tasks and to observe how they improve or fail to improve over time.

Cognitive retraining activities should include tasks with both an arousal and orientation component. The treatment day begins with these tasks to help patients increase their arousal/attention level. The therapies also help orient them to what they are doing and why they are doing it. Frequently, patients will perform a series of tasks with a speed-of-information-processing component. They are asked to monitor their performance on various tasks, which include scoring and plotting a learning curve. In this manner, patients can see how they progress with time.

Patients also are helped to recognize that there is a point beyond which they will not improve even with extensive practice. This information gives them an opportunity to learn about their strengths and limitations. Within the context of this work, patients observe how the therapists perform various cognitive tasks. If therapists are not too threatened by revealing their own cognitive strengths and weaknesses, such mirroring gives patients a more realistic view of what normal performance is. Collectively, various cognitive experiences are aimed at helping patients progressively have a more realistic view of themselves and their relationship to others (Prigatano et al., 1986).

Thus, the initial focus of cognitive retraining is to engage patients in rehabilitation and improve their self-awareness of their impairments and disabilities (Figure 16.1) (see Ben-Yishay & Prigatano, 1990; Prigatano, 1995).

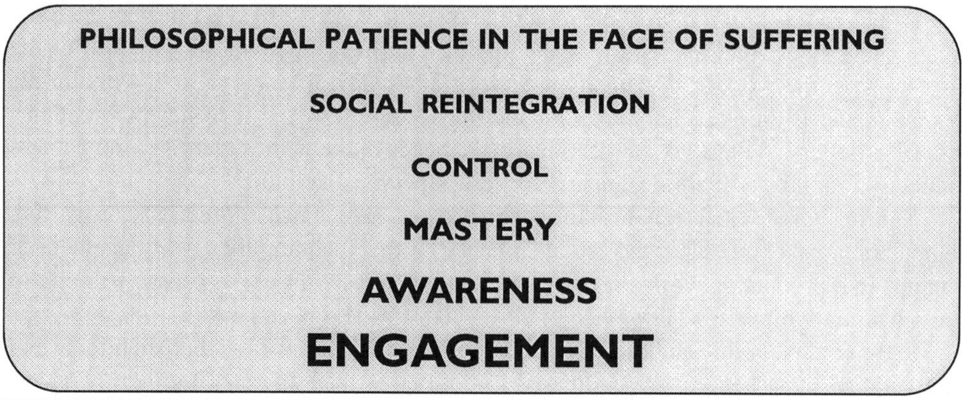

PHILOSOPHICAL PATIENCE IN THE FACE OF SUFFERING

SOCIAL REINTEGRATION

CONTROL

MASTERY

AWARENESS

ENGAGEMENT

Figure 16.1: Global components of neuropsychologically oriented rehabilitation (adapted with permission from Ben-Yishay & Prigatan, 1990. Cognitive remediation. Published in this adapted form in Prigatano, 1995).

Since cognitive rehabilitation inevitably produces an affective reaction (Prigatano, 1987), it is extremely important that some form of psychotherapeutic intervention be available to patients during the course of neuropsychologically oriented rehabilitation. The emphasis is on "availability." Not all patients should automatically be seen in psychotherapeutic consultation. The purpose of psychotherapeutic consultation is two-fold. First, it may help patients engage the rehabilitation activities if they are having problems in the engagement process (Prigatano, 1989b, 1991b, 1994). Second, it may help patients deal with emotions that are disruptive to adjusting to the effects of brain injury. If patients are adequately engaging the rehabilitation process and show no disruptive emotional reactions in their adjustment to their injury, psychotherapy is not needed. Forcing patients into psychotherapy is a major mistake in some settings that advocate psychotherapy for brain-injured individuals. Clinicians may be too eager to begin the process of psychotherapy when, in fact, it is unnecessary.

It is beyond the scope of this chapter to discuss what psychotherapy is and how it should be applied after brain injury, but this topic has been considered in detail elsewhere (Prigatano et al., 1986; Prigatano, 1991, 1994, 1995). Typically, psychotherapy is the process by which individuals begin to understand their own emotional and motivational reactions and, in so doing, avoid actions that can further complicate their adjustment after brain injury. This process can be done in both individual and group formats. Because brain dysfunctional patients often lack many verbal skills and have difficulties remembering what was said or done, nonlinguistic methods for coping with their affective reactions can be useful. Sometimes spontaneous drawings of the patients or various art forms (including choosing their favorite music) can help the therapist and patients better understand the patient's personality disturbances (Prigatano, 1991).

In addition to cognitive retraining and psychotherapy, which is done in the context of a milieu environment, active involvement of patients in some form of productive work is important. This has long been recognized as important for the goals of rehabilitation (Goldstein, 1942). Individuals need a sense of productivity to feel a sense of mastery over their life (Figure 16.1). These two components, mastery and control, are extremely important to the rehabilitation process and should not be forgotten. In fact, the whole focus of trying to develop a rehabilitation program that engages patients is precisely to foster self-awareness so individuals can achieve a more realistic view of what they can and cannot do. As they achieve some sense of mastery in life, they have more control over what happens to them. With mastery and control comes greater capacity, or potential, for social reintegration. Here, the work-trial experience allows patients to see how they can integrate with others.

Ingredients of the work trial are complex. The basic goal is to place the individual in a protected work environment so that he/she has an opportunity to perform some job responsibilities and get feedback about his/her performance. The term *protected* is used because sometimes individuals demonstrate behavioral or cognitive deficits that might normally result in their dismissal. By having a therapist work closely with patients in the work environment, the therapist attempts to provide the needed support so that the patient can carry out responsibilities without being terminated.

In the context of a protected work trial, patients' behavior concerning their ability to meet various responsibilities at work is monitored, and feedback is given to patients. In this way, patients receive a true sense of how they are doing in relationship to others at work.

Finally, work with the patient's family is crucial. Families will either support or not support the rehabilitation activities suggested to a patient. Also, patients have to interact with family members as well as with others. Without this help, social isolation is common after a severe TBI (Kozloff, 1987). Work with families can be difficult. Family members are often upset and emotionally overwhelmed by the consequences of a brain injury in a loved one. Yet, if these family members are worked with consistently to develop a realistic understanding of how the patient has been affected, they can begin to cope with the patient's cognitive and behavioral problems in a more reasonable way. They can follow the guidelines that have been established within the context of a neuropsychologically oriented rehabilitation program.

As this process unfolds, both the patient and family are faced with the hard realities of the aftermath of the brain injury. This process of facing the problem of lost normality and developing philosophical patience in the presence of suffering is described in Figure 16.1. The latter phase is borrowed from the work of Carl Jung, who emphasized that the goal of psychotherapy was precisely the development of philosophical patience (see Prigatano, 1991, 1994). Psychotherapy does not eliminate the sadness or frustrations of life; rather, it helps individuals cope with these problems in a more reasonable way. The focus of neuropsychologically oriented rehabilitation (which includes psychotherapeutic interventions) is to help in this regard.

Against this background, one can ask a legitimate question: "What is the evidence that such a form of rehabilitation makes a difference for brain dysfunctional patients?"

THE EFFECTIVENESS OF NEUROPSYCHOLOGICALLY ORIENTED REHABILITATION

A few studies that appeared between 1984 and 1994 documented the usefulness of neuropsychologically oriented rehabilitation and also attempted to identify the key variables that relate to a successful outcome. Typically, a successful outcome is defined as return to a productive lifestyle and often includes gainful employment. Prigatano et al. (1984) showed that 50% of TBI patients involved in a neuropsychologically oriented rehabilitation program returned to gainful employment after their rehabilitation. These patients were 1–2 years post-TBI and failed to establish adequate psychosocial adjustment on their own and after various forms of inpatient and outpatient rehabilitation. In that study, however, 36% of the control patients were able to work without receiving such rehabilitative efforts. The establishment of a protected work-trial as a part of this form of rehabilitation seemed to increase the number of individuals who were productive. Interestingly, it seemed to affect the number of individuals who were able to maintain voluntary work as opposed to gainful employment (Prigatano et al., 1994).

Ben-Yishay, Rattok, Lakin, Piasetsky, Ross, Silver, Zide, and Ezrachi (1985) also reported that 50% of patients undergoing neuropsychological rehabilitation were able to return to gainful employment. Unfortunately, no control group was used in this study. In an extended study by Prigatano et al. (1986), similar percentages for returning to work were recorded for TBI patients and other brain dysfunctional individuals. The neuropsychological and behavioral problems that separated those who returned to work compared to those who did not were documented. Memory and speed-of-information-processing deficits were more severe in those who did not return to work. Impaired self-awareness was identified as a major deterrent for returning to a productive lifestyle.

Ben-Yishay and Prigatano (1990) summarized the major ingredients of cognitive rehabilitation and the work that Ben-Yishay and other colleagues have done in predicting return to a productive lifestyle after brain injury. Severity of coma (for the patients that they treated) accounted for less than 10% of the variance. Neuropsychological deficits such as verbal abstract reasoning skills and visuospatial problem-solving skills accounted for another 12% of the variance. The most powerful combination of variables that predicted outcome (about 46%) centered on patients' ability to control their emotional reaction and to interact with others in a socially appropriate manner. It also included the patients' capacity to demonstrate good awareness/acceptance of their disabilities.

Follow-up work by Rattok et al. (1992) further clarified these earlier observations. Patients who had received rehabilitation that emphasized small-group interaction compared to purely cognitive retraining showed better interpersonal adjustment and greater appreciation of their deficits. These individuals also exhibited greater self-control over their affective responses. Data by Christensen, Pinner, Pedersen, Teasdale, and Trexler (1991) further cross-validated the usefulness of the methods described by Ben-Yishay et al. (1985) and Prigatano et al. (1984) using a European sample.

Finally, a recent controlled study (Prigatano et al., 1994) again showed that neuropsychologically oriented rehabilitation was effective: 48% of patients returned to gainful employment, and an additional 25% obtained and maintained meaningful voluntary work. This finding is an important contribution, because patients with severe TBI often are precluded from being competitively employed. In our culture, productivity is a major symbol that provides meaning for both brain-injured and nonbrain-injured individuals (Prigatano, 1989; Prigatano, 1991).

IMPROVING AWARENESS AND DEPRESSION AFTER BRAIN INJURY

In the course of working with different types of brain dysfunctional patients, some of these individuals eventually become depressed. The argument is often made that as patients recognize or develop better insight into their impairments and disabilities, depression naturally occurs. Certainly, depression can occur after any major loss. Also, denial as a psychological defense is common with major losses (Prigatano, 1995).

However, one should be cautious about the idea that increased awareness after brain injury automatically leads to depression. This author's experience has been different.

Patients who show true impaired self-awareness (i.e., a loss of information about the self) are often perplexed about why they are behaving the way they do. They may lose friends or jobs and, as a consequence of those losses, become depressed, but they may not link their own impairments to their losses. As true self-awareness is enhanced, patients' perplexity often is reduced, and they are able to "see something" that they had not recognized before. This increased self-knowledge does not automatically lead to depression. In fact, it gives some patients a better appreciation of the problems they face, and, with that knowledge, they may feel better prepared to cope with life's difficulties. The literature on anosognosia after a cerebrovascular accident (CVA) suggests that anosognostic patients are no more or no less depressed than CVA patients who do not demonstrate anosognosia (Starkstein, Fedoroff, Price, Leiguarda, & Robinson, 1992).

Patients who exhibit denial of disability may become depressed as their previous methods of coping fail them. In this instance, they are attempting to deal with partial information about themselves using old coping skills. As they can no longer effectively apply their coping (and defensive) maneuvers, they may lose hope and move from normal sadness about a loss to true depression. This dichotomy has not been considered when attempting to explain why some TBI patients report greater depression with the passage of time after TBI (Godfrey, Partridge, Knight, & Bishara, 1993).

As the problem of impaired self-awareness versus denial of disability is better understood and dealt with, perhaps better methods of neuropsychological rehabilitation will be developed.

SUMMARY AND CONCLUSIONS

This chapter has attempted to highlight the problem of impaired self-awareness after brain injury as a legitimate neuropsychological disturbance and one that is not primarily psychiatrically mediated. It is extremely important to understand the problems of self-awareness and denial of disability. Perhaps methods that attempt to study these phenomena as negative and positive symptoms after brain injury will ultimately prove useful in this form of care.

This chapter also outlined the problems of frustration and cognitive confusion after brain injury and how they might be approached within the context of a neuropsychologically oriented rehabilitation program aimed at returning patients to work. The empirical evidence supporting this form of rehabilitation was summarized.

It is hoped that this chapter will allow clinicians to better recognize problems of impaired insight after brain injury and what a key role they play in neuropsychologically oriented rehabilitation. As strange as it may be, when the brain is injured, it does not always recognize that fact. The ability to help patients see how their brain has been injured and to guide them in the process of coping with disorders of higher cerebral functions becomes an extremely important and useful goal of neuropsychologically oriented rehabilitation.

REFERENCES

Ben-Yishay, Y., & Prigatano, G.P. (1990). Cognitive remediation. In M. Rosenthal, E.R. Griffith, M.R. Bond, & J.D. Miller (Eds.), *Rehabilitation of the adult and child with traumatic brain injury* (pp. 393–409). Philadelphia: F.A. Davis Company.

Ben-Yishay, Y., Rattok, J., Lakin, P., Piasetsky, E.D., Ross, B., Silver, S., Zide, E., & Ezrachi, O. (1985). Neuropsychological rehabilitation: Quest for a holistic approach. *Seminars. Neurol., 5,* 252–258.

Bisiach, E., & Geminiani, G. (1991). Anosognosia related to hemiplegia and hemianopia. In G.P. Prigatano and D.L. Schacter (Eds.), *Awareness of deficit after brain injury: Clinical and theoretical issues* (pp. 17-39). New York: Oxford University Press.

Christensen, A.-L., Pinner, E.M., Moller Pedersen, P., Teasdale, T.W., & Trexler, L.E. (1991). Psychosocial outcome following individualized neuropsychological rehabilitation of brain damage. *Acta Neurol Scand., 85*, 32–38.

Crosson, B., Barco, P.P., Velozo, C.A., Bolesta, M.M., Cooper, P.V., Werts, D., & Brobeck, T.C. (1989). Awareness and compensation in post-acute head injury rehabilitation. *Journal of Head Trauma Rehabilitation, 4*, 45–54.

Gainotti, G. (1975). Confabulation of denial in senile dementia. *Psychiatry Clin., 8*, 99–108.

Godfrey, H.P.D., Partridge, F.M., Knight, R.G., & Bishara, S. (1993). Course of insight disorder and emotional dysfunction following closed head injury: A controlled cross-sectional follow-up study. *Journal of Clinical and Experimental Neuropsychology, 15*, 503–515.

Goldstein, K. (1942). *Aftereffects of brain injuries in war.* New York: Grune and Stratton.

———. (1952). The effect of brain damage on the personality. *Psychiatry, 15*, 245–260.

Klonoff, P.S., O'Brien, K.P., Prigatano, G.P., Chiapello, D.A., Cunningham, M., & Shepherd, J. (1989). Cognitive retraining after traumatic brain injury and its role in facilitating awareness. *Journal of Head Trauma Rehabilitation, 4*, 37–45.

Kozloff, R. (1987). Network of social support and the outcome from severe head injury. *Journal of Head Trauma Rehabilitation, 2*, 14–23.

Lebrun, Y. (1987). Anosognosia and aphasics. *Cortex, 23*, 251–263.

Logue, V., Durward, M., Pratt, R.T.C., Piercy, M., & Nixon, W.L.B. (1968). The quality of survival after rupture of an anterior cerebral aneurysm. *British Journal of Psychiatry, 114*, 137–160.

Oddy, M., Coughlan, T., Tyerman, A., & Jenkins, D. (1985). Social adjustment after closed head injury: A further follow-up seven years after injury. *Journal of Neurology, Neurosurgery, and Psychiatry, 48*, 264–268.

Prigatano, G.P. (1987). Recovery and cognitive retraining after craniocerebral trauma. *Journal of Learning Disability, 20*, 603–613.

———. (1989a). Bring it up in milieu: Toward effective traumatic brain injury rehabilitation interaction. *Rehabilitation Psychology, 34*, 135–144).

———. (1989b, September). Work, love, and play after brain injury. *Bulletin of the Menninger Clinic, 53*, 414–431.

———. (1990). Effective traumatic brain injury rehabilitation: Team/patient interaction. In E.D. Bigler (Ed.), *Traumatic brain injury* (pp. 297–311). Austin: Pro-ed.

———. (1991a). Disordered mind, wounded soul: The emerging role of psychotherapy in rehabilitation after brain injury. *Journal of Head Trauma Rehabilitation, 6*, 1–10.

———. (1991b). Disturbances of self-awareness of deficit after traumatic brain injury. In G.P. Prigatano & D.L. Schacter (Eds.), *Awareness of deficit after brain injury: Theoretical and clinical issues* (pp. 111–126). New York: Oxford University Press.

———. (1992). Neuropsychological rehabilitation and the problem of altered self-awareness. In V. von Steinbuchel, D.Y. von Cramon, & E. Poppel (Eds.), *Neuropsychological rehabilitation* (pp. 55–65). New York: Springer-Verlag.

———. (1994). Individuality, lesion location and psychotherapy after brain injury. In A.-L. Christensen & B. Uzzell (Eds.), *Brain injury and neuropsychological rehabilitation: International perspective* (pp. 173–199). Hillsdale: Lawrence Erlbaum Associates.

———. (1995). 1994 Sheldon Berrol, MD, Senior Lectureship: The problem of lost normality after brain injury. *Journal of Head Trauma Rehabilitation, 10*, 97–95.

———. (in press). Behavioral limitations TBI patients tend to underestimate: A replication and extension to patients with lateralized cerebral dysfunction. *The Clinical Neuropsychologist.*

Prigatano, G.P., & Altman, I.M. (1990). Impaired awareness of behavioral limitations after traumatic brain injury. *Archives of Physical Medicine and Rehabilitation, 71*, 1058–1064.

Prigatano, G.P., & Klonoff, P.S. (1995). *Impaired awareness and denial of disability: Negative and positive symptoms after brain injury.* Paper presented at the 10th Anniversary Meeting of the Section of Neuropsychology, Barrow Neurological Institute, Scottsdale, AZ, May 4–5.

Prigatano, G.P., & Leathem, J.M. (1993). Awareness of behavioral limitations after traumatic brain injury: A cross-cultural study of New Zealand Maoris and non-Maoris. *The Clinical Neuropsychologist, 7,* 123–135.

Prigatano, G.P., & O'Brien, K. (1991). Awareness of deficit in patients with frontal vs. parietal lesions: Two case reports. *BNI Quarterly, 7,* 17–23.

Prigatano, G.P., & Schacter, D.L. (Eds.). (1991). *Awareness of deficit after brain injury: Theoretical and clinical issues.* New York: Oxford University Press.

Prigatano, G.P., & Weinstein, E.A. (in press). Edwin A. Weinstein's contributions to neuropsychological rehabilitation. *Neuropsychological Rehabilitation.*

Prigatano, G.P., Altman, I.M., & O'Brien, K.P. (1990). Behavioral limitations that brain injured patients tend to underestimate. *The Clinical Neuropsychologist, 4,* 163–176.

Prigatano, G.P., Fordyce, D.J., Zeiner, H.K., Roueche, J.R., Pepping, M., & Wood, B. (1984). Neuropsychological rehabilitation after closed head injury in young adults. *Journal of Neurology, Neurosurgery, and Psychiatry, 47,* 505–513.

Prigatano, G.P., Klonoff, P.S., O'Brien, K.P., Altman, I.M., Amin, K., Chiapello, D., Shepherd, J., Cunningham, M., & Mora, M. (1994). Productivity after neuropsychologically oriented milieu rehabilitation. *Journal of Head Trauma Rehabilitation, 9,* 91–102.

Prigatano, G.P., et al. (1986). *Neuropsychological rehabilitation after brain injury.* Baltimore: The Johns Hopkins University Press.

Rattok, J., Ben-Yishay, Y., Ezrachi, O., Laking, P., Piasetsky, R., Ross, B., Silver, S., Vakil, E., Zide, E., & Diller, L. (1992). Outcome of different treatment mixes in a multidimensional neuropsychological rehabilitation program. *Neuropsychology, 6,* 395–415.

Starkstein, S.E., Fedoroff, J.P., Price, T.R., Leiguarada, R., & Robinson, R.G. (1992). Anosognosia in patients with cerebrovascular lesions: A study of causative factors. *Stroke, 23,* 1446–1453.

Weiller, C., Ramsay, S.C., Wise, R.J.S., Friston, K.J., & Frackowisk, R.S.J. (1993). Individual patterns of functional reorganization in the human cerebral cortex after capsular infarction. *Annals of Neurology, 33,* 181–189.

Weinstein, E.A., & Kahn, R.L. (1955). *Denial of illness.* Springfield: Charles C. Thomas Publishing Company.

Zimmerman, R.A., & Bilaniuk, L.T. (1989). CT and MRI: Diagnosis and evolution of head injury, stroke, and brain tumors. *Neuropsychology, 3,* 191–230.

17 Aphasia Rehabilitation

José L. Miralles

INTRODUCTION

It is possible to consider, generally speaking, that aphasia exists with a language disorder caused by cerebral damage. It is, therefore, a neurological and linguistic disorder. As language is a cognitive activity, aphasia must also be considered a neurocognitive disorder. Finally, and according to Benson (1993), as it is a function loss, a therapeutic point of view derives from it.

The need, then, of a variety of approachs to the problem which consider the complexity of a disorder of the symbolic activity, requires, from the beginning, a description of the special features of the aphasic disorder and a discussion of the different theoretical frameworks of interpretation.

Nevertheless, it is necessary to make some preliminary comments before starting the development of the contents of this chapter. Specific and particular strategies of intervention for each aphasic syndrome and symptom will not be explained here. This level of detail is beyond the scope of this book. The general approach is focused on the rehabilitation of oral language. The treatment of the disorders of written language is examined in other parts of this book.

Language disorders, independently of whether their manifestation also affects oral structure and linguistic organization, are basically of a cognitive nature. There has neither existed throughout history nor exists now a single paradigm to explain cognitive processes. Consequently, we will begin by developing the different interpretations of aphasias in accordance with historical criteria and continue with a semiological description of these aphasias.

THE APHASIA CONCEPT

Aphasia is understood as the loss of the use of a once acquired language due to localized damage (i.e., aphasic disorders are caused by an alteration in the symbolic code). Therefore, this does not include motor disorders produced by injury to neural structures not involved in language areas. Also excluded are those language disorders that are a consequence of general damage or of a degenerative process such as dementia.

The most frequent cause of aphasic disorders is a stroke that affects the middle brain artery of the left hemisphere. These disorders are also produced, to a lesser extent, by trauma and tumors. Affected in all these cases are the cerebral areas that directly participate in the language processes.

Since the treatment of a disorder should principally be derived from the conception of such a disorder and there exist different interpretations and models of both normal language and its deficiencies, reference to the theoretical framework of interpretation is needed.

NEUROLINGUISTIC MODELS

The Traditional Neurolinguistic Model: Theories of Localization and Association

Between 1830 and 1840, Gall and Spurzheim's phrenology, despite the heterodoxy it assumed within the medical sciences of the era, proposed that the qualities of human beings and their psychological or moral characteristics were located in precise regions of the brain. Broca's work appears within the realm of this viewpoint that is partly influenced by the last century's physiology. Broca, after a postmortem examination of a patient whose linguistic production was limited to extremely reduced and stereotyped oral expressions, laid the foundations of a neurolinguistic tradition based on anatomical locations of linguistic functions. This he did by relating the linguistic deficiencies of this patient to an injury in the third frontal circumvolution of the left hemisphere.

In accordance with Broca, these neuroanatomical structures should be considered as "the faculty of articulated speech," which is not a synonym for the faculty of general linguistic representation. Consequently, Broca names the deficiency associated with damage in this area as "aphemia," or the loss of the faculty of speech.

Continuing along the same lines initiated by Broca, Wernicke discovered other types of language disorders that fundamentally impair language comprehension without any apparent impairment to production. In these cases, the anatomical damage is found in the structures of the superior circumvolution of the temporal lobe. In 1874, in a paper entitled "The Complex Symptom of the Aphasia: A Psychological Study Based on Neurology," Wernicke gathers all the neuroanatomical knowledge elaborated until then and formulates what could be considered the first neurolinguistic model.

Wernicke identifies the existence of two significant centers intervening in language production and comprehension, respectively. The former corresponds to Broca's area, located in the third left frontal circumvolution, and the latter to Wernicke's temporal lobe area. Since oral production is preceded by a cognitive programming of the message to be formed in Wernicke's areas, a connecting path must be introduced in the model. This path guarantees an adequate transmission of information between Wernicke's and Broca's areas. This connection is made by the fasciculus arcuatus.

This model of location and connection is characterized by the association between linguistic functions and specific neuroanatomical structures. To each structure corresponds a function, and the different structures themselves are connected in a way that information elaborated in one is sent to the following center for further processing. The model is typified by Lichteim (1885) as a network of nodes and directional vectors. The nodes represent neural centers, and the vectors are equivalent to paths of connection. From this functional location, the model should efficiently predict the alterations caused by an injury in each element of the structure.

The following years in neurolinguistics witness what Caplan called "the diagram-makers generation." All the interest is centered around the anatomical locations of functions and the connections between them.

The Holistic Models

From the beginning, nonetheless, the locationist model has received severe criticism. Pierre Marie, in 1906, defended a holistic concept claiming that there is only one aphasia, namely the disintegration of the processes of language comprehension. Comprehension, Marie believed, becomes affected due to a deficiency in general intelligence. This deficiency is related to an injury at the rear of the brain in the region of temporal and parietal union.

A similarly holistic posture is also defended by Goldstein (1948), but, under the influence of Gestalt psychology, he carried the interpretation of the disorder into the domain of personality. Goldstein established a dichotomy between specific and abstract language. *Specific language*, which can be related to the automation of processing, corresponds to emotional expressions, sounds, words, and all those usually very familiar linguistic segments executed without conscious control. On the contrary, *abstract language* is a purposeful and intentional language.

These language types are one particular case of a more general rivalry between two forms of *adaptive attitude* or two types of intelligence. *Specific attitude* is shown when the mechanisms of rational adaptation, such as thought, automatically respond to the immediate demands of the situation. *Abstract attitude*, Goldstein believes, implies a detachment from the specific aspects of the stimulus in order to act upon the conceptual representation of this stimulus. This facilitates adaptation in terms of symbolic representations. The aphasia shows itself as an incapacity to adopt an abstract attitude or disposition, impeding symbolic processing.

Hierarchical Models

Hughlings Jackson considers behavior as being formed by a series of functions of increasing complexity. These functions are hierarchically arranged within neural complexity, with the most elemental positioned at the base of the system. As behavior evolves, more complex functions and structures appear. The neurological interpretation of Jackson's conception states that structures of greater evolution control those of a lesser evolution.

Along the same lines, the microgenetic theory (Brown, 1972, 1977) considers language as a code organized in different levels of related representation. The performance of linguistic behaviors implies the simultaneous activation of the different levels of neural activity. The most primitive neural structures are responsible for the execution of simpler linguistic levels, and the most evolved structures are the ones that perform the levels of greater linguistic complexity. This concept assumes that the language processing is carried out by vertically disposed structures from an evolutionary view but not by horizontally disposed ones, as in classical associationism. According to Brown, the nervous tracts maintain in phase the different levels of processing instead of connecting the processing centers in a series among themselves.

In accordance with this interpretation, functional disorders are due to a defect in the working of the underlying structures, as it is thought to occur in locationist models. However, while, in these latter models, the system only partially works, in the case of the hierarchical models, it is assumed that the system acts as a whole only for those more automatic and stereotyped behaviors, since the higher order has been lost.

The Cognitive Interpretation of Language

There exist, however, many phenomena observed in clinical practice that cannot be explained by any of the above models. The difficulty in finding pure models, the variability of the symptoms assumed to be characteristic of a particular disorder, and the complexity of the disorders of written language must all be considered, along with both the implied neuroanatomical structures, their functionality, and the cognitive nature of the process. The cognitive interpretation of language has not only added a new dimension but has also offered an adequate frame of reference so that both levels of explanation, neurological and cognitive, can be integrated into one.

From a cognitive perspective, behavior is the result of successive transformations undergone by the information as it is processed in the mind. The mind can be compared to a structural processor functionally composed of modules. As Fodor stated (1883), a module consists of a specific unit of processing (i.e., it responds to only one definite type of signal or signal part). A second characteristic of the modules is encapsulation, which is where modules form closed and autonomous units of processing (i.e., they work independently from the system). However, modularity does not imply isolation but rather a functional specificity.

Processing in stages, a characteristic of cognitive interpretations, allows for explanation of aphasia aspects that were unresolved by the previous theory of connection. Agrammatism, anomia, and the various types of reading disorders are examples of this cognitive interpretation of language.

Certain comprehension disorders in which the comprehension of the first linguistic segment is lost or in which the impairment affects the end of the sentence, can only be interpreted within a cognitive frame of reference such as attention or memory disorders. In the first case, it can be thought that the patient has difficulties in focusing his/her attention and that is why he/she loses the information contained in the first segment of the message. The comprehension difficulties of the last part of the message could be associated with limitations in the capacity and performance of the working memory.

Agrammatism, which is the loss of the particles of syntactic connection, is primarily associated with motor aphasias. The language produced in these cases has a schematic, telegraphic structure without any loss of meaning. If the injuries in Broca's region appear as a loss of the functional particles and this same region is the memory of the motor representation of words, it seems paradoxical that those words demanding less processing are the first to be lost.

On the other hand, agrammatism does not appear as a homogeneous symptom but produces a high variability associated to the linguistic system, to the severity of the damage, or to the complexity of functional forms. Goodglass and Berko (1960) observed that the "s" morpheme of third person in English present tense or of possessive forms is more easily lost than the "s" indicating plural. These differences in lexical production have been partially explained by the fact that the functional particles are usually syntactically ambiguous, so their processing needs the support from contextual content words. This relevance within the text is the reason for which the latter show themselves more resistant to impairment.

Apart from this linguistic relevance, the lexical units of language are charged with a psychological relevance produced by certain properties of the word such as stress, phonetic structure, and affective interest (Goodglass, 1973). These characteristics make content words less affected by aphasic lesions than functional particles.

Schwarz, Safran, and Marin (1980) observed that subjects with grammatical deficiencies have problems with the word order in the sentence. This could be due to the limitations in working memory, namely, in the articulatory loop that plays an important role in maintaining word order.

Generally speaking, various theoretical approaches attempt to explain agrammatism in terms of an economical processing of information. Nonetheless, this disorder could also be explained as a defect in the language production within a model such as that of Garret (1980). This model suggests that language production is a process of a serial construction of sentences through different levels of programming, initially of a conceptual nonlinguistic character, and finally, of an articulatory nature. A general syntactic and semantic representation of the sentence occurs at an intermediate, functional stage. The positional level is where the more formal representation is executed with the election of the lexical terms and specific syntactic relations to be used in the sentence. The existence of these levels or modules could explain why the syntactic structure of the sentence is lost in agrammatism, while the meaning and intention are not affected. The lesion would only damage the syntactic processing module but not the semantic processing one.

With regard to the symptom's complexity and variability, Badecker and Caramazza (1985) believe that agrammatism should not be considered as a single and homogeneous disorder. In this sense, a modular interpretation could explain this variability.

The importance of the cognitive models needs to be emphasized. Cognitivism suggests that the processes are formed by a series of subprocesses. The processing of information can be divided up into a series of stages, each carrying out a particular function. Undoubtedly, this vision of the processes is similar to the one of the last century, when language was considered as a unifying series of nodes and vectors. However, there are important differences in the conceptualization of modules working independently and in parallel. Language disorders, in this case, can be explained at a microscopic level. At the same time in each disorder, one or some modules are disorganized but not necessarily the whole of the system.

Suitable treatment implies investigating each situation, model, or theory. In linguistic analysis, the symptoms must be observed and treated in accordance with the cognitive models; the treatment could be aimed at each of the subskills. Since this is difficult, however, all the treatments agree in using the organic base as the common treatment area. Here, the importance of the neurological substratum in the recovery of cognitive functions can be seen.

SYMPTOMATOLOGY AND APHASIA TYPES

Throughout the history of aphasiology, different classifications have been proposed. Some authors have adopted clinical and anatomical criteria, and others have based classifications on linguistic criteria, especially those based on Jacobson's research. Faced with the difficulty of clearly differentiating syndromes, a less rigid classification has also been attempted with a wide spectrum and two types of aphasias structured around the maintaining or loss of the fluency of language. The non-fluent aphasias are characterized by a decrease in the number of linguistic elements making up the sentence, with slow production and articulatory suppression but not failing to maintain a good level of comprehension. On the contrary, in fluent aphasias, the fluency is maintained at a high level and even appears to accelerate; comprehension, however, is deficient.

Due to the variability of the symptomatic manifestations in aphasia and the inconsistency of them, the utility and convenience of a classification based on groups of symptoms has been questioned. In clinical practice, nevertheless, the syndromes usually treated are those that can be considered more or less specific or pure organized groups of distinct symptoms. In this sense, a classification of aphasic disorders in base to big patterns becomes a principle of structuring something that appears, first of all, ambiguous and confused (Marshall, 1982).

On the basic, the following explanation follows the classification of Benson and Geschwin that, along with the later review carried out by the Aphasia Research Center at the Boston Veterans Administration Hospital, is perhaps the most widespread in the clinical field. A brief explanation of aphasic syndromes follows. More detailed expositions can be found in specialized literature on neurology and neuropsychology such as Benson (1988) or Kertesz (1985).

Broca's Aphasia

The clinical characteristics of Broca's aphasia are perhaps the most clearly identified. Verbal production in all cases lacks fluency; words are slurred, unclear, and pronounced with great effort. Sentences are short, and dysprosodia appears. The phonemes are distorted, and paraphasias are apparent. The repetition, although nearly always irregular, is much better than with the spontaneous language. Naming objects is also difficult, although it is made considerably easier when the subject is given phonetic or contextual clues. A limited production means that the patient restricts verbal expressions to words that require less effort and are more automatic, resulting in a good production of familiar words and a stereotyped appearance.

Patients with motor aphasia usually have a good level of reading comprehension of isolated words, but sequential reading presents difficulties associated with deficiencies in grammatical processing.

Agrammatism, along with fluency loss, are the most interesting characteristics of oral production in Broca's aphasia. The loss of functional particles, whether isolated or linked, leads to a telegraphic style of speech.

Comprehension, although generally good, is also affected due to the fact that the loss of the binding elements of the sentence impedes the appropriate links being made between words. Added to this is the problem stemming from dysprosody. Prosodic variables, which are basically variations in the acoustic intensity of oral production relative to time, bear the affective content of language. Thus, difficulties of production impede the use of information contained in, for example, intonation and rhythm for understanding expressive language.

Wernicke's Aphasia

Anatomically, Wernicke's aphasia is characterized by an injury in the rear temporal region of the left hemisphere. Speech is fluent with good articulation, and the rhythm, prosody, and length of the sentence are adequately maintained. Sometimes these parameters are exaggerated, resulting in logorrhea. The message content, on the contrary, usually lacks meaning. Verbal and semantic paraphasias appear frequently as do literal and phonetic paraphasias, but to a lesser extent. In the most serious impairment, speech consists of a jargon, where the language becomes unintelligible due to the simultaneous presence of neologisms, paraphasias, and a breaking of syntactic rules. The ability of naming is also considerably reduced in direct relation to comprehension deficiencies.

Reading and writing are also affected, although, to a variable degree, depending on the location and extension of the injury. When structures behind Wernicke's region are affected, such as the angular gyrus, breaks in reading and writing are produced. Dejerine indicates the fundamental role of the angular gyrus in reading processes.

Subjects with Wernicke's aphasia are more prone to develop clinical histories affecting personality integration. Comprehension defects can occasionally generate a certain paranoia which, combined with language disorders, can be confusing in the diagnosis of these patients.

Conduction Aphasia

This was originally defined by Wernicke in 1974 as a logical and necessary consequence of his proposed neurolinguistic model. Once the two major language centers were defined—one intervening in the tasks of comprehension and the other in those of production, as previously proposed by Broca—both centers had to be connected to guarantee the coherence and consistency between both processes. In other words, the subject performs as a transmitter and receiver of the communication. This path of connection corresponds to the fasciculus arcuatus.

Generally speaking, subsequent research has confirmed Wernicke's fundamental assumptions. Speech is fluent with the appropriate use of grammatical elements. Nonetheless, phonemic paraphasias appear, as do verbal and neologisms to a lesser extent. Comprehension is adequate, while Wernicke's region is not affected.

The most characteristic symptom of the aphasia of conduction is the extreme difficulty shown by the patient in tasks of repetition, which clashes with the efficiency of comprehension evidenced by appropriate descriptions and circumlocution.

In classic neurolinguistics, all these symptoms are interpreted as being a result of the disconnection between the centers operating language comprehension and production. The fact that the damage is occasionally located in the supramarginal gyrus allows for the proposal of other hypotheses in relation to the cognitive subprocesses participating in the activation and recovery of lexical information.

Anomic Aphasia

This is the most benign manifestation of language disorganization. The patient is incapable of finding the appropriate naming situation, whether in written or spoken language. Oral production is fluent with good repetition and adequate comprehension. It is frequently seen as the final stage of a more serious aphasia. Being unable to find the appropriate name in a difficult situation, the patient uses substitutes and circumlocutions, showing a good level of both language production and comprehension.

In this aphasia, there is no well-defined anatomical location. The processes intervening in naming tasks involve many anatomical structures, and, at the same time, anomia is very often is a residual expression of other aphasias. For this reason, the neuroanatomical location is not precise. In fact Goodglass (1994) indicates different types depending on their symptoms.

Sensory Transcortical Aphasia

The term was initially introduced by Wernicke in 1886 and was used for those patients whose spontaneous language was impaired but who were capable of correct repetitions. As shown in Lichteim's neurolinguistic model, comprehension processes imply the connection between Wernicke's area to a so-called center of concepts with the anatomical location spread throughout the peripheric associative cortex to the perisylvian region. The associations between the auditory cortex and this conceptual center are required, at first, to complete comprehension tasks. At the same time, coherent spontaneous language demands the activation of connections from this conceptual center to the region of Broca. Based on research on damage in this region, three types of transcortical aphasias have been proposed: sensory, motor, and mixed.

The sensory transcortical aphasia produces symptoms similar to those of Wernicke's aphasia, but repetition is maintained. Speech is fluent, but comprehension is poor; reading and writing, especially comprehensive reading, are seriously affected.

The location of brain regions associated with this kind of damage are not clearly defined. Nonetheless, it is possible to associate this disorder with injuries of the temporo-occipital and angular gyrus regions.

Motor Transcortical Aphasia

The most outstanding characteristic of this syndrome is the patient's difficulty in producing spontaneous language. The production is dysartric and intermittent. However, in repetition tasks, the patient shows a good performance, and at the same time, a good level of comprehension is maintained. The capacity of naming, also found to be slightly affected, shows an interesting phenomenon of "warm-up," in which the subject is capable of using the phonetic linguistic indications given in rehabilitation to facilitate his/her oral production. Speech falls, again, to the primitive levels of performance.

Mixed Transcortical Aphasia

This is a disorder that combines the symptoms of sensory and motor transcortical aphasias. It appears simultaneously in production and comprehension difficulties. Repetition is preserved. In communication, the speech of the patient consists of a compulsive imitation of the therapist's speech or in stereotypes. Reading and writing are also damaged.

Global Aphasia

This aphasia is characterized by extensive injury in both front and rear regions of the brain, which seriously damages language production and comprehension. The patient also has serious difficulty in repetition, denomination, reading, and writing. When the language problems are accompanied by right hemiplegia, the prognosis is not very optimistic.

In cases of generalized aphasia, the patient is only capable of very short stereotyped productions that are usually reduced to a single word or syllable. These reduced transmissions, together with the maintaining of certain rhythmic patterns, constitute the basis upon which the therapy of melodic intonation operates.

Subcortical Aphasias

Thanks to the use of neuro-imaging techniques, it has been possible to relate injuries in the basal ganglia, in the internal capsule, and in the thalamus with aphasic manifestations (Mohr, Watters, & Duncan, 1975). The associated symptomatology is variable and basically depends on the location of the damage. At least three different anatomical areas affected can show different symptoms.

APHASIA REHABILITATION

Brain damage due to stroke, tumor, or trauma provokes defects in brain matter and functioning. This is why language recovery in aphasias must be considered as a specific case of recovery of a brain function, and the recovery of these lost functions relies, to a great extent, upon the recuperation of the corresponding neural tissue.

However, it is clear that aphasic disorders are a result of a loss of brain matter and functioning. Consequently, it is logical to assume that recovery from the aphasia is closely related to neural regeneration and functional restoration. This regeneration may be produced by a process of spontaneous or natural recovery immediately after the damage has occurred.

During the first days post-onset, there are changes in the cellular metabolism, a decrease in the edema, a reabsorption of blood, etc. that have as a consequence a certain recovery of the altered functions. This process may be stimulated by means of adequate treatment.

Therefore, there is a double recovery route of linguistic function: that directly related to the regeneration of the appropriate neural structures and that related to the action which could lead directly to the restoration of certain structures or indirectly to the incorporation of the lost functions in the brain.

This partially spontaneous recovery is perhaps the reason why treatment techniques of aphasias have not been developed as one might have hoped. Nonetheless, numerous studies show the positive correlation between treatment and language recovery if certain conditions prevail (Basso, Capitani, & Vignolo, 1979).

Treatment, naturally, always comes after the evaluation of the disorder and its characteristics. Without providing more detail, it can be said that after a neurological exploration, adequate information of the patient's linguistic behavior must be available. Among the most widespread and used tests in the evaluation of aphasic disorders are the Boston Diagnostic Aphasia Examination, the Token Test, the Porch Index of Communicative Abilities, the Western Aphasia Battery, the Minnesota Test for the Differential Diagnosis of Aphasia, the Functional Communication Profile, and Communicative Abilities in Daily Living.

In accordance with the above, a brief explanation will be made here of certain neural regeneration processes that occur in the spontaneous recuperation of language. A more detailed explanation is found elsewhere in this book.

Spontaneous Language Recovery

Shortly after suffering brain damage and the subsequent loss of language, a certain recovery is produced without any therapeutic intervention. Usually this spontaneous recovery begins one or two months after the injury has happened and may continue for up to six months, although the majority of the recuperation occurs in the first three months

(Kertesz & McCabe, 1977; Sarno & Levita, 1971; Vignolo, 1964; Wade, Hewer, David, & Enderby, 1986).

Observation of this recovery allows certain authors (Weigel & Bierwisch, 1970) to conclude that in aphasic disorders, the patient loses linguistic "performance" while "competence" remains intact. The severity and the persistency of the linguistic functions in some aphasias certainly do not allow for the fact that in these disorders, linguistic competence remains completely untouched.

Immediately after the event of injury, changes in the affected region are produced upon which functional recovery depends. A decrease in the edema, the reabsorption of lost blood, the reestablishing of the activity of neurotransmitters, and effects of diaschisis are all indicated by Rubens (1977) as being sufficient explanation of the recovery processes. In any case, neural plasticity would appear to be at the root of functional recuperation.

The mechanism of neural plasticity is as yet only partially understood, and a great deal of research is still to be carried out. However, this mutability and flexibility depends, among other factors, upon the reactive processes of the intact axon, which can generate branches of collateral connection; on neural scarring, when the injury partially affects the axon; and on the modification of synapsis and the increase in the sensitivity of the neurotransmitters.

Kertesz (1993) distinguishes two different phases in the language recovery. In the first one, which occurs during the first days or weeks immediately after the damage, take part mechanisms that restore the cellular metabolism and performance begin to recover. The second phase has firmer and more balanced effects in the function recovery and reaches a maximum between the second and sixth months after the damage. In this phase, the recovery is associated with compensation mechanisms where take part neural ipsilateral structures close to or connected to the ones damaged establish homologous contralateral mechanisms or subcortical systems related to the damaged ones.

Also to be considered as recuperation mechanisms, although rather slower, are the phenomena of neural regeneration, diaschisis, functional compensation, and the vicarious action of other structures of the brain.

Independent of those neurological mechanisms leading to the recovery of cognitive functions, language recovery depends on the following variables:

1. *Type and severity of the damage.* It would be logical to expect that if functional losses are related to neuroanatomical injuries, then the greater the amount of brain matter affected, the more dramatic the effects on behavior. Furthermore, different kinds of damage will follow a different post-traumatic course. Rubens (1977) explains the differences in the initiation of spontaneous recuperation between subjects with brain hemorrhage and those having suffered ischemic infarction. Aphasias produced by trauma evolve better than those produced by a stroke. Nonetheless, it is difficult to come to any conclusions by means of these observations since these effects may be due to the interaction of variables. Traumatic aphasias, for example, usually affect a younger population, while those of vascular origin are seen more frequently with older patients. Age is a variable that is directly related to neural plasticity.

2. *Location of the damage and aphasia type.* Linguistic differences have been observed among the processes of spontaneous recuperation and the type of damage suffered. Although, generally speaking, different aphasias evolve towards

anomia in a terminal phase, it is possible to discover very diverse and variable routes in each syndrome. Patients suffering from Wernicke's aphasia with jargonaphasia end up with anomia after an intermediate phase of paraphasias and substitutions. Non-fluent aphasias also evolve towards anomia but through intermediate phases where fluency is also affected. It can be seen that deficiencies of auditory comprehension recover better than those of production (Lomas & Kertesz, 1978).

3. *Age.* As a general rule, it can be said that recovery is achieved ,to a lesser extent, with the increase of age (Vignolo, 1964; Wepman, 1951). Fast and significant progress does not seem to be so common in disorders suffered in adult life as with those suffered in childhood. Of course, injuries that occur when the nervous system is maturing can expect total or partial recovery due to the greater plasticity of the system. When the damage appears in adulthood, on the other hand, it is necessary to take into account the interaction of age with other variables in order for recovery to be achieved.

4. *Emotional state.* In the event of brain damage, the emotional state of the patient may be affected for two reasons. First, a depressive state usually appears several days after the injury that affects those patients with motor aphasia in a particular way. Difficulty in communication may produce social withdrawal and depression. In the clinical description of Wernicke's aphasia, agitation and paranoid behavior can also develop, so it is not surprising that depressions related to the limitation of social life also appear. On the other hand, there is a closer correlation between the depressive state and the affected organic base in the cases where the damage has a frontal location. In these cases, Robinson and Price (1982) have observed that the effects of spontaneous recovery are less than when the patient maintains a normal emotional state.

5. *State before damage.* A negative correlation has been found between spontaneous recovery and disorders in the nervous system prior to injury (Yarnell, Monroe, & Sobel, 1976).

6. *Other variables* such as sex, brain dominance, and cultural level are not seen to be of particular importance in the process of spontaneous recovery. In cases where differences could arise that might be associated with these factors, those differences have to be interpreted carefully.

Treatment of Aphasic Disorders

Observation of spontaneous recovery, to a certain extent independent from external control and intervention, has not exactly contributed towards stimulating the design of intervention and treatment techniques of aphasic language. Nonetheless, since World War II, with a new concept of welfare and quality of life and the development of theoretical systems in the health sciences, certain therapeutic techniques for the treatment of aphasias have been designed. In general, these techniques are theoretically either based on systems concentrating on the study of language, as in the techniques originating in the psychological concept of language, or derived directly from the pragmatic action on the patient in rehabilitation.

It has already been stated that since there does not exist either a psycholinguistic or a neurolinguistic model, therapeutic orientations are multiple and diverse in nature. All the same, the characteristics of the different rehabilitation techniques depend upon the neurolinguistic and psycholinguistic theoretical frame of reference.

Generally speaking, a possible classification can be based on three major groups of therapies:

1. Therapies based on the knowledge and performance of linguistic behavior in accordance with the traditional interpretations of linguistics.
2. Therapies based on the communication function of language.
3. Therapies based on a neurocognitive concept of language.

In the first group of therapies, the linguistic behavior of the patient is the starting point for the therapist. Errors in linguistic performance are seen as a series of violations of the code regulating language at its different levels: phonetic, phonological, morphological, lexical, syntactic, and semantic. These cases may also be interpreted in relation to defects in competence and execution. However, the rules of a specific linguistic system determine, in each case, the degree of language deterioration.

On other occasions, the aim has been to preserve more the possibility of language communication than the symbolic representation. For this reason, the elements considered in therapy are more oriented towards pragmatism and paralinguistic structure of language upon which the functions of communication are organized.

The principles of cognitive neuropsychology have been previously established. The treatment must take into account the modular character of the process and especially, the phase in which this process has been deteriorated. In fact, some therapies responding to the basic principles of either of the above classes illustrate, unintentionally, the modular conception and composition of the linguistic process. This is how Melodic Intonation Therapy, for example, works on the existence of a module of prosodic processing in the right hemisphere, which acts autonomously and from where other linguistic modules can be activated. These therapies, however, require better verification of the different cognitive subprocesses making up a particular linguistic behavior. Until now, it would seem that they have been applied in a more effective and developed manner in the treatment of problems of written language. It may be because this area has developed its own field of research based on experimental data that it has appeared in a proliferation of theoretical models. Also to be considered is the fact that in the research of subprocesses such as lexical access, working memory, inferential processes, and others which, presumably, integrate any model of language processing, written language has been used more than oral language.

From these three major theoretical frameworks, numerous intervention techniques have been designed responding to the classification shown in the following rather eclectic presentation:

- stimulation therapies
- behavioral therapies
- functional therapies
- cognitive therapies
- compensatory approaches

Stimulation Therapy

Stimulation techniques share two assumptions: aphasia does not mean a loss of linguistic abilities but a more or less transitory interference impeding the use of these abilities. In the aphasia, there is a disintegration of a generalized skill due to the disorganization of auditory comprehension (Schuell, Jenkins, & Jimenez-Pabon, 1964).

In accordance with these assumptions, the objective of therapeutic intervention would consist of achieving the reactivation of these abilities that are not lost but simply blocked. For this reason, the facilitation of verbal behavior through auditory stimulation is used as a rehabilitation technique. Language, presumably, acts in relation to particular neural activations formed during the acquisition period. These networks of neural connection have become blocked due to damage. The aim of therapy is to reactivate these networks by means of exercise and practice.

The principles of therapy naturally originate in their theoretical bases. At first, it is established that the treatment will act directly and immediately on oral language. As claimed by Schuell (1973), the most natural task of language is the comprehension of the message. Thus, and far from a cognitive framework, Schuell relegates the other psycholinguistic abilities to the processes of oral comprehension. The suitable path for this stimulation is, consequently, auditory.

Schuell et al. (1964) concentrate on a series of principles to guide therapy. The first establishes the need for a wide-ranging and adequate sensory stimulation, especially of the auditory type, in order for rehabilitation to be carried out. It is assumed that the more clues given to the subject, the more his/her linguistic behavior will be facilitated; at the same time, these clues must be relevant to the desired behavior. Therefore, determined characteristics of stimulus must be taken into account such as intensity, significance, color, realism, etc. that can be easily perceived by the subject.

According to this principle, the following establishes that the response must not appear forced but naturally evoked by the stimulus. In order for this association to take place, the tasks of facilitation must be suitable for the response desired.

The following principle naturally completes the former. In order for a stimulus to facilitate a linguistic response, it must be presented repeatedly. Not to be forgotten is the assumption that language is not lost but blocked, and it is understood that repeated stimulation may be necessary to reestablish the functionality of these blocked centers and paths.

Behavioral Therapies

In accordance with the behavioral conception, language is the result of a process of associative learning (Skinner, 1957). Therefore, any alteration in this process is contemplated as a loss or weakening of the association between the situations and linguistic behavior emitted. In this case, the disorder is interpreted as a weakening of habit. The aim of therapy is to reestablish this habit by means of reinforced practice.

In general, the application of techniques of behavioral modification implies a first phase, where a base line of behavior to be modified is established. In this first phase, an inventory of behaviors is made that must be sufficiently consistent to be able to determine the base line. The determination of this base line poses the empirical problem of defining the criteria of which behaviors are to be included. Secondly, the techniques of behavior modification are applied with the final hope that the necessary transfer in other similar situations will occur.

Once the base line is determined, the technique proceeds in successive stages of stepwise complexity, beginning with the simplest and leading up to the most complex, thus modulating the desired behavior. From the behaviors forming the base line, a criteria of increasing difficulty is established and used as an objective by the patient. Rehabilitation begins with those behaviors with a high probability of successful execution, thus reinforcing the behavior from the onset.

Apart from the theoretical problems underlying the associationist concept, these techniques are characterized by their lack of sensitivity towards individual variations. It is understood that the success of the treatment depends on the correct methodological application of the technique. It can be equally well applied to the treatment of syntactic problems, comprehension problems, or a variety of linguistic problems. In this sense, the method is of universal value, but its efficiency depends on its correct administration.

Emphasis is placed on explicit behavior (i.e., on the analysis of linguistic content more than on the strategies of use). Consequently, there is sometimes a certain lack of motivation on the part of the subject.

Functional Therapies

This includes a group of therapies centered around the pragmatic aspects of language with the aim of recovering their communicative function. They have many elements in common with the techniques of stimulation and facilitation, but they differ in that the latter concentrate on the treatment of the formal aspects of language, while the former focus on the use of language as an instrument of communication.

Aphasic disorders also imply alterations that affect personality, social behavior, etc. Immediately following an injury, it is not unusual for depressions and emotional instability to appear. For this reason, it is advisable to maintain an adequate level of social contact.

The starting point for this group of therapies is the communication situation. In this situation, the subject uses, as well as linguistic components, some paralinguistic levels that bear part of the meaning of the message. This viewpoint on language reveals the two main characteristics of these therapies. First, and differing from the stimulation techniques, the linguistic exercise, as a source of transference, is not an objective in itself. The patient, instead, has to try to adjust his/her linguistic behavior to the situation, which distinguishes this approach from the stimulation technique. Second, the paralinguistic elements, being of a different nature and associated with different brain structures that remain intact after injury, become the basis for the initiation of treatment.

In accordance with these premises, various therapeutic techniques have been designed. The majority of them use the accompanying gestures of language or alternative systems of communication as therapeutic resources.

Davis and Wilcox (1981) proposed the PACE technique (Promoting Aphasic's Communication Effectiveness). The basic principles of the technique follow:

1. Patient and therapist must exchange the functions of transmitter and receiver in such a way that during the treatment, real situations of communication are reproduced.
2. In a natural situation of communication, the adequate use of language requires constructing a scheme of mental representation. Given that only one part of the information is explicit in speech, the use of contextual keys is needed to elaborate the required inferences in comprehension (Bransford & Johnson, 1973). PACE uses graphic representations of objects unseen by the receiver as messages. This forces the patient to use different strategies of communication and to introduce new elements into the message with the aim of facilitating comprehension. Thus the patient achieves a more integrated development of language whether acting as transmitter or receiver.
3. As a consequence of the above, the technique allows the use of different forms of communication, fulfilling its aim of increasing communication skills.

4. Finally, the patient must receive adequate and punctual feedback of his communication efficiency.

PACE has been criticized for its excessive dependence on a communication system of mime and gestures rather than on verbal communication. Naturally, the relevance of criticism depends on the objectives established in therapy and on the theoretical viewpoint of language. Currently, there is an open debate on other areas of speech therapy, specifically between oralist theories and those supporting specific communication systems of gestures in the re-education of auditory deficiencies.

Considering PACE as a complement to other techniques and the fact that communication is a generalized skill, this technique can be used, according to the authors, in any type of aphasic disorder.

Helm-Esterbrooks et al. (1982) developed a therapeutic program for the treatment of generalized aphasic disorders, having failed with traditional rehabilitation techniques. Arising from an early work by Gardner, Zurif, Berr, and Baker (1976) where aphasic subjects worked with a system of visual communication, favorable conclusions were obtained on the possibilities of patients with generalized aphasia in the treatment of symbolic material. The system of knowledge representation of these patients is actually less affected than would appear from their linguistic performance.

The technique created by Helm-Esterbrooks and colleagues, called Visual Action Therapy (VAT), aims at the patient's producing symbolic gestures. The VAT was originally designed to treat generalized aphasias but has undergone many modifications. The latest version, besides treating symbolic aspects of communication, uses subprograms for the rehabilitation of apraxia that may appear with the aphasic disorder.

When practicing the technique, real basic objects are used, along with drawings of these objects and images. The technique progresses through a series of stages from a simple reproduction and manipulation of objects to the comprehension of the concept and production of gestures and mimes representing these objects. In the same way within this framework of progressive tasks, the patient begins to work with objects and images in front of him/her and finishes with hidden objects. Efficiency in the development of these tasks shows the power of the generalization of the technique and the facilitation of particular subprocesses such as training in tasks of spacial orientation and the restoration of the system of conceptual representation.

Cognitive Techniques

Techniques of cognitive orientation are not characterized as much for the type of tasks proposed as for the theoretical conception they have of language and its alterations. Language, from a cognitive point of view, is considered to be made up of a series of subprocesses. These subprocesses are linked to the functioning of processing modules, but their processing does not impede their action of coordination and interaction in any way. From this perspective, aphasic syndromes, as defined by traditional neurolinguistics, are not considered as valid for the diagnosis and classification of language disorders (Caramazza, 1984). If linguistic processes depend on the functioning of specific modules, an injury within the system may affect one or several of them without necessarily affecting the system as a whole. The function of assessment and diagnosis consists of determining the affected module or subprocess. Consequently, therapy has to be aimed at the restoration of this phase of processing and its integration with the rest of the system.

This theory at present, nonetheless, is not exempt from problems. First, since the cognitive models are detailed representations of a series of subprocesses, it is necessary to find an adequate correspondence between each subprocess and the tasks needed to improve it. Until now, this correspondence has not been well established. The cognitive models, on the other hand, cannot be built as simple formal representations of mental processes but must be capable of making certain predictions about the functioning of the neuroanatomical structures underlying the cognitive processes.

Although, at present, a greater development of cognitive rehabilitation techniques is needed along with an assessment of their efficiency, a considerable number of intervention strategies have been generated, particularly with reading and writing disorders. It should be remembered that the cognitive paradigm has preferred written language in its research, and this is where the most developed models have been elaborated.

As these models show, the comprehension processes can be considered to be made up of a series of subprocesses including, among others, phonetic-phonological transformations, lexical access, syntactic assignation, and semantic interpretation. At the same time, the integration of the information at different levels is carried out.

Language production, in turn, can be explained as the result of a series of mental operations from the activation of an abstract representation to its motor execution. At higher levels, the process is guided by the plans, aims, and objectives of the subject. At this first level of generic representation, context knowledge is incorporated as a pragmatic variable in order to elaborate the translation from the first cognitive structure into another of linguistic nature. A semantic structure is compiled through successive phases, and lexical units and grammatical rules are selected. Linguistic planning of speech at a central level is carried out, which corresponds to the activity of cortical structures from similar cortical activation levels. The next stage is the programming of the motor execution of speech.

Kremin (1993) and Lesser (1989) demonstrated the possibility of using the cognitive interpretation of language in the treatment of anomia. Howard and Patterson (1989) developed the basic characteristics of cognitive neuropsychological models applied to therapy.

Specific Techniques

The techniques included here could equally fit in some of the above groups. Generally speaking, they are called specific because only one particular aspect of language is considered as a motive of therapy. The idea is that, by means of phases of gradual complexity, the benefits of partial treatment can be extended throughout language as a whole.

Perhaps the most widespread of these techniques is the Melodic Intonation Therapy (MIT) proposed by Albert, Sparks, and Helm-Esterbrooks (1973). The technique is based on the contribution of prosody in language organization and on the lateralization in the right hemisphere of these patterns.

Prosody consists of variations in intensity within the speech in relation to time and shows itself in the rhythm and intonation of language. At the same time, prosody bears the affective and emotional information of the message. If we consider that this is a suprasegmental variable and that prosodic variations share acoustically the nature of musical variations, it is possible to make some hypothesis about its lateralization in the right hemisphere. As the structures in the right hemisphere are supposed to not be affected in aphasic disorders, it is possible to design an intervention technique that, starting from the stimulation of these structures, is able to facilitate the speech of the patient.

MIT consists of a series of hierarchically organized activities. In the first levels, patients have to follow with beats of their hand the rhythmical pattern of the intonation of a verbal structure of the therapist. Patients change progressively from a motor behavior to another of verbal character where they try to assimilate their performance to that of the therapist. The therapy continues with the modulation of variable intonational and rhythmical patterns where the patient must be able to follow the structure. Patients progressively free their behavior from that of the therapist, focusing more on stimuli of a linguistic character and releasing themselves from solely rhythmical structures. Finally, patients must be capable of verbal repetitions and of giving an answer to a question.

According to Sparks, Helm, and Albert (1974), the treatment with this technique is suitable for patients with severe difficulties in oral production, repetition, good comprehension, and emotional stability.

CONCLUSION

The rehabilitation of aphasic disorders still shows, at present, serious theoretical, methodological, and application problems. First, there is a lack of psycholinguistic and neurolinguistic theories that are scientifically tested. In addition, there is a great proliferation of formal models in psycholinguistics that lack a well-founded anatomic and neural basis. Thus, it is difficult to find good correlations between linguistic functions and neuroanatomic structures where it is possible to intervene to improve the linguistic processes.

On the other hand, the variability of aphasic disorders and the need for a quick clinical intervention after the damage hinders a slower and more systematic investigation about treatment techniques and their application.

Another problem arises related to the difficulty of evaluating the therapy effects. First, it is difficult to separate the effects of the spontaneous recuperation and the treatment, as both can overlap in time in the same patient or group of patients. Many comparisons among different types of treatment have not included control groups, or the procedure has not allowed for isolation of the different factors that contribute to the recuperation of the aphasia.

In any case and despite these problems, deontological and pragmatic reasoning justifies the therapeutic intervention in aphasias. It must be taken into account that the aphasic patients often suffers personality disorders associated with their linguistic problems. The therapist's presence in the aphasic treatment, as well as producing a positive effect on the linguistic behavior of the patient, will help to achieve a better individual and social adaptation after the damage suffered.

REFERENCES

Albert, M., Sparks, R., & Helm-Esterbrooks, N. (1973). Melodic intonation therapy for aphasia. *Archives of Neurology, 29*, 130–131.

Badecker, B., & Caramazza, A. (1985) On considerations of method and theory governing the uses of clinical categories in neurolinguistics and cognitive psychology: The case against agrammatism. *Cognition, 20*, 97–125.

Basso, A., Capitani, E., & Vignolo, L. (1979). Influence of rehabilitation of language skills in aphasic patients: A controlled study. *Archives of Neurology, 36*, 190–196.

Benson, D.F. (1988). Classical syndromes of aphasia. In F. Boller & J. Grafman (Eds.), *Handbook of neuropsychology* (Vol. 1) (pp. 267--280). Amsterdam: Elsevier.

————. (1993). Aphasia. In K.M. Heilman & E. Valenstein (Eds.), *Clinical neuropsychology* (pp. 18–36). New York: Oxford University Press.

Bransford, F.D., & Johnson, M.K. (1973). Consideration on some problems of comprehension. In W.G. Chase (Ed.), *Visual information processing* (pp. 383–438). New York: Academic Press.

Brown, J.W. (1972). *Aphasias, apraxis and agnosia: Clincial and theoretical aspects.* Springfield: Charles C. Thomas.

————. (1977). *Mind, brain and consciousness.* New York: Academic Press.

Caramazza, A. (1984). The logic of neuropsychological research and the problem of patient classification in aphasia. *Brain and Language, 21,* 9–20.

Davis, G.A., & Wilcox, M.J. (1981). Incorporating parameters of natural conversation aphasia treatment. In R. Chapey (Ed.), *Language intervention strategies in adult aphasia* (pp. 169–193). Baltimore: Williams and Wilkins.

Fodor, J.A. (1983). *The modularity of mind.* Cambridge: MIT Press.

Gardner, H., Zurif, E., Berry, T., & Baker, E. (1976). Visual communication in aphasia. *Neuropsychologia, 14,* 275–292.

Garrett, M.F. (1980). Levels of processing in sentence production. In B. Butterworth (Ed.), *Language production* (pp. 177–220). New York: Academic Press.

Geschwind, N. (1965). Disconnection syndromes in animals and man. *Brain, 88,* 237–294, 585-644.

Golstein, K. (1948). *Language and language disturbances.* New York: Grune and Stratton.

Goodglass, H. (1973). Studies on the grammar of aphasics. In H. Goodglass & S. Blumstein (Eds.), *Psycholinguistics and aphasia.* Baltimore: John Hopkins University Press.

————. (1994). *Understanding aphasia.* New York: Academic Press.

Goodglass, H., & Berko, J. (1960). Agrammatism and inflectional morphology in English. *Journal of Speech and Hearing Research, 3,* 257–267.

Helm-Estabrooks, N., Fitzpatrick, P.M., & Barresi, B. (1982). Visual action therapy for aphasia. *Journal of Speech and Hearing Disorders, 47,* 385–389.

Holland, A. (1991). Pragmatic aspects of intervention in aphasia. *Journal of Neurolinguistics, 6,* 197–211.

Howard, D., & Patterson, K. (1989). Models for therapy. In X. Seron & G. Deloche (Eds.), *Cognitive approaches to neuropsychological rehabilitation* (pp. 39–64). Hillsdale: Lawrence Erlbaum Associates.

Kertesz, A. (1985). Aphasia. In J.A.M. Frederiks (Ed.), *Clinical neuropsychology.* Amsterdam: Elsevier.

————. (1993). Recovery and treatment. In K.M. Heilman & E. Valenstein (Eds.), *Clinical neuropsychology* (pp. 647–674). New York: Oxford University Press.

Kertesz, A., & McCabe, P. (1977) Recovery patterns and prognosis in aphasia. *Brain, 100,* 1–18.

Kremin, H. (1993). Therapeutic approaches to naming disorders. In M. Paradis (Ed.), *Foundations of aphasia rehabilitation* (pp. 261–292). Oxford: Pergamon Press.

Lesser, R. (1989). Some issues in the neuropsychological rehabilitation of anomia. In X. Seron & G. Deloche (Eds.), *Cognitive approaches in neuropsychological rehabilitation* (pp. 66–104). Hillsdale: Lawrence Erlbaum Associates.

Lichteim, L. (1885). On aphasia. *Brain, 7,* 434–484.

Lomas, J., & Kertesz, A. (1978). Patterns of spontaneous recovery in aphasics groups: A study of adult stroke patients. *Cortex, 5,* 388–401.

Marshall, J.C. (1982) What is a symptom-complex? In M.A. Arbib, D. Caplan, & J.C. Marshall (Eds.), *Neural models of language processes* (pp. 389–410). New York: Academic Press.

Mohr, J.P., Watters, W.C., & Duncan, G.W. (1975). Thalamic hemorrhage and aphasia. *Brain and Language, 2,* 3–17.

Robinson, R.G., & Price, T.R. (1982). Post-stroke depressive disorders: A follow-up study of 103 patients. *Stroke, 13,* 635–641.

Rubens, A.B. (1977). The role of changes within the central nervous system during recovery of aphasia. In M. Sullivan & M.S. Kommers (Eds.), *Rationale for aphasia adult therapy* (pp. 28–43). Lincoln: University of Nebraska Press.

Sarno, M.T., & Levita, E. (1971). Natural course of recovery in severe aphasia. *Archives of Physical Medicine and Rehabilitation, 52,* 175–189.

Schuell, H. (1973). *Differential diagnosis of aphasia with the Minnesota Test.* Minneapolis: Lund Press.

Schuell, H., Jenkins, J., & Jiménez-Pabón, E. (1964). *Aphasia in adults.* New York: Harper & Row.

Schwartz, M., Saffran, E., & Marin, O.S.M. (1980). The word order problem in agrammatism. I: Comprehension. *Brain and Language, 10,* 249–262.

Shewan, C.M., & Kertesz, A. (1984). Effects of speech and language treatment on recovery from aphasia. *Brain and Language, 23,* 272–299.

Skinner, B.F. (1957). *Verbal behavior.* New York: Appleton-Century-Crofts.

Sparks, R., Helm-Esterbrooks, N., & Albert, M. (1974). Aphasia rehabilitation resulting from melodic intonation therapy. *Cortex, 10,* 303–316

Sparks, R.W., & Holland, A.L. (1976). Method: melodic intonation therapy for aphasia. *Journal of Speech and Hearing Disorders, 41,* 287–297.

Vignolo, A. (1964). Evolution of aphasia and language rehabilitation: A retrospective exploratory study. *Cortex, 1,* 344–367.

Wade, D.T., Hewer, R.L., David, R.M., & Enderby, P.M. (1986). Aphasia after stroke: Natural history and associated deficits. *Journal of Neurology, Neurosurgery and Psychiatry, 49,* 11–16.

Weigel, E., & Bierwisch, M. (1970). Neuropsychology and linguistics: Topics of common research. *Foundations of Language, 6,* 1–18.

Wepman, J. (1951). *Recovery from aphasia.* Chicago: Ronald Press.

Wertz, R.T. (1987). Language treatment for aphasia is efficacious, but for whom? *Topics in Language Disorders, 8,* 1–10.

Yarnell, P., Monroe, P., & Sobel, L. (1976). Aphasia outcome in stroke: A clinical neuroradiological correlation. *Stroke, 7,* 516–522.

18 Reading and Writing Impairments and Rehabilitation

Teresa Boget and Teodor Marcos

Neuropsychology and Rehabilitation of Cognitive Functions Unit
Hospital Clínic i Provincial, Barcelona, Spain

INTRODUCTION

Reading impairments were originally associated with language impairments. Later, however, it was established that reading impairments could develop independently of oral expression disorders and even independently of writing disorders.

Charcot notes that Grendin, in 1838, published various clinical observations of certain patients who could not read but could write without the slightest difficulty. Trousseau (1865) and Broadbent (1872) provided more precise data about this phenomenon. Nonetheless, it was Charcot who in 1887 described in detail a characteristic case of total alexia with conservation of spontaneous and dictated writing and inability to copy in a patient with hemianopsia.

In 1892, the first anatomical-clinical case of "pure word blindness" was recorded (i.e., with no writing impairment except copying) and attempts began to systematize the various forms of reading impairments clinically, physiopathologically, and anatomically. According to Déjerine, pure alexia was a *specialized aphasia*; Marie considered it to be only a *specialized agnosia*.

The study of reading impairments has increased greatly since then, and, in spite of differences in theoretical viewpoints, the various forms of impairment described clinically have provided data on the normal psychophysiology of reading that have made it possible to define the basic visuo-oral and semantic links in the process.

The longitudinal neuropsychological study of various types of alexia, incorporating exploration and rehabilitation, is of considerable interest. It aids in detecting the patterns that may emerge as developmental evidence of reversibility/irreversibility and provides information that contributes to understanding the patient's specific deficits in this complex process through which the graphic signs of written language are "decoded" and reach the semantic plane that the signs represent.

The reading process starts at the level of the visual system and goes on to reach the symbolic and semantic senses and the oral motor systems. However, this description is oversimplified and insufficient. Clearly, the reading skill is related to the oral language system and to the acoustic organization of language in general.

Alexia can be defined as an acquired inability to understand and verbalize written language due to a focal general lesion.

EXPLORATION OF READING

As in all neuropsychological deficits, in order to adequately examine the diagnosis, prognosis, and rehabilitation of reading impairments, a thorough neuropsychological exploration is required, evaluating quantitatively and qualitatively the higher cortical functions that are affected and those which are not.

The term *alexia* denotes the partial or complete loss of the ability to understand written language. The exploration of reading should, therefore, analyze the deficit in detail, studying the specific characteristics of each case. As Bagunya (1987) notes, in the exploration of an alexic patient, a distinction should be made between the difficulties presented by the act of reading aloud and those encountered in understanding written material. The two functions may be affected in different ways. Reading aloud is of interest in the analysis of linguistic errors and in studying reading mechanisms, but the ability to read written texts has a greater functional value for the individual.

The linguistic component includes the choice of the correct letter (spelling) and the choice of the correct word (meaning). The motor component comprises the neuropsychological functions required to reproduce the correct form of the letters and words.

Learning to read is a stage-by-stage process, which eventually becomes an automatic skill. At the moment it becomes automatic, reading follows a characteristic course of its own—the reverse of that taken by the process of writing in that the process goes *from* the word *to* cognition.

Christensen (1974) reported the exercises used by Luria in his clinical procedure and suggested that the exploration of reading should be preceded by a study of the patient's analysis and synthesis of sounds. The *analysis of phonemic audition* involves identifying the number and the position of sounds and their synthesis to compose a syllable or word.

The assessment of reading also incorporates preliminary examinations of visual acuity and range and of eye movement. The neuropsychological exploration of reading should include the *analysis of letter perception* (i.e., naming isolated handwritten and printed letters, identifying letters written with a stencil), *reading syllables and words* (i.e., simple and complex syllables, simple and more complicated words, ideograms, words with complex structures, and unusual words), and *reading sentences and texts* (i.e., short sentences, complex sentences, and passages from a clearly printed text).

The examiner observes patients' eye movements, the agility of pronunciation, and the strategies they use to pass from one line to another and notes whether they begin to read in the middle of a line or only the part of the text in the right visual field. Examiners can use a wide range of variations: they can present words written in different styles, words written incorrectly, or can alternate between having patients read aloud or to themselves. The length of time that the words are presented can also be varied.

Many neuropsychological and aphasia assessment batteries lend themselves to the exploration of reading expression and comprehension. The Luria-Nebraska Battery (Golden et al., 1980), the Barcelona-PIENC Test (Peña, 1986), and aphasia test batteries such as the Boston Test (Goodglass & Kaplan, 1974) or the Western Aphasia Battery (Kertesz & Poole, 1974) are examples. For the recognition of forms and visual scanning, tests that evaluate spatio-visual inattention, cancellation, and visual search (Lezak, 1995) can be used.

CLINICAL FORMS OF ALEXIA

In spite of certain theoretical divergences, the following forms of alexia are generally recognized:

- Pure alexia (alexia without agraphia); also agnosic alexia
- Aphasic alexia
- Alexia-agraphia
- Spatial alexia

Pure Alexia

Pure alexia, also considered to be a specialized optical agnosia due to the loss of recognition of the forms of letters, differs from other reading impairments of cortical origin in that (1) pure alexics show no language impairment—they retain fluency of discourse and conversation—except for a certain deficit in naming, (2) they conserve the perceptual strategy for reading, and (3) their writing and spelling are unaffected, or at least there is a considerable difference between the intensity of the reading impairment and that of the dictated or spontaneous writing impairment. In contrast, copying is always affected. Acalculia is frequent, although, in general, mild, and visual agnosias (e.g., objects, colors, images) are not constant; when they exist, they are usually of low intensity. *Right homonymous lateral hemianopsia* is observed in all cases.

Hécaen (1977) reports that three differentiated aspects of pure alexia have been described in the literature. In each, one particular ability is the most affected: in literal alexia, it is the ability to read letters; in verbal alexia, the ability to read words; in global alexia, a combination of both; and in sentence alexia, the inability to read sentences.

The topographies involved in agnosic alexia, according to Déjerine and Vialet (1893), result from a disconnection of the calcarine region *from the left angular circumvolution and from a lesion causing a right homonymous lateral hemianopsia*. Nonetheless, as the excellent and comprehensive review of Orgogozo and Péré (1991) indicates, many authors hold that for alexia to exist, there must be a double lesion—in the splenius of the corpus callosum, on the one hand, and in the white substance of the lingual and fusiform lobes of the left hemisphere as well.

According to Orgogozo and Péré's review, verbal alexia is associated with a lesion of the lingual and fusiform lobes (of the left hemisphere), with conservation of the corpus callosum. Global alexia is held to be caused by this same lesion in combination with a lesion of the corpus callosum (i.e., a double lesion). Literal and sentence alexia are attributed to extended occipital lesions, toward the temporal lobe in the former case and toward the parietal lobe in the latter.

Aphasic Alexia

Aphasic alexias are characterized by the loss of understanding of the semantic value of the signs of written language. They are more literal than verbal. In this form of alexia, a dissociation between the verbalization and the comprehension of written words may be found; the patient may understand the meaning of the words or sentences but be unable to produce them verbally. This dissociation is not observed in pure alexia. In aphasic alexia, agraphia is found.

In Broca's aphasia, written comprehension is slightly more affected than oral comprehension, but comprehension of simple written instructions may be possible.

In Wernicke's aphasia, there is frequently a deficit in the comprehension of written language that may be proportional to the impairment of comprehension of spoken language; this may be linked to a certain element of word deafness and may improve with evolution.

Alexia-Agraphia

In the third form of alexia, also associated with agraphia, the patient is unable to read but retains the capacity to spell words orally and to recognize words spelled aloud. In alexia-agraphia the impairment of reading is fundamentally verbal. Letters can be read, and short instructions can be understood and carried out. Long words and long sentences are not read with complete understanding. Writing impairments are considerable and are observed in all types of writing (spontaneous, dictated, and copied). This disorder presents other symptoms associated with apraxia and other language impairments.

Spatial Alexia

Right hemisphere lesions can involve an alexic defect related to left negligence and spatial deficits (spatial alexia). The patient starts reading in the middle of the line and leaves out the text at the extreme left of the page.

Spoken language is generally preserved in these cases, except for a number of deficits associated with the right hemisphere syndrome. In alexics with left lesion, the defects may predominate on the right side of words, while in cases with right lesions, the deficits predominate on the left side.

REHABILITATION OF READING: METHODOLOGY

In a child's development, reading is an analytical and synthetic process; subjects analyze letters, translate them into sounds, combine them in syllables, and with these syllables, synthesize the word. In later stages of reading, the process is more complex. The expert reader only perceives a reduced set of letters (the root of the word) that contain the essential information and through this set of sounds/letters establishes the meaning of the word. During the development and automating of the habit of reading, understanding gradually begins to overtake the process of perception.

The reading process can be disturbed at different stages, and the psychological structure of the disturbances may vary according to the localization of the impairment. For the reading flow to be normal, the visual images of the literal signs and the ability to correlate the optical representations of the letters with their acoustic characteristics must remain unimpaired.

Patients suffering from optical alexia have difficulty recognizing letters. They confuse them with similar optical signs, misunderstand their spatial orientation, or completely fail to recognize them. In reading impairments caused by disorders in the temporal areas of the left hemisphere (such as aphasic alexia), visual identification may remain intact, but the process of analyzing and synthesizing the sounds of the word read is affected, thus making its recognition impossible. Finally, reading may be hampered if eye movement is impaired.

Each form of alexia has its own psychological structure and a particular methodology for rehabilitation. We will now briefly examine the range of rehabilitation programs used as described by Tsvétkova (1977).

Rehabilitation of Reading in Optic Alexia

Optic alexia is always connected with the *syndrome of optic or optic/spatial impairments*. In the process of reading, optic alexics misinterpret literal signs due to their visual perception deficit. They cannot distinguish between similar letters, nor can they separate the elements inside letters that characterize them. Any feature of the letter can become a global feature, and patients misunderstand the meaning of the sign itself. Methods for rehabilitating reading in all cases of optical alexia bear resemblances to each other, as they aim to redress the deficits in the optical perception of the sign.

First Stage

The first stage attempts to rehabilitate the patient's ability to perceive letters in isolation and to recognize them. Initially, letters that vary greatly in terms of optical design (i.e., O–H and A–B) are used. To recognize and name letters, the patient must perform a series of successive tasks: (1) with eyes closed, the patient draws the motor image of the letter in the air, (2) writes the letter in a notebook, (3) identifies it among others presented three-dimensionally, (4) touches it, (5) compares it with others visually and kinesthetically, and (6) names it.

This learning is consolidated by means of exercises with words and texts in which the patient looks for the correct letter, compares it with its prototype and underlines it, or underlines the words that begin with the letter in question.

From analyzing the shape of letters whose optical design differs greatly, patients move on to analyzing letters whose structure is very similar (i.e., O–C, H–N, etc.). They note what is common to the shapes of the letters being compared and also what distinguishes them. To reinforce this analysis, patients are asked to feel the corresponding letters with their hands and to look for them among others with their eyes closed. The examiner asks questions such as, "What do you have to do to change a 'b' into a 'p' or a capital 'B' into a capital 'P'?" Patients then work on reproducing the form of the letter, and, in this way, recover the generalized image of the literal sign.

Second Stage

The second stage involves the recovery of the ability to read syllables and letters. It incorporates the "multi-colored word reading procedure" in which each letter has a different color. This diversity allows patients to distinguish between letters more clearly; the colors represent an additional tool for optically discriminating between the letters inside the words.

Third Stage

The third stage aims to reestablish automatic reading. Patients are given a time limit for reading (understanding and assimilating) a text. Gradually, the time allowed to read texts of a similar length becomes shorter. The method, known as "movable text," also contributes to the automating process. Patients are presented with a text that moves across the screen before their eyes at a preset speed that increases as the learning process progresses. This procedure helps to establish the speed of eye movement necessary for reading.

The methodology aiming to create conditions for an active, discriminant perception of literal signs ensures the recovery of a precise, consistent, and generalized image of letters and contributes towards making the process automatic when deficiencies in the optical-perceptual link exist.

Methodology for the Recovery of Reading in Cases of Impaired Eye Movement

The process of reading involves coordinated eye movement. While reading, the eye goes from one place in the text to another following a straight line. In impairments of occipital-parietal areas of the cerebral cortex, the synthetic perception of whole structures is altered. The patient sees only one point and is unable to simultaneously perceive groups of signs. The organization of eye movements is disturbed, and during reading, the line of vision may jump from one printed line to another.

First Stage

In the first stage, the "framed reading" method is used. This involves a type of cardboard ruler with a sliding part that can increase or reduce the "framed" space when it is placed on top of a word. The text as a whole is hidden, and only the word that the patient is to read is visible. The ruler moves gradually along the line from word to word.

Second and Third Stages

The second stage involves the use of an ordinary ruler. Patients follow the line they are reading by using a ruler that stops them from jumping to another line. In the third stage, patients follow the line with their finger. Through these stages, they learn to move the ruler along the line, to move it from line to line, and to discriminate between the beginning and end of a line with their finger.

Rehabilitation in Cases of Alexia-Aphasia

Disturbances in the temporal areas of the cortex of the left hemisphere affect the analysis of sounds and the synthesis of words. Patients with sensorial alexia can visually identify very familiar words, but the process of sound analysis and word synthesis may be seriously impaired. They may be unable to read an isolated letter or an unfamiliar syllable or word because they have no perception of the *sonic-literal scheme*. For this reason, one of the main aims of rehabilitation is to recover this capacity to analyze sounds and letters. The process takes as its starting point the two unimpaired capacities: (1) visual and (2) kinesthetic analysis.

First Stage

The rehabilitation process starts by changing and limiting patients' tendency to attempt to read by directly identifying the word and gradually tries to implant analysis and synthesis. In this stage, it is essential for patients to correlate letters with their corresponding sounds and to identify and name them inside syllables and later inside words.

To reduce patients' tendency to read globally, this stage incorporates certain external methods that limit the possibility that they will recognize words immediately. Patients must center their attention on the individual letters that make up the structure of the word. The "framed reading" method (described above)) is used; this method trains patients to analyze the word by reading only the letter or syllable that is visible.

Second Stage

The second stage centers on the recovery of the ability to read syllables and words by analyzing sounds and letters. "Framed reading" is replaced by words and texts broken down into syllables.

Third Stage

Making reading automatic (both reading aloud and reading to oneself) is the objective of the final stage. Here patients begin to read without external props (the ruler, texts separated by syllables, following syllables with the finger, etc.).

NEUROPSYCHOLOGICAL REHABILITATION OF A CASE OF ALEXIA WITHOUT AGRAPHIA

The longitudinal neuropsychological study of individual cases can provide information that is extremely helpful in planning clinical studies and more general research. The use of neuropsychological rehabilitation techniques and control explorations can reveal psychometric patterns that may emerge as developmental indices of reversibility/irreversibility and can contribute to a qualitative understanding of the nature of the deficits. This, in turn, makes it possible to formulate or create specific rehabilitation exercises.

The basis of a rehabilitation program is a thorough, detailed evaluation. As Walsh (1982) suggests, the implicit objective of the evaluation is to establish rehabilitative, educational, and vocational programs. In addition, the general improvement in quality of life, the increase in life expectancy, and technological progress all mean that individuals who have suffered cranial trauma, and their families, demand a course of treatment that is as integrated as possible (León-Carrión, 1994).

Neuropsychological rehabilitation is the combination of knowledge, techniques, and technology that aims to ensure that the deficits caused by brain damage should have as limited an effect as possible on the individual's life (León-Carrión, 1994).

Clinical Case Study

The subject was a 20-year-old male patient, a second year technical engineering student referred to the Neuropsychology and Rehabilitation of Cognitive Functions Unit of the Hospital Clínic i Provincial of Barcelona by the Neurosurgical Service of the same hospital four months post-trauma and three months post-discharge. There was no pathological history of interest; the patient was admitted in a coma with traumatic shock level 5 on the Glasgow scale, anisicoria, and left *otorrhagie* after a car crash. Cranial radiography revealed a left parietal fracture, and the CAT showed left occipital and right frontal contusion with moderate cerebral edema. Neurological evolution was slow but toward a state of relative arousal with partial response to verbal stimuli. At the moment of discharge, the patient could hold simple conversations, although a certain level of aphasia and left facial paralysis (without electromyographic signs of reinnervation) were reported. Motor and neuropsychological rehabilitation were recommended.

The TAC revealed a fracture of the left *horn*, focus of bilateral subcortical hemorrhagic contusion, predominantly left frontotemporal, and moderate cerebral edema (Figure 18.1).

Neuropsychological Exploration

The first exploration was performed four months post-trauma. The WAIS subtest and the Luria-Nebraska Battery were administered.The first profile of WAIS (Figure 18.2)

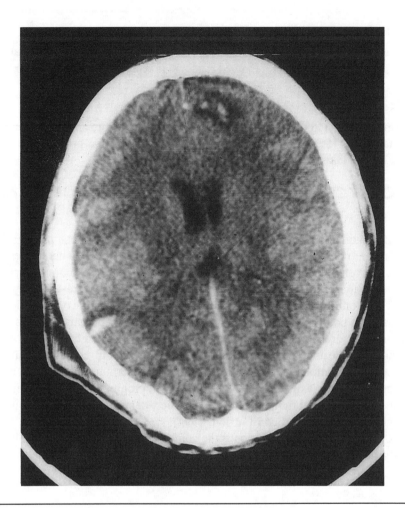

Figure 18.1: TAC of the clincial case study.

revealed heterogeneity in the various subtests. The patient was in the mid-range in the Similarities, Digits, and Kohs Block Design Tests. His fluency was low in the Vocabulary subtest, with presence of perseverations, stereotypy, circumlocutions, some anomia, and loss of school-acquired information. However, the most striking result of the profile was the patient's deficient performance on the Digit Symbol subtest. He understood the instruction quickly but had difficulty copying, as he was unable to represent and copy the spatial position of the symbols. It is interesting to observe the qualitative performance on this subtest in Figure 18.3.

The profile of the Luria-Nebraska Battery (Figure 18.4) was, in pathological terms, above the estimated critical level (i.e., the number of errors expected on the basis of his chronological age and years of schooling, which, in common with the other scales, were converted into T scores). Although the profile revealed disorders in all scales, the most marked deficits were found on the scales that require the identification of symbols with the involvement of the visual channel (e.g., Reading and Arithmetic scales and also the Expressive Language scale, as it contains a considerable number of items that require subjects to pronounce phonemes and to read syllables and words from written stimuli).

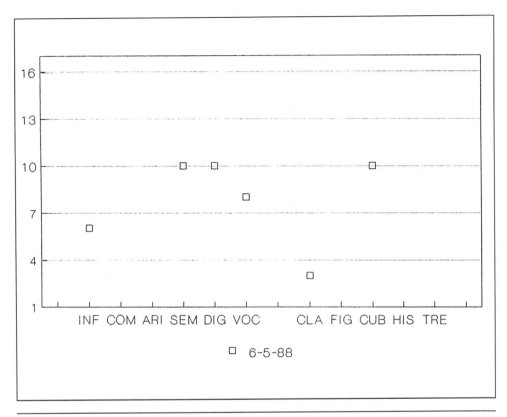

Figure 18.2: Profile of WAIS.

On the Reading scale, the subject was unable to recognize any of the letters, pho-nemes, syllables, ideograms, or words. On the Arithmetic scale, although the deficit was not as complete, the patient read certain numbers incorrectly, causing acalculia; he wrote all numbers correctly when they were dictated to him and recognized mathematical symbols. On the Expressive Language scale, he made mistakes in all items that required reading and showed a deficit in naming objects presented in photographs. On the Memory scale, he showed a certain deficit in immediate retention when presented with verbal and visual stimuli, with a positive but stagnant learning curve. On the Intellectual Processes scale, he showed a deficit in cause and effect, vocabulary, and arithmetic.

The qualitative performance on the Writing scale item is shown in Figure 18.5, which makes clear the discrepancy between the deficient writing in the copying exercise and the unimpaired production in the spontaneous or dictated writing tasks.

The psychometric and neuropsychological exploration described highlighted reduced verbal fluency, difficulty copying both symbols and writing, difficulty in spatial praxis, moderate presence of nominative-mnesic aphasic errors, agnosia of colors, and global alexia. These deficits required an immediate intervention program based on neuropsycho-logical rehabilitation. In the first phase, the program was carried out in the Neuropsychol-ogy and Rehabilitation of Cognitive Functions Unit with three sessions per week.

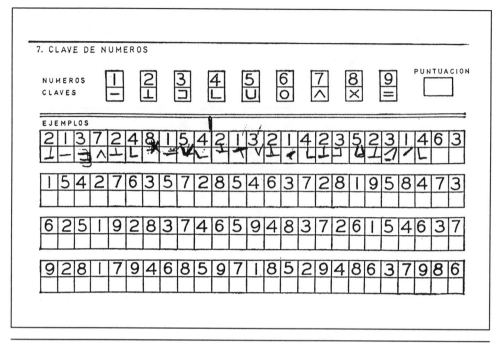

Figure 18.3: Digit Symbol subtest—WAIS.

Rehabilitation Exercises

The neuropsychological rehabilitation program for this alexic patient had three basic aims: (1) discriminatory perception of symbols, (2) automating processes, and (3) mechanical speed and comprehension.

1. *Discriminatory perception of symbols.* Given the patient's inability to recognize letters through the visual channel, the rehabilitation program began with exercises that involved vision only minimally. The patient was asked to

   - Feel the shape of letters cut out of fiberglass or wood with his index finger. The neuropsychologist traced the shapes of letters on the patient's hand; the patient had to identify them. The exercise continued with the examiner tracing the same letters as before in the air.
   - Simultaneously begin working on skills involving spatial coordinates (recognizing right and left, recognizing mirror-writing, drawing sketches of the room in the hospital or of rooms in the patient's home, identifying coordinates, including simple orders for placing objects).
   - Identify and memorize the shapes of letters (initially with letters that varied considerably in shape, and later, with letters that greatly resembled each other), and simplify these forms and associate them with others that the patient knew (e.g., "the letter *m* is formed by two bridges," "the letter *b* is a stick with a ball at the bottom on the right hand side," and "the letter *d* looks like the letter *b* but the ball is on the left").
   - Copy the letters studied. In each session two or three letters were proposed for study; the patient copied them several times, described their forms, and associated them with other forms that he knew. The previous

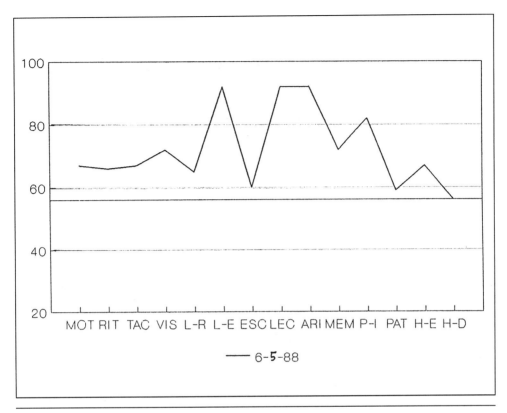

Figure 18.4: Profile of Luria-Nebraska Battery.

exercises of identification, reproduction in the air, memorizing shapes, and spatial coordinates were essential to the success of this copying exercise.

- Identify one of the letters studied. In a visual scan of a range of symbols mixed among letters that the patient had not studied and others that he had worked on in previous sessions, he had to identify certain specific letters.

These exercises became gradually more difficult as the program advanced, accommodating the patient's individual learning rhythm and incorporating the possibility of reinforcement at all times.

2. *Automating processes.* When the patient began to identify letters, the next step was to join the letters together into syllables and words. Since any links between letters disoriented the patient, the syllables or letters were initially written in different colors, until the patient could automatically identify them in only one color. In the same way, words were initially presented in multi-color and subsequently in one color only. This process began with words that were the most automatic for the patient such as his first name, his surnames, the name of the street on which he lived, days of the week, etc.

3. *Mechanical speed and comprehension.* The patient's right homonymous hemianopsia interfered markedly with reading speed. Three types of exercises were devised to address this problem:

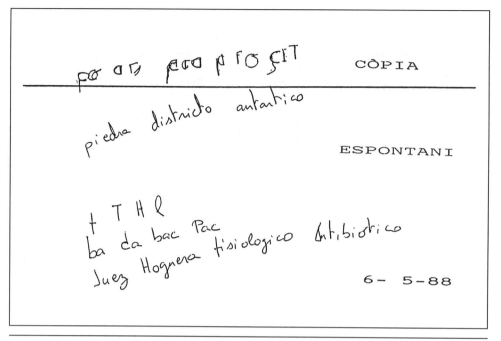

Figure 18.5: The Writing scale item.

- The patient had to become accustomed to following words (and later sentences) "at a glance" and to see that words and lines continued outside his limited field of vision. The examiner drew lines on a piece of paper and then longer lines on a blackboard; the patient had to "follow" them with his eyes. The time that he was allowed for the task decreased gradually as the test advanced.
- Using moving text and following the exercises described by Tsvétkova (1977), we constructed an imitation *cimometer* in order to accelerate the patient's eye movement and to increase his reading speed. This instrument consisted of two rotating cylinders moving at a constant speed, powered by a small homemade motor. A roll of paper was inserted showing prepared sentences and lined newspaper cuttings. The patient took an active part in producing this material. As the speed was constant, in order to increase the difficulty of the task, the size of the letters and headlines was gradually reduced.
- The exercise to intensify the movement of the right eye provided an activation of the visual field affected. A screen was used to limit the visual field to the right eye only.

Longitudinal Control

Control explorations of the test batteries administered in the first assessment were carried out. The first test-retest was performed four months after the start of the sessions and the second, nine months after the start of the program.

The longitudinal control of performance on the WAIS (Figure 18.6) shows a significant improvement. The subtests that predominantly saturated on the intelligence 'g' factor

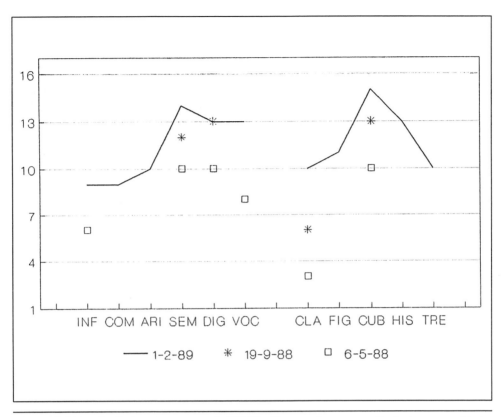

Figure 18.6: Longitudinal performance on the WAIS. □ = performance on the first assessment (prior to rehabilitation sessions). * = performance after four months of rehabilitation. ———— = performance nine months after the start of the sessions.

(Vocabulary, Similarities, Kohs' Blocks) tended to be at the upper limit of normality. There was a gradual, moderate improvement in performance on the Digit Symbol subtest; execution of the task was still slow, but there was a significant qualitative improvement.

In the Luria-Nebraska Battery (Figure 18.7), the different scales tended longitudinally to be at or below the critical level in the final test.

The Reading scale shows a positive evolution. The global alexia indicated in the first assessment evolved into a form of slow reading, mostly of polysyllabic words. Reading of monosyllables and frequently used words improved significantly.

Finally, Figures 18.8 and 18.9 show the evolution of the patient's ability to copy. Figure 18.8 refers to a copying exercise performed after a month of the program; in this task, the patient identified a letter that he had already studied. Clearly, the writing is very childish.

As recovery progressed, hospital rehabilitation sessions became less frequent, and during the maintenance phase, sessions took place in his home. These sessions included reading exercises, reading comprehension, verbal memory, and color association and identification. Various ways of resuming academic studies were considered, such as taking at courses at night schools, since the patient was not able to continue his university

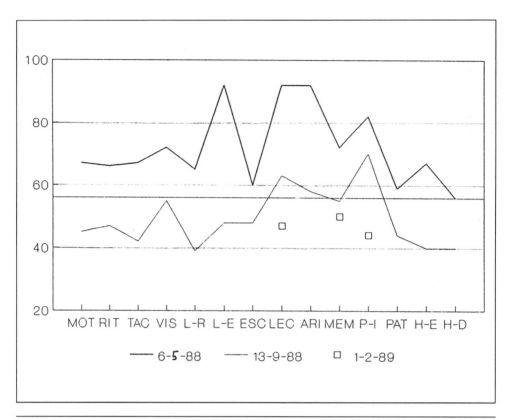

Figure 18.7: Longitudinal performance on the Luria-Nebraska Battery. The upper profile (————) indicates the first assessment prior to the start of the rehabilitation sessions. The ——— shows performance after four months of the rehabilitation program. The □ shows performance on some of the most critical scales (Reading, Memory, and Intellectual Processes) after nine months of sessions.

studies. After a number of false starts, he joined the fourth and fifth year courses in the Professional Training syllabus, studying electronics. His performance was satisfactory.

This account has not mentioned the psychological support that obviously is involved in all processes of rehabilitation. The patient, as in many cases of cranial trauma, was left by his girlfriend and often felt ignored by his group of friends. Although the rehabilitation of reading represented a psychological reinforcement, as he improved, the patient became aware that he would have to face radical changes in his studies, professional life, and personal life as well. A rehabilitation program, according to Luria (1947), is based on an awareness of the nature of the disturbed function and is adapted to the normal course of its development. Auxiliary techniques, modifications of forms in which the functions are usually performed, are used. Nonetheless, Luria warns, the process rarely culminates in the complete automatic recovery of the reorganized function.

WRITING IMPAIRMENTS AND REHABILITATION

In Spanish, there are various tools available for the exploration of writing ability: items from the TALE, the Reading and Writing Analysis Test (Cervera & Toro, 1980); from the PIENC, the Integrated Program of Computerized Neuropsychological Exploration

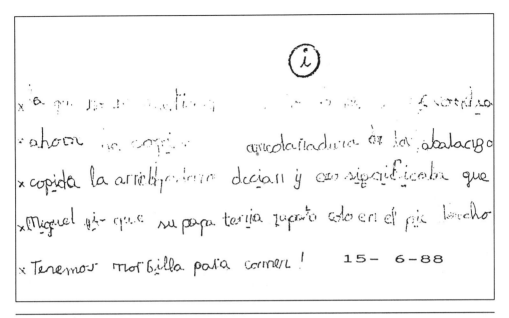

Figure 18.8: Handwriting in a copying exercise during rehabilitation.

(Peña, 1986); and the Luria-Nebraska Neuropsychological Battery (in its Spanish version by Boget, Hernández, & Marcos, 1988). The exploration should distinguish between mechanical and *praxic* disorders on the one hand, and neurolinguistic disorders such as *writing* agrammatism, paragrammatism, *paragraphias*, and *jargonagraphias* on the other. For a general review of these "writing" tests, see Lezak (1995).

The exploration uses materials of progressively increasing complexity: syllables, *logatomas*, words, phrases, and paragraphs. It includes several different methods: dictation, copying, and spontaneous writing.

Writing impairments are commonly associated with aphasia and alexia, as in the case of reading impairments. Pure agraphia is very rare (Peña & Pérez Pamies, 1984). The opposite, though rare, is more frequent (Marcos, 1986).

Obviously, it is necessary to distinguish between the various forms of dysgraphia, which, in general, are the consequence of craneoencephalic traumas, cerebral vascular accidents, cerebral tumors, and sequelae of other cerebral or systemic illnesses leading to disorders in learning to write (well described by Monfort, 1988). Cervera and Toro's Reading and Writing Analysis Test (TALE) (1980) facilitates this important task as it presents standardized materials in accordance with normal teaching levels (of the first through fourth years of Primary Education, ages 6–10). This material lends itself to a three-way analysis through dictation, copying, and spontaneous writing. Its level of complexity increases gradually, going from syllables to paragraphs, making it possible to determine the level of maturity of the subject's reading and writing.

The first task when taking on a writing rehabilitation program is to establish, as far as possible, the subject's premorbid level. Even in an environment with compulsory schooling, the existence of subjects with serious reading and writing difficulties due not to the sequelae of cerebral lesions but to deficiencies in the process of learning the corresponding skills should not be a cause for surprise. It is not only a characteristic of the postwar generation. These deficiencies can be seen only too often in television and

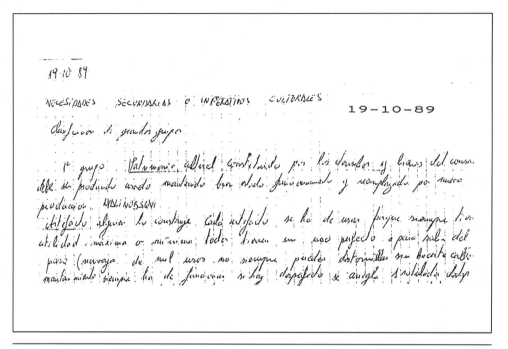

Figure 18.9: Handwriting in a copying exercise during patient's academic reintegration.

radio programs in which the audience participates, and in school classrooms throughout the educational system, even at the university level. There are a multitude of studies of dyslexias—a term which is, incidentally, a controversial one—and so they need not concern us here.

As in cases of normal development, we can say that, in general, subjects who have not reached a sufficient reading maturity are unlikely to be able to write well. In the field of dysgraphias, writing disorders are not usually considered to be independent of reading disorders or even language disorders. However, all authors report clinical cases that call into quesion the traditional models and, in a continuous feedback process, oblige cognitive and ecological neuropsychology to reformulate the processes of learning and acquiring the skills in particular environmental conditions other than those considered normal and call for specific strategies for the rehabilitation of the writing skill.

Sánchez Bernardos (1992) speaks of written language, including reading and writing disorders, under this heading. Although perhaps slightly simplistic, his division of dysgraphia into deep and surface phonology in the same way as the model proposed by cognitive neuropsychology for dyslexias is of considerable use in teaching. It lacks, in our view, some correlation with the corresponding organic cerebral impairments in each clinical case reported.

Types of Dysgraphias

By (phonological) dysgraphia is meant a writing impairment consisting of the inability to spell—to transcribe letters—in response to a sound stimulus. When we write spontaneously (this is not the case with dictated writing), we recover the meaning of the words that we wish to write (i.e., the semantic representation from a kind of "memory" or "graphemic system of word production" that contains many individual units of production

[Morton, 1980]). This model reveals the difference in performance of patients (Shallice, 1981) who can spell real words correctly in dictation but cannot spell pseudo-words.

A semantic writing error is to write "correctly" the word "moon" instead of "star"; a semantic reading error is to read "pixie" instead of "gnome," as did a patient reported by Marshall and Newcombe (1973), cited by Sánchez Bernardos (1992).

Although it may appear surprising, a "deep" dysgraphia may be found in a patient who maintains a good level of understanding of both spoken and written words, speaks in *telegraphic language,* and writes "table" instead of "chair," "watch" instead of "time," "give" instead of "take"—typical semantic errors—as observed in a patient reported by Bub and Kertesz (1982), also cited by Sánchez Bernardos (1992). According to this author, "surface" dysgraphia is a complex syndrome in which less frequent words do not have access to the units of production. If patients can recover the complete spelling of a word, they can write it correctly; if they cannot recover the word completely, access to a part of it helps them to write that part correctly and, by filling in the gaps, patients may occasionally be able to complete the entire word.

In our view, this background constitutes a good basis for programs designed to rehabilitate the ability to write. If patients can use elementary correspondences between phonemes and graphemes, they will be able to assemble a possible spelling for a particular word. In any case, as we said above, cerebral lesions rarely leave the channels needed for recovering the writing skill unharmed; indeed, patients' disorders normally affect reading as well.

The model of cerebral functionalism, *in practice antilocalizationism,* described by A. R. Luria (1973) and L.S. Tsvétkova in the field of language, reading, and writing retention (1977), continues to offer useful clues for the development of increasingly comprehensive models for the cognitive neuropsychology of language and for strategies of rehabilitation, in this case, of the ability to write.

We next outline Luria's methodology, as described in Tsvétkova (1977), for the rehabilitation of the writing skill. This is the methodology that has been used as a general framework in the Neuropsychology and Rehabilitation of Cognitive Functions Unit at the Hospital Clínic i Provincial in Barcelona.

REHABILITATION OF WRITING: METHODOLOGY

Writing, like reading and arithmetical calculation but unlike speaking, is the result of special training. It does not emerge spontaneously as a result of individual maturity or in imitation of the environment, as it is not a natural form of communication between children and the adults around them.

For this reason, the rehabilitation of writing begins with an attempt to reestablish concrete *sonic-literal operations,* and, at the same time (or very shortly afterwards), bases itself on the semantic regime of the discourse and the meaning of the word. The reconstruction of the functional system is a vital step in which an unharmed analyzer substitutes for the one that is affected, and writing can be produced in spite of the existence of a profound topical lesion of the brain.

This may appear hard to understand to someone who has not performed exercises aimed at the rehabilitation of writing (or of some other function) in patients (see Marcos, 1994).

In cases of *aneurysm breakdown of the anterior communicating artery* and in other serious vascular disorders, a wide range of sequelae affecting the functions of speaking, reading, writing, and arithmetic are often observed. Frequently, the patient retains little more than rudimentary ideogrammatic writing and sometimes not even this. Our first patient, JMVL, age 31, a policeman studying the third year of a university law degree, could only "draw" the five vowels by copying.

The first large-scale disturbance in these cases is the serious impairment of the auditive analysis of language, interfering with writing due to problems in the analysis of the sounds of the words.

The basic element in the rehabilitation of writing is the use of the unharmed analyzers: visual, kinesthetic, or articulatory-motor. The central task in cases of "sensorial agraphia" (following the terms used by the Soviet school for aphasic disorders; see Luria, 1947) is to reestablish a clear perception and awareness of each individual sound and the ability to separate it from the sound of the word as a whole. In practice, as the treatment includes both speaking and writing, the two functions reinforce each other.

In the initial stage, the treatment involves (though not to an excessive degree) the semantic sphere, which is generally intact. The ability to listen to speech has to be rehabilitated, as well as the ability to distinguish between and identify whole sentences or individual words. The length of this stage varies with each case, and no work is done on "writing" as such at this point. The therapist pronounces syllables and words slowly, loudly, and clearly, progressing gradually to short and then long sentences, ensuring at all times that the patient's *repetition is always followed by the establishment of the detailed relation of the visual and kinesthetic afferent* of the objects and actions. At all stages of the rehabilitation of writing (and of language in general), cue cards and other aids can be prepared to suit the specific characteristics of the patient.

In the second stage, patients are taught letters and sounds, and the treatment concentrates on increasing their ability to distinguish between sounds inside the words. The qualitative and quantitative structure of the word is externalized (Tsvétkova, 1977):

> the patient is given a sheet showing an object (a phenomenon, or an action) the name of which is a simple one- or two-syllable word. Below there is a quantitative diagram of the word in the form of small squares or lines, as in a crossword. The patient first hears the name of the object and then repeats it. S/he then begins to break down the word into individual sounds, using the mirror, the oral image. One after the other s/he writes down the separate sound in the square that corresponds to it. Initially words with the same first syllable are used, then words with the same two first syllables. This aids the patient's analytic work and focuses attention on the semantic and discriminatory role of sounds. The process continues with words beginning with the same sound, but followed by a different vowel. Later, to emphasize the interpretation of the positional relations of the phoneme, the sounds to be practised appear in the middle or at the end of the word. With time, the patient divides the word into syllables, counts the number of syllables, breaks down each syllable into different sounds, designs the right quantitative diagram and then fills it with the corresponding sounds....

With each word, the patient is asked, "What is the first sound of the word...? What is the fifth sound of the word? What sound comes after the '*a*' in the word '___'?" This type of exercise is found in the sections on reading and writing in Christensen's *Luria's Neuropsychological Investigation* (1974). The exercises are carried out aloud and use no external material resources.

At the end of this stage, a tape recorder is used to rehabilitate discrimination between sounds. The patient is presented with two different pronunciations of the same word and must choose the correct one. Sound and word dictations are used for the purposes of checking; the mistakes are analyzed and written correctly.

The third stage involves writing complete sentences. In the first two stages, resources extrinsic to writing in itself were used, such as touching the cheeks and throat during the phonation of unvoiced and voiced sounds; noting the air flow when pronouncing lisping and sibilant sounds; touching three-dimensional shapes of letters; using dermolexia and other essential aids to understanding spoken language and writing at these stages. Subsequently, the need for this backup gradually falls as the process becomes automatic and the productive flow increases. Sight and phonation are still the driving forces of the process, even when the patient has progressed to writing short dictated sentences.

As one would imagine, the total duration of the rehabilitation process varies greatly. In serious cases, it may easily surpass one year.

Although the methodology varies to an extent according to the lesions and disorders of each individual case, we have outlined what are in practice the most useful rehabilitation procedures on the basis of the specific guidelines proposed by the Soviet school and which, in our experience, function well.

We should stress again that patience is an essential quality for any psychologist interested in neurofunctional rehabilitation. Progress is slow, at times nonexistent, producing feelings of frustration in both the patient and the therapist. Therapists must transmit optimism to the patient and give their "classes" in an atmosphere that is relaxed and conducive to progress, even though they are aware that the success of the project may well only be relative.

REFERENCES

Bagunya, J. (1987). La exploración de la lectura y la escritura. In J. Peña (Ed.), *La exploración neuropsicológica*. Barcelona: MCR.

Boget, T., Hernández, E., & Marcos, T. (1988). Versión castellana de la batería neuropsicológica Luria-Nebraska. *Rev. Psiquiatría. Fac. Med. Barna., 15(3),* 121–132.

Bub, D. & Kerstesz, A. (1982). Deep agraphia. *Brain and Language, 17,* 146–165.

Cervera, M. & Toro, J. (1980). *Test de análisis de lectoescritura: TALE.* Madrid: Pablo del Rio.

Christensen, A.L. (1973). *El diagnóstico neuropsicológico de Luria.* Madrid: Pablo del Rio Editor.

Dejerine, J., & Vialet, N. (1893). Contribution à l'étude de la localisation anatomique de la cécité verbale pure. *CR Hebd. Séances Mém. Soc. Biol., 5,* 790–793.

Golden, C.J., Hammeke, T.A., & Purish, A.D. (1980). *The Luria-Nebraska Neuropsychological Battery.* Los Angeles: Western Psychological Services.

Goodglass, H., & Kaplan, E. (1974). *Evaluación de la afasia y trastornos similares.* Buenos Aires: Panamericana.

Hecaen, H. (1977). *Afasias y apraxias.* Buenos Aires: Paidos.

Kertesz, A., & Poole, E. (1974). The aphasia quotient: The taxonomic approach to measurement of aphasia disability. *Can. J. Neurol. Sci., 1,* 7–16.

León-Carrión, J. (1994). *Daño cerebral: Guía para familiares y cuidadores.* Madrid: Siglo XXI de España Editores.

Lezak, M.D. (1995). *Neuropsychological assessment: Verbal functions* (pp. 312–341). New York: Oxford University Press.

Luria, A.R. (1947). *Traumatic aphasia: Its syndromes, psychology and treatment* (Russian). Moscow. (English trans. 1970, The Hague: Mouton).

———. (1973). *The working brain: An introduction to neuropsychology.* Harmondsworth: Penguin Books, Ltd.

Marcos, T. (1986). Alexia sin agrafia: Evolución neuropsicológica de un caso en tratamiento. *Rev. Psiquiatría Fac. Med. Barna., 13(3),* 153–154.

_____. (1994). *Neuropsicología clínica: Más allá de la psicometría.* Barcelona: Doyma Libros.

Marshall, J. & Newcombe, F. (1973). Patterns of paralexia. *Journal of Psycholinguistics Research, 2,* 175–199.

Monfort, M. (1988). Los trastornos del aprendizaje del lenguaje escrito. In J. Peña (Ed.), *Manual de logopedia.* Barcelona: Masson S.A.

Morton, J. (1980). The logogen model and orthographic structure. In U. Frith (Ed.), *Cognitive processes in spelling.* London: Academic Press.

Orgogozo, J.M., & Péré, J.J. (1991). *L'alexie sans agraphie.* Rapport de Neurologie. LXXXIX e Session. La Rochelle, June.

Peña Casanova, J. (1986). *Programa integrado de exploración neuropsicológica computadorizada.* PIENC-Barcelona, 86. Tesis, Universidad de Navarra, Pamplona.

Sánchez, M.L. (1992). Lenguaje escrito: Trastornos de la lectura y la escritura. In L. Manning (Ed.), *Introducción a la neuropsicología clásica y cognitiva del lenguaje: Teoría, evaluación y rehabilitación de la afasia.* Madrid: Trotta.

Shallice, T. (1981). Phonological agraphia and the lexical route in writing. *Brain, 104,* 413-429.

Tsvetkova, L.S. (1977). *Reeducación del lenguaje, la lectura y la escritura.* Barcelona: Fontanella.

Walsh, K.W. (1982). Neuropsychological aspects of rehabilitation following brain injury. In J.F. Garret (Ed.), *International exchange of information in rehabilitation* (Vol. 19) (pp. 36–40).

19 Rehabilitation of Calculation Disorders

Mónica Rosselli and Alfredo Ardila

Miami Institute of Psychology
Miami, Florida

INTRODUCTION

The ability to calculate is highly sensitive to brain injury. The loss of the ability to perform calculation tasks resulting from a cerebral pathology is called *acalculia* or *acquired dyscalculia*. The defects in learning numerical dexterities are usually known as *developmental dyscalculia* or simply, *dyscalculia*.

According to the DSM-IV (American Psychiatric Association, 1994), the Mathematics Disorder is diagnosed when an individual receives significantly lower scores on standardized calculation tests or on numerical reasoning. These difficulties are found to be below what they should be for the age, education, and intellectual capability of the subject and interfere with his/her academic achievements and his/her daily life activities. Mathematics Disorder, as defined in DSM-IV, corresponds to both developmental dyscalculia and acquired acalculia.

HISTORICAL DEVELOPMENT OF THE CONCEPT OF ACALCULIA

The term *acalculia* was proposed by Henschen (1925) and defined as "the impairments in mathematical skills resulting from brain injury." The distinction between primary and secondary acalculia was introduced by Berger in 1926. Primary acalculia corresponds to the loss of numerical concepts and to the ability to understand or execute basic arithmetic operations. Secondary acalculia refers to the defect in calculation derived from a different cognitive deficit: memory, attention, language, etc. Some authors have questioned the existence of acalculia as an independent cognitive deficit (Goldstein, 1948; Collington et al., 1977).

Gerstmann (1940) proposed that primary acalculia is associated with agraphia, right-left disorientation, and digital agnosia, forming a single syndrome that since then has been known as "Gerstmann syndrome." Imaginological methods have shown a correlation between the Gerstmann syndrome and left posterior parietal injuries (Mazzoni et al., 1990).

Lindquist (1936) identified different types of acalculia associated with lesions in different brain areas. As a result, several classifications of acalculias have been presented (Hecaen, Angelergues, & Houillaer, 1961; Ardila & Rosselli, 1990, 1992). Different types of errors in the performance of arithmetic operations have been observed in patients with right and left hemispheric injuries (Rosselli & Ardila, 1989; Levin, Goldstein, & Spiers, 1993).

Boller and Grafman (1983) believe that calculation skills can be altered as a result of (1) inability to appreciate the significance of the names of numbers, (2) visual-spatial defects that interfere with the spatial organization of the numbers and the mechanical aspects of the operations, (3) inability to remember mathematical facts and to appropriately use them, and (4) defects in mathematical thought and in the comprehension of the underlying operations. Perhaps the ability to conceptualize quantities (numerosity) and invert operations (adding and subtracting) could be added (Ardila & Rosselli, 1992).

The concept of numbers can be associated with the presence of at least four factors: (1) immediate representation of quantity, implicit in the number; (2) understanding the numerical position within the system of other numerical symbols (i.e., its position in the series of digits and its place in class); (3) understanding the relationships between a number and other numbers; and (4) understanding the relationships between numerical symbols and their verbal representations (Tsvetkova, 1996).

McCloskey and collaborators (1985, 1986, 1991) and McCloskey and Caramazza (1987) have proposed a cognitive model regarding the processing of numbers and the relationship of arithmetic operations. This model includes a distinction between the processing system of numbers that includes the understanding mechanism and the production of numbers, in addition to the numerical calculation system that includes the necessary processing components to accomplish mathematical operations. In the event of brain injury, these components can be disassociated (Dagenbach & McCloskey, 1992; Pesenti, Seron, & Van Der Linden, 1994). The principles (multiplication tables), rules (N $\times 0 = 0$), and procedures (right to left multiplication) form part of the numerical calculation system. Errors of calculation observed in patients with brain injury and in normal subjects can result in inappropriate recall of principles, inadequate use of rules, and/or errors in procedures. The cognitive models have helped to establish similarities between acquired acalculias and developmental dyscalculias (Temple, 1991).

CLASSIFICATION OF ACALCULIAS

Several classifications have been proposed for acalculias (Ardila & Rosselli, 1990; Grafman, 1988; Grafman et al., 1982; Hecaen et al., 1961; Levin, Goldstein, & Speirs, 1993). The most traditional classification distinguishes between primary acalculia and secondary acalculia. Luria (1977) establishes a distinction between optical acalculia, frontal acalculia, and primary acalculia. Hecaen, Angelergues, and Houiller (1961) consider three types of disorders in calculation: alexia and agraphia for numbers, spatial acalculia, and anarithmetia.

Integrating the classifications mentioned above, the following six types of acalculia can be distinguished: (1) anarithmetia, (2) aphasic acalculia, (3) alexic acalculia, (4) agraphic acalculia, (5) frontal acalculia, and (6) spatial acalculia (Ardila & Rosselli, 1990). Primary acalculia corresponds to anarithmetia. The other forms of acalculia represent secondary acalculias (Table 19.1).

Table 19.1: Classification of Acalculias

PRIMARY ACALCULIA	Anarithmetia
SECONDARY ACALCULIAS	Aphasic Acalculia
	In Broca's aphasia
	In Wernicke's aphasia
	In conduction aphasia
	Alexic Acalculia
	In central alexia
	In pure alexia
	Agraphic Acalculia
	Frontal Acalculia
	Spatial Acalculia
DEVELOPMENTAL DYSCALCULIA	Anarithmetia
	Alexic-agraphic
	Attentional-sequential (Frontal)
	Spatial
	Mixed

Diverse groups of defects have also been noted in children with developmental dyscalculia: (1) dyscalculia secondary to alexia and agraphia for numbers, (2) sequential-attentional dyscalculia, (3) spatial dyscalculia, (4) developmental anarithmetia, and (5) mixed dyscalculia (Bandia, 1983; Shalev, Weirtman, & Amir, 1988). Kosc (1970) describes six types of difficulties observed in developmental dyscalculia: (1) in the verbalization of numbers and mathematical procedures, (2) in the management of mathematical symbols/objects, (3) in the reading of numbers, (4) in the writing of numbers, (5) in the understanding of mathematical ideas, and (6) in the "carrying over" when performing arithmetic operations.

It is common to find developmental dyscalculia associated with dyslexia (Rosselli & Ardila, 1992). Some authors still believe that dyscalculia does not appear as an isolated manifestation of cerebral dysfunction but as a part of developmental Gerstmann syndrome (PeBenito, 1987; PeBenito et al., 1988).

ANARITHMETIA

Anarithmetia corresponds to primary acalculia. The patient with anarithmetia presents a loss of numerical concepts, an inability to understand quantities, deficits in the execution of basic mathematical operations, inability to use syntactical rules in calculation (such as "carrying over"), and frequent confusion of arithmetic signs (Ferro & Botelho, 1980). Hécaen, Angelergues, and Houiller (1961) found a superposition between anarithmetia and alexia and agraphia for numbers. In a sample of 73 patients with anarithmetia, they found that 62% had aphasia, 61% constructional errors, 54% visual field defects, 50% general cognitive deficits, 39% verbal alexia, 37% somatosensory defects, 37% right-left confusion, and 33% ocumolomotor defects. Their sample, however, was too heterogeneous, and acalculia could easily be correlated with other neurological and neuropsychological defects.

It is not easy to find cases of pure anarithmetia without additional aphasic defects. The patient must present errors in the performance of both oral and written arithmetical operations. Usually, the patient presents errors in the management of mathematical concepts and incorrectly uses arithmetic symbols. Rosselli and Ardila (1989) analyzed the errors made by patients with left parietal injuries. These patients exhibited defects in oral and written calculations, 75% of the patients confused symbols, and all made errors in transcoding tasks, in successive operations, and in solving mathematical problems. Although it is uncommon to find cases of pure anarithmetia caused by focal lesions in the brain, in cases of dementia, it is routine to find at least a certain degree of anarithmetia (Ardila & Rosselli, 1987; Grafman et al., 1989; Parlato et al., 1992).

APHASIC ACALCULIA

Calculation difficulties are generally found in aphasic patients, correlated with their linguistic defects. As a result, patients with Wernicke's aphasia exhibit their verbal memory defects in the performance of numerical calculations. Patients with Broca's aphasia have difficulties handling the syntax when applied to calculations. In conduction aphasia, repetition defects affect mental successive operations and counting backwards. This means that the calculation defects are correlated with general linguistic difficulties in aphasic patients (Grafman et al., 1982).

Acalculia in Broca's aphasia

Dahmen et al. (1982) observed that patients with Broca's aphasia presented disorders in numerical-symbolic calculations derived from their linguistic defects. Deloche and Seron (1982, 1987) found syntactical errors in patients with Broca's aphasia. They presented errors in counting backwards and in mental successive operations (e.g., 100,93,87...; or 1,4,7...). They also exhibited hierarchy (e.g., 5–50, especially in reading) and order (e.g., 5–6, especially in writing) errors. In transcoding tasks, the omission of grammatical particles was also observed. In addition, "carrying over" was difficult for them.

The use of grammar and syntax is difficult in patients with Broca's aphasia, and this is reflected in transcoding from a verbal to a numerical code. The patient presents difficulties reading and interpreting indicative grammatical elements of the numerical position within a class (e.g., when reading three-hundred-fifty-thousand-two-hundred [350,200], they have difficulty reading and understanding the words "hundred" and "thousand," consequently presenting hierarchy mistakes [e.g., 30050000200]). Broca's aphasia can be interpreted as a disorder in the sequencing of language. The production of numerical sequences is impaired in these patients (Rosselli & Ardila, 1989).

Acalculia in Wernicke's Aphasia

Patients with Wernicke's aphasia present semantic and lexical errors in reading and writing numbers. Dahman and collaborators (1982) suggest that calculation errors in Wernicke aphasics are correlated with their defects in visual-spatial processing. Luria (1977) suggests that calculation errors in patients with acoustic-amnesic aphasia depend on their defects in verbal memory. This is particularly noticeable in the solution of numerical problems, when the patient has to remember certain conditions of the problem. When the patient is asked about numerical facts (i.e., "How many days are there in a year?"), paraphasic errors are evident. The meaning of the words is weakened, and this is also valid for the meaning of numbers. Lexical errors are abundant in different types of tasks. Benson and Denckla (1969) stress the presence of verbal paraphasias as an important source of calculation errors in these patients. When writing dictated numbers, patients with Wernicke's aphasia may write completely irrelevant numbers (e.g., the patient is given the number 257, repeats 820, and finally, writes 193), exhibiting a loss of the sense of language. In reading, they show errors by decomposition (463 —> 46, 3). Mental operations, successive operations, and the solution of numerical problems appear equally difficult for these patients (Rosselli & Ardila, 1989).

Acalculia in Conduction Aphasia

Patients with conduction aphasia (afferent motor aphasia or verbal apraxia) present very important calculation errors. They may fail in the performance of both mental and written operations. They have serious flaws in performing successive operations and in problem solving. In reading numbers, errors of decomposition, order, and hierarchy appear. They usually fail in "carrying over," in the general use of calculation syntax, and even in the reading of arithmetic signs (Rosselli & Ardila, 1989). All of this together could be interpreted as anarithmetia. However, it should be addressed that the topography of the damage in conduction aphasia can be similar to the topography of the damage in anarithmetia. Conduction aphasia, as well as anarithmetia, have been correlated with left parietal brain injury. The association is not coincidental.

ALEXIC ACALCULIA

Defects in calculation can be correlated with general difficulties in reading. This represents an alexic acalculia or alexia for numbers. Four basic types of alexia have been described: central alexia, pure alexia, frontal alexia, and spatial alexia. Calculation errors observed in frontal alexia were analyzed when describing acalculia in the Broca's aphasia, and errors in calculation in spatial alexia will be analyzed when describing spatial acalculia.

Acalculia in Central Alexia

Parietal-temporal alexia (central alexia or aphasic alexia) includes the inability to read numbers or other symbolic systems (such as musical notes). However, in these patients, reading digits is usually superior to reading letters. Occasionally, the patient may be unable to decide if a symbol corresponds to a letter or a number. Written mathematical operations are seriously impaired, and mental execution is superior. Although the distinction between alexia with number agraphia and anarithmetia is conceptually valid, in practice, it is difficult to establish. The brain topography of the two syndromes is similar, corresponding to the left angular gyrus. Usually alexia for numbers and arithmetic signs is associated with alexia for letters, certain agraphia, and some aphasic disorders.

Acalculia in Alexia without Agraphia

Alexia without agraphia or occipital alexia is mainly a verbal alexia in which there is recognition of letters but not of words. The patient, therefore, presents greater difficulties in reading numbers composed of several digits (compound numbers) than in reading single digits. When reading compound numbers, the patient exhibits decomposition

(27 becomes 2,7) and hierarchy errors (50 becomes 5). When reading words, letters placed on the left are generally understood better than letters placed on the right. Likewise, in reading numbers, only the first or first digits are read correctly, and a certain degree of right hemi-neglect is observed (5637 becomes 563). Due to the alexia, performing written operations is difficult and even impossible. As a result of visual exploration and attention defects, listing numbers in columns and "carrying over" are tasks in which the patient usually fails. It is important to stress that reading is performed from left to right (in Western languages, at least), but the performance of arithmetic operations goes from right to left. This disparity may create problems in patients with visual attention problems.

AGRAPHIC ACALCULIA

Calculation errors may appear as a result of an inability to write quantities. The calculation deficit may be a function of the type of agraphia. In the agraphia associated with Broca's aphasia, the writing of numbers will be non-fluent, with some perseveration and order errors. In transcoding tasks, from the numerical code to the verbal code, grammatical and letter omissions appear. The patient presents difficulties in the production of written numerical sequences (1,2,3...), particularly backwards (10,9,8...) (Ardila & Rosselli, 1990).

In Wernicke's aphasia, there is a fluent agraphia for numbers. Due to verbal comprehension defects, the patient presents errors in writing number dictation and even writes totally irrelevant numbers (428 becomes 2530). Lexical errors (numerical verbal paragraphias) and fragmentation (25 becomes 20,5) are observed. In conduction aphasia, there is a very significant agraphic defect is in the writing of numbers. The patient seems unable to convert the number that he/she has heard and even repeated to himself/herself in graphic form. Order, hierarchy, and inversion errors are observed (Rosselli & Ardila, 1989).

Apraxic agraphia impairs the performance of motor sequences required to write letters. Writing numbers becomes slow and difficult, and permanent self-corrections appear.

In cases of motor agraphia, the difficulties observed in writing letters and words are also going to be observed when writing numbers. In paretic agraphia, numbers are large and clumsily formed. In hypokinetic agraphia, difficulties in starting the motor activity are evident, as micrography and progressive narrowing of numbers appear. In hyperkinetic agraphia, numbers are usually large, hard to read, and distorted; frequently the patient is unable to write.

FRONTAL ACALCULIA

Patients with prefrontal injuries frequently develop calculation difficulties that are not easily detected. These patients show difficulties in performing mental (written operations are superior) and successive operations, and in the solutions of mathematical problems. The pattern of errors in frontal acalculia includes attention defects, perseveration, and the loss of complex mathematical concepts. Attention deficits are reflected in the patient's difficulty in maintaining concentration on the problem. Perseveration is observed in the tendency to continue presenting the very same response to different conditions. Perseveration also appears in writing and reading numbers. When trying to solve mathematical problems the patient may present difficulties in simultaneously handling diverse information from the same problem and may even be unable to understand the nature of the problem. Instead of solving the mathematical problem, the patient with frontal acalculia may simply repeat it. The above defects are reflected in the abnormal handling of complex mathematical concepts.

SPATIAL ACALCULIA

Spatial acalculia is observed in patients with right hemispheric damage, particularly parietal. It frequently coexists with hemi-spatial neglect, spatial alexia and agraphia, constructional difficulties, and other spatial disorders. Mental calculation is superior to written calculation in these patients No difficulties are in counting nor in performing successive operations. A certain degree of fragmentation appears in the reading of numbers (523 becomes 23) resulting from left hemi-spatial neglect. Reading complex numbers, in which the spatial position is critical, is affected (1003 becomes 103), and inversions are noted (32 becomes 23) (Ardila & Rosselli, 1990, 1994).

The difficulties observed in writing numbers are common across all written tasks: exclusive use of the right half of the page, digit iterations (227 becomes 22277) and feature iterations (particularly in the number 3), inability to maintain the direction in writing, spatial disorganization, and writing over segments of the page already used. When performing written arithmetic operations, the patient understands how much should be "carried over" (or "borrowed") but cannot find where to place the carried over quantity. Also, the inability to align numbers in columns prevents such patients from performing written arithmetic operations. When performing multiplication, the difficulty in remembering multiplication tables becomes obvious, a defect correlated with the general difficulty in making use of automatic levels of language. These patients frequently mix procedures up (e.g., when they should subtract, they add). This is related to another frequently found defect: they do not seem surprised by impossible results (reasoning errors). For instance, the result of subtraction is larger than the original number being subtracted. This type of error in arithmetical reasoning has also been noted in children with developmental dyscalculia.

Ardila and Rosselli (1994) studied calculation errors in a sample of 21 patients. Spatial defects that interfered with the reading and writing of numbers and with the loss of arithmetic automatisms (e.g., multiplication tables) were found. The processing system seems changed in these patients while the numerical calculation system is partially preserved. Difficulties in calculation procedures and problems in the recall of arithmetic principles were observed; however, arithmetic rules were intact. The authors conclude that the numerical changes observed in patients with right hemisphere injury are due to (1) visual-spatial defects that interfere with the spatial organization of numbers and mechanical aspects of the mathematical operations, (2) inability to evoke mathematical facts and remember their appropriate uses, and (3) inability to normally conceptualize quantities and to process numbers.

In summary, in the case of cerebral pathology, it is possible to find very different types of disorders in calculation skills. Some of them represent a disability derived from defects (oral and written) in language. Others are closely correlated with spatial defects (spatial acalculia), frontal deficits (frontal acalculia), or primary defects in the performance of arithmetic tasks (anarithmetia).

DEVELOPMENTAL DYSCALCULIA

The term developmental dyscalculia refers to a difficulty learning to perform arithmetic operations that prevents an adequate academic performance. Usually, the general intellectual capability of these children is normal. It is estimated that approximately 6% of school-age children in the United States suffer from this disorder (Grafman, 1988). It is often the case that children with difficulties in writing and reading present problems in mathematical learning as well (Rosselli, 1992).

Ronsenberger (1989) found that visual-perceptual and attention disorders were evident in children who had specific difficulties in mathematics. Strang and Rourke (1985) not only support the presence of difficulties in visual-perceptual organization in children with dyscalculia, but they also describe difficulties in the tactile analysis of objects, particularly with the left hand, as well as in the interpretation of facial and emotional expressions (Rourke, 1987). Children with dyscalculia also present an inadequate prosody in verbal language (Rourke, 1988), difficulties in the interpretation of nonverbal events (Loveland et al., 1990), and emotional adaptation problems. These neuropsychological findings have suggested the presence of a functional immaturity of the right hemisphere as a structural fact underlying the acalculia.

The errors found in children with dyscalculia can be classified into seven categories (Strang & Rourke, 1985): (1) errors in spatial organization, (2) errors in visual attention, (3) procedural errors, (4) graphic-motor errors, (5) judgment and reasoning errors, (6) memory errors, and (7) perseveration.

CALCULATION EVALUATION

The assessment of calculation abilities in a patient with brain injury usually has three objectives:

1. To determine if sufficient difficulties in calculation exist to confirm acalculia.
2. To establish what type of acalculia patients exhibit and if the underlying deficit compromises the number system (positional and ordinal value) or their processing system (mathematical relations and arithmetic operations).
3. To determine the profile of mathematical errors in order to be able to develop a rehabilitation plan.

Although the majority of neuropsychologists agree that a cognitive evaluation would not be complete without considering mathematical skills (Lezak, 1995), there are few of the standardized tests that evaluate calculation. Generally, the most frequently used test is the arithmetic subtest of the Wechsler Intelligence Scale for Children (WISC) (Wechsler, 1991) and for adults, the Wechsler Adult Intelligence Scale (WAIS) (Wechsler, 1955, 1981). This subtest has two limitations: it evaluates only one aspect of the numerical processing (problem solving), and it also is difficult to give to patients with language problems since it is administered verbally. Some authors (Grafman et al., 1982; Deloche et al., 1994; Rosselli & Ardila, 1989; Warrington, 1982) have developed evaluation procedures directed to populations with brain injury. The demographic effects of age, sex, and educational level on calculation skills in a normal population are carefully analyzed by Deloche and his collaborators (1994).

The principle points to be considered in developing a test battery to evaluate calculation skills are as follows:

1. Oral counting forward and backwards.
2. Writing numbers forward and backwards.
3. Reading simple and complex numbers.
4. Writing simple and complex numbers of different levels of complexity.

5. Transcoding numbers from verbal code to numerical code and vice versa.
6. Establishing the number value: relationships between "larger" and "smaller" numbers.
7. Recognizing and writing arithmetic symbols.
8. Performing mental arithmetic operations given orally (including the four arithmetic operations).
9. Executing written arithmetic operations (including the four arithmetic operations).
10. Executing successive arithmetic operations (addition and subtraction).
11. Organizing numbers in columns so they can be added.
12. Solving of numerical problems.
13. Demonstrating numerical knowledge (days of the week, months of the year, etc.).

A detailed description of each one of these subtests goes beyond the objectives of this chapter and can be found in Deloche and collaborators (1994) and in Rosselli and Ardila (1989).

REHABILITATION OF CALCULATION ABILITIES

The majority of brain-injured patients (especially in vascular and traumatic injury cases) present some spontaneous cognitive recovery during the first months after the injury. Afterwards, the spontaneous recovery curve becomes slower and requires the implementation of rehabilitation programs to achieve some additional improvement (Lomas & Kertesz, 1978).

Two strategies have been proposed to achieve the rehabilitation of cognitive difficulties: the reactivation of the lost function and the development of an alternative strategy that achieves the same result through an *alternative* procedure. The majority of rehabilitation models for aphasias, alexias, and agraphias have emphasized the second strategy, which implies a cognitive reorganization (Seron, 1982) or a "functional system" reorganization (Luria, 1977). A solid model applicable to calculation rehabilitation still does not exist. Rehabilitation of calculation abilities is treated frequently in a superficial way or even ignored by many neuropsychological clinics. There are few investigative efforts directed at studying diverse procedures in calculation rehabilitation. Acalculia is usually evaluated and rehabilitated as a function dependent on language.

A test battery developed specifically to evaluate acalculia should be used to analyze the disturbances of calculation in a patient with brain injury. Variables such as the patient's educational level and occupational activity should be carefully considered.

Once the presence of acalculia is determined, a quantitative and qualitative analysis of the patient's errors in different sections of the test battery should be performed. Table 19.2 presents a description of the most frequent types of errors observed in patients with different types of acalculia.

The reorganization of the procedures that underlie a calculation defect requires clarity about the altered numerical process and how the latter interacts within normal behavior. The justification of the rehabilitation plan should be based on the limitation that acalculia has in the patient's occupational and social life. The patient should preserve sufficient cognitive capability that will allow him/her the reorganization of a new behavior or alternative strategy (Seron, 1984; De Partz, 1986).

In the following sections, techniques that have been developed in order to rehabilitate patients with primary and secondary acalculias are presented. The majority of the methods

Table 19.2: Classification of the Types of Errors in Acalculias (adapted from Ardila & Rosselli, 1994; Levin et al., 1993; Rosselli & Ardila, 1989; Spiers, 1987)

Type of Error	Description	Type of Acalculia
1. Errors in digits		
Number value	Inability to distinguish the larger of two numbers, due to flaws in differentiating between tens, hundreds, etc... (Ex: 97 vs. 306)	Anarithmetia
Number expansion (Lexicalization)	Numbers are written as they sound without integrating tens, hundreds, etc. (Ex: 3620 is written 300060020)	Aphasic (Wernicke's)
Decomposition	Numbers are read without considering the number as a whole (Ex: 127 is read as 12, 7)	Anarithmetia Aphasic (Wenicke and Conduction)
Mirror rotation or inversions	Numbers are copied, written and repeated in the reverse order (Ex: 21 is written as 12). This rotation can be partial (Ex: 2456 is written as 2465)	Spatial Posterior Aphasias
Substitutions	A number is substituted by another due to paralexia, paraphasia or paragraphia, affecting the result of an operation	
	1. Hierarchy errors; the number is substituted by another from a different position of series (Ex: 5 -> 50)	Posterior aphasics
	2. Order errors: The substitution is by another from the same series (Ex: 5 -> 6)	Aphasia (Posterior and Anterior) Anarithmetia
Omission	One or several digits are omitted (can be on the left or right side)	Spatial Pure alexia
Additions	A digit is inappropriately repeated upon writing it (Ex: 23 -> 233) Addition of traits to a digit (Usually 3) Addition of numbers previously presented can be a perseveration	Spatial Frontal
Errors in transcoding	When numbers are passed from one code to another code (numerical to verbal or vice versa), decomposition, order, omission or addition errors are noted.	Aphasic Anarithmetia
2. Errors in "carrying over"		
Omission	The patient does not "carry over"	Anarithmetia
Incorrect "carrying over"	Any "carrying over" error with acalculia (Ex: 254+189=41413)	All acalculias
Incorrect placement	"Carries over" correctly but adds in the wrong column (Ex: 254+119=463)	Spatial
3. Borrowing errors		
Borrowing zero	Difficulties or confusion if the arithmetic operation has a zero	Anarithmetia
Omits borrowing	The last digit on the left is not reduced despite verbalizing the loan (Ex: 524–92=532)	Frontal acalculia
Defective borrowing	Adding the borrowed quantity incorrectly; borrowing unnecessarily	Anarithmetia
4. Errors in basic principles		
Multiplication tables	Incorrect recall; usually, the patient tries to correct it with additions in series	Spatial
Zero	Fundamental errors are observed when a zero is present	Anarithmetia Aphasic
5. Errors in Algorithms		
Incomplete	Initiates operation correctly but is not capable of finishing	Frontal
Spatial:	a. Inappropriate use of space on the paper limiting the correct response	Spatial

Table 19.2: Classification of the Types of Errors in Acalculias Cont.

	b. Inappropriate use of columns in arithmetic operations	Spatial

	Ex: 678 825
	    +32 x15
	    998 4125
	         825
	        4950	

Incorrect sequence	Initiates the operation from left to right	Anarithmetia
Inappropriate algorithms	Numbers are organized spatially on the page for a different operation than the desired one (Ex: In multiplication, the numbers are placed to be divided)	Anarithmetia Spatial
Mixed procedures	Different operations are used in the same problem. (Ex: Adds in one column and multiplies in another)	Spatial
Reasoning errors	The subject does not realize that the result is impossible (Ex: The result is larger than what was subtracted)	Spatial
6. Errors in symbols		
Forgetting	The patient cannot remember nor write the four arithmetic signs	Anarithmetia
Substitution	The sign is substituted by another that is different from what was asked	Spatial Acalculia

described have been implemented in individual cases. Until now, no study exists that evaluates the effectiveness of these techniques in large samples of patients.

Primary Acalculia Rehabilitation

Primary acalculia or anarithmetia is associated with parietal or parietal-occipital injuries (Ardila & Rosselli, 1992). Tsvetkova (1996) considers that underlying primary acalculia is an alteration in the spatial perception and representation of numbers along with defects in verbal organization of spatial perception. The alteration in spatial coordination systems constitutes a central underlying defect in this type of acalculia (Luria, 1977; Tsvetkova, 1996). These patients present defects in numerical concepts, in understanding number positions, and in the performance of arithmetic procedural sequences and often make mistakes in recognizing arithmetic symbols.

In patients who have primary acalculia combined with semantic aphasia (and according to some authors, this combination is constant) (Luria, 1977; Ardila, 1993; Ardila, Lopez, & Solano, 1989), the comprehension defects extend themselves to logic-grammar relationships in language. In cases of semantic aphasia, numbers lose their relationship with the conceptual system and are perceived in a concrete and isolated manner (Tsvetkova, 1996).

These patients present numerous errors in the "larger than" and "smaller than" tests (Table 19.2), perceiving the number 86 as larger than 112, since they consider the independent value of each number. Although the concrete denomination of digits (reading digits) is preserved, it is impossible for them to use abstract numerical concepts. They are unable to recognize the number of tens and hundreds included in the number (e.g., in 800) or of understanding the content of relationships such as 30 = 10 + 10 +10. According to Tsvetkova (1996), anarithmetia is characterized by the loss of the numerical system and of the internal relationships of numbers within the decimal system.

Tsvetkova proposes a structured rehabilitation plan for anarithmetia aimed at recovering the understanding of the composition of numbers and their positional value. Initially, the patient relearns the concept of numbers by performing tasks consisting of putting together real objects (tokens or sticks) and illustrations that contain the corresponding numbers. The tasks consist of dividing the objects into groups (initially, alike, and afterwards, different), counting the number of objects in each group, finding the illustration that represents the corresponding number, placing it in each group, deciding how many of these numbers are found in the given amount, and finally, writing the number on a sheet of paper.

Once the patient has reacquired the concept of digits and tens, he/she moves on to developing the concept of numerical composition, interrelationships between numbers, and the possibility of operating with them. Then, numerical denomination exercises (beginning with the second tenth) and comprehension exercises between the name of the number and its position are initiated. The patient begins to understand that the name of the number indicates its positional value and the left to right reading indicates to him/her a decreasing positional value (e.g., 154: one-hundred and fifty-four). During this time, the positional composition of the numbers and their quantitative significance depending on their place in the series is worked on. Tsvetkova emphasizes the importance of using concrete mediators like tokens. When the patient also presents anomia for numbers, one should work on the reestablishment of the naming of numbers.

The understanding of numbers constitutes a recurring learning process in order to relearn the arithmetic operations. This relearning should always be initiated in the most explicit and concrete way possible, using external aides such as outlines, drawings, etc. Verbalizing aloud the steps that should be followed is generally useful. As patients improve, they go from speaking aloud to murmuring, then to "speaking to themselves." Training for particular problems (i.e., 9×0) can lead to the recuperation of arithmetic rules ($n \times 0 = 0$) (McCloskey, Aliminos, & Sokol, 1991). The training for particular problems or operations within the rehabilitation sessions leads then to the comprehension of arithmetic principles and rules.

Understanding calculation direction should be worked on simultaneously with the relearning of arithmetic operations. If the patient with anarithmetia also presents aphasic problems, language should be rehabilitated first. Calculation rehabilitation can be implemented once an appropriate level of linguistic comprehension and production is achieved (Tsvetkova, 1996).

In conclusion, the patient with anarithmetia should relearn the basic concepts that underlie the numerical system. These basic concepts range from knowing numbers to handling them within the system of operations.

Rehabilitation of Secondary Acalculias

In patients with difficulties in recognizing numbers as a result of a perceptual deficit, the rehabilitation process is directed at the recovery of steadfastness and the generalization of visual perception. These patients frequently present low scores on reading numbers tests and on the transcoding of numbers from one code to another, with numerous rotation errors. (Rosselli & Ardila, 1989). The visual-perceptual difficulties affect the execution of written numbers tasks, in contrast to an adequate performance of mental arithmetic operations. When writing is preserved in these patients (as is the case of alexia without agraphia), writing numbers in the air helps their recognition.

Tsvetkova (1996) proposes using the "number reconstruction" technique with these patients. The technique includes number reconstruction by starting from certain visual elements (e.g., completing eight, starting from the number three), looking for certain elements within a number (e.g., looking for the number one in the number four), and finally, performing a verbal analysis of the similarities and differences that can be observed between numbers. At the same time that the "number reconstruction" technique is used, spatial orientation exercises, comprehension of the right-to-left relationship, and visual analysis of geometrical objects and forms should be developed.

Patients with alexia without agraphia generally present spatial integration difficulties (simultanagnosia) and inaccuracy in visual-motor coordination (optical ataxia). Treatment should then include exercises that permit spatial analysis and visual-motor ability training. Rehabilitation tasks are implemented following a program that progressively increases difficulty, beginning with simple movements designed for reaching for or indicating objects followed by copying figures in two dimensions, and concluding with the construction of three-dimensional figures (Sohlberg & Mateer, 1989). The training in the reproduction of designs of different forms, colors, and sizes can be initiated with aides. For instance, the patient is asked to finish a design already started until he/she can finally perform the task completely and independently (Ben-Yishay, 1983). Sohlberg and Mateer (1989) propose, as a procedure to evaluate the generalization of the task, obtaining a base line over the performance of ten designs, noting the accuracy, time of execution, and the number of aides required. The therapist can choose five out of ten designs for training. When the execution desired from these five designs is achieved, the performance in the five unused designs during training is evaluated, with the goal of observing the effects of training. This generalization should be looked for in untrained visual-motor tasks that require the same underlying skill (Gouvier & Warner, 1987). When a visual search defect (ocular apraxia) exists, visual pursuit tasks may help to compensate. Rosselli and Ardila (1996) describe the writing and reading rehabilitation of a patient with Balint syndrome, with severe ocular apraxia. They used visual movement exercises such as (a) demonstrating the visual pursuit of objects, (b) placing the index fingers at a distance of 15 cm from the sides of the face and requiring the patient to look towards the left and right index fingers ten times consecutively, and (c) practicing convergence exercises—from a central point at a distance of 30 cm, the patient must bring the right or left index finger towards his/her nose, permanently maintaining visual contact. In addition, visual-kinesthetic exercises are included in the rehabilitation plan; the patient was shown letters he had to reproduce in the air, and, later, he had to say the name of the letters. Likewise, when following words, the patient should simultaneously perform the movements of writing these words. In place of letters, numbers may be used. Within the visual searching exercises described by Rosselli and Ardila (1996), looking for words and letters in letter groups that progressively become more complex is included. Time and precision are recorded.

Patients with aphasic acalculia that receive therapy for their oral disorder usually improve significantly and in parallel fashion with the improvement of the calculation disturbance (Basso, 1987). Acalculia rehabilitation in these patients parallels language rehabilitation using denomination techniques, auditive verbal memory techniques, and semantic conceptual classification techniques. When acalculia is fundamentally derived from defects in phonological discrimination, prominent errors in oral numerical tasks are found. Therefore, within the rehabilitation program, visual stimuli should be used initially (Tsvetkova, 1996).

Patients with frontal lesions generally present perseverations and attention difficulties that prevent an adequate performance on calculation tests. These patients usually do not present errors in naming or in the recognition of numbers. Tsvetkova (1996) proposes the idea of providing control strategies to patients that will allow them to direct their attention and reduce perseveration. These control strategies refer to descriptions of the steps that the patient should follow in order to satisfactorily complete the task. When faced with the problem of forming the number twelve, by starting from other numbers, the following steps can be described to the patient: (1) forming the number twelve by starting from other numbers with the help of addition, the patient is asked to use the maximum number of combinations; (2) achieving the same number by starting from other numbers with the help of subtraction, the patient is asked to use the maximum number of combinations; and (3) achieving the same number starting from other numbers with the help of multiplication. The maximum number of combinations should be used. The patient is trained to verbalize and follow the necessary steps. Since these patients do not generally present defects in mathematical procedures, it is not necessary to provide them with special instructions for the execution of each operation. The use of permanent verbalization is a useful technique with patients with visual-perceptual difficulties.

Spatial acalculia is associated with hemi-inattention (unilateral spatial neglect), which can be observed in right as well as left injuries (Rosselli et al., 1986). Although it is notoriously more frequent and severe in cases of right brain injury, unilateral spatial neglect or hemi-inattention refers to the inability to respond (attend to stimuli) presented in the contralateral visual field to the brain injury. These patients tend to present number omissions on the opposite side of the brain lesion. The hemi-spatial neglect constitutes one of the factors that interferes most with an adequate cognitive recovery. Although hemi-spatial neglect is frequently associated with hemianopsia (visual loss in the contralateral field to the lesion), it should be evaluated independently. Frequently, cancelation tasks, copies of drawings, visual search tasks, bisection of a line, and a drawing of a clock are used, as well as tasks that help to overcome the neglect.

Based on the hypothesis that patients with unilateral spatial neglect present difficulties in adequately exploring their environment, several rehabilitation programs have been directed to develop this ability (Weinberg et al., 1977). Within the rehabilitation techniques for hemi-inattention during reading, the following is discussed: (1) placing a vertical line on the left margin of the paragraph to be read, and (2) numbering the beginning and end of each line. As the treatment advances, the clues are eliminated until the patient is finally capable of reading without help. Upon diminishing the hemi-spatial neglect in general, spatial defects in reading diminish simultaneously (Ardila & Rosselli, 1992). In the recovery of spatial agraphia, it has been suggested using sheets of lined paper, which limit the writing space. It is also suggested to draw vertical lines that mark spaces between letters and words.

Rosselli and Ardila (1996) describe the rehabilitation of a 58-year-old woman with alexia, agraphia, and spatial acalculia secondary to a vascular injury in the right hemisphere. The rehabilitation process was based in the rehabilitation of unilateral spatial neglect and associated spatial difficulties. The patient could adequately perform oral calculations but was completely incapable of performing written arithmetic operations with numbers composed of two or more digits. In a special test of arithmetic operations (additions, subtractions, multiplications, and divisions), an initial score of 0/20 was obtained. Left hemi-inattention, a mixing up of procedures and the impossibility of adequately orienting the columns were observed. The rehabilitation techniques implemented included:

1. Using short paragraphs with a red vertical line placed on the left margin and with the lines numbered on the left and right sides, the patient, using her index finger, had to look for the numbers corresponding to each line. The clues (vertical line and numbers) were progressively eliminated.
2. In a text with no more than twelve lines, the patient had to complete the missing letters (i.e., perform sequential and ordered spatial exploration).
3. Letter cancellation exercises were repeated constantly, and clues to facilitate their execution were included. Time and precision were recorded.
4. In spontaneous writing exercises using lined paper with a thick colored line in the left margin, the patient had to look for the vertical line when finishing each line. Later, the line was eliminated, but the patient had to verbalize (initially aloud and later to herself) and explore to the extreme left before beginning to read the next line.
5. To facilitate relearning of numbers through dictation, squares were used to place the numbers in space, and the concepts of hierarchy were practiced permanently (units, tens, hundreds, etc.).
6. To provide training in arithmetic operations, she was given in writing additions, subtractions, multiplications, and divisions with digits separated in columns by thick colored lines, and the tops of the columns were numbered (from right to left). The patient had to verbalize the arithmetic procedures and, with her right index finger, look for the left margin before she could pass to the next column. Later, the patient herself would write the operations she was dictated.

The techniques described above were proven useful eight months after the treatment was started. The patient presented significant recovery but in no way a complete recovery.

Rehabilitation of Developmental Dyscalculia

Strang and Rourke (1985) recommend that the remedial programs for children with dyscalculia include, when possible, systematic and concrete verbalizations of the operations and arithmetical procedures. The operations that involve mechanical arithmetic should be converted into verbal tasks that permit the child to take apart the operations, and, in this way, facilitate his/her learning. The teaching method should be clear, concrete, precise, and systematic.

Once the child has developed an adequate recognition of the numbers, one should begin to work with calculation difficulties. Initially, one should choose an arithmetic operation that presents a problem and describe it verbally in such a way that the child can repeat the description independently of whether or not he/she understands the underlying mathematical concept. Later, the child should verbalize the steps that should be followed in order to perform the operation in question (e.g., Step 1, name the mathematical sign; Step 2, direct eyes toward the right, etc.). Once the different steps have been verbalized, the child should write them and repeat them orally as many times as needed. Then, the instructor should use concrete aides (table, equipment, places) to explain the mathematical concept.

Squared sheets of paper should always be used. At times, the use of colors helps the discrimination of the right-left idea. Each time the child is presented with an arithmetic problem, it should be read out loud to minimize the possibility of his/her forgetting visual details. It is useful to have an adding machine at hand so that the child can revise the results of the operations. It is very important that the instructor record all errors committed by the child, with the purpose of analyzing the cognitive processing steps that have problems (Rosselli, 1992).

The child's parents should be taught about the learning strategy that is being used so that in family activities (e.g., shopping), the practice of the same arithmetic activities can be included, and the generalization of the remedial program can be promoted. Since these children present attention and visual-perceptual discrimination difficulties, it is convenient to involve the child with developmental discalculia in tasks that involve a detailed description of visual stimuli. In addition, one should work on the parts in an organized manner. Difficulties in the interpretation of social situations can be improved by creating artificial situations (e.g., movies, photographs, etc.) so that the child can interpret the images and the context. The instructor can give clues to appropriately perceive the fictional circumstances and the meanings of the gestures (Ozols & Rourke, 1987).

The prognosis of developmental dyscalculia depends on variables such as the severity of the disorder, the degree of the child's deficiency in the execution of neuropsychological tests, the promptness of the initiation treatment, and the collaboration of the parents in the remedial program.

REFERENCES

American Psychiatric Association. (1994). *Diagnostic and statistical manual of mental disorders, DSM-IV*. Washington, DC: American Psychiatric Association.

Ardila A. (1993). On the origins of calculation abilities. *Behavioural Neurology, 6,* 89–98.

Ardila, A., & Rosselli, M. (1986). *La vejez: Neuropsicología del fenómeno del envejecimiento*. Medellin (Colombia): Prensa Creativa.

———. (1990). Acalculias. *Behavioural Neurology, 3,* 39–48.

———. (1992). *Neuropsicología clínica*. Medellin (Colombia): Prensa Creativa.

———. (1994). Spatial acalculia. *International Journal of Neuroscience, 78,* 177–184.

Ardila, A., Lopez, M.V., & Solano, E. (1989). Semantic aphasia reconsidered. In A. Ardila & F. Ostrosky-Solis (Eds.), *Brain organization of language and cognitive processes*. New York: Plenum Press.

Badian, N.A. (1983). Dyscalculia and nonverbal disorders of learning. In H.R. Miklebust (Ed.), *Progress in learning disabilities* (Vol. 5). New York: Grune & Stratton.

Basso, A. (1987). Approaches to neuropsychological rehabilitation: Language disorders. In M. Meier, A. Benton, & L. Diller (Eds.), *Neuropsychological rehabilitation*. New York: Guilford Press.

Benson, D.F., & Denckla, M.B. (1969). Verbal paraphasias as a source of calculations disturbances. *Archives of Neurology, 21,* 96–102.

Ben-Yishay, Y. (1983). Working approaches to the remediation of cognitive deficits in brain damaged persons. *Rehabilitation Monographs, 6,* New York: NYU Medical Center Institute of Rehabilitation Medicine.

Berger, H. (1926). Uber Rechenstorunger bei Herderkraunkunger des Grosshirns. *Archives Psychiatrie und Nervenkr, 78,* 236–263.

Boller, F., & Grafman, J. (1983). Acalculia: Historical development and current significance. *Brain and Cognition, 2,* 205–223.

Collington, R., LeClerq, C., & Mathy, J. (1977). Estude de la semologie des troubles du calcul observes au cours des lesions corticales. *Acta Neurologique Belgique, 77,* 257–275.

Dagenbach, D., & McCloskey, M. (1992). The organization of arithmetic facts in memory: Evidence from a brain-damaged patient. *Brain and Cognition, 20,* 345–366.

Dahmen, W., Hartje, W., Bussing, A., & Sturm, W. (1982). Disorders in calculation in aphasic patients: Spatial and verbal components. *Neuropsychologia, 20,* 145–153.

Deloche, G., & Seron, X. (1982). From three to 3: A differential analysis of skills in transcoding quantities between patients with Broca's aphasia and Wernicke's aphasia. *Brain, 105,* 719–733.

———. (1987). Numerical transcoding: A general production model. In G. Deloche & X. Seron (Eds.), *Mathematical disabilities: A cognitive neuropsychological perspective.* Hillsdale: Lawrence Erlbaum Associates.

Deloche, G., Seron, X., Larroque, C., Magnien, C., Metz-Lutz, M.N., Riva, I., et al. (1994). Calculation and number processing: assessment battery: role of demographic factors. *Journal of Clinical and Experimental Neuropsychology, 16,* 195–208.

De Partz, M.P. (1986). Re-education of a deep dyslexic patient: Rationale of the method and results. *Cognitive Neuropsychology, 3,* 149–177.

Ferro, J.M., & Botelho, H.M. (1980). Alexia for arithmetical signs: A cause of disturbed calculation. *Cortex, 16,* 175–180.

Gerstman, J. (1940). The syndrome of finger agnosia, disorientation for right and left, agraphia and acalculia. *Archives of Neurology, Neurosurgery and Psychiatry, 44,* 398–408.

Goldstein, K. (1948). *Language and language disturbances.* New York: Grune & Stratton.

Gouvier, W., & Warner, M. (1987). Treatment of visual imperception and related disorders. In J.M. Williams & C.H. Long (Eds.), *The rehabilitation of cognitive disabilities.* New York: Plenum Press.

Grafman, J. (1988). Acalculia. In F. Boller, J. Grafman, G. Rizzolatti & H. Goodglas (Eds.), *Handbook of neuropsychology* (Vol.1). Amsterdam: Elsevier.

Grafman, J., & Boller, F. (1987). Cross-cultural approaches to the study of calculation processes. In G. Deloche & X. Seron (Eds.), *Mathematical disabilities: A cognitive neuropsychological perspective.* Hillsdale: Lawrence Erlbaum Associates.

Grafman, J., Passafiume, D., Faglioni, P., & Boller, F. (1982). Calculation disturbances in adults with focal hemipheric damage. *Cortex, 18,* 37–49.

Grafman, J., Kampen, D., Rosenberg, J., Salazar, A.M., & Booler F. (1989). The progressive breakdown of number processing and calculation ability: A case study. *Cortex, 25,* 121–133.

Hecaen, H., Angelergues, T., & Houiller, S. (1961). Les vrietes cliniques des acalculies au cours des lesions retrorolandiques. *Revue de Neurologie, 105,* 85–103.

Henschen, S.E. (1925). Clinical and anatomical contributions on brain pathology. *Archives of Neurology and Psychiatry, 13,* 226–249.

Kosc, L. (1970). Psychology and psychopatology of mathematical abilities. *Studies of Psychology, 12,* 159–162.

Levin, H., Goldstein, F.C., & Spiers, P.A. (1993). Acalculia. In K.M. Heilman & E. Valenstein (Eds.), *Clinical neuropsychology* (3rd ed.). New York: Oxford University Press.

Lezak, M.D. (1995). *Neuropsychological assessment* (3rd ed.). New York: Oxford University Press.

Lindquist, T. (1936). De l'acalculie. *Acta Médica Scandinávica, 38,* 217–277.

Lomas, J., & Kertesz, A. (1978). Patterns of spontaneous recovery in aphasic groups: A study of adult stroke patients. *Brain and Language, 5,* 388–401.

Loveland, K.A., Fletcher, J.M., & Bailey, B. (1990). Verbal and nonverbal communication of events in learning disabilities subtypes. *Journal of Clinical and Experimental Neuropsychology, 12,* 433–447.

Luria, A.R. (1977). *Las funciones corticales superiores en el hombre.* La Habana: Editorial Orbe.

McCloskey, M., & Caramazza, A. (1987). Cognitive mechanisms in normal and impaired number processing. In G. Deloche & X. Seron (Eds.), *Mathematical disabilities: A cognitive neuropsychological perspective.* Hillsdale: Lawrence Erlbaum Associates.

McCloskey, M., Aliminosa, D., & Sokol, S.M. (1991). Facts, rules, and procedures in normal calculation: evidence from multiple single-patient studies of impaired arithmetic fact retrieval. *Brain and Cognition, 17,* 154–203.

McCloskey, M., Caramazza, A., & Basili, A. (1985). Cognitive processes in number processing and calculation: Evidence from dyscalculia. *Brain and Cognition, 4,* 313–330.

McCloskey, M., Sokol, S.M., & Goodman, R.A. (1986). Cognitive processes in verbal number processing: Inference from the performance of brain-damaged subjects. *Journal of Experimental Psychology: General, 115,* 313–330.

Ozols, E., & Rourke, B.P. (1985). Dimensions of social sensitivity in two types of learning disabled children. In B.P. Rourke (Ed.), *Neuropsychology of learning disabilities*. New York: Guilford Press.

Parlato, V., López, O., Panisset, M., et al. (1992). Mental calculation in mild Alzheimer's disease: A pilot study. *International Journal of Geriatric Psychiatry, 7,* 599–602.

PeBenito, R. (1987). Developmental Gerstmann syndrome: Case report and review of literature. *Developmental and Behavioral Pediatrics, 8,* 229–232.

PeBenito, R., Fisch, B.C., & Fisch, M.L. (1988). Developmental Gerstmann syndrome. *Archives of Neurology, 45,* 977–982.

Presenti, M. Seron, X., & Van Der Lider, M. (1994). Selective impairments as evidence for mental organisation of arithmetical facts: BB, a case of preserved subtractions. *Cortex, 25,* 661–671.

Rosemberger, P.B. (1989). Perceptual-motor and attentional correlates of developmental dyscalculia. *Annals of Neurology, 26,* 216–220.

Rosselli, M. (1992). Discalculia. In M. Roselli & A. Ardila (Eds.), *Neuropsicología infantil.* Medellin (Colombia): Prensa Creativa.

Rosselli, M., & Ardila, A. (1989). Calculation deficits in patients with right and left hemisphere damage. *Neuropsychologia 27,* 607–618.

———. (Eds.). (1992). *Neuropsicología infantil.* Medellin (Colombia): Prensa Creativa.

———. (1996). Rehabilitación de la alexia y la agrafía. In F. Ostrosky, A. Ardila, & R. Dochy (Eds.), *Rehabilitación neuropsicología.* Mexico: Trillas.

Rosselli, M., Rosselli, A., Vergara, I., & Ardila, A. (1986). Topography of the hemi-inattention syndrome. *International Journal of Neuroscience, 27,* 165–172.

Rourke, B.P. (1987) Syndrome of non verbal learning disabilities: The final common path of white matter disease disfunction. *The Clinical Neuropsychologist, 1,* 209–234.

———. (1988). The syndrome of nonverbal learning disabilities: Developmental manifestation in neurological diseases, disorders and dysfunctions. *The Clinical Neuropsychologist, 2,* 293–330.

Seron, X. (1984). Re-education strategies in neuropsychology: Cognitive and pragmatic approaches of the disorders. In F.C. Rose (Ed.), *Advances in neurology: Progress in aphasiology* (Vol. 4). New York: Raven Press.

Shalev, R., Weirtman, R., & Amir, N. (1988). Developmental dyscalculia. *Cortex, 24,* 555–561.

Sholberg, M.M., & Mateer, C.A. (1989). *Introduction to cognitive rehabilitation: theory and practice.* Hillsdale: Lawrence Erlbaum Associates.

Spiers, P. (1987). Acalculia revisited: Current issues. In G. Deloche & X. Seron (Eds.), *Mathematical disabilities: A cognitive neuropsychological perspective* (pp. 1–25). Hillsdale, NJ: Lawrence Erlbaum Associates.

Strang, J.D., & Rourke, B.P. (1985). Arithmetic disability subtypes: The neuropsychological significance of specific arithmetical impairment in childhood. In B.P. Rourke (Ed.), *Neuropsychology of learning disabilities*. New York: Guilford Press.

Temple, C.M. (1991). Procedural dyscalculia and number fact dyscalculia: double dissociation in developmental dyscalculia. *Cognitive Neuropsychology, 8,* 155–176.

Tsvetkova, L.S. (1996). Acalculia: Aproximación neuropsicológica al análisis de la alteración y la rehabilitación del cálculo. In F. Ostrosky, A. Ardila, & R. Dochy (Eds.), *Rehabilitación neuropsicología.* Mexico: Trillas.

Warrington, E.K. (1982). The fractionation of arithmetical skills: A single case study. *Quarterly Journal of Experimental Psychology, 34A,* 31–51.

Wechsler, D. (1955). *WAIS manual.* New York: The Psychological Corporation.

———. (1981). *WAIS-R manual.* New York: The Psychological Corporation.

———. (1991). *Weschler Intelligence Scale for Children* (3rd ed.). San Antonio, TX: The Psychological Corporation.

Weinberg, J., Diller, L., Gordon, W.A., Gerstmann, L., Lieberman, A., Lakin, P., Hodges, G., & Ezrachi, O. (1977). Visual scanning training effect on reading related tasks in acquired right brain damage. *Archives of Physical Medicine and Rehabilitation, 58,* 479–483.

20 Rehabilitation of Memory

José León-Carrión

Facultad de Psicología
Universidad de Seville, Seville, Spain

INTRODUCTION[1]

Memory is not an easy-to-delimit unitary phenomenon; therefore, it is not possible to expect that any attempt to treat or rehabilitate the deficits associated with it be unique. On the other hand, different nervous system disorders and different types of brain damage are also capable of affecting and producing different memory flaws; different brain zones play a relevant role in the process of recall, evoking, and fixation of traces. Additionally, different classifications related to memory exist, and not all of them are valid from the anatomical-functional point of view. Nevertheless, despite all the complexity that its study implies, memory is perhaps the best studied of all the neurocognitive sequela derived from brain damage.

However, despite possibly being the best studied higher function by psychologists and neuropsychologists, that is not the case with its treatment. Few studies have been published regarding rehabilitation of memory processes, although in the last ten years the studies centered on the repair of organic memory deficits have increased considerably (Ryan & Ruff, 1988; Schachter, Rich, & Stampp, 1985; Sholberg & Mateer, 1989; Wilson & Moffat, 1984; Wilson, 1987a, b; Berg, Koning-Haanstra, & Deelmon, 1991). Well controlled studies with a large number of cases are not abundant.

The importance of memory rehabilitation becomes manifest, therefore, in that it is one of the easiest to locate sequela in patients who have suffered some type of brain damage. In a study by Levin, Grossman, Rose, and Teasdale (1979), it was stated that 36% of the patients with severe brain damage presented information recovery problems a year after the accident. It seems appropriate to examine what happens with these disorders.

PROGNOSIS AND COURSE OF MEMORY DEFICITS

Some investigations have tried to establish the prognosis of memory deficits; however, little is known regarding the long-term prognosis of severe memory disorders (Wilson, 1991). In a study in which a large group of head injury patients were studied, Dirkmen, Temkin, McLeant, Wyler, and Machamer (1987) found that in this type of patient, memory deterioration depended on the type of task used to evaluate them, the time lapsed since the injury, and the evaluation and the severity of the trauma. In a year's time, the data that will predict a greater severity of memory deficits in the patients are closely related to three fundamental variables: (1) having been in a coma for over a day, (2) having obtained a score of 8 or less on the Glasgow Coma Scale, and (3) having suffered post-traumatic amnesia for over two weeks.

In another study, Gronwall and Wrightson (1981) maintain that closed brain damage has at least three different effects on memory. First, it brings with it a deficit in the ability to process information, especially when the process required is complex or there is a time limitation in its performance. Second, there is a deficit in the ability to place material in the long-term memory, and, third, there seems to be a deficit in the recovery of material from the memory once it has been stored.

For Levin (1989), one of the main characteristics of the first moments of recovery of closed brain trauma patients is the retrograde and the post-traumatic amnesia. For them, although residual memory deficits are normally resolved within three months after moderate brain damage, the deterioration in learning and retention persists in almost a fourth of the patients that survive severe closed brain trauma, and it is a normally disabling sequela.

To determine the long-term prognosis of patients with severe memory disorders, Wilson (1991) studied a group that had quit rehabilitation 5–10 years before. She found that the majority of the subjects lived independently of institutional care. Fifteen of them had a paying job (Table 20.1), fewer than a third of them seemed to show improvement in the mnesic functioning according to test results, a small number had worsened, and around 60% showed little or no change since they had quit rehabilitation. What the majority of subjects had done was to learn coping mechanisms, or they had compensated their deficits with the help of memory aids and strategies.

In light of this data, one can say that the severity of the injury will condition the prognosis of memory deficits in traumatic brain-injured patients. The majority of them will experience memory deficits within the year following the brain injury, over a third will suffer them a year after, with the duration depending on the time they had remained in coma, its severity, and the period of time they suffered post-traumatic amnesia. Recovery possibilities are complex, and benefits can be obtained with neuropsychological treatment, but well controlled studies are still needed to gauge the effects of this treatment. Consequently, our proposal is that the rehabilitation program applied should have the greatest theoretical, technological, and imaginative soundness.

Therefore, keeping in mind this data and before going into the demands that the rehabilitation of mnemonic deficits presents, from our point of view, when trying to create a design and plan of treatment of the problems that affect memory, it is convenient to know from what premise one starts. We will review broad aspects that seem fundamental to consider when proposing a treatment plan.

Table 20.1: Pre- and post-injury occupation of a group of subjects in paid employment (from Wilson, 1991, p. 122)

Diagnosis*	Sex	Age at Insult	Previous Occupation	Occupation Now	Full or Part Time
THI	M	15	Schoolboy	Shelf filler	Part
THI	M	15	Schoolboy	Owns and lets property	Full
THI	F	17	Bank clerk	Microfilm technician	Full
THI	M	18	Schoolboy	Clerk	Full
THI	M	19	Trainee car mechanic	Driver for father's firm	Full
THI	M	19	University student	Administrative officer	Full
Near drowning	M	19	University student	Salesman in book shop	Full
THI	M	22	Draughtsman	Helper in warehouse	Part
THI	M	24	River boat pilot	Dishwasher	Full
THI	F	27	Social worker	Social worker	Part
THI	M	29	Journalist	Journalist	Full
THI	M	29	Clerk to House of Commons	Running own business with wife	Full
SAH	M	36	Engineer	Engineer	Full
SAH	F	39	Hairdresser	Hairdresser	Part
SAH	M	42	Entertainment officer	On bookbinding course	Full

*THI, traumatic head injury; SAH, subarachnoid hemorrhage.

THE THEORETICAL FIELD OF MEMORY

The majority of authors indicate that memory is not a simple entity (Squire, 1992; Schacter & Tulving, 1982; Squire & Knowlton, 1995), that it is, instead, composed of different, separate systems. For Tulving (1985), memory is composed of a number of interrelated systems, of operating structures with a definite organization of its cognitive and behavioral correlates. Luria (1975) already indicated, in this sense, that memory was a higher psychological process and that, therefore, it cannot be isolated in a specific location of the brain since it is a functional system. This functional system is complex and is organized at different levels; it is active by nature and develops itself in a temporal space through the links of the brain interconnections network which defines that functional system (León-Carrión, 1995). Therefore, to try to understand memory as a narrow, localized function is impossible.

Thus, when Tulving talks about systems, he is referring to a set of correlated processes, to structures with elemental, organized operative components. Each operative component is composed of a neural substratum and its behavioral correlate and/or cognitive correlate.[2] Some components of a system may be shared by other systems, or according to Luria, a link in the functional system may participate in different functional systems. In any event, the components of each system do not all have the same functional equivalence, but, instead, some of them may participate in different systems, given their functional, anatomic, physiological characteristics; others, for the same reasons, only participate in a few functional systems, and a few others still probably only participate in one functional system.

It is very important to keep all of the above in mind. Thus, for example, we know that the frontal lobe participates in memory as well as in other cognitive processes; that does not imply it is the central organ or seat of memory but, instead, that it forms part of the functional systems of the different memory systems. In this sense, different and distant zones of the brain work in conjunction in order that a certain memory functional system may operate.

Some authors have tried to explain the reason for the existence of the functional systems, such as Tulving (op. cit.), who justifies his multiple memory systems as follows:

1. It is not possible to generalize about memory as a whole.
2. Human memory has its present configuration as a result of a long evolutionary period, and the structures and the cerebral mechanisms that make memory possible also have to reflect the adjustments and the mechanisms which evolution has been developing.
3. Memory, as well as other psychological functions, is subserved by separate neurocognitive systems. The fact that it appears as a unit is due solely to the absence of evidence to the contrary.
4. Sooner or later, we will find better ideas and theories on the mental processes that will be more in accord with nature. We must find other alternatives.
5. Researchers need more imagination; it does not appear reasonable that the different varieties of memory and learning that appear to be so different, at first view, share the same set of structures and processes.

Because of the above reasons, as well as others which could be given, it appears that we should accept that memory is a complex functional system, and, therefore, the idea of the existence of distinct memory systems. As researchers, we must have more imagination and be more critical of the accepted concepts which scientific evidence is demonstrating do not hold up. In order to try to convince us of the existence of multiple systems, Tulving (op. cit., p. 386) states:

> *If we reflect on the limits of generalizations about memory, think about the twists and turns of evolution, examine possible analogies with other biological and psychological systems, believe that most current ideas we have about the human mind are wrong, and have great difficulty apprehending sameness in different varieties of learning and memory, we might be ready to imagine the possibility that memory consists of a number of interrelated systems.*

Throughout the chapter, we are going to refer to the memory types and classifications presently accepted by the research community in this field. We will summarize them briefly.

Short-term memory, primary memory, active memory, or *work memory* refers fundamentally to the volume of information that a subject can simultaneously retain while developing a task; this kind of memory is indispensable in order to carry out complex cognitive tasks. For Baddeley and Hitch (1974), work memory is the space in which information is maintained and is manipulated while it is being processed. Thus, for example, while we are speaking, we maintain an active memory that corresponds to the capacity we have to handle a volume of information at one time. When an excess of information is offered, the subject feels blocked and incapable of handling it all—people will, therefore, stop and divide the information into manageable blocks.

Miller (1956), in a classic article, presented the limited capacity of short-term memory as 7 ± 2 units of information. He stated: "...the span of absolute judgement and the span of immediate memory impose severe limitations on the amount of information that we are able to receive, process, and remember. By organizing the stimulus input simultaneously into several dimensions and successively into a sequence of chunks, we manage to break (or at least stretch) this informational bottleneck." According to Baddeley (1994), this work is still cited because the underlying ideas in it are still valid when stressing the importance of re-encoding and developing the concept of chunking.[3] A chunk is an item of information. Later research stated that there could exist multiple work memories (Monsell, 1984), a set of temporary work capabilities of distributed processing subsystems of information.

Long-term memory, *inactive memory*, or *secondary memory* is a storing of unlimited persistence and capacity, in which the stored information may remain inactive or latent during an indefinite period of time; it can only be recovered as a function of the demands of the medium. Since it is not a unitary system, we need to consider the different types of long-term memory that can be established.

First, there is a distinction between episodic memory and semantic memory. With the term *episodic memory*, we refer to knowledge stored about episodes or events dated temporarily and to the space-time relations between them. *Semantic memory* refers to learned organized knowledge that is needed, for example, in order to use language, mathematical formulas, to know the names of the European capitals, etc., and it does not have the capability of dating that knowledge in time.

Another important distinction between the types of memory in the design of the neuropsychological rehabilitation of patients with brain damage is between declarative memory and procedural memory. *Declarative memory (explicit)* is the ability to inform explicitly about something known. It is that memory directly accessible to conscience which is related with events and facts acquired through learning. *Procedural (implicit) memory* makes reference to skills and habits—it is the capacity to learn through rules, learning skills, habits, behavioral conditionings, etc. Many times, patients do not know that they possess this type of learning.

It is important to consider the "priming" effect during the rehabilitation process, because it will indicate whether the patient has preserved this aspect of memory. It has to do with the patient having a type of evocation, when provoked, that he/she is not conscious of having. It is a non-conscious memory of certain specific information possibly regulated by relatively automatic mechanisms and which can be observed very well through memory tests (Mayes, 1992). Thus, for example, if we show subjects the word "airplane" and, after some time, we ask them to complete words, if they retain this effect when we ask them to complete the word "air —," they will say "airplane" and no other word.

MEMORY FUNCTIONS[4]

Several concepts regarding memory functions, according to cognitive psychology, should be considered.

Encoding is the process through which the information received is placed in an adequate format so that it may be used later, thus eliminating the superfluous and marking significantly that which is relevant for the subject. In addition, the format of the information will be significant. An event, fact, or information presents itself before the subject in visual, auditive/semantic, gustatory, olfactory form, etc.—that presentation format has to be reformatted so that it may be retrieved later (i.e., fundamentally, one uses a mechanism capable of storing and/or making lasting registers of experience). In the encoding process, there is what Craik and Lockhart (1972) called different *levels of processing*, meaning that not all traces are encoded in the same manner. For example, the encoding of information based on repeating it many times is not the same as if the encoding strategy is performed by means of outlined sketches, having the subjects construct them as they proceed to understand them.

An aspect that has become very important in the encoding process is the situation, what Anderson and Pichest (1978) called *context*. Any type of perception, sensation, or thought that occurs simultaneously while certain information is being encoded will also be encoded. On the other hand, there are also other variables—the principles of association, contiguity, and frequency. The most classic and extreme type of association by contiguity is flashbulb memory (Brown & Kulik, 1977) (i.e., unimportant events that occur simultaneously with strong events tend to be remembered, perhaps due to emotional aspects). On the other hand, there is preparedness (Seligman, 1970), which refers to experiences that are memorized or learned before others; those that are biologically or socially important for the survival of the individual are learned first. Finally, the other important principle is that of frequency or practice (Crowder, 1976). The more frequently two events, facts, or elements of information occur together, the stronger will be the association between them.

Of course, the event by which the effectiveness of memory is best noticed is during the *evocation* or *recovery* process of consolidated memories. If we assume that memory is not a unitary entity but that, instead, it is a functional system, we have to accept a connective point of view for the evocation. Evocation, therefore, is the process whereby the functional network is activated to which memory belongs and to which we wish to gain access. Placing this network into action is a function of the contents of the processing levels and of the organization of the general processing of knowledge.

There are different theories about *forgetfulness* that try to explain why there are events that are not remembered, traces of events and facts that we have lived but which do not return to our memory. But, do we really forget? It is possible that nothing that has entered into the memory gets lost; what may be lost is the ability to access the connections that lead to those memories (León-Carrión, 1995). Cognitive psychologists propose four theories to explain why things are forgotten: non-use, interference, emotional factors, and organizational factors.

The **theory of non-use** is the oldest of the four and maintains that information which is not used is lost. Thus, facts that are not brought back in the memory with a certain degree of frequency tend to weaken and, in extreme cases, to be forgotten. However, although this theory has a good deal of truth to it, it does not explain why certain older persons with organic disorders have very vivid recollections of their youth or childhood but forget recent events. The **interference theory** states that memory weakens as a result of the interference generated by newer learning processes. There is a proactive interference that takes place when already acquired knowledge makes it difficult for new memories to take place. There is also a retroactive interference that occurs when new knowledge interferes, making it difficult to recover old memories. From our point of view, the interference theory seems to bring forth the complexity of the ecphoric processes.

The **emotional factors theory** maintains that the moods of the individual interfere with the process of evoking experiential events and facts. For example, subjects who are depressed have problems remembering, and recollection is distorted by their emotional state. The **organizational levels theory** states that forgetting is due to poor or inadequate organization of the memorization process.

An interesting aspect related to quasi-forgetfulness is what is recognized as a feeling of knowing. This is such a common phenomena that it can happen to anyone—the feeling of knowing the answer to a question but of not being able to remember it (e.g., if you are asked for the name of a person with whom you went out during last summer's vacation, it is possible that you may not remember it but at the same time, you are convinced that you know it and that if you are given several names, you will recognize it from among them).

BRAIN SYSTEMS ASSOCIATED WITH MEMORY

Any event or action interior or exterior to us has been registered by the adequate brain systems so that it may become memory. The brain systems manipulate that registry by means of encoding and decoding mechanisms so as to be able to handle it and introduce it into the set of knowledge that the individual already has. The type of encoding and decoding that takes place is complex, especially at the level of the significance of the registries.[5] Such engrams may have a strong visual, verbal, tactile, olfactory, or gustatory content in which the different brain zones (temporal, visual, parietal, and subcortical levels) play their own role. This entire process is regulated and controlled by the brain's executive system—the frontal lobe and, especially, the prefrontal cortex—and regulated emotionally by the amigdala.

Therefore, in memory processes, practically the entire brain intervenes through the different functional systems. First, the attentional system intervenes, a system that shares links with the decoding and re-encoding processes. But, in this first phase, the part controlled by the brainstem and the diencephalon intervenes, especially the reticular formation and the thalamus. Obviously, an injury at this level prevents the entire process from going ahead. Brain zones also intervene where exterior information arrives and is analyzed—these are the retrorolandic areas of the brain. All is controlled and programmed by the executive system, the prefrontal zone, which is what plans and organizes relevant information and determines what is its convenience for the system. The prefrontal zone plays an important role in the placing into play the previous knowledge that the subject has and in designing and programing the memorization processes.

The hippocampus codifies as files the memory traces and is related to the consolidation processes and reducing interference. Once the memory traces have been consolidated, a simultaneous registry of previous knowledge takes place; it is in this knowledge that the new trace is incorporated and, at the same time, causes a readjustment of that previous knowledge. This is what Tulving (1983) called ecphoria,[6] the process that takes place when a cue internally or externally generated interacts with a memory trace. Ecphoric processes, like any other modular processes, once acquired, are quick, obligatory, informationally encapsulated, and cognitively impenetrable (Moscovitsch, 1995). In these processes, the hippocampus and related structures play a very relevant role, but the frontal lobe does not seem to play a less significant role.

The amigdala, another central component of the limbic system, plays a central role in the memory processes (Sarter & Markowitsch, 1985; Tranel & Hayman, 1990; Markowitsch, Von Cramon et al., 1990). The amigdala is probably the formation which

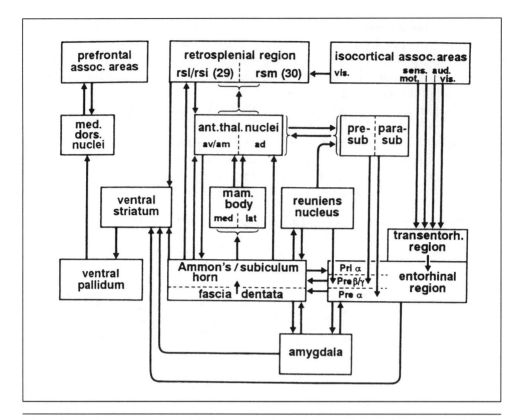

Figure 20.1: Limbic and associated brain structure involved in memory processing (from Braak & Braak, 1992).

regulates the emotional-affective component of memory. Some studies have shown that injury to the amygdala affects emotional reactivity. While injuries to the hippocampal formation or to the related cortex only affect the memory, combined injuries affect both emotions and memory (see Zola-Morgan, Squire, Alvarez-Royo, & Clower, 1991). Therefore, the role the amygdala seems to play in memory is emotional, possibly assessing the motivational and affective significance of the events and stimuli that come from the exterior (Gloor, 1960; Fuster & Uyeda, 1971; LeDoux, 1993). Studies conducted on monkeys have shown that the amygdala responds selectively to significant visual social scenes (Brothers & Ring, 1993). Therefore, the amygdala seems to play a central and fundamental role in regulating memory, since all that is stored, coded, and also recovered is done as a function of the emotional content of the memories (Figure 20.1). Table 20.2, adapted from Squire and Knowlton (1995), presents a taxonomy of long-term memory and of the associated brain structures.

Any memory process requires, above all, an intact attention system that keeps open the channels so that the information considered emotionally significant by the amygdala can reach the retrorolandic zones of the cortex. The hippocampus will help, fundamentally, by reducing the interference and by helping in the consolidation. The retrorolandic lobes will analyze the information received from their functional mode and will serve it to the prefrontal cortex, which will, in turn, organize the implementation of the entire process (Figure 20.2).

Table 20.2: Long-Term Memory and Associated Brain Structures

TYPE OF MEMORY	BRAIN STRUCTURE	
Declarative (Explicit)	Facts	Medial temporal lobe
	Events	Diencephalon
Non declarative (Implicit)	Skills and habits	Striatum
	"Priming"	Neocortex
	Emotional responses	Amigdala
	Simple classical conditioning	Skeletal musculature Cerebellum
	Non-associative learning	Reflex Pathways

MEMORY REHABILITATION PRINCIPLES

The rehabilitation of memory problems derived from brain damage is not an easy task.[7] All to the contrary, there is broad agreement in considering that amnesic patients are difficult to rehabilitate, especially in the learning of new semantic or factual information. Levin (1989) finds that survivors of severe brain damage have a passive manner of learning.[8] This was also the finding of a study conducted by Hayman, Macdonald, and Tulving (1993, pp. 375–376) with the appropriate estimates. According to these authors, there are several aspects that characterize the learning of new information in amnesic patients:

1. The learning of new semantic information in these patients is typically slow and inefficient, compared to the learning by normal subjects, but they can learn new factual information.
2. The learning and retention of new semantic information takes place despite the amnesic patient's inability to remember extensively the source of the new acquired information, for which reason implicit learning is used.
3. Once the information has been retained, long-term retention is as good as that of normal subjects.

The implications for neurorehabilitators are that subjects with memory deficits can be trained and learning will again be possible for them. The job will not be easy—it will be laborious. But by using the proper strategies and the proper time, new learning can be achieved. Therefore, as the cited authors have suggested, it is not justified to say that amnesic subjects have deficiencies or absences of new semantic learning. Their results suggest that at least some amnesic patients can acquire it and retain it, depending on the conditions under which the rehabilitation process occurs.

Once convinced that the memory rehabilitation work is worthwhile, there are three basic principles required for successful rehabilitation: (1) the natural rehabilitation principle, (2) the especificity principle, and (3) the central regulation principle.

The *natural rehabilitation* principle refers to the fact that the rehabilitation of the mnesic processes must start from those processes that are least deteriorated (i.e., that memory must be reconstructed from that which is left). It is possible that, in many cases,

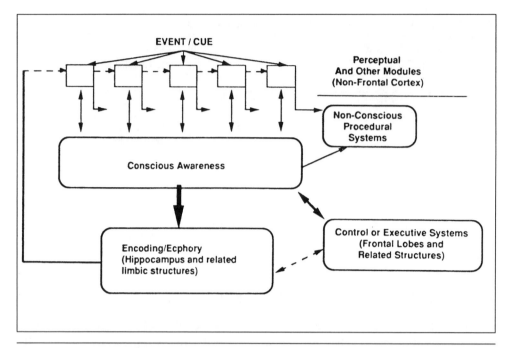

EVENT / CUE

Perceptual
And Other Modules
(Non-Frontal Cortex)

Non-Conscious
Procedural
Systems

Conscious Awareness

Encoding/Ecphory
(Hippocampus and related
limbic structures)

Control or Executive Systems
(Frontal Lobes and
Related Structures)

Figure 20.2: A neuropsychological model of memory showing the interaction of the cortico-subcorical systems (from Moscovitch, 1989).

work may have to start as if we were dealing with a small child. One should start from the mechanical memory that the patient retains and convert it slowly into logical memory. The process goes from natural memory to mediatized memory. Many authors start their rehabilitation process with complex learning procedures. An essential principle of rehabilitation, which cannot be forgotten, is that one cannot build from nothing. What can help the most in the reconstruction process is to start by reinforcing what still stands in the memory; this is a natural process, similar to the way in which a child builds, from the mechanical to the complex. Rehabilitation should try to facilitate the creation of new brain functional systems.

Another principle which must be considered when planning the rehabilitation process of memory problems of patients who have suffered brain damage is that of *specificity*. Generally speaking, as Luria (1974) indicates, the memory deficits that they present can be of two types—specific and nonspecific. The specific type alterations are those that take place as a result of focal lesions or lesions localized in the brain and which, consequently, may be limited to only one sensory mode. Therefore, alterations in audio-verbal memory could take place as a result of left temporal lesions. However, nonspecific mode alterations of memory are related fundamentally to lesions of the limbic system and usually manifest themselves in alterations in the memorization of any of the sensory modes, which are also accompanied by disturbances of consciousness (León-Carrión, 1995).

The *central regulation principle* refers to the executive mode, to the consequences of lesions caused in the prefrontal lobe, which lead actually not to a memory problem but instead to a problem of disorganization of the entire mnemonic process. We refer below to this principle.

NEUROPSYCHOLOGICAL REHABILITATION IN ENCODING PROCESSES

The Role of the Processing Levels

Rehabilitation centered on the processing levels refers to the design of the memorization strategies. It has to do with the design of how the subject is going to approach the memorization process. In this manner, for example, semantic encoding levels will be more effective, robust, and permanent than those of non-semantic levels. On the other hand, memory problem subjects who have a good ability in specific domains (mathematics, physics, agriculture, soccer, movies) will benefit if rehabilitation starts with recovery procedures related to these domains (see Adelson, 1984; Chase & Ericsson, 1981; De Groot, 1965). Consequently, for our rehabilitation purposes

- Any memorization strategy for patients must begin with tasks of a specific previous domain in which they had great skills. For example, if they had great knowledge of soccer, start by encoding elementary aspects of soccer, beginning with basic points and progressing to the more complex.
- Any memorization strategy will center itself fundamentally on the content and the meaning of the measure to be remembered. Thus, for example, it will be easier for the subjects to remember a story if we manage to explain it to them at their own level so that they understand it, rather than if we ask them to repeat it many times.
- Repetition is sometimes a necessary exercise in order to establish stimulation and neuronal connectivity, for which reason all rehabilitation must include memorization exercises by repetition in order to establish a favorable climate for long-term potentation.
- In any memory mode—visual, verbal, tactile, auditory, or olfactory—the subjects will tend to remember better if the direct information they receive is connected to its significance.
- Patients should be encouraged to remember the most significant information about a task.
- The task to be remembered will be easier if it is contained and expressed several times, in different fashions, in the reminder exercise itself. Thus, for example, if we want subjects to remember the name of a river of a certain city, we will give them a context of greater or lesser length in which the river's name will appear several times or in which it plays an important role.
- A task will be better remembered if it is focused from different vantage points. For example, when a subject has to remember the fundamental aspects of a story about two lovers, if he/she is given, first, a general view of the situation, then the story from the point of view of one of the lovers, and, finally, from the point of view of the other lover, the details and the informational content of the story will be remembered better.

The Role of Context in Memory Rehabilitation

The role of context in memory rehabilitation refers to the fact that when subjects have to evoke a stimulus, they have to reconstruct the context in which that stimulus found itself (Anderson & Pichest, 1978). Consequently, any task or event to be remembered will be encoded in a different manner in different contexts. For example, if subjects have to remember a specific story, the encoding of it will vary if we change the internal context. For example, we could tell a patient with memory problems a story about "John, the bridge builder" or change its intrinsic context and tell it as the "bridges that John built." It is the same story but with two different contexts. In the first case, John is the protagonist, and the story is centered on the man; in the second version, the protagonists are the bridges. Therefore, the memories will be very closely related with the context with which they were encoded.

When the episode to be evoked has to do with events that the subjects have lived themselves, it will be recalled as a function of the contextual situation in which the subjects have placed themselves and will depend, therefore, on how the scene was lived, what understanding was derived from it, and how it was elaborated once it was over. Thus, if subjects have to remember the first date they had, the recollections will be different if the narrator encoded based only on his/her own feelings and on his/her mood; in this case, he/she will make few references to anything that is not him/herself and his/her emotional recollections. Nothing else happened for him/her, and if he/she does think that something else happened, it may possibly be his/her own elaboration rather than an exact or real recollection of the events. He/she will have difficulty remembering important aspects of the date and of his/her partner on that occasion. If what was encoded, however, was based on situational aspects of the date, on the reactions of the couple, etc., the recollections will be different. Although the events will be the same, there will be two different "scripts." Ask a couple, for instance, to describe their first dates, and you will get two different accounts.

Therefore, in neuropsychological rehabilitation, one must consider the intrinsic context of the memories, since the patients will elaborate their recollections as a function of the encoding contexts.

1.   The rehabilitating neuropsychologist has to consider and be aware of the design and execution of the treatment, of the context of the facts, events, tasks etc., and of encoding.
2.   The rehabilitation of any memory will be carried out by helping the patient to reconstruct it from the context in which it was encoded.
3.   If, in the course of the memory reconstruction process, contamination or interference from other memories appears, the neuropsychologist must help the patient remove them from the process that is being carried out.
4.   When a therapist is encoding new memories, he/she should facilitate the interactive context by helping the patient construct and elaborate the story from the context he/she chooses. The context can later be changed if that is desired from the rehabilitation point of view.

There is also another external context in which encoding is produced—the environment. All that we have advocated previously could fail or be facilitated as a result of the environment in which the encoding was done. In this sense, at the moment of planning the rehabilitation from this contextual point of view, the following influences must be considered:

•   Environments that are very charged up from the informational standpoint may interfere in the encoding processes. Rehabilitation must start in lightly charged information environments.
•   The environments chosen for rehabilitation must be emotionally neutral for the patient. For example, a male patient with problems controlling his impulses and

with difficulty controlling his sexual appetites will not be able to perform his memory rehabilitation exercises if he is surrounded by women.

Association Principles in Memory Rehabilitation

When rehabilitating deficits in memory encoding, one needs to consider association principles—knowing how ideas or facts are associated during encoding. During the encoding process, it is possible that what is being encoded is not only the memory that the rehabilitator has proposed but also others associated that the latter does not control. That is why the central encoding task must be stressed. It is possible that the types of associations that are being made during encoding are idiosyncratic, and, consequently, of difficult to control experimentally or contextually. The neuropsychologist may try to neutralize this interference by manipulating the environment and the intrinsic context of the task. However, as the patient improves the encoding, the association principles may be useful in the encoding of more complex memories.

REHABILITATION PRINCIPLES FOR MEMORY STORAGE AND CONSOLIDATION DEFICITS

It appears that it was Ramon y Cajal (1923) who first pointed to the possibility that neuronal connections, which must be established so that information may be stored in the brain, are stimulated with activity and exercise. According to them, when we write, read, play the piano, or perform any activity with a certain degree of frequency, the contacts between the nerve cells in the brain are quite efficiently improved. This potentiation is brought about through the creation of new cell appendixes and also by reorganizing and/ or creating new neural networks. Years later, D.O. Hebb (1949, p. 62) presented his famous neuropsychological principle about synaptic modification in the memory. He explained how contacts between nerve cells can favor memory:

> *When an axon of cell A is near enough to excite cell B and repeatedly or persistently takes part in firing it, some growth process or metabolic change takes place in one or both cells such that A's efficiency, as one of the cells firing B, is increased...some memories are both instantaneously established and permanent. To account for the performance, some structural change seems necessary, but a structural growth presumably would require an appreciable time.*

These influential principles begin to get experimental support with the studies done by Bliss, Lomo, and Gardner-Medwin (1973) in which they demonstrated that a brief, high frequency electrical stimulation on the dentate gyrus of the hippocampus would result in a lasting improvement in the synaptic transmission of this pathway, which will last for days or weeks. The physiological characteristics of these improvements have been called long-term potentiation (LTP). LTP is an electrophysiological phenomenon of persistent changes in the strength of the synapse due to the transmission of impulses through the synapse. However, the cell mechanisms and the intracellular reactions of the LTP are still not well known, although several hypotheses exist that have not been consistently proven. The LTP can be obtained in different structures of the brain and in the hippocampus (Bliss, Lomo, & Gardner-Medwin, 1973), as well as in the amygdala, in the neocortex, and in the cerebellum.

The implication, in terms of memory theory and in the rehabilitation of memory deficits, is that changes occur in the synapse as a result of their use (see Fuster, 1995). Nevertheless, some studies have shown that even when restricted to a simple monoaminergic pathway, the LTP has certain characteristics that are useful to memory mechanisms. According to Abraham, Corballis, and White (1991), these characteristics are persistence, input specificity, cooperativity/associativity, ubiquity, and saturability and are incremental.

Neuropsychological rehabilitation, following these characteristics, should try to achieve LTP in the undamaged brain synapse with the goal of creating new functional networks for memory. The rehabilitation process will progress to the extent that the therapist is capable of creating, through neuropsychological techniques, this progress in the patient.

Consequently, we describe below the characteristics and their implication for the rehabilitation of memory storage and consolidation disorders:

- **Persistence.** LTP may last for days or weeks, independent of the brevity (hundredths of a millisecond) of the stimulation, although it has not been shown that it causes a permanent change in the synaptic transmission. Anything that happens around us can be memorized, no matter how fleeting its presentation or appearance is. In the case of patients with brain damage, adequate neuropsychological stimulation can produce LTP, and the latter may persist in time. The question lies in knowing what comprises adequate stimuli.
- **Input specificity.** The LTP is produced in those synapses that are active during the electrical stimulation period. The inactive synapses of the same post-synaptic nerve cells are not potentiated. Therefore, rehabilitation must begin with very clear and specific tasks and not with non-specific tasks. If at all possible, the tasks should only involve one sensory mode (e.g., tasks involving auditory memory should not be mixed with visual memory, etc.) at least initially in the rehabilitation program and not until a notable progress has been achieved that would indicate moving to more complex tasks.
- **Cooperativity/associativity.** The input fibers interact in order to induce the LTP in such a way that more LTPs are generated due to the co-activity of inputs than when they are generated only by means of the stimulation of individual entry pathways. In our opinion, this characteristic in patients with organic memory deficits must follow the previous indication. In normal persons, memorization will be reinforced by presenting information through sensory multimodes, because, in addition to being better understood, it will cause better insights. In our patients, uncontrolled multistimulation could favor cognitive activity but not the functional organization of the system. Therefore, multimode stimulation must always follow progress achieved in specific stimulation and must be implemented gradually.
- **Ubiquity.** LTP is found in many pathways throughout the brain; however, it seems to be found more preeminently in the limbic and neocortical zones.
- **Saturability.** LTP seems to have a saturation effect reaching its highest at levels that represent a 50–100% increase in the size of synaptic potentiation.
- **Incremental quality.** LTP is incremental; thus, for example, a couple of small electrical stimuli produce 5–10% of the increase in the synaptic responses. When these stimuli occur separated by an optimum interval, the increments seem to be quite stable. When additional pairs of stimuli continue to be given, the same increments are produced until the response reaches saturation or has reached its peak.

The Role of Repetition in the Rehabilitation of Memory Deficits[9]

Repetition seems to be the most primitive, effective, and natural mechanism to produce memories. It is a matter of trying to obtain what has been called long-term potentitation and of stimulating to the maximum viable nerve cell connections in the subject. It seems that this would be one of the most natural ways of learning. It has to do with strengthening mechanical memory. In our opinion, it is from this point that any rehabilitation strategy of organic storage and memory consolidation problems should begin. Glysky, Schacter, and Tulving (1986, p. 326) state that their results "indicate that with the use of an effective technique and extensive repetition, even severely impaired patients can acquire a good deal of new knowledge, perhaps more than would have been expected on the basis of previous research."

The Priming Effect on the Rehabilitation of Memory Processes

What is known as *priming* is a form of indirect memory and refers to those times when a person has been exposed to a determined stimulus that influences in the later memory process. In a study performed by Mayes and Gooding (1989, p. 1068) on the enhancement of word completion priming, they reached three conclusions that have implications for the rehabilitation of amnesic patients:

1. Amnesic patients failed in any new association word completion priming effect; they had only a normal effect.
2. There was a great deal of variability in the results obtained by the patients: for some, there were negative effects; for others, normal effects; and for still others, there was some improvement.
3. Although priming did not correlate with any cognitive or memory variable, the best results were obtained by those who had the greatest verbal fluency and by those who performed guided evocation in the priming tasks.

The findings of these authors clearly indicate that not all amnesic patients present improvements with priming and, instead, it seems that only those patients with moderate amnesia show improvement (Graf & Schacter, 1985), although those with greater levels of intelligence seem to get better results (Cermak, Blackford, O'Connor, & Bleitch, 1988). Therefore, the pre-exposure to stimuli in order to later remember them seems to make some sense in those patients with a premorbid level of intelligence above the normal and which at the time of rehabilitation do not have it greatly deteriorated.

On the other hand, Schacter, Cooper, Tharan, and Rubens (1991) found that patients with organic memory disorders showed a robust priming effect in the implicit memory exam for new visual objects impossible to have existed in tridemensional form. Although the priming effect and its magnitude was the same as with the control group subjects or with the student group, explicit memory was deteriorated. For them, priming was obstructed by a subsystem of perceptive representation that functions at a presemantic level and that is preserved in amnesic patients.

REHABILITATION OF EVOCATION AND RECOVERY PROCESSES

People can tell that they have a memory problem when they try to remember something and cannot, or when someone close to them tells them about an event they lived together and they cannot remember it, or when after having studied something for a long time cannot remember it several days later. People, therefore, become alarmed when they cannot recall at will under the same conditions in which they were able to do so at other times. Sometimes, they are not even aware that they have memory problems.

The fundamental characteristics of the amnesic syndrome were summarized by Baddeley (1982a, b). The profile of the post-traumatic amnesia patient is that of a person who has difficulty learning and remembering new information of almost any sort. Although these patients may seem to have an acceptable short-term memory, they may have serious difficulties when trying to evoke memories prior to the beginning of the amnesia, and they may also have other cognitive skills with a near normal functioning level.

There are several hypotheses regarding the functional deficits that underlie in the memory, from among which we will stress the two we consider most relevant for rehabilitation purposes:

- Patients with evocation problems have some type of problem in consolidating and storing information, and, therefore, cannot recover what they have not stored (Zola-Morgan & Squire, 1990).
- Amnesic patients are capable, normally, of storing and consolidating information, but they cannot gain access to it (Schachter, 1990).

The first case is that of an anterograde amnesia (i.e., patients are unable to consolidate new experiences in their memory, although the memory prior to the accident is intact, and they can access it; in addition, they are capable of immediate repetition of new information at the same level as subjects without brain damage [Cohen & Squire, 1981; Squire, 1986]). Temporal disorientation is a common event among these patients. Numerous studies have been conducted on the effects of brain damage on the consolidation and storage of information in the memory (Newcombe, 1969; Grafman et al., 1986), which demonstrate that these deficits exist. These subjects are unable to recall new information, although they can understand and express themselves adequately, resolve more or less complex problems, and carry out other mental activities that do not require memory.

In retrograde memory, the patients are unable to remember episodes in their lives that took place before the brain damage. This lack of memory can run from a few seconds before the accident that produced the brain damage and can last minutes, months, or years. Some authors make a distinction between retrograde amnesia and remote memory deficit. For them, while the former usually is present in any type of amnesia, the deterioration of remote memory would be a different entity related to superimposed cognitive deficits (Cohen & Squire, 1981, p. 353). These authors reach the following conclusions regarding amnesia and the neuropsychology of memory:

- Amnesia is a unitary disorder.
- Brief retrograde amnesia and the extensive deterioration of remote memory are two different entities.
- The place and extent of the brain lesion determine the characteristics of the amnesia. The location (diencephalic or temporal) is related to the nature of the anterograde deficit, and the extent, to the degree of the remote memory deterioration.
- The brain region damaged in the amnesia appears to be specialized in the formation of new memories and in the elaboration and maintenance during later years of learning with adequate storage.
- As time passes after learning, some memories become more resistent to disruption in a process that continues for years.

Therefore, from the rehabilitation point of view, if we are faced with an encoding and consolidation topic, we make reference to those subjects treated previously; if we have an evocation problem, the rehabilitation strategies must be focused in accordance with the type of memory that has the deficit.

REHABILITATION ACCORDING TO THE TYPES OF MEMORY

Different authors and research groups have attempted to study the underlying factors in the rehabilitation processes for the different types of deficits corresponding to the different types of memory, not all of which are conclusive. In addition, it is not possible to believe that the rehabilitation of these deficits is based solely on the characteristics of the type of deficit but rather that one has to consider that the rehabilitation of organic disorders of memory must be done in a multimode and integrated manner. We have been examining throughout this chapter the rehabilitation process as a series of separate entities; however, all the headings of the chapters are perfectly linked together in such a fashion as to offer a complete and clear image of the puzzle. Therefore, any partial approach would result in not seeing the whole picture but rather only a part of the problem.

The Rehabilitation of Short-Term Memory

The rehabilitation of short-term memory, work memory, or active memory deficits is very important. If the patients reflect these deficits, the situation is quite important for the acquisition of new learning, to be able to follow the course of a conversation, or in the solving of problems that have an important propositional content.

There is an entire series of conditions that must be controlled when designing the rehabilitation program for short-term memory deficits:

- Knowledge of the availability of short-term storage space. This will be achieved by means of short-term memory tests. The results will indicate what is the real space, and it is from here that more space will be built.
- Knowledge of the operative space that the subject has available for the purpose of carrying out intellectual functions.
- Awareness of the total processing space, the sum of the volume of the two previous spaces. These, after all, are the central processing resources possessed by the subject.

Some studies indicate that the important goal is to gain storage space (Case, Kurland, & Goldberg, 1982), and that is achieved in a natural manner with children when the operational speed and efficiency increases. With the goal of rehabilitating the work memory, this seems to be achieved by attempting to go beyond the patient's current capacity of storage units more than by remaining just at the capacity he/she is showing. Thus, for example, a subject with an immediate storage capacity of four units will have to start working with five units and move on quickly to working with six and seven units and, as efficiency increases, with eight or more.

A short-term memory training (as well as a long-term memory one) is presented by Gianutsos (1981). The design consisted of a series of seven phases of four sessions each in an intensive rehabilitation program, each session being for two hours three times per week. The first phase was meant to establish the free recall baseline. The second phase focused on the initiation of memory span practice by means of computer-generated word-lists.

The third phase emphasized the initiation of mnemonic elaboration training. The fourth phase was a continuation of the training. In the fifth phase, the session's sequence was changed, and it began with free recall. In the sixth phase, memory span training was discontinued and included unrelated tasks. Finally, in the seventh phase, there was a discontinuation of mnemonic elaboration training.

Another important factor to consider is that of interference, which makes work memory extremely vulnerable; this is especially present in patients with lesions in the hippocampus. The techniques considered most appropriate will have to be used in order to minimize or to eliminate the interference or interferences that might be produced. It is a matter of teaching the patient to internally inhibit by offering him/her attractive tasks that will require his/her concentration. One should start with the simplest tasks he/she can handle, making them more complex later.

The Rehabilitation of Long-Term Memory Deficits

The rehabilitation of declarative or explicit memory disorders requires the use of diverse strategies and techniques. It is a question of bringing to the level of consciousness events having taken place in the past (episodic deficit) or of data acquired through training (semantic deficit). Amnesic patients and demented patients have a deterioration of the capability to acquire and evoke material associated with temporal and spatial contexts (i.e., they show evidence of deterioration of episodic memory, although only the demented patients show a serious deterioration of the evocation of general knowledge or of semantic memory [Butters, Granholm, Salmon, et al., 1987]). These facts seem to show that the underlying processes in the failures of both memory systems may vary from one patient to another, although Zola-Morgan, Cohen, and Squire (1983) do not show evidence of a selective deficit in episodic memory in amnesia. Similarly, Ostergaard (1987) finds it inconsistent that the amnesic syndrome represents a selective deterioration of the episodic memory that leaves semantic memory practically unaffected. In our rehabilitation program, therefore, we do not contemplate including demented patients.

Episodic memory is fundamentally autobiographical memory, among other things, because it contains information on facts and events temporally dated. The rehabilitation goal is, therefore, two-fold. First, there is an attempt to have patients recover the information and, second, to be able to date it temporally so that they place it chronologically in their own autobiography. Some techniques used to study autobiographical memory with demented patients have been used (Crovitz & Schiffman, 1974; Kopelman, Wilson & Baddeley, 1989).

From the standpoint of our program, we believe that the Crovitz technique could serve as an initial point of departure for rebuilding patients' autobiographies because it offers them a list of key words and then asks them to associate each one with a key episode of their lives. It is possible that patients might invent, therefore, as much as possible, and some of the data will have to be compared. When the episodes related are partial and are full of inventions and fiction in order to complete them, patients should try to rebuild them gradually with the help of persons who shared those episodes. It may happen that patients may accept the rebuilding of the facts without having remembered them; this is not advisable, although it might be good from the standpoint of effectiveness for social life and for self-identity.[10]

Consequently, patients' accounts should be accompanied by personal videos and photographs when the episode to be remembered has been completed in its basic structure.

It can be of great help, once the episode has been located in time, to have this exercise accompanied by music of significance to subjects of the period of the episode.

The rehabilitation of semantic memory deficits, such as the multiplication tables, grammar rules, the capitals of the nations of the world, the most important rivers of a home country, etc., will probably require new training. Thus, if patients have to learn to read again, they will have to do it following the reading learning system considered most adequate. Clinical evidence seems to indicate that patients relearn much more rapidly than they did the first time around. One should proceed in the same manner with the other types of semantic information that have to be reestablished.

INTERVENTION IN THE MEMORY ORGANIZATION DEFICITS

One of the most important aspects to consider in the rehabilitation of memory problems is to know what the integrity is of the executive system resident in prefrontal areas. Although frontal lobe lesions normally do not cause amnesia, they do affect the internal organization and control of the mnesic process itself. The studies by Moscovitch (1982) and Squire (1982) were the first in the West to indicate that the memory of amnesia patients may be strongly influenced by an injury in the frontal lobes. As Schacter (1987) indicates, the amnesia patients who also suffer from frontal damage represent an amnesic syndrome that shows qualitative differences from those shown by patients with no frontal damage. Therefore, the memory functions of these frontal patients are different from those noted in "pure" amnesic patients.

The functions of the prefrontal zones of the brain are extensively described, and it is widely accepted that they especially have an executive function. This part of the brain is in charge of organizing, planning, executing, and controlling any of the brain's functional systems, and, consequently, also of the memory as a complex functional system. The prefrontal cortex is in charge of organizing the information received in a manner that will be useful in order to reach the most correct strategy for mnemonic processing; it starts the adequate execution mechanisms so that the tasks may be carried out, determining the temporal sequence and the correct execution pathways, and, subsequently, it monitors and makes sure that the entire process is carried out correctly (Figure 20.3).

Therefore, any lesion that affects the anterior areas of the brain will cause memory deficits related to the organizing, planning, and executing of the process that has to be carried out, especially because there will be a disorganization of the entire process, and its control will not be assured. As Moscovitch (1995, p. 1353) indicates (Figure 20.4):

> ...memory disorders following frontal lesions are not related to deficits in storage and retention, which are hippocampical functions. Instead, they are associated with impaired organizational and strategic processes that, at the extreme, result in confabulations in which accurately remembered elements of one event are combined with those of another without regard to their internal consistency and plausibility...if the hippocampical complex can be considered to consist of "raw memory" structures, then the frontal lobes are "working-with-memory" structures that operate on the input to the hippocampal component and the output from it.

According to Shimamura (1995), patients with frontal lobe lesions usually have many memory problems, among which are free evocation, word-finding, metamemory, memory for temporal order, and source memory. However, these patients do not usually present serious deterioration on standard tests of new learning ability (see Janowsky, Shimamura,

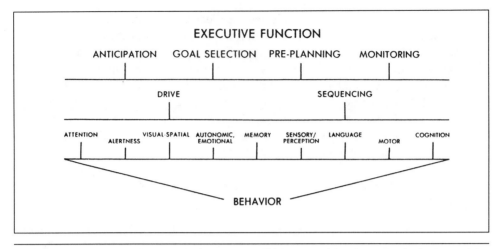

Figure 20.3: Executive control functions. They establish how and in what order the basic cognitive functions of a fixed system are to be used to achieve a specific goal (from Stuss & Benson, 1986).

Kritcheusky, & Squire, 1989). These patients are not able to control the processing of irrelevant information due to a failure in the inhibition of previous memory associations. This same point is made by Luria (1974, p. 533), for whom the mechanisms of serious memory disorders derived from frontal lesions are not due so much to the extinction of the traces but rather to their inhibition augmented by factors of interference that take place against a background of a strong pathologic inertia of the stereotype traces which have emerged once. All of this provokes a very notable alteration of the selection of the emerging linkup systems, the results of which are that the patient mixes up the information of the different systems causing a contamination phenomena.

In another article, Shimamura, Jurica, Mangels, Gershberg, and Knight (1995), in working with frontal patients, suggest that the on-line control of competitive or irrelevant memories is altered in frontal lobe lesions. This alteration could be indicative of a deteriorated gating or filtering mechanism that affects not only the memory functions but also other cognitive functions. From this standpoint, the frontal lobe is seen as a dynamic filter mechanism that modulates other activities and inhibits strange activities. Therefore, the frontal lobe would be implicated in the inhibiting control of the posterior cortical activity in such a manner that a lesion in those areas would provoke a disinhibition of these activities. This seems logical if we keep in mind that one of the most clear effects of frontal lesions, according to Luria (1966, 1974), besides what has already been stated, is that of disinhibition. Patients are impulsive and not very reflexive when required to give an answer or perform an act; it is as if they acted upon impulse, although others have problems in voluntarily initiating an action or a determined task.

Consequently, patients with a frontal lesion will exhibit peculiarities in the rehabilitation of memory problems. In the first place, we could find that patients are uninhibited or, on the contrary, have difficulties in beginning or carrying out any task.

In the case of subjects with a clear difficulty in inhibiting impulses, the rehabilitation task will be complicated, since it will be very difficult for them to maintain a sufficient attention span on the task they have been given. The first rehabilitation objective will be just that—making it possible for them to maintain their attention spans for a sufficient period of time. The second objective is to get them to establish an organization system

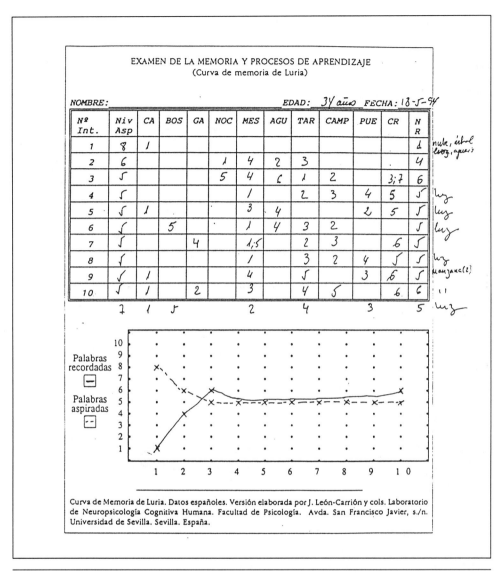

Figure 20.4: Luria's Memory Word Test (LMW) from a frontal lobe patient 34-years-old. The patient doesn't control the memory and learning processes. There are no learning strategies or planning (from León-Carrión, 1995).

for the information they have to learn. For that purpose, they will have to be taught how to organize themselves with the tasks; in this sense, it will help that they express themselves verbally to the rehabilitator how they expect to do it. Verbalization helps organization. Patients should not be allowed to perform any task if they have not first explained how they plan to do it, why they have decided to do it in such a fashion, and what the objectives are that they are pursuing. Frontal patients with initiative deficits will be helped in starting tasks, and later the procedure outlined before will be followed. It is important to teach these patients to recognize the consequences of their actions (prospective, anticipation) by asking them to say what it is that is going to happen if they do something, and then, after the action, compare what has happened with what they said was going to happen.

THE ROLE OF COMPUTERS IN THE REHABILITATION OF MEMORY DEFICITS

Different studies have tried to show how the use of computers is an excellent external aid in the rehabilitation of patients with memory deficits. The suggestions that some of these authors have made in this regard, especially the Glisky and Schacter group, follow.

In a study published by Glisky, Schacter, and Tulving in 1986, they state that patients with memory disorders of different severity can be helped with computer programs to learn and handle relatively complex information. They are capable of learning to handle information on the screen—write, edit, and execute simple computer tasks—store information on the diskettes, and even recover it. These authors also indicate that these patients require time, since their learning is slower than with subjects who have no memory problems.

That same year, these authors presented a technique using computers that they considered very adequate for mnesic patients (Glysky, Schacter, & Tulving, 1986b). It taught the learning and retention of vocabulary through the use of the computer by means of vanishing cues. It involved a system of presenting words, which the subjects had to learn, during which letters are gradually being removed. The authors indicate that the learning of these patients is slow and strongly dependent on first letter cues. The results showed that all the patients were capable of learning a large volume of vocabulary that could be retained for weeks.

Regarding the long-term retention of what is learned by computer, Glysky and Schacter (1988) indicate that the vanishing cues method is an effective technique to teach the acquisition of complex knowledge to patients with organic memory disorders and that the knowledge acquired by this means is retained by the patients for a long time (which does not mean that the rhythm and amount of learning is normal). This method, also by means of a computer, has been used by these authors (Glysky & Schacter, 1987) to train in the acquisition of domain-specific knowledge in organic amnesia. It trained for work with a computer in real life. In order for this method to be successful, these authors indicate that training techniques, extensive repetition of all procedures, and specific and direct training in all work components are required.

THE ROLE OF PSYCHOPHYSIOLOGIC SLEEP IN THE REHABILITATION OF MEMORY DEFICITS

From the moment that sleep was studied from the psychophysiological standpoint, more and more evidence has been found of its importance in psychological functions, since we know that during sleep, the nervous system is quite active. This activity is both qualitative and quantitative. From the memory's theoretical field, it is coherent to propose that it is during psychophysiological sleep that all the information received during the day is placed in order. With a sense of cognitive economy and efficiency, it is during sleep that the information which is considered biologically or psychologically relevant and significant to the subject is stored and filed in some place in the brain by means of specific mechanisms. The other information that is not considered relevant for him/her at that time in the life of the subject is not stored, and, if it is, it is done so under other parameters and with other access or recovery codes different from those for normal recollection. It is probably stored as unorganized or unelaborated information as second level transformations. This all is produced fundamentally during REM sleep.[11]

Therefore, from our point of interest, it is important to understand what it is that happens from the cognitive point of view if a person does not sleep. One effect seems to be the non-dating of the events which took place during that period of time, confusion in the sequential development of the events, and, at times, even invention and contamination with other events that took place. Subjects are often unable to give dates for events that took place, understand which events came first and which came after, and events become confused and intermixed for them. The subjects try to order their recollections based on their sense of logic, and, for this reason, the accounts are usually full of errors, fiction, and invention. It could be compared with what is called the "state of dependent learning phenomenon" (i.e., the learning that is acquired under the effects of drugs or altered mental states cannot be remembered effectively in a normal state).

REM sleep increases after a period of learning, as has been shown in studies by Oswald (1969) and Lucero (1970). Bloch (1973) indicates that learning encourages the appearance of mechanisms triggering REM sleep, and the trigger is much more likely to be tripped during sleep. Recently, Smith and Lapp (1991), when studying students after an exam, found an increase in the number of REMs compared with other controls and with a baseline, in addition to an increase in the REM density in the fourth REM period of the night. According to these authors, findings seem to indicate that REM sleep is involved in memory even several days after the study period. In a study by Arons (1990), the subjects had to memorize and recreate a text previously unknown and after sleeping. He found a redistribution of the REM phases of those nights, with increases in the second cycle of sleep and its corresponding decrease at the end of the night. The subjects' difficulties in memorization were noted in the REM latency.

In order to *consolidate* and *store* information, it is classically accepted that both functions improve after sleep. The first known study was that of Jenkin and Dallenbach (1924). It showed how two subjects learned from lists without meaning, which they later had to recreate; they remained awake or asleep during the time between the learning and the recreation. The results showed that retention was better after sleeping for a period of time equal to the time they were awake. Later it was found that when the subjects slept right after the learning session, retention was quite good compared with the retention of those who, instead of sleeping, remained awake and performed other activities.

Studies conducted by Fishbein (1970) showed that REM sleep deprivation produces a permanent amnesic effect on long-term memory without impaired learning. His data suggested that what happens is that a deficit takes place in the process of converting short-term storage into long-term storage. Also, Fishbein (1971) found that the suppression of REM sleep interferes with the normal fixation of memory traces. Rotenberg also found (1992a, b) that a long deprivation of REM sleep before learning may cause learned helplessness and alter the learning process. When sleep is removed after learning, retention problems appear.

Therefore, it is important to consider the regulation of the sleep of patients with brain damage and with memory problems (see also Chapter 14) as follows:

- It is advisable to have an 8-hour registry of the psychophysiological sleep of the patient with brain damage in the baseline (i.e., it is necessary to know how his/her sleep phases are distributed).

- In the event that the REM phases were few, it would be advisable to verify with each patient whether the learning exercises increase the amount and density of the sleep phases.
- In the event that that happens, the rehabilitation program should continue. If it does not, pharmaceuticals may be required in order to promote REM sleep.
- It would be advisable, in general terms, that patients sleep a normal period of from 7–8 hours daily.
- It might be advisable that in the two hour period before going to sleep, the patients work on some type of memory exercise.
- After the rehabilitation sessions, it might be advisable, if the sessions are not at night, that they take a 45- to 100-minute nap, preferably closer to the 100- than to the 45-minute duration.

COMPENSATION TECHNIQUES IN THE REHABILITATION OF MEMORY DEFICITS

One of the most frequent approaches in the rehabilitation of memory disorders is the use of compensation techniques. Perhaps this is so because it is a natural response to a complex problem such as memory deficits, and it is within the reach of anyone with any type of formation or condition. The compensation techniques are not meant to directly improve memory deficits; their objective is to try to make the effects of the lack of memory be less disabling by using external aids such as agendas, electronic organizers, alarms, or environmental modification. Thus, patients deposit their memory outside of themselves, for example, in an electronic agenda programmed for this purpose, which notifies them and reminds them of what to do at every moment. Today, one can find such electronic organizers in the market place, which, at the programmed time, will indicate by means of a sound or a phrase what has to be done at that moment.

In these cases, patients do not have to worry about their memory for the activities of daily life; the electronic organizer will do it for them. From our point of view, these techniques are interesting and are very useful for patients who need them, but they are not in themselves rehabilitation techniques nor do they have scientific support behind them. They are ultimately compensation techniques. Our doubt lies in knowing whether it is advisable to do simultaneously the rehabilitation and the compensation. It is possible that it might not be advisable to carry out both efforts, especially since the compensation techniques might interfere with the necessary effort required by all neuropsychological rehabilitation processes of the patients who are doing them. To further study compensation techniques, see Sholberg and Mateer (1989), Glisky and Schacter (1987), and Wilson (1987a, b).

ENDNOTES

1. The design of the rehabilitation of memory disorders following brain damage that is proposed in this chapter is one used at the Human Neuropsychological Laboratory of the University of Seville (Spain). It is experimental and, consequently, it could be improved. We will also present the theoretical basis upon which it was developed, convinced as we are that it is from the current framework of knowledge about memory and its deficits that we can improve treatment strategies. Possibly neuropsychological treatment combined with pharmacological treatment may bring forth, in coming years, greater advances which will make easier today's complex and laborious organic memory deficits rehabilitation chores.

2. This systems definition by Tulving is identical to the functional system proposed almost 20 years before by Luria in 1962. A functional system is, for Luria, a group of different and distant cerebral zones with a common task.

3. For Miller, (1956, p. 94), the process of memorization may simply be the formation of chunks or groups of items that go together until there are few enough chunks to recall all the items.

4. We will briefly review the functions of memory because we are convinced that all neuropsychologists are familiar with them. There are excellent works on psychology and cognitive neuropsychology that may be consulted. But we have thought it necessary to include in this chapter a brief overview of the subject so that the reader may have a clear and coherent point of reference. This will serve as the starting point for constructing our rehabilitation design for organic memory disorders.

5. We shall call "engram" the informational contents of the registries.

6. The term "ecphoria" was coined by Richard Simon in 1904 in *Die Mneme als erhaltendes Prinzip im Wechsel des organischen gesechehens.* Leipzig: William Engelman.

7. During the 1970s and 1980s, there was a strong feeling that the restoration of the mnesic functions was an impossible goal (Miller, 1978; Schacter & Glysky, 1986; Wilson & Moffat, 1984).

8. This same author had previously suggested that survivors of severe closed brain injury exhibit frequent persistent deterioration of memory despite intensive rehabilitation (Levin, Handel, Goldman, Eisenberg, & Guinto, 1985).

9. Some researchers believe, in a deceptive manner, that repetition as a technique is quite simplistic. This may be true but only for the memorization of complex information. Even so, once that information has been ecphorized, it has to be brought back to the memory periodically so that it can be well retained. All of which is much easier with normal persons without memory deficits.

10. When personal videos and photographs are used as central techniques for the treatment of evocation problems, patients may end up rebuilding their lives and accepting it as their own without having recollections of it (i.e., they have created new memories). However, these are not rehabilitation or treatment techniques, but rather compensation techniques.

11. The relation between REM sleep and memory was reinforced when it was discovered that the amount of REM sleep is greater at youth when learning is central to mental development and life.

REFERENCES

Abraham, W.C., Corballis, M.C., & White K.G. (1991). *Memory mechanisms: A tribute to G.V. Goddard* (Introduction) (pp. XV–XXIII). Hillsdale: Lawrence Erlbaum Associates.

Adelson, B. (1984). When novices surpass experts: The difficulty of a task may increase with expertise. *Journal of Psychology: Learning, Memory and Cognition, 10,* 483–495.

Anderson, R.C., & Pichest, J.W. (1978). Recall of previously unrecallable information following a shift in perspective. *Journal of Verbal Learning and Verbal Behavior, 17,* 1–12.

Arons, E.K. (1990). The effect of memorization processes on the structural organization of natural human sleep. *Zh-Vyssh-Nerv-Deiat, 40,* 419–425.

Baddeley, A.D. (1982a). Amnesia: A minimal model and an interpretation. In L. Cermak (Ed.), *Human memory and amnesia.* Hillsdale: Lawrence Erlbaum Associates.

———. (1982b). Domains of recollection. *Psychological Review, 89,* 708–729.

———. (1994). The magical number seven: Still magic after all these years? *Psychological Review, 101,* 353–356.

Baddeley, A.D., & Hitch G. (1974). Working memory. In G.H. Bower (Comp.), *The psychology of learning and motivation* (Vol. 8). New York, Academic Press.

Berg, I.J., Koning-Haanstra, D., & Deelmon, B.G. (1991). Long-term effects of memory rehabilitation: A controlled study. *Neuropsychological Rehabilitation, 1,* 97–111.

Bliss, T.V.P., Lomo T., & Gardner-Medwin, A.R. (1973). Long-lasting potentation of squaptic transmission in the dentate area of the anesthesized rabbit following stimulation of the perforant path. *Journal of Psychology, 232,* 331–374.

Bloch, V. (1973). L'activation cérébrale et la fixation mnésique. *Arch. Ital. Biol., 111,* 577–590.

Braak, H., and Braak, E. (1992). The human entorninal cortex: Normal morphology and lamina specific pathology in various diseases. *Neuroscience Research, 15,* 6–31.

Brothers, L., & Ring, B. (1993). Mesial temporal neurons in the macaque monkey with responses selective for aspects of social stimuli. *Behav. Brain. Res.*, *57*, 53–61.

Brown, R., & Kulik, J. (1977). Flashbulb memories. *Cognition*, *5*, 73–99.

Butters, N., Granholm, E., Salmon, D.P., Grant, I., & Wolfe, J. (1987). Episodic and semantic memory: A comparison of amnesia and demented patients. *Journal of Clinical and Experimental Neuropsychology*, *9*, 479–497.

Case, R., Kurland, D.M., & Goldberg, J. (1982). Operational efficiency and the growth of short-term memory span. *Journal of Experimental Child Psychology*, *26*, 386–403.

Cermak, L.S., Blackford, S.P., O'Conner, M., & Bleich, R.P. (1988). The implicit memory ability of a patients with amnesia due to encephalitis. *Brain and Cognition*, *7*, 145–156.

Chase, W.G., & Ericsson, K.A. (1981). Skilled memory. In J.R. Anderson (Ed.), *Cognitive skills and their acquisition*. Hillsdale: Lawrence Erlbaum Associates.

Cohen, N.J., & Squire, R. (1981). Retrograde amnesia and remote memory impairment. *Neuropsychologia*, *19*, 337–356.

Craik, F.I.M., & Lockhart, R.S. (1972). Levels of processing: A framework for memory research. *Journal of Verbal and Learning Behavior*, *11*, 671–684.

Crovitz, H.F., & Schiffman, H. (1974). Frequency of episodic memories as a function of their age. *Bulletin of the Psychonomics Society*, *4*, 517–518.

Crowder, R.G. (1976). *Principles of learning and memory*. Hillsdale: Lawrence Erlbaum Associates.

De Groot, A.D. (1965). *Thought and choice in chess*. The Hague: Mouton.

Dirkmen, S., Temkin, N., Mcleant, A., Wyler A., & Machamer, J. (1987). Memory and head injury severity. *Journal of Neurology, Neuroscience and Psychiatry*, *50*, 1613–1618.

Fishbein, W. (1970). Interference with conversion of memory from short-term to long-term storage by partial sleep deprivation. *Commun. Beh. Biol.*, *5*, 171–175.

———. (1971). Disruptive effects of rapid eye movement sleep deprivation on long-term memory. *Physiol. Behav.*, *6*, 279–282.

Fuster, J.M. (1995). *Memory in the cerebral cortex*. Cambridge: MIT Press.

Fuster, J.M., & Uyeda, A.A. (1971). Reactivity of limbic neurons of the monkey to appetitive and aversive signals. *Electroencephalogic. Clin. Neurophysiol.*, *30*, 281–293.

Gianutsos, R. (1981). Training the short- and long-term verbal recall of a post-encephalitic amnesic. *Journal of Clinical Neuropsychology*, *1*, 117–135.

Glisky, E.L., & Schacter, D.L. (1987). Acquisition of domain-specific knowledge in organic amnesia: Training for computer-related work. *Neuropsychologia*, *25*, 839–906.

———. (1988). Long-term retention of computer learning by patients with memory disorders. *Neuropsychologia*, *26*, 173–178.

Glisky, E.L., Schacter, D.L. & Tulving, E. (1986a). Computer learning by memory-impaired patients: Acquisition and retention of complex knowledge. *Neuropsychologia*, *24*, 313–328.

———. (1986b). Learning and retention of computer-related vocabulary in memory-impaired patients: Method of vanishing cues. *Journal of Clinical and Experimental Neuropsychology*, *8*, 292–312.

Gloor, P. (1960). Amigdala. In J. Field & M.W. Magoun (Eds.), *Handbook of physiology and neurophysiology* (pp. 1395–1420). Washington, DC: American Physiological Society.

Graf, P., & Schacter, D.L. (1985). Implicit and explicit memory for new associations in normal and amnesic subjects. *Journal of Experimental Psychology: Learning, Memory and Cognition*, *11*, 501–518.

Grafman, J., Salazar, A.M., Smutok, M.A., Vance S., & Brown, H.R. (1986). Factors in community adjustment following penetrating brain wounds. Paper presented at INS meeting, Denver.

Gronwall, D., & Wrightson, P. (1981). Memory information processing capacity after closed head injury. *Journal of Neurology, Neurosurgery and Psychiatry*, *44*, 889–895.

Hayman, C.A., MacDonald, C.A., & Tulving, E. (1993). The role of repetition and associative interference in new semantic learning in amnesia: A case experiment. *Journal of Cognitive Neuroscience*, *4*, 375–389.

Hebb, D.O. (1949). *The organization of behavior*. New York: John Wiley and Sons.

Janowsky, J.S., Shimamura, A.P., Kritcheusky, M., & Squire C.R. (1989). Cognitive impairment following frontal lobe damage and its relevance to human amnesia. *Behavioural Neuroscience*, *103*, 289–303.

Jenkin, J., & Dallenbach, K. (1924). Obliviscence during sleep and waking. *Answer J. of Psychology, 35,* 605.

Kopelman, M.D., Wilson, B.A., & Baddeley, A.D. (1989). The autobiographical memory interview: A new assessment of autobiographical and personal semantic memory in amnesic patients. *Journal of Clinical and Experimental Neuropsychology, 11,* 724–744.

Le Doux, J.E. (1993). Emotional memory system in the brain. *Behavi. Brain. Res., 39,* 203–215.

León-Carrión, J. (1995). *Manual de neuropsicologia.* Madrid: s.XXI.

Levin, H.S. (1989). Memory deficit after closed head injury. *Journal of Clinical and Experimental Neuropsychology, 12,* 129–153.

Levin, H.S., Handel, S.F., Goldman, A.M., Eisenberg, H.M., & Guinto, F.C. (1985). Magnetic resonance imaging after "diffuse" nonmissile head injury. *Archives of Neurology, 42,* 963–968.

Levin, M.S., Grossman, R.G., Rose J.E., & Teasdale, G. (1979). Long-term neuropsychological outcome of close head injury. *Journal of Neuropsychology, 50,* 412–422.

Lucero, M. (1970). Lengthening of REM sleep duration consecutive to learning in the rat. *Brain Res., 20,* 319–322.

Luria, A.R. (1966). *Higher cortical functions in man.* London: Tabistock. (*Las funciones corticales del hombre,* La Habana, Orbe, 1976).

———. (1974). *Neuropsicologia Pamiati.* Moscow: Nauta.

———. (1975). Neuropsychology: Its sources, principles and prospects. In F.G. Worden, J.P. Swazey, & G. Adelman (Comps.), *The neurosciences: Paths of discovery* (pp. 335–361). Cambridge: The MIT Press.

Markowitsch, H.J., Von Cramon, D.V., Hoffmann, E., et al. (1990). Verbal memory deterioration after unilateral infarct of the internal capsula in adolescents. *Cortex, 26,* 597–609.

Mayes, A.R. (1992). What are the functional deficits that underlie amnesia? In L.R. Squire and N. Butters (Eds.), *Neuropsychology of memory* (2nd ed.) (pp. 23–36). New York: Guilford Press.

Mayes, A.R., & Gooding, P. (1989). Enhancement of word completion priming in amnesics by cueing with previously novel associates. *Neuropsichologia, 8,* 1057–1072.

Miller, E. (1978). Is amnesia remediable? In M.M. Gruneberg, P.E. Morris, & R.N. Sykes (Eds.), *Practical aspects of memory.* New York: Academic Press.

Miller, G.A. (1956). The magical numbers, plus or minus two: Some limits on our capacity for processing information. *Psychological Review, 63,* 81–97.

Monsell, S. (1984). Repetition and the lexicon. In A.W. Ellis (Comp.), *Progress in the psychology of language* (pp. 147–195). London: Lawrence Erlbaum Associates.

Moscovitch, M. (1982). Multiple dissociation of function in amnesia. In L.S. Cermak (Ed.), *Human memory and amnesia* (pp. 337–370). Hillsdale: Lawrence Erlbaum Associates.

———. (1989). In H.L. Roediger III and F.I.M. Vraik (Eds.), *Varieties of memories and consciousness: Essays in honor of Endel Tulving* (pp. 133–156). Hillsdale: Lawrence Erlbaum.

———. (1995). Models of consciousness and memory. In M.S. Gazzaniga (Ed.), *The cognitive neuro-science* (pp. 1341–1356). Cambridge: The MIT Press.

Newcombe, F. (1969). *Missile wounds of the brain.* London: Oxford University Press.

Ostergaard, A.L. (1987). Episodic, semantic and procedural memory in a case of amnesia at an early age. *Neuropsychologia, 25,* 341–357.

Oswald, I. (1969). Human brain protein, drugs and dreams. *Nature* (London), *223,* 893–897.

Ramon y Cajal, S. (1923). *Recuerdos de mi vida.* Madrid: Pueyo.

Rotenberg, V. S. (1992a). Sleep and memory. I: The influence of different sleep stages on memory. *Neuroscience and Biobehavioral Reviews, 16,* 497–502.

———. (1992 a). Sleep and memory. II. Investigations on humans. *Neuroscience and Biobehavioral Reviews, 16,* 503–505.

Ryan, T.V., & Ruff, R.M. (1988). The efficacy of structured memory retaining in a group comparison of head trauma patients. *Archives of Clinical Neuropsychology, 3,* 165–179.

Sarter, M., & Markowitsch, H.J. (1985). Involvement of the amygdala in learning and memory: a critical review, with emphasis on anatomical relations. *Beh. Neursci., 99,* 342–380.

Schacter, D.L. (1987). Memory amnesia and frontal lobe dysfunction. *Psychobiology, 15,* 21–36.

————. (1990). Perceptual representation systems and implicit memory: Toward a resolution of the multiple memory system debate. In A. Diamond (Ed.), *Development and neural bases of higher cognitive functions* (pp. 543–571). New York: New York Academy of Sciences.

Schacter, D.L., & Glisky E.L. (1986). Memory remediation: Restoration, alleviation and the acquisition of domain-specific knowledge. In B. Uzzell & Y. Gross (Eds.), *Clinical neuropsychology of intervention.* Boston: Martinus Nijhoff.

Schacter, D.L., & Tulving, E. (1982). Memory, amnesia and the episodic semantic distinction. In R.L. Isaacson & N.E. Spear (Eds.), *The expression of knowledge* (pp. 35–65). New York: Plenum Press.

Schacter, D.L., Rich S., & Stamp A. (1985). Remediation of memory disorders: Experimental evaluation of the speed retrieval technique. *Journal of Clinical and Experimental Neuropsychology, 7,* 79–96.

Schacter, D.L., Cooper, L.A., Tharan, M., & Rubens, A.B. (1991). Preserved priming of novel objects in patients with memory disorders. *Journal of Cognitive Neuroscience 3,* 117–130.

Seligman, M.E.P. (1970). On the generality of the laws of learning. *Psychological Review, 77,* 406–418.

Shimamura, A.P. (1995). Memory and frontal lobe function. In M.S. Gazzaniga (Ed.), *The cognitive neurosciences.* Cambridge: MIT Press.

Shimamura, A.P., Jurica, P.J., Mangels, J.A., Gershberg, F.B., & Knight, R.T. (1995). Susceptibility to memory interference effects following frontal lobe damage: Findings from test of paired-associated learning. *Journal of Cognitive Neuroscience, 7,* 144–152.

Sholberg, M.M., & Mateer, C.A. (1989). *Introduction to cognitive rehabilitation.* New York: Guilford Press.

Smith, C., & Lapp, L. (1991). Increases in number of REMS and REM density in human following on intensive learning period. *Sleep, 14,* 325–330.

Squire, L. (1982). The neuropsychology of human memory. *Annual Review of Neuroscience, 5,* 241–73.

————. (1986). The neuropsychology of memory disfunction on its assessment. In I. Grant & K.M. Adams (Comps.), *Neuropsychological assessment of neuropsychiatric disorders* (pp. 268–299). New York: Oxford University Press.

————. (1992). Declarative and non-declarative memory: Multiple brain system supporting learning and memory. *Journal of Cognitive Neuroscience, 3,* 232–240.

Squire, L.R., & Knowlton, B.J. (1995). Memory hippocampus and brain systems. In M.S. Gazzaniga (Ed.), *The cognitive neuroscience (pp.* 825–837). Cambridge: MIT Press.

Tranel, D., & Hayman, B.T. (1990). Neuropsychological correlates of bilateral amygdala damage. *Archives of Neurology, 47,* 349–355.

Tulving, E. (1983). *Elements of episodic memory.* Oxford: Clarendon Press.

————. (1985a). *Elements of episodic memory.* New York: Oxford University Press.

————. (1985b). How many memory systems are there? *Am. Psycholo., 40,* 385–398.

Wilson, B.A. (1987a). *Rehabilitation of memory.* New York: Guilford Press.

————. (1987b). Identification and remediation of everyday problems in memory-impaired patients. In O.A. Parsons, N. Butters, & P.E. Nathan (Eds.), *Neuropsychology of alcoholism: Implications for diagnosis and treatment* (pp. 322–338). New York: Guilford Press.

————. (1991). Long-term prognosis of patients with severe memory disorders. *Neuropsychological Rehabilitation, 1,* 117–134.

Wilson, B.A., & Moffat, N. (1984). Rehabilitation of memory for everyday life. In J.E. Harris & P. Morris (Eds.), *Everyday memory: Actions and absent-mindedness.* London: Academic Press.

Zola-Morgan, S.M., & Squire, L.R. (1990). The primate hippocampal formation: Evidence for a time-limited role in memory storage. *Science, 250,* 288–290.

Zola-Morgan, S.M., Cohen N.J., & Squire, L.R. (1983). Recall of remote episodic memory in amnesia. *Neuropsychologia, 21,* 487–500.

Zola-Morgan, S.M., Squire, L.R., Alvarez-Royo, P., & Clower R.P. (1991). Independence of memory functions and emotional behavior: Separate contributions of the hippocampal formation and the amygdale. *Hippocampus, 1,* 181–194.

21

From a Componential Analysis to a Cognitive Rehabilitation of Everyday Planning

T.M. Sgaramella,[1] P.S. Bisiacchi,[1] and M. Zettin[2]

[1]Dipartimento di Psicologia Generale, Padova, Italy
[2]Presidio Ospedaliero Ausiliatrice, Torino, Italy

INTRODUCTION

The distinctive role of the frontal region in cognition has been brought to light by a series of studies that dates from the last century. The work of Stuss and Benson (1986) is one of the most interesting contributions in understanding the possible role of the frontal lobes in behavior. This contribution can be summarized by four basic operations: *sequencing*, the ability to maintain information in meaningful bits that can be serially interrelated; *driving*, the ability to initiate, modulate, or inhibit cerebral activities; *controlling*, the capacity to adjust the ongoing modular activity; and *self-analysis*, the ability to reflect upon what elements and processes of cognition themselves may mean for the organism. Control ability consists of several operations including anticipation, planning and plan monitoring, and response and response monitoring. The executive control is, instead, thought of as a superordinate capacity to both the frontal and the posterior functional systems. In a further analysis (1987) the authors describe the behavioral deficits following frontal lobe pathology as follows:

- an inability to translate knowledge of specific facts into appropriate action.
- a problem in shifting from one concept to another and in changing a specific behavior, once started.
- a tendency to respond to a fragment (of data) while failing to grasp the totality or the key feature.
- a deficit in relating or integrating isolated details.
- a deficiency in handling simultaneous sources of information.

© GR/St. Lucie Press CCC 1-57444-039-X 1/97/$100/$.50

The process of plan formulation and evaluation has been often ascribed to frontal lobe systems (Penfield & Evans, 1935; Luria, 1966) as goal articulation (Duncan, 1986) and, together with marker creation and triggering (Shallice, 1994), these processes are key elements in the temporal integration of behavior, the basic function of the frontal lobes (Fuster, 1980).

In current neuropsychological research, terms such as "executive control function," "supervisor system," and "dysexecutive syndrome" relate directly to the psychological concept of frontal system function, and recently, many findings on the decline of such functions either in frontal lobe patients, in older adults, and in closed head injury (CHI) patients have been reported (see Stuss & Gow, 1992; Daigneault, Braun, & Whitaker, 1992). In particular, the CHI patients are often characterized by a mild difficulty in laboratory frontal lobe tests and by a more marked difficulty when frontal lobe abilities are required in order to accomplish everyday activities such as planning a meal or choosing a travel program.

It is crucial, therefore, to study the performance of CHI patients in tasks requiring planning in order to design a proper treatment aimed at improving their everyday life performance. First, it is necessary to understand what planning is.

SOME DEFINITIONS AND PSYCHOLOGICAL MODELS OF PLANNING

Planning consists of the ability to organize behavior in order to achieve a goal. It has been defined as "the predetermination of a course of action aimed at achieving some goals" (Hayes-Roth & Hayes-Roth, 1979) or as "a mental simulation which envisages the circumstances and runs possible actions evaluating the consequences and selecting the optimal order for executing them" (Cohen, 1988).

A useful general model of planning is suggested by Hayes-Roth and Hayes-Roth (1979), who developed an errand-planning task in which subjects were given a list of errands to run in a limited amount of time. As in real life, in order to organize their errands, they had to acquire information about the errands and prioritize and sequence errands or action alternatives, taking into account spatio-temporal factors. Several heuristics used by the subjects were also identified by the authors.

The problem of accounting for everyday planning is also a central interest for environmental psychologists who deal with people's memory representations of the spatial structure of the environment. The travelling salesman's problem (Simon, 1957), in which one decides which order between a given number of locations minimizes total travel distance, is often used as an analogue of spatial decisions in a large-scale environment. Within this framework, the "gravity" model represents a general class of models that have been developed to predict aggregated data on shopping trips and work journeys and to describe individuals' spatial decision making. Spatial preference results from a function of psychological attractiveness, memorized distance to it, and familiarity. Cadwallader (1975, 1981) states that a person's spatial preferences and choices are based on information represented in a cognitive map of the environment and are guided by the attractiveness given by its memorized distance.

Models of this sort do not take into account that when people travel, they often combine several purposes and make a sequence of spatial decisions that are likely to embody decisions about the travel, routing, and scheduling.

Gärling et al. (1984) and Gärling (1986) have constrained a model of planning formation, focusing their attention on planning as sequencing hierarchically organized spatial decisions. Their starting point is the idea that the subject is constrained by a limited-capacity short-term memory; hence, the process of plan formation is assumed to be serial and characterized by the use of heuristic rules. Plan formation would include, then,

- forming a list of errands to be run,
- retrieving information about the locations from the cognitive map and representing them in short-term memory,
- making decisions about the order to visit the place, and
- making decisions about which paths to travel between the locations in the order specified in the preceding stage.

These decisions also involve selective retrieval of additional information about how to connect destinations. To reduce cognitive complexity and load, several heuristics may be adopted by the subjects. Minimization of distance is the general criteria used in order to choose between paths; decisions will, then, be guided by minimal local distance (MLD), a heuristic based on the choice from a given location of the nearest location (Hayes-Roth & Hayes-Roth, 1979; Gärling, Säisä, Böök, & Lindberg, 1986), or by the straight-line heuristics (SLH). With increasing complexity of the plan to be formed, information about spatial locations needs a hierarchical organization. In this case, choices about the order will require

- finding clusters of destinations (i.e., analyzing the entire plan in order to identify which goals are to be executed in succession,
- ordering clusters into a global plan, and
- ordering destinations within clusters and by using MLD (Hirtle & Gärling, 1992).

Besides deciding about spatial locations, an everyday errand-planning task requires subjects to choose when to perform a number of errands; time constraints need to be taken into account. Gärling (1995) has recently shown, in fact, that in a usual errand-planning task, subjects frequently confuse travel distance with time. He also found that, in any case, they minimized time accurately when there are time constraints, whether or not distance minimization was required. Sometimes subjects ignored opening hours; wait time was minimized even though it did not lead to time minimization. This behavior has been interpreted as an example of the "realism principle" and introduces in the model a sort of superordinate criteria, invariably important, at the stage of making decisions about the plan.

These models do not consider the finding that in normal human activity, plans, when originally developed, do not correspond to completely worked out courses of action. A consequence is that planning as a whole needs to be viewed as a more opportunistic process carried out on-line when opportunities arise or difficulties occur (Hayes-Roth & Hayes-Roth, 1979; Ellis, 1989). It implies, also, that it could be thought of as "an ordered set of control statements to support the efficiency of actions and the preparation of alternative actions for the case of failure" (Cohen, 1988). It follows the need for a continuous monitoring of the activity; serial models are, then, insufficient in order to understand and describe planning.

NEUROPSYCHOLOGICAL MODELS OF PLANNING

A neuropsychological model that has shown to be relevant in studying planning derives from Luria's (1966) theory of frontal lobes as a system for the programming, regulation, and verification of activity.

Luria, analyzing the performance of frontal lobe patients, identified several possible behaviors deriving from deficit in frontal lobe functions and affecting planning ability. These patients did not face problems with a preliminary evaluation of the situation to be planned; they tended to produce several attempts without performing any active analysis. Because they showed a marked difficulty in focusing on the crucial points of the action to be planned, their performance resulted in the absence of a plan. Finally, they also showed a difficulty in monitoring the verbal plan produced, as shown by the absence of self-corrections.

Later, Ben-Yishay and Diller (1983), starting from the analysis of the effects of frontal lobe lesions, identified four processing stages involved in planning: specification of one or more goals, sketch of a plan, execution of a provisional solution, and assessment of a provisional solution.

Some authors (Duncan, 1986; Vikki & Holst, 1991) have emphasized the stage of goals specification in planning (or programming), which they view as the goal-based search for action structure. Planning involves, then, the selection of sub-goals that would match the subjects' capabilities to the task requirements in a way leading to the final goal. Following this view, the selection of sub-goals is the process that transforms the preliminary plan representation into a pattern of activation and inhibition of available lower level schemata so that the resulting action structure is adjusted to the specific task conditions.

A formalized model that may explain most of the planning activity (and which the authors view as one possible realization of Luria's theory in information processing terms) is the Supervisor Attention System (SAS) proposed by Norman and Shallice (1986) and Shallice (1982, 1988, 1994) in order to account for the different levels of control needed to carry out various sequences of actions or thoughts.

The model involves three levels. The lowest level consists of a psychological processing structure whose operation is controlled by action or thought schemas. Then, the model distinguishes between two modes of action control: an automatic mode via a "contention scheduling" mechanism and a deliberate attentional control via a supervisory attentional system (SAS) that operates by biasing the contention scheduling selection process. The first control is involved in the execution of overlearned or routine actions and skills. Action schemas, well defined sets of responses associated with specific environmental stimuli or triggers, are selected when a threshold specific to that schema is activated. The second component is a general planning unit or a supervisory system needed to solve non-routine problems. It provides conscious control to modulate performance.

The role of the SAS in planning would be in controlling processes such as goal articulation, provisional plan formulation, marker creation, and triggering (a marker is created to trigger the right behavior and eventually inhibit an ongoing activity). In addition, an evaluation process is postulated at any stage to modify a provisional plan.

While the contribution of psychological models consists of the identification of the variables affecting planning and of the role of different strategies in order to formulate and execute an efficient plan, neuropsychological studies have shed more light on the components involved in planning. In particular, besides the formulating and sequencing components, the role of on-line processes, such as modulating and controlling operations, has been emphasized.

PLANNING AND CLOSED HEAD INJURY

It is well recognized that frontal lobe lesions can grossly alter the performance of everyday life activities other than routines, even though neuropsychological tests do not evidence gross cognitive changes. This is particularly true in the case of CHI patients.

Shallice and Burgess (1991b) have studied the performance of three CHI patients with severe problems in spontaneously organizing everyday activities. These patients performed well on cognitive tests, with the exception of "frontal lobe" tests; here, their performance showed a large variation. In order to study their planning ability, the authors developed two tests. In the "six-element test," subjects were asked to carry out six open-ended tasks (dictating a route, carrying out arithmetic problems, and writing down the names of approximately 100 pictures of objects) in 15 minutes in a way that maximized their overall score. In the Multiple Errands Test, undertaken in the area near the hospital and unknown to the patients, they had to carry out a number of tasks of various difficulty following some rules specified in the instructions (e.g., they had to buy a brown loaf, be to a certain place at a given hour, and obtain a set of instructions to be written on a postcard). The authors believed it did not seem possible to explain the poor performance of these patients in terms of memory, motivational, or posterior cognitive problems, although the authors recognized the possible role of these processes. They analyzed and interpreted the performance in light of the Supervisory Attentional System account (Norman & Shallice, 1986; Shallice, 1982, 1988, 1994). Following this view, while one patient showed a more general difficulty that seemed to affect all the components suggested by the model, a second patient showed a more severe difficulty in marker creating and in triggering processes; a third patient, instead, showed a more relevant difficulty in plan formulation and modification; all the patients studied showed difficulties in evaluating and articulating goals. This study provides support for the possibility of specific dissociations within planning disturbances (which the authors call deficits in strategy application) in CHI patients.

Following the same line (i.e., studying everyday life difficulties in planning and looking to the strategic behavior), Bisiacchi and Sgaramella (1992) have built up an everyday type of errand-planning task in which subjects had to organize their morning in a new town with some shopping to do. Subjects were presented with a map of a town and asked to move around this hypothetical town. They were asked to perform an ideal journey for completing as many as possible of ten errands proposed in the instructions, using the shortest way. The subjects' task was to sequence errands, time actions, and logically order goals (Cohen, 1988; Hayes-Roth & Hayes-Roth, 1979). They were also given some constraints: the starting and return times (respectively, 9:00 and 12:30 A.M.), the opening hours of shops and public offices (from 9:00 to 12:30 A.M.), and of the hospital (from 11:00 A.M. to 1:00 P.M.). Furthermore, subjects might ask the experimenter how long it took to reach each goal from whatever point.

The scores were calculated considering the number of performed errands (goals) and the type of errors made by the subject. Errors were categorized as follows: omissions, rule breaking (i.e., not considering the given constraints like, for instance, going to the post office before taking money from the bank), changes in directions that determined going back and forth on the same route, perseverations (i.e., going more than once to the same place), and intrusions (i.e., executing errands that were not present in the instructions). The authors also considered a global score, which took into account the total number of errors and indicated with a value of 100 the best way to perform the task (i.e., achieving all the goals with no errors), and the optimization score, which consisted of the ratio between goals and moves. This last score indicated with a value of 100 the best way to perform the task (i.e., achieving the goals, with no attention to the number, with the minimum of moves). A study on normal subjects of different age ranges (Sgaramella, Bisiacchi, & Falchero, 1995) has shown that subjects from 20- to 40-years-old are able to perform this task with almost no errors (i.e., they are able to choose the right sequence and the optimal spatial organization in order to perform the task and to take into account the spatio-temporal and logical constraints given).

We used this task in order to study the performance of CHI patients. First, we studied an unselected group of 19 CHI patients. Their ages ranged from 16 to 30 (mean age = 24.8); all had presented coma for at least one week. Their I.Q. ranged from 78 to 126. CT scan showed a wide range of localization of damage. Most of the patients showed mild difficulties in memory tests, either with working memory and long-term memory. In frontal lobe functions, they showed a variable degree of deficit.

The analysis of their performance at the planning task (see Table 21.1) showed that CHI patients were able to select and execute the goals as shown by the mean number of goals reached, which did not differ from the one accomplished by controls. CHI patients showed, instead, relevant difficulties in organizing the plan according to the logical rules (e.g., going to the bank to take money before paying the bill at the post office) and to the spatio-temporal constraints (e.g., going to the hospital during the opening hours or performing all the possible goals on the way). This finding was evidenced by the move/goals ratio, by the global score, and by an increased number of changes in direction and rule breaks.

Sometimes, as a compensation for the difficulty in dealing with the task, they also tended to produce intrusions from their daily routines in the task (i.e., they selected actions they were used to performing in their everyday life). Finally, some perseverations could be evidenced (i.e., some patients forgot they had already accomplished an errand). Both of these last types of errors remained, most of the time, undetected.

Table 21.1: Summary of the Mean Performance at the Planning Task in an Unselected Group of CHI Patients and in Normal Controls

Subjects	Goals	Changes	Goals/Moves Ratio	Rule Breaks	Time Errors	Perseverations	Intrusions	Global Score (%)
CHI patients	9.4	1.46	.88	.72	.81	.18	.05	58
Controls	9.72	0.51	.93	.16	.23	.09	.02	94

As a whole, the patients' performance could be interpreted as the result of a difficulty in keeping active all instructions required in order to correctly perform the task and in monitoring their own performance. They tended to produce organized groups of goals (clusters in Gärling's terms), but they failed to organize these clusters into an efficient global plan.

In a subsequent analysis (Zettin, Sgaramella, Bisiacchi et al., 1994), we have tried to isolate the influence of the length of the coma, the distance from the trauma, and the involvement in a training program on planning ability of CHI patients. The analyses were carried out on a more homogeneous group of 11 patients, all of whom were characterized by normal I.Q. and a mild disturbance either in memory or frontal lobe functions. First, it is worth noting that this selected group showed the predominance of two types of errors: time errors and rule-breaking errors (Table 21.2). As a whole, these patients did not show particular problems in the spatial organization of the plan, as shown by the goals/moves ratio which is close to the controls value. Only the presence of a rehabilitation program for a period longer than one year seemed to positively influence the performance.

Table 21.2: Summary of the Mean Performance at the Planning Task in a Selected Group of CHI Patients and in Normal Controls

Subjects	Goals	Changes	Goals/Moves Ratio	Rule Breaks	Time Errors	Global Score (%)
CHI patients	9.3	1.54	.90	.72	.81	60
Controls	9.7	.51	.93	.16	.23	94

AN ATTEMPT OF TRAINING

There is no doubt about the preeminence of frontal dysfunction in CHI patients and about the role deficits in planning, perhaps more than in other cognitive processes, may play in determining the extent of the recovery. Although impairment in such functions as anticipation, goal selection, planning, monitoring, and completing intended activities are prevalent following head injury, remediation efforts have been fairly minimal (Prigatano, 1986; Sohlberg & Mateer, 1989).

The flexibility of the performance, the sensibility to improve after training, although not specifically tied to the planning ability, and the possibility of selective problems in the organization of the plan suggested to us the usefulness of an attempt to directly train specific components of planning.

Two patients were selected for this attempt, NO and PI. Their performance and change were compared with that of TR and AL, who were trained using a non-specific rehabilitation program.

All the patients studied (Table 21.3) were at a post-acute recovery phase, insofar as they were tested at least six months after the injury. These patients were comparable for age and schooling. They were all characterized by a CT scan evidence of focal frontal lobe damage, except for TR.

Table 21.3: Performance of the Four Patents at the Neuropsychological Examination Before Treatment

SUBJECTS	Age	TC	QI	RAVENs	WCST	Stories	Digit span	Prose memory	Corsi span
NO	19	bilaterial frontal and right temporal	103	36	89	6	5	16	7
PI	17	bilateral occpital	77	28	50	4	4	12.07	4
TR	24	right temporal	102	44	83	9	5	24.5	6
AL	18	bilateral frontal	113	42	78	12	5	19.2	7

Only PI had a low I.Q. and a low performance at other intelligence and reasoning tests such as Raven Matrices (Raven, 1938) and the WCST (Nelson, 1975), showing a significant overall intellectual impairment. All showed a difficulty in sequencing stories. All were characterized by a reduction in verbal short-term memory but performed well within normal range on long-term memory tests. Visuospatial short-term memory was reduced only in PI.

All these patients reported difficulties in spontaneous organization in everyday life. They were, then, given the planning task in order to detail the reported difficulty. The analysis of their performance is summarized in Table 21.4. All patients were characterized by a difficulty in forming an efficient plan, as shown by rule-breaking errors and by the presence of changes. Besides these problems, PI and TR also showed a difficulty in selecting and executing all the goals.

Table 21.4: Summary of Patients' Performance at the Planning Task before Treatment

SUBJECTS	Goals	Changes	Goals/Moves Ratio	Rule Breaks	Global Score(%)
NO	10	1.00	.91	2.00	70
PI	8	1.00	.88	1.00	60
TR	9	1.00	.90	0.00	80
AL	10	1.00	.91	1.00	80
Controls	9.7	0.51	.93	0.16	96

It did not seem possible to explain their performance in terms of memory or deficits in cognitive processes other than planning—first, because they had available throughout all the tasks the list of the errands to be performed and the map, and, second, because of their mild deficits on memory tests.

PI and TR had problems in selecting and executing the goals, and also, to a varying degree, they showed problems in dealing with logical and spatial constraints in forming the plan. While the rule-breaking errors could underlie a more general, cognitive difficulty in linking bits of information and be the expression of a general overload while trying to accomplish the task, the problems in dealing with the spatial constraints suggest some relevant thoughts.

In terms of the model of Gärling et al., change errors show that they are able to organize goals following a clustering strategy, but they sometimes fail to link them together using a more global strategy. In agreement with neuropsychological studies, they had a difficulty in dealing with all the constraints, more specifically, in considering all of them. Their performance could underlie a difficulty relative to on-line control processes. Within this framework, there are at least two possible sources for this behavior: a weak marking of key information or a difficulty in monitoring the plan produced.

RATIONALE OF THE TREATMENT

Because, at that time, no further specification was possible for the origin of the disturbance (which probably was two-fold, in any case), two patients—PI and NO— were involved in training aimed at either finding and marking rules or monitoring the plan produced.

The marking rules task was performed by teaching strategies for finding and underlining key points; monitoring was performed by helping find errors on their own production, thus improving their level of control of their output.

PROCEDURE

Their performance was evaluated in a first session, without giving any cues, by performing a series of exercises consisting of sequencing pictures of stories, describing the rules and the sequence of card games (e.g., material used, aim of the game, specific rules, actions performed by the players), and solving problems of everyday life (i.e., what to do and in which order).

At the beginning of the training, their behavior was characterized by the absence of a schema or anchor points in the descriptions, by the use of irrelevant information, and by a lack of self-correction during and after the production. Besides the specific difficulties in performing the tasks, a low level of awareness of their performance characterized these patients.

After the first session, once the patients had performed each exercise, they were directly cued by the trainer on finding a schema—on where to look in order to find and correct logical errors or to find the information they did not consider during the execution.

For four months, with three 1-hour sessions per week, they were given three sets of exercises of each type (Figure 21.1).

POST-TREATMENT EVALUATION

At the end of the training, PI and NO were able to correctly execute the exercises or at least to self-correct the errors during or after the execution.

All the patients were again submitted to a neuropsychological examination in order to evaluate the recovery of the general cognitive abilities. They all had improved, as shown by the higher IQ. A relevant improvement was evidenced at sequencing stories, more marked in PI and NO; given the nature of the training, this improvement could be more directly linked to the treatment these two patients received. However, they did not show a relevant improvement at performing the Raven matrices and the WCST. A mild improvement was also evidenced in their memory ability, both in short- and long-term memory tests.

Finally, they were again tested on the planning task. As shown in Table 21.5, patients PI and NO were found to be able to select and execute all goals in the right order, taking into account all the relevant information.

Table 21.5: Summary of Patients' Performance at the Planning Task after Treatment

SUBJECTS	Goals	Changes	Goals/Moves Ratio	Rule Breaks	Global Score(%)
NO	10	0	1.00	0	100
PI	10	0	1.00	0	100
TR	10	1	0.91	0	90
AL	10	1	0.91	0	90

<u>Sequencing pictures:</u> Going for a picnic.

The subject is asked to describe each picture, telling a reasonable story about what is going on.

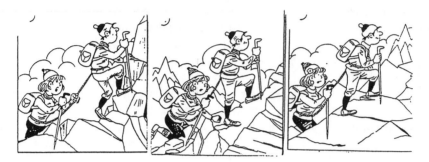

<u>Card games:</u> Master mind

The aim is to use deductive processes to guess four-five numbers or letters (D G S Z L) of the alphabet, in their correct order, thought of by experimenter. The numbers or letters must not be repeated during the sequence.

The experimenter writes a sequence of numbers, or letters, hidden out of sight of the subject. The subject is asked to try to guess the sequence.

If one of the numbers or letters is the same as the one in the hidden sequence, the experimenter indicates it with:

-a cross, if it is in the right place,

-a circle, if it is correct but in the wrong place on the right of the subject s sequence.

The examiner notes the number of circles or crosses corresponding to the quantity of the numbers or letters guessed.

The subject is allowed up to twelve attempts. The game ends when he/she manages to guess the sequence.

<u>Everyday Problem solving:</u> The light has gone off.

The subject is asked to describe what you do and in which order.
The examiner notes all the informations and the order given by the subject.

Figure 21.1: Example of the types of exercises used for the training.

TR and AL still showed a difficulty in forming an efficient plan performing all the goals on the way (i.e., without going back and forth on the map). Although not quantitatively evaluated, they still showed, then, a difficulty in taking into account all the information needed. Independent of the training in which patients were involved, rule breakings disappeared, providing, therefore, further evidence for the general cognitive deficit nature of these types of errors—changes disappeared only after a more focused rehabilitation.

CONCLUSIONS

As the group and single case studies have shown, the problems CHI patients often demonstrate in organizing a plan can affect various components and to a various degree. More specifically, these problems seem to be relative to taking into account all the information relevant for developing a plan and in dealing with spatio-temporal organization of the plan.

The two patients treated for planning difficulties showed both types of problems. The effectiveness of the training comes directly from the fact that it followed from a theory-based analysis of planning processes. The treatment presented here, in fact, is similar to the approach proposed by Gärling et al., which emphasizes the role of strategy choice and decision making. But it mostly derives the rationale from the neuropsychological studies on frontal lobe functions that underlie the role of on-line processing required when subjects need to consider alternative courses of action, that stress evaluating them against the ongoing feedback and goals, and that emphasize the role of intervention of specific executive processes (Shallice & Burgess, 1991a). The neuropsychological studies have, in fact, supplied two possible sources for the planning disturbances evidenced on which the training was focused (i.e., marker creating while forming a provisional plan and monitoring during the execution).

Although the training was successful in tapping the level of the disturbance so that the performance improved, a limitation of this study comes from the impossibility of deciding the specific role played by marker creating and by monitoring deficits in explaining the performance of the two patients.

A further limitation, and a question still open at the end of the treatment, is whether the patients have really automated the strategies trained to face complex, either occasionally or routinely, situations in their own real life. At the end of the training, we observed a spontaneous transfer to their spontaneous speech production, which appeared more organized and tied to transmit relevant information during communication.

This study provides support for the possibility of dissociations within the planning deficits in CHI patients. In order to separate problems in marker creating and maintenance or in monitoring processes, it is important to find patients showing a more selective pattern of disturbance, deriving from one of the two sources evidenced or with more specific deficits in the spatio-temporal organization of the plan. From the rehabilitation point of view, this study might be considered as a starting point for further theory-based interventions and for building up other treatment programs specific for different levels of difficulty highlighted in CHI patients.

REFERENCES

Ben Yishay, Y., & Diller, L. (1983). Cognitive remediation. In E. R. Griffith, M.R. Bond, & J.D. Miller (Eds.), *Rehabilitation of the head injured adult.* Philadelphia: FA Davis Company.

Bisiacchi P.S., & Sgaramella T.S. (1992). La memoria prospettica negli anziani. *Psicologia e Societa' XVII, 1,* 77–94.

Cadwallader, M. (1975). A behavioral model of consumer spatial decision making. *Economic Geography, 51,* 339–349.

———. (1981). Towards a cognitive gravity model: The case of consumer spatial behavior. *Regional Studies, 15,* 275–284.

Cohen, G. (1988). *Memory for the real world.* London: Lawrence Erlbaum Associates.

Daigneault, S., Braun, C.M.J., & Whitaker, H.A. (1992). Early effects of normal aging on perseverative and nonperseverative prefrontal measures. *Developmental Neuropsychology, 8,* 99–114.

Dalla Malva, C.L., Stuss, D.T., D'Alton, J., & Willmer, J. (1993). Capture errors and sequencing after frontal brain lesions. *Neuropsychologia, 4,* 363–372.

Duncan, J. (1986). Disorganization of behavior after frontal lobe lesions. *Cognitive Neuropsychology, 9,* 271–290.

Ellis, J.A. (1989). *Memory for naturally occurring intentions.* Doctoral dissertation, University of Cambridge.

Fuster, J.M. (1980). *The prefrontal cortex.* New York: Raven Press.

Gärling, T. (1989). The role of cognitive maps in spatial decisions. *Journal of Environmental Psychology, 9,* 269–278.

———. (1994). Processing of time constraints on sequence decisions in a planning task. *European Journal of Cognitive Psychology, 7,* 399–416.

Gärling, T., Böök, A., & Lindberg, E. (1984). Cognitive mapping of large-scale environments: The interrelationships of action plans, acquisition, and orientation. *Environment and Behavior, 16,* 3–34.

Gärling, T., Säisä, J., Böök, A., & Lindberg, E. (1986). The spatiotemporal sequencing of everyday activities in the large-scale environment. *Journal of Environmental Psychology, 6,* 261–280.

Hayes-Roth, B., & Hayes-Roth, F. (1979). A cognitive model of planning. *Cognitive Science, 3,* 275–310.

Hirtle, S.C., & Gärling, T. (1992). Heuristic rules for sequential spatial decisions. *Geoforum, 23,* 227–238.

Luria, A. R. (1966). *Higher cortical function in man.* (D. Haigh, trans., 1st ed.). New York: Basic Books and Plenum Press.

Nelson, H. E. (1976). A modified card sorting test sensitive to frontal lobe defects. *Cortex, 12,* 313–324.

Norman, D., & Shallice, T. (1986). Attention to action: Willed and automatic control of behavior. In R.J. Davidson, G.E. Schwartz, & D. Shapiro (Eds.), *Consciousness and self-regulation* (Vol. 4). New York: Plenum Press.

Penfield, W., & Evans, J. (1935). The frontal lobe in man: A clinical study of maximum removal. *Brain, 58,* 115.

Perozzo, Paola. (data collection).

Prigatano, G.P. (1986). *Neuropsychological rehabilitation after brain injury.* Baltimore: Johns Hopkins University Press.

Raven, J.C. (1938). *Standard progressive matrices.* London: H.K. Lewis.

Sgaramella, T.M., Bisiacchi, P.S., & Falchero, S. (1995). Ruolo dell'eta' nella pianificazione di azioni in un constesto ambientale. *Ricerche di Psicologi, 19*(2), 165–181.

Shallice, T. (1988). *From neuropsychology to mental structure.* Cambridge: Cambridge University Press.

———. (1994). Multiple levels of control processes. In C.A. Umilta & M. Moskovitch (Eds.), *Attention & performance XV.* Hillsdale: Lawrence Erlbaum.

Shallice, T., & Burgess, P.W. (1991a). Higher-order cognitive impairments and frontal lobe lesions in man. In H.S. Levin, H.M. Eisenberg, & A.L. Benton (Eds.), *Frontal lobe function and dysfunction.* New York: Oxford University Press.

———. (1991b). Deficits in strategy application following frontal lobe damage in man. *Brain, 114,* 727–741.

Simon, H. (1957). *Models of man.* New York: John Wiley & Sons.

Sohlberg, M.M., & Maater, C.A. (1989). Introduction to cognitive rehabilitation: Theory and practice. New York: Guilford Press.

Stuss, D.T., & Benson D. F. (1986). The frontal lobes. New York: Raven Press.

Stuss, D.T., & Gow, C.A. (1992). Frontal dysfunction after traumatic head injury. *Neuropsychiatry, Neuropsychology, and Behavioral Neurology, 5,* 272–282.

Wechsler, D. (1955). Wechsler adult intelligence scale. New York; Sidkup, Kent: Psychological Corporation.

Wilkki, J., & Holst, P. (1991). Mental programming after frontal lobe lesions: Results on digit symbol performance with self-selected goals. *Cortex, 27,* 203–211.

Zettin, M., Sgaramella, T.M., Bisiacchi, P.S., Verné, D., & Rago, S. (1994). *I disturbi di pianificazione nei traumi cranici.* Abstracts of the "Simposio Alpino Adriatico," Lucerne.

PART IV:

REHABILITATING PERSONALITY AND RETURNING TO COMMUNITY

22

An Approach to the Treatment of Affective Disorders and Suicide Tendencies after TBI

José León-Carrión

Facultad de Psicología
Universidad de Seville, Seville, Spain

INTRODUCTION

The consequences of cerebral damage are multiple and varied and can affect any sphere of an individual's life—personal, family, or social. People develop their daily lives in these three spheres where the neurocognitive and affective components play an important role. When any of these three components or systems are altered or injured by some means, human activity is altered, as is the case in traumatic brain injury (TBI). Numerous studies are being carried out in which the effects of brain injury concerning cognition (i.e., attention, memory, language, reasoning, solving problems, mental images, and executive functions) are shown (León-Carrión, 1994). Nevertheless, the affective and emotional aspects have been studied less despite the fact that the affective factors play a relevant role in the neurocognitive recovery after brain injury. As Prigatano (1988) indicates, this is so because emotions and motivations are tightly interconnected with arousal disorders, perception, and, finally, with self-awareness. We know much more of the processes fundamentally regulated by the cortex (cognitive functions) than about those regulated by the subcortex (affective functions). Nevertheless, relatives and patients complain more frequently about the post-traumatic affective and emotional deterioration than about the cognitive impairment. The affective and emotional problems derived from brain injury are more visible because they can make interpersonal, family, and work relations unbearable.

In short, patients' affective and emotional disorders directly affect their quality of life, that of their relatives, and that of those that surround them, provoking strong family stress and making difficult the successful return to social life and relationships of persons with brain injury. The consequences of brain injury that relatives and close friends of patients with TBI refer to—those that interfere the most in the adjustment and equilibrium in the home—are

1. Impairment of the capability of awareness and the capability to respond.
2. Learning and memory problems.
3. Emotional changes (anxiety and depression).
4. Personality changes (aggressiveness, paranoia, dependence, impulsiveness, lack of control, etc.).

The reactions from relatives and close friends who confront these problems go from denial and feeling trapped and isolated to jealousy and feelings of guilt. Depression, changes in family roles, changes in family expectations (see Miller, 1991), intrafamily problems, problems in parental relations, and changes in the way life is seen (see León-Carrión, 1994) also occur, and it is normal that these reactions appear after a family member suffers a TBI.

In the majority of the patients who have suffered a TBI, to a greater or lesser degree, changes in the manner of expressing their emotions or feelings can be observed. These changes have to be carefully considered at the time of planning the patient's integral rehabilitation. It should not be forgotten that human beings not only live by cognition but also by their feelings. A person is a person in the measure of his/her ability to maintain his/her intelligence integrated with his/her emotions. A neuropsychological rehabilitation program that is only designed to approach the cognitive deficits will reap important failures, in the same way that a rehabilitation program will fail if centered only on improving the emotional and affective aspects. Through rehabilitation, it is possible that a person suffering from TBI can succeed in functioning correctly from the cognitive point of view. Nevertheless, this success will be inefficient if cognition does not integrate or modulate affectively and emotionally. Similarly, the opposite can occur—people may be capable of modulating their affects but be incapable of leading them on the effective part by maintaining their cognitive deficits. In any event, in the rehabilitation design, one should plan that both aspects be treated simultaneously—it is difficult enough to obtain results in the affective area if achievements are not attained in the cognitive area.

Another of the problems or questions asked of the neuropsychologist is whether these disorders, also called personality disorders, are disorders similar to those suffered by persons without TBI. The answer is not totally clear. However, there is a tendency to recognize that the nature of the affective alterations and the changes in emotional expressions differ from the classically described psychopathological cases. In addition, there is increasing evidence that the treatments are different. This possibility is described by Prigatano (1987), when he suggests as an important study area the relation between certain metabolic and endocrinologic changes that occur in TBI and in depression.

This chapter will fundamentally focus on the two signs that usually, with more or less frequency, accompany as sequelae the chronic phase of patients with TBI: depression and suicidal tendency.

DEPRESSION AFTER TBI

The possibility of depressive episodes appearing after a TBI exists. The prevalence of depression after TBI has been studied by different authors. For Schoenhuber, Gentilin, and Orlando (1988), 39% of patients suffer from depression a year after the trauma. Diamond, Bacth, and Zillmer (1988) found 26% suffering from depression three months after the TBI. For Oddy, Couglan, Tyerman, and Jenkins (1985), 10% of the patients suffered depressions 10 years after the trauma. Kinsella, Moran, Ford, and Ponsford (1988) found that 33% of the patients suffered depressions two years after the trauma. Brooks, Campsre, Symington et al. (1986) found 57% of patients depressed, according to relatives, five years after the trauma.

In the study done by Jorge, Robinson, Arndt, and Starkstein (1993), after evaluating 66 hospitalized patients for closed brain injury in four periods (upon admission and at 3, 6 and 12 months later), it was found that 46.6% of the subjects could be diagnosed with major depression during the follow-up year. The duration of the period of depression averaged 4.7 months. Nevertheless, it should be noted that less than half (41%) of the subjects that suffered from depression in the hospital were not depressed three months after leaving the hospital. Likewise, these authors showed that the depression had a strong correlation to poor social performance. The location of the brain injury was associated with the development of major depression only in the acute state. The transitory depressive syndromes were associated with left frontal dorso-lateral lesions and/or left lesions in the basal ganglia.

These same authors (Jorge, Robinson, & Arndt, 1993) asked themselves if there are specific symptoms for the depressive mood of the patients with TBI. After studying the specificity of the vegetative and psychological symptoms of depression in subjects with TBI, they found that the frequency average of these symptoms among depressed subjects was three times the respective rates found in subjects who were not depressed. At the end of six months, the symptoms that distinguished both groups were precocious awakening and difficulty in concentration, which lead to the conclusion that there were almost no subjects with depressive symptoms without a depressive mood.

Some authors advise looking for certain characteristics when assessing the symptoms of a patient who appears depressive after TBI. The patients may have a depressive mood without experiencing the typical somatic symptoms of a major depressive disorder diagnosis. The mood lability may occur with rapid changes from crying to laughter. This lability may be caused by limbical-temporal and basal ganglia lesions (Ross & Stewart, 1987).

For Silver, Yudofsky, and Hales (1991), apathy can be seen as depression due to the lack of happiness or desire. Patients with TBI are generally slow in thought and in the cognitive processing, aspects that could be considered negative symptoms and can be associated with a dysfunction of the dorsal lateral frontal cortex (Berman, Illowsky, & Weinberger, 1988).

A group of subjects with closed brain injury but without damage in the spinal cord or other organs was studied by Federoff, Starkstein, Forrester, Fred et al. (1992) through a semi-structured psychiatric interview, the Hamilton Rating Scale for Depression, scales assessing the deterioration of daily life activities, and social and intellectual performance in addition to CT scans. The results of the neuro-images showed who the subjects that had a higher probability of developing depression were those that had suffered dorso-lateral frontal injuries and/or left injuries in the basal ganglia, as well as parietal-occipital lesions of the right hemisphere. When they compared depressed subjects with those of the groups that did not show depression, they found that the group with major depression had a higher frequency of previous psychiatric disorders and showed evidence of worse social performance.

On the other hand, Dunlap, Udewanhelwi, Stedem, O'Connor et al. (1991) compared the clinical histories of patients who showed clear signs of emotional deterioration beyond the six months after the brain trauma with those of another group of patients with identical severity of neuropsychiatric deterioration, but who had not shown such emotional deterioration. The group with emotional deterioration was more susceptible to be implicated in assaults, less likely to be involved traffic accidents, and more likely to have had a prior history of alcohol abuse and to have suffered a cranial fracture with damage in the left parietal lobe than the other group. The symptoms that worsened with time were agitation, hostility, apathy, lability of mood, emotional reactivity, and depression.

With the idea of finding causal factors of the mania after brain injury, Starkstein, Pearlson, Boston, and Robinson (1987) studied patients with bi-polar affective disorders, control subjects with brain injury, and normal control subjects. They found that the subjects with mania had focal cerebral injuries involving the limbic structures and significantly associated with damage in the right hemisphere, superior bi-frontal injuries, and damage in the third ventricle. These patients frequently had bi-polar disorders with prior depressive episodes, and nearly half had a family history of affective disorders in first degree relatives.

Trying to delve deeper into the subject, Robinson, Boston, Starkstein, and Price (1988) found that the group of patients who developed mania after TBI were those with lesions in the right hemisphere connected with the limbic system significantly when they were compared with a group of patients with cerebrovascular disorders with major depression who had an injury fundamentally in the left frontal cortex in the basal ganglia.

In another group of patients without mood disturbances after TBI, the location of the injury was not significant. They also found that the patients with secondary mania also had a significantly higher frequency of family history of affective disorders than the other two groups. The authors interpreted their findings as indicating interaction between brain injury in certain areas of the right hemisphere and genetic factors or other neuropathological conditions that produce secondary mania. The possibility of there being seasonal effects on affective disorders resulting from brain injury is considered by Hunt and Silverton (1990), with depression occurring during the winter and hypo-mania occurring in the summer.

The duration of the affective and emotional disorders has been studied by Jorge, Robinson, Starkstein, and Arndt (1993). These authors find that the average duration of non-anxious depressions is 1.5 months, 7.5 months for anxious depression, and 1.5 months for generalized anxiety disorders. The anxious depressions were associated with injuries in the right hemisphere, while the major depressions were only associated with left anterior lesions. These authors conclude that major depressions with anxiety and major depressions that follow a TBI may be different disorders with different underlying etiological mechanisms and perhaps with different responses to treatment.

They have also tried to find sexual differences in the emotional state of patients with TBI. A distress syndrome characterized by impulsiveness, depression, anxiety, and reports of unusual experiences has been found in men. The authors do not relate these finding with localized brain injury but, instead, suggest that it can be due to an emotional reaction to the trauma or due to certain premorbid personality characteristics (Burton & Volpe, 1988).

POST-TRAUMATIC AFFECTIVE DISORDERS TREATMENT

A therapeutic approximation to the affective disorders appearing after a TBI is not easy, since, as we have shown in the previous review, there are different types of depressive patterns—not all of the mood changes of these patients have the same etiology or the same course. On the other hand, it is not clear that the post-traumatic organic affective disorders should be treated in the same way as those of subjects without TBI. In any case, we can say that two approximations exist: (1) pharmacological and (2) neuropsychological.

The *pharmacological approximation*[1] is, at this time, the most common. Up to this time, researchers have tried to give a psychopharmalogical answer or psychiatric type to the affective disorders that patients with TBI present. In the majority of the cases, this opinion has been chosen in centers that attend to these patients without taking into account the specific identity of the organic post-traumatic affective patterns.

For Glenn and Wroblewsky (1989), the best possible psychopharmacological treatment option for patients with TBI who present depression are the Nonmonamine Oxidase Inhibitor (Non-MAOI) and antidepressants (ADs); since the MAOI/ADs have disadvantages in as much as they are non-anticolinergic, they generally do not produce a reaction. These authors also recommend lithium and carbamazepine in combination with antidepressants.

For Wroblewski, Guidos, Leary, and Joseph (1992), the control of future dysfunction in subjects with TBI can be performed with fluoxetine together with anti-convulsive medication. Anti-convulsive medication is also used by Shedlack and Pope (1992), with which they treat an anorexic and affective syndrome connected with brain injury in the right hemisphere. On the other hand, Santos and Ballenguer (1992) warm to the possibility that triciclical antidepressants as treatment for organic affective disorders could trigger maniac episodes and a rapid cyclical bi-polar process. In the same manner, Zwill, McAllister, Cohen, and Halpern (1993) report a case of a 32-year-old woman who developed an ultra-rapid cyclical bi-polar affective disorder after moderated brain injury. The patient did not have a previous history of affective disorders and was marginally *responsive* to the psychotropic medication.

For Zahn and Littman (1989), treatment for depression of survivors of TBI should be designed as a function of two etiopathological dimensions: the structural changes having taken place in the brain and the personality changes related with a narcissistic damage to the prior "I" of the patient. For these authors, a psychopharmacological therapy, especially desipramine or nortriptiline, can be used effectively to stabilize the neurochemical aspects of depression in these patients. With psychotherapy, patients should reorganize the basic constructs through which they define themselves, their place in the world, and their future personal performance predictions.

Other authors present lithium as a possible option. Thus, Glenn and Joseph (1987) review and find that it is used especially for acute treatment for mania and as a prophylaxis for bipolar affective disorders. Nevertheless, lithium can have collateral effects such as aphasia, confusion, hallucinations, and incontinence. For Stewart and Hemsath (1988), treatment with lithium for TBI should be accompanied by carbamazepine.

On the other hand, Prigatano (1987) points out that it is important

to consider the relationship between changes in cognitive recovery and cortisol serum changes. If the patient becomes aware of his or her deficits, this insight results in increased cortisol serum and, during this time, potentially an increase in depression. If the patients are treated with antidepressant drugs and the cortisol serum decreases, then the pharmacological correlates of depression could be more clearly explored. Also, if the drugs do not lower serum cortisol, then either there is a faculty neurofeedback mechanism or one is using the wrong medication.

To conclude, and according to Perino (1993), the pharmacological therapy cannot be carried out alone but should rather form part of a complex and integral system of intervention. On the other hand, in the application of pharmacological treatment, the cost/benefits ratio should be taken into account. *Some medications that seem to be indicated for the improvement of the emotional and affective disorders worsen, slow down, or impede the progress and cognitive rehabilitation.* For this reason, one has to consider what is the goal of the pharmacological therapy, its benefits, and its undesired effects. A pharmacological therapy that impedes the cognitive recovery should be seriously questioned by the team that attends the patient and should be shared with relatives, involving them in the decision to be made.

The neuropsychological approach to the treatment of affective disorders that follow TBIs involves the simultaneous treatment of the cognitive, emotional, and affective deficits. In our experience, it is very difficult to obtain affective improvements without attending to the cognitive problems that the patient presents. The affective sequelae are often linked to the different cognitive deteriorations. However, one should not expect that affective deficits improve without treatment only because the deteriorated cognitive functions are improving. If the affective aspects are not attended to simultaneously, it is possible that they worsen as the cognitive aspects continue improving.

The treatment of the emotional and affective disorders should be directed, from the first moment, to *support* the patient's basic *necessities* and should be centered on the following:

1. Offering *hope,* always.
2. Offering affection *explicitly,* especially on the part of relatives and close friends.
3. Promoting *self-esteem.* Some studies of TBI have demonstrated that self-esteem and depression are negatively correlated (Garske & Thomas, 1992).
4. Seeing to what is affectively relevant for patients. If what they need is *not* coherent, it should be worked on therapeutically in order to make it disappear as a necessity, without provoking nontherapeutic discussion and confrontations.
5. Providing, in so far as patients can, opportunities for participation in group therapy, group discussion, or group activities. It is convenient to begin this last.
6. Providing some weekly individual therapy sessions where patients can express their most intimate feelings or needs, etc., which can and should be worked on at the individual level more than at the group level.
7. Carrying out adjustment therapies to reality rather than interpretative or figurative therapies of reality. In the therapy, reality *should be clear.* Therapy should favor "awareness," not confusion.
8. Involving the family in treatment. In case it may be necessary, it is convenient to carry out family therapy with the first objective being the *rebuilding of the family affective system.*
9. Trying to find *the patient's strong side*, that which he/she has preserved best and what he/she does best, reinforcing it and, from this point, expanding to other areas. Finding motivation points and areas.
10. Developing the *expression of emotions* so that they are socially adequate and not socially disabling.

SUICIDAL TENDENCIES IN PERSONS WHO HAVE SUFFERED A BRAIN INJURY

The possibility that persons who have suffered a TBI can have some tendency to commit a suicidal act has to be contemplated. In our experience, not all patients with TBI run the risk of committing a such as act; however, the percentage of those that run this risk is high and can reach 30%. Therefore, in the planning of these patients' neuropsychological treatment, this possibility has to be contemplated. The neuropsychological characteristics of subjects with TBI who commit suicide are variable, and there is still no agreement on this issue. In Table 22.1, the characteristics of 10 adolescents who survived a suicidal attempt upon admission into a rehabilitation hospital 6–9 months after brain injury are shown. (Parmalee, Kowadt, Sellman, & Pavidow, 1989).

The worrisome incidence of suicide attempts among the general population and among patients with certain neurological disorders has been the reason for looking further into this issue. The classic dynamic approximation has been abandoned, and studies concerned with exploring the biological factors that can be present in a person when he/she commits suicide have increased (Edmand, Asberg, Mils et al., 1986; Maris, 1986). Some authors point out that the cognitive component of the suicidal conduct *is not* the central aspect to consider but rather that the behavioral act of committing suicide is linked to biochemical and neuroendocrine dysfunctions (Naes, Vanderwonde, Schotte et al., 1989). Different studies about neurobiology of emotional control have shown that brain injury, by itself, can increase emotional disorders (Cullum & Bigler, 1988), while Ross (1985) has suggested that the right hemisphere plays an important role in the emotional control similar to the role the left hemisphere plays in the control of expressive and receptive language. An injury in the right frontal region increases the levels of anxiety and depression (Grafman, Vance, Weingaratner et al., 1986), although one should not think that the left hemisphere plays no role in emotional control.

Different studies have been carried out to try to find a biological basis for suicidal conduct. For Scarone, Gambini, Calabrese, and Saurdete (1990), suicidal behavior could be related with lateralized mechanisms of mood control. They suggest this after evaluating the levels of Beta endorphines in different symmetrical cerebral regions of people who commit suicide. Their findings revealed a decrease in concentration of these substances in the left temporal and frontal cortex, as well as in the caudate nucleus in relation to a control group. The Beta endorphine concentrations in symmetrical cerebral regions showed an asymmetrical concentration in suicidal persons (left < right) in the frontal cortex and in the caudate nucleus. In another work by Paermentier, Cheetham, Carom010 et al. (1990), they found that in suicidal persons, the number of Beta-adrenoceptors and Beta-sub-1-andrenoceptors is significantly lower in the temporal cortex compared to the controls. The suicidal people who died in a violent way had significantly lower rates of total adrenoceptors (l Beta and Beta-Sub-1 in the frontal cortex) than the control subjects and the nonviolent suicidal persons. The violent suicidal persons also had a lower number of Beta-Sub-1 adrenoceptors in the temporal cortex than the control subjects (deaths not by suicide). The suicidal people who died in a nonviolent way had a lower rate of the total Beta adrenoceptors in the occipital cortex than the controls and the violent suicidal persons.

Through auto-X-rays, Arango, Ernsbager, Marzuk et al. (1990) found that there is a selective regional increase 5-HT-sub-2 in the prefrontal cortex of suicide victims in comparison with the controls. Likewise, they also found a Beta-adrenergical increase in

Table 22.1: Characteristics of Suicide-Surviving Adolescents on Admission to Rehabilitation Hospital 6–9 Months after Injury (from Parmalee, Kowadt, Selman, & Davidlow, 1989)

Case	Sex	Age at Injury	Method	Premorbid Features	Coma Duration (in days)	6–9 Months Post-injury
1	F	18	Gun, R temporal	3 years drug/alcohol abuse, suicide attempts, runaway, truancy	14	Blind, no short-term memory, labile, violent
2	F	19	OD insulin	5 years drug/alcohol abuse, suicide attempts, school drop out	5	Severe, short-term memory deficit, depressed, suicidal
3	M	17	Gun, R temporal	4 years drug/alcohol abuse, truancy, delinquency	9	Psychotically paranoid and suicidal, impulsive
4	M	17	Hanging	5 years drug/alcohol abuse, truancy, delinquency, school drop out	6	Severe short- and long-term memory deficits, cognitive deficits, amotivational, aprosodic
5	M	18	Electrocution, fall	5 years drug/alcohol abuse, truancy, delinquency, school drop out	6	Spastic quadraparesis, dysarthria, depressed, suicidal, violent rages
6	M	13	3-story leap, head	1 year minor delinquency, excellent school performance	7	Quadraplegic, seizures, short-term memory problems, amotivational
7	M	14	Gun, R temporal	6 months moderate drug abuse, preoccupied with Dungeons & Dragons, 6 months school decline	10	g-Tube, L-hemiparesis, dysarthric, delusional, suicidal
8	M	16	Gun, R frontal	6 months drug abuse, truancy, defiance, "risk-taker" as child	42	L-Hemiplegia, global aphasia
9	M	18	Carbon monoxide	Suicide attempt 4 months before, in therapy, 6 year combative relationship with family, good in school	7	Global intellectual impairment (IQ in 50's), perseverative
10	M	19	Drove into oncoming truck	4 years alcohol abuse, behavior and academic problems in school	14	L-Hemiplegia, anhedonic, sleep disturbance, perserverative

the pre-frontal cortex of those who committed suicide. Also, through the quantitative auto-X-ray studies, Dilon, Gross-Isseroff, Israeli, and Biegon (1991) found specific regional decreases in the 5-HT-sub(1A) receptors in several cortical and hippocampical regions, as well as in the raphe nucleus. According to these authors, the receptors have a limited neuroanatomical distribution in the human brain fundamentally located in brain zones most closely linked to cognition, the cortex, and hippocampus. They did not find a correlation between 5-HT-sub(1A) receptor binding and accidental death or suicide.

The possibility that biochemical asymmetries exist in the brain that are related to suicidal behavior has also been studied by several authors. Thus, Laurence, de-Parmentier, Cheethan et al. (1990) carried out a post-mortem examination of frontal cortex, putamen, and black substance of suicide victims with previous diagnoses of depression. They did not find marked hemispherical asymmetries of 5-HT uptake sites with respect to the controls. However, Arato, Tekas, Tothfalusi et al. (1991) found a pronounced asymmetry of the serotonergical mechanisms. The suicide victims showed reversed asymmetries with significantly high B-sub(max) levels in the left frontal lobe; this finding was much more pronounced in the violent suicide victims. The nonviolent suicide victims did not differ from the control group. According to these authors, the facts demonstrated the significance of serotonergical mechanisms in suicides. Likewise, Arato, Frecska, MacCrimmon et al. (1991), through post-mortem neurochemical investigations, found inter-hemispheric asymmetries in the median-frontal region. They observed higher levels of 5-HIAA in the right hemisphere than in the left. The pharmaco-electroencephalographic results tended to support the post-mortem neurochemical facts.

A study of the post-mortem brain of 10 suicide victims who were not taking anti-depressive medication compared with 10 control subjects was carried out by Hardina, Deureter, Vu, Sotonyi et al. (1993). The data showed that the density of the 5-HT-sub2 labeled with (-3-sup-3H) Ketaserin receptors was significantly increased in the pre-frontal cortex (67%) and in the amygdala (97%) of the suicide victims in comparison with the control subjects. Their data suggest that an abnormality in the brain serotoninergical system is associated with depression and suicidal behavior. In a group of patients diagnosed with Multiple Sclerosis (Sandyk & Awerbuch, 1993), it was found that the medium level of melatonina in those who had tried to commit suicide was significantly lower than the nonsuicidal group (Figure 22.1).

That serotonin (5-HT) is linked to suicide has also been stated by Nordstrous and Asberg (1992). These authors suggest the existence of a relation between suicide and 5-HT; it has been demonstrated in post-mortem studies. Different studies with cerebro-spinal fluid (CSF) have indicated a decrease of (5-HIAA) in patients who had tried to commit suicide recently. Likewise, follow-up studies have confirmed the original hypothesis that a low CSF 5-HIAA predicts a suicide risk after trying to commit suicide. Mann, Arango, Marzuk, Theccanar et al. (1989) arrived at identical conclusions when they studied the post-mortem brain tissue of suicide victims. They found low rates of 5HT and 5-HIAA in the post-mortem exam of the brainstem tissue in suicide victims, while the levels of the cortical tissue were generally normal. Likewise, they found an increase in the number of 5-HT-sub-2 receptors in the pre-frontal cortex of suicide victims as well as an increase in the 5-HT-sub(1A) receptors. In any event, they note that the population of receptors may be altered by the chronic use of psychotropic medication.

Traskman-Bendz, Asberg, Nordstrom, and Stanley (1989) also state that suicidal patients display a decrease of 5-HIAA. In depressive patients, a low rate 5-HIAA in the CSF and low concentration of metabolite of the dopamina homovanillic acid (HVA) is

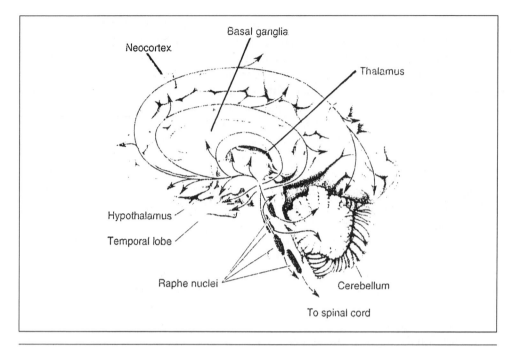

Figure 22.1: The serotonergic diffuse modulatory system. Each nucleus projects on different regions of the brain (from Bear, Connors, & Paradiso [Eds.], 1996).

associated with suicide. Likewise, in the work of Ohmori, Arora, and Meltzer (1992), it was found that homicidal and suicidal persons have a significantly higher cortical concentration of HVA than the subject who died from physical causes and not as a result of an accident. HVA/5-HIAA was also significantly higher in suicidal persons compared to deaths by other nonviolent causes.

On the other hand, Linnoila, Markku, and Vikkunen (1992) suggest that a high probability of committing suicide exists in those persons with a profile of violent and impulsive behavior, alcohol abuse, low CSF of 5-HIAA concentrations, low blood glucose, and low serotonin. This clinical pattern may represent a physical and behavioral manifestation of an underlying defect in the serotoninergical function, specifically in the serotoninergical regulation of the suprachiasmatic nucleus.

In general, we can agree with Coccaro (1992) when he suggests that the reduction of the function of the central serotoninergical system in patients with major mood disorders and/or personality disorders is associated with the deregulation of the impulse controls. When this deregulation appears, there is an increases in the probability of aggressive behavior directed towards oneself or others if the appropriate environmental trigger mechanisms are present.

THE TREATMENT OF PERSONS WITH SUICIDAL TENDENCIES AFTER TBI

The explanation to the question related to the fact that 30% of patients with TBI may have suicidal ideas or try to commit suicide may be answered in the studies presented above (i.e., depending on whether the brain injury affects, to a greater or lesser degree, certain brain systems, the risk of suicide can be greater or lesser). As a hypothesis that emerges from the revised literature, the risk of suicidal tendency in patients with brain injury will be more probable when the following conditions exist: (1) the serotoninergical system is affected, (2) there is injury to the right hemisphere, and (3) injury to the right frontal region exists.

Another important question remains: Is there a dynamic or purely psychological interpretation to the suicide attempts in persons who have suffered TBI? In our judgement, there exists the possibility of an attempt or suicidal ideation as a consequence of an emotional reaction when faced with an event difficult to adapt to by the individual. In the case of the subject with TBI who does not accept the deficits caused by the injury and who tries to commit suicide, the problem will be the same as that of a subject without brain injury who tries to commit suicide because he/she has suffered the amputation of his/her leg or because his/her partner has left (i.e., the suicidal tendency in the TBI subject would not be a direct consequence of profound alterations in the nervous system resulting from brain injury, and further, it is possible that the strong emotional reaction existed in the subject prior to the trauma).

However, in the case of subjects with severe TBI, the problem of awareness exists and persists for a long time (i.e., subjects are not capable of realizing their situation during a long period of post-traumatic time). Therefore, in those cases, it is difficult to react to something that is not perceived as totally unacceptable. However, in our experience (León-Carrión, 1994), *the subjects with suicidal ideas or who try to commit suicide after the brain injury are those who have recovered the ability of being aware* (i.e., as subjects improve cognitively, those that run the risk of committing suicide will have more possibilities of trying it, and this fact is very important to consider when planning the neuropsychological intervention with these patients).

Therefore, the design of the neuropsychological treatment for these persons should emphasize the following:

1. Locating the damage
2. Gradation of the cognitive treatment
3. Personalized psychotherapeutic treatment
4. Group therapy
5. Family counseling
6. Daily life activities

In any event, these steps are nothing more than strategies that form part of an integral neuropsychological treatment program. *One should never carry out a cognitive therapy isolated* from the rest of the complete rehabilitation program. At least the cognitive therapy should be carried out jointly, at its level of complexity, with the emotional and affective psychological treatment. The risk of focusing the rehabilitation on the cognitive aspects and forgetting the emotional aspects may cause patients with suicide risk to make an attempt.

Locating the damage is fundamental in determining the level of the patient's suicide risk (changes in the serotoninergic system, right hemisphere injury, right frontal injury). The greater the risk, the more careful the planning of the rehabilitation process must be.

From the pharmacological point of view, Mann, Arango, Marzuk et al. (1989) point out that antidepressants can be effective in preventing patients from committing suicide who do *not* show depressive syndromes but who exhibit suicidal behavior. On the other hand, Slabby (1994) suggests the use of antidepressants "which are specific serotonin uptake inhibitions" together "with other mood-stabilizing agents." For him, it is important to continue the use of antidepressants for weeks or months and use psychotherapy combined with the medication, as well as support therapy in the event the family needs it.

The **gradation of the cognitive treatment** means that cognition and affects should be treated simultaneously but in the measure that one permits the treatment of the other.

The **personalized psychotherapeutic treatment** refers to the fact that each subject has his/her own personal and injury characteristics. The treatment designed should be the one that fits him/her specifically and not a standard one. A standard treatment should be formed by the particular treatments of the subjects who make up the groups. Therefore, it should be adaptable. That will require individual therapy sessions held simultaneously with group therapy sessions.

In the individual, group, and family therapies, the *suicidal episode or attempt must be accepted as fact.* It should be discussed naturally and calmly as one would speak about any other negative or positive episode in the individual's life. Patients should be able to easily and freely express themselves, their anguish, fears, expectations, dreams, etc. in order to work on them psychotherapeutically. Avoiding talking about suicide, using euphemisms (Parmalee, Kowatch, Sellman, & Davidow, 1989), talking in an embarrassed manner with feelings of guilt, etc. will not make the therapeutic process easier nor will patients be able to integrate that episode into their lives, accepting it as one more episode that has taken place at a certain moment in their biographies equal to other disagreeable events that have also occurred which they have had to accept and integrate.

In our life, many episodes occur, both good and bad, and all of them form part of our personal lives, and, if *integrated properly*, will contribute acceptably to our future. It can be just as damaging not to know how to accept a positive episode in one's personal trajectory as not to know how to accept a negative episode. Life offers hope always if we know how to integrate all of our biographical events, and the therapist should never forget that *building or bringing forth the patient's feeling of hope is the key to building a healthy future for the patient.*

Group therapy allows patients to connect with other realities and to step outside themselves in an adequate space and time. **Family counseling** is essential in order for the family to become involved in the treatment and to work at the patient's affective level and family system. **Daily life activities** should be centered on socialization and develop social skills and adaptation to the patient's environment.

CONCLUSIONS

People who have suffered a TBI will suffer, through their recovery process, affective disorders whose severity will depend on the specific recovery phase in which they find themselves and on the type and location of the brain injury that has caused it. In these disorders, one may observe behavior from mild mood variations to major depressions, maniac states, and/or bi-polar disorders. Frontal lesions together with those of the limbic system and of the right hemisphere are associated with a higher possibility of the appearance of these disorders. Two therapeutic options exist that can be applied jointly or as an alternative to each other. The pharmacological approach will always be adequate as long as the therapeutic benefits obtained are greater than drawbacks (interferences in the cognitive recovery). The neuropsychological treatment will always be suitable, especially, because it mobilizes the patient's own and intact resources, allowing a reconfiguration of the process, to actively face the new situations.

ENDNOTES

1. The pharmacological data disclosed here are for the reader's information. The reader who decides to apply them or is interested in them should refer directly to the bibliographical source provided. We do not recommend that it be done only through this review.

REFERENCES

Arango, V., Ernsberger, P., Marzuk, P.M., Chen, J., et al. (1990). Autoradiographic demonstration of increased serotonin 5-HT-sub-2 and b-adrenergic receptor binding sites in the brain of suicide victims. *Archives of General Psychiatry, 47*, 1038–10477.

Arato, M., Frecska, E., MacCrimmon, D.J., Guscott, R., et al. (1991). Serotoninergic interhemispheric asymmetry: Neurochemical and pharmaco-EEG evidence. *Progress in Neuro-Psychopharmacology and Biological Psychiatry, 15*, 759–764.

Arato, M., Tekas, K., Tothfalusi, L., Magyar, K., et al. (1991). Reserved hemispheric asymmetry of imipramine binding in suicide victims. *Biological Psychiatry, 29*, 699–702.

Bear, M.F., Connors, B.W., and Paradiso, M.A. (1996). *Neuroscience: Exploring the brain*. Baltimore: Williams and Wilkins.

Berman, K.F., Illowsky, B.P., & Weinberger, D.R. (1988). Physiological dysfunction of dorsolateral prefrontal cortex in schizophrenia. IV. Further evidence for regional and behavioral specificity. *Arch. Gen. Psychiatry, 45*, 616–622.

Bigler, E.D. (1989). On the neuropsychology of suicide. *Journal of Learning Disabilities, 22*, 180–185.

Brooks, N., Campsie, L., Symington, C., Beattie, A., & McKinley, W. (1986). The five-year outcome of severe blunt head injury: A relative's view. *J. Neurol. Neurosurg. Psychiatry, 49*, 764–770.

Burton, L.A., & Volpe, B.T. (1988). Sex differences in emotional status of traumatically brain-injured patients. *Journal of Neurologic Rehabilitation, 2*, 151–157.

Charlton, B.G., Wright, C., Leake, A., Ferrier, I.N., et al. (1988). Somatostatin immunoreactivity in postmortem brain from depressed suicides. *Archives of General Psychiatry, 45*, 597.

Coccaro, E.F. (1992). Impulsive aggression and central serotonergic system function in humans: An example of a dimensional brain-behavior relationship. *International Clinical Psychopharmacology, 7*, 3–12.

Cullum, C.M., & Bigler, E.D. (1988). Short form MMPI findings in patients with predominately lateralized cerebral dysfunction: Neuropsychological and CT-derived parameters. *Journal of Nervous and Mental Disease, 176*, 332–342.

de-Parmentier, F., Cheetham, S.C., Crompton, M.R., Katona, C.L., et al. (1990). Brain b-adrenoceptor binding sites in antidepressant-free depressed suicide victims. *Brain Research, 525*, 71–77.

Diamond, R., Barth, J.T., & Zillmer, E.A. (1988). Emotional correlates of mild closed head trauma: The role of the MMPI. *Int. J. Clin. Neuropsychology, 10*, 35–40.

Dillon, K.A., Gross-Isseroff, R., Israeli, M. & Biegon, A. (1991). Autoradiographic analysis of serotonin 5-HT-sub(1A) receptor binding in the human brain postmortem: Effects of age and alcohol. *Brain Research, 554*, 56–64.

Dunlop, T.W., Udvarhelyi, G.B., Stedem, A.F., O'Connor, J.M., et al. (1991). Comparison of patients with and without emotional/behavioral deterioration during the first year after traumatic brain injury. *Journal of Neuropsychiatry and Clinical Neurosciences, 3*, 150–156.

Edman, G., Asberg, M., Miles, E., Levander, S., & Schalling, D. (1986). Skin conductance habituation and cerebrospinal fluid 5-Hydroxyindoleacetic acid in suicidal patients. *Archives of General Psychiatry, 43*, 586–592.

Fedoroff, J.P., Starkstein, S.E., Forrester, A.W., Geisler, F.H., et al. (1992). Depression in patients with acute traumatic brain injury. *American Journal of Psychiatry, 149*, 918–923.

Garske, G.G., & Thomas, K.R. (1992). Self-report self-esteem and depression: Indexes of psychosocial adjustment following severe traumatic brain injury. *Rehabilitation Counseling Bulletin, 36*, 44–52.

Glenn, M.B., & Joseph, A.B. (1987). The use of lithium for behavioral and affective disorders after traumatic brain injury. Special Issue: Psychopharmacology. *Journal of Head Trauma Rehabilitation, 2*, 68–76.

Glenn, M.B., & Wroblewski, B. (1989). The choice of antidepressants in depressed survivors of traumatic brain injury. *Journal of Head Trauma Rehabilitation, 4,* 85–88.

Grafman, J., Vance, S.C., Weingartner, H., Salazar, A.M., & Amin, D. (1986). The effects of lateralized frontal lesions on mood regulation. *Brain, 109,* 1127–1148.

Hrdina, P.D., Demeter, E., Vu, T.B, Sotonyi, P., et al. (1993). 5-HT uptake sites and 5-HT-sub-2 receptors in brain of antidepressant-free suicide victims/depressives: Increase in 5-HT-sub-2 sites in cortex and amygdala. *Brain Research, 614,* 37–44.

Hunt, N., & Silverstone, T. (1990). Seasonal affective disorder following brain injury. *British Journal of Psychiatry, 156,* 884–886.

Jorge, R.E., Robinson, R.G., & Arndt, S. (1993). Are there symptoms that are specific for depressed mood in patients with traumatic brain injury? *Journal of Nervous and Mental Disease, 181,* 91-99.

Jorge, R.E., Robinson, R.G., Arndt, S.V., Starkstein, S.E., et al. (1993). Depression following traumatic brain injury: A 1-year longitudinal study. *Journal of Affective Disorders, 27,* 233–243.

Jorge, R.E., Robinson, R.G., Starkstein, S.E., & Arndt, S.V. (1993). Depression and anxiety following traumatic brain injury. *Journal of Neuropsychiatry and Clinical Neurosciences, 5,* 369–374.

Kay, S.R., Fiszbein, A., & Opler, L.A. (1987). The Positive And Negative Syndrome Scale (PANSS) for schizophrenia. *Schizophr. Bull., 13,* 261–276.

Kinsella, G., Moran, C., Ford, B., & Ponsford, J. (1988). Emotional disorder and its assessment within the severe head injured population. *Psychol. Med., 18,* 57–63.

Lawrence, K.M., de-Parmentier, F., Cheetham, S.C., Crompton, M.R., et al. (1990). Symmetrical hemispheric distribution of sup-3H-paroxetine binding sites in postmortem human brain from controls and suicides. *Biological Psychiatry, 28,* 544–546.

León-Carrión, J. (1994). *Daño cerebral: Guía para familiares y cuidadores.* Madrid: Siglo XXI.

Linnoila, V.M., Markku, V., & Virkkunen, M. (1992). Aggression, suicidality, and serotonin. Symposium: Brain serotonin and its relation to psychiatric diseases. *Journal of Clinical Psychiatry, 53,* 46–51.

Maes, M., Vanderwoude, M., Schotte, C., Martin, M., et al. (1989). Hypothalamic pituitary adrenal and thyroid axis dysfunction and decrements in the availability of L-tryptophan as biological markers of suicidal ideation in major depressed females. *Acta Psychiatrica Scandinavica, 80,* 13–17.

Mann, J.J., Arango, V., Marzuk, P.M., Theccanat, S., et al. (1989). Evidence for the 5-HT hypothesis of suicide: A review of post-mortem studies. *British Journal of Psychiatry, 155* (Suppl. 8), 7–14.

Maris, R. (1986). *Biology of suicide.* New York: Guilford Press.

Miller, L. (1991). Significant others: Treating brain injury in the family context. *Cognitive Rehabilitation, 9,* 16–25.

Nordstrom, P., & Asberg, M. (1992). Suicide risk and serotonin. *International Clinical Psychopharmacology, 6,* 12–21.

Oddy, M., Coughlam, T., Tyerman, A., & Jenkins, D. (1985). Social adjustment after closed head injury: A further follow up seven years after injury. *J. Neurol. Neurosurg. Psychiatry, 48,* 564–568.

Ohmori, T., Arora, R.C. & Meltzer, H.Y. (1992). Serotonergic measures in suicide brain: The concentration of 5-HIAA, HVA, and tryptophan in frontal cortex of suicide victims. *Biological Psychiatry, 32,* 57–71.

Parmalee, D.X., Kowatch, R.A., Sellman, J. & Davidow, D. (1989). Ten cases of head-injured, suicide-surviving adolescents: Challenges for rehabilitations. *Brain Injury, 3,* 295–300.

Perino, C. (1993). Il trattamento neuropsicofarmacologico del danno celebrale post-traumatico (Neuropharmacological treatment of TBI). In R. Rago & C. Perino (Eds.), *La riabilitazione dei T.C.E. nell'adulto* (pp. 209–220). Milano, Italy: Ed. Ghedini.

Prigatano, G. (1987). Psychiatric aspects of head injury: Problems areas and suggested guidelines for research. In H.S. Levin, J. Grafman, & H.M. Eisenberg (Eds.), *Neurobehavioural recovery from head-injury* (pp. 215–231). New York: Oxford University Press.

———. (1988). Emotion and motivation in recovery and adaptation after brain damage. In S. Finger, T.E. leVere, C.R. Robert Almli, & D.G. Stain (Eds.), *Brain injury and recovery: Theoretical and controversial Issues* (pp. 335–350). New York: Plenum Press.

Robinson, R.G., Boston, J.D., Starkstein, S.E., & Price, T.R. (1988). Comparison of mania and depression after brain injury: Causal factors. *American Journal of Psychiatry, 145,* 172–178.

Ross, E.D. (1985). Right-hemisphere lesions in disorders of affective language. In A. Kertesz (Ed.), *Localization in neuropsychology* (pp. 493–508). New York: Academic Press.

Ross, E.D., & Stewart, R.S. (1987). Pathological display on affect in patients with depression and right frontal brain damage: An alternative mechanism. *J. Nerv. Ment. Dis., 170,* 165–172.

Sandyk, R., & Awerbuch, G.I. (1993). Nocturnal melatonin secretion in suicidal patients with multiple sclerosis. *International Journal of Neuroscience, 71,* 173–182.

Santos, A.B., & Ballenger, J.C. (1992). Tricyclic antidepressant triggers mania in patient with organic affective disorder. *Journal of Clinical Psychiatry, 53,* 377–378.

Scarone, S., Gambini, O., Calabrese, G., Saurdete, P., et al. (1990). Asymmetrical distribution of beta-endorphin in cerebral hemispheres or suicides: Preliminary data. *Psychiatry Research, 32,* 159–166.

Schoenhuber, R., Gentilini, M., & Orlando, A. (1988). A prognostic value of auditory brainstem responses for late postconcussion symptoms following minor head trauma. *J. Neurosurg., 68,* 742–744.

Shedlack, K.J., & Pope, H.G. (1992). Anticonvulsant response in a case of anorexia nervosa and bipolar disorder associated with right-sided brain injury. *International Journal of Eating Disorders, 12,* 333–336.

Silver, J.M., Yudofsky, S.C., & Hales, R.E. (1991). Depression in traumatic brain injury. *Neuropsychiatry Neuropsychology, and Behavioral Neurology, 4,* 12–23.

Slaby, A.E. (1994). Psychopharmacotherapy of suicide. Special Issue: Clinical and legal issues in suicide assessment. *Death Studies, 18,* 483–495.

Starkstein, S.E., Pearlson, G.D., Boston, J., & Robinson, R.G. (1987). Mania after brain injury: A controlled study of causative factors. *Archives of Neurology, 44,* 1069–1073.

Stewart, J.T., & Hemsath, R.H. (1988). Bipolar illness following traumatic brain injury: Treatment with lithium and carbamazepine. *Journal of Clinical Psychiatry, 49,* 74–75.

Traskman-Bendz, L., Asberg, M., Nosdstrom, P. & Stanley, M. (1989). Biochemical aspects of suicidal behavior. *Progress in Neuro-Psychopharmacology and Biological Psychiatry,* 13(Suppl.), S35–S44.

Wroblewski, B.A., Guidos, A., Leary, J.M., & Joseph, A.B. (1992). Control of depression with fluoxetine and antiseizure medication in a brain-injured patient. *American Journal of Psychiatry, 149,* 273.

Zahn, B.S., & Littman, S.I. (1989). Depression in survivors of severe traumatic brain injury: Issues in assessment and management. *Psychiatric Forum, 15,* 6–10.

Zwil, A.S., McAllister, T.W., Cohen, I.H., & Halpern, L.R. (1993). Ultra-rapid cyclingbipolar affective disorder following a closer-head injury. *Brain Injury, 7,* 147–152.

23 Management of Aggression

Peter D. Patrick and David W. Hebda

Learning Services Corporation
Manassas, VA

INTRODUCTION: DESCRIPTION OF THE PROBLEM

What we are to describe is not a new problem. The story of Phineas Gage is a part of brain-injury folklore and depicts the events following the passing of a tamping iron through the frontal lobes of this construction worker. In 1868, Harlow described a situation all too prevalent in our care of the brain-injured today:

> *The equilibrium of balance, so to speak, between his intellectual faculties and animal propensities, seems to have been destroyed. He is fitful, irreverent, indulging at times in the grossest of profanity (which was not previously his custom), manifesting but little deference for his fellows, impatient or restraint of advice when it conflicts with his desires, at times pertinaciously obstinate, yet capricious and vacillating, devising many plans of future operations, which are no sooner arranged than they are abandoned in turn for others...his mind is radically changed, so decidedly that his friends and acquaintances said he was "no longer Gage" (p. 327).*

Following brain injury, disturbances to conduct and behaviors, especially angry and aggressive behaviors, continue to have the most disqualifying influence on the person's membership at home, at work, and throughout social systems at large.

Since the time human beings banded together to live in communities for the mutual benefit of all, pro-social behaviors such as cooperation and self-control have been essential for both the survival of the individual and the community. Disturbances to conduct and behavior were most likely to disqualify individuals from the community for membership and affiliation, and it became imperative that unmanageable, antisocial, or incomprehensible behaviors be eliminated, cured, or managed. The effect of unrestrained behaviors had consequences for quality of life for each of the members of that group and especially for that individual.

Muriel Lezak (1978) identified a series of complex behavioral symptoms that were previously ignored symptoms of brain injury. These now commonly recognized signs had to do with the complex changes to personality and character. Among the characterologic alterations following brain injury are included the following:

1. Loss of social perceptiveness
2. Impaired self-regulation
3. Stimulus bound behaviors
4. Emotional lability
5. Failure to prosper from experience

With the development of trauma services and with the prevalence of strokes in any given population, there has been a rapidly growing group of patients that not only presents with sensory-motor deficits but with being challenged to live successfully with alterations in cognition and personality. Although the ability to survive brain injuries has greatly improved, learning to live again with the complex alterations associated with the injury still seeks solution.

A particularly noticeable aspect of these personality and characterologic changes is the alteration in mood and self-regulation (Lezak, 1978). In particular, the brain-injured person's inability to manage anger and frustration rapidly becomes a central complaint from family members, work colleagues, and those who socially interact with the brain-injured person. Frequently, the presence of uncontrolled anger and aggression disqualify the person from opportunities of living. Housing, vocational/educational, and social life opportunities are frequently undermined by the presence of anger and aggression.

Changes in personality, along with reduced cognition, limitations in emotional expression, and the loss of executive functioning combine to render a picture of loss of control. Within the context of the brain injury, the onset of aggression and destructive anger has been, for some, part of the overall change in personality. However, it has been the expression of anger, in particular, that greatly interferes with the person's ability to collaborate in therapies, to participate in social settings, and to generally allow for group membership. Without success in restoring management of anger and aggression, the person remains chronically disqualified for opportunity, regardless of the degree of recovery in other areas.

VARIANTS OF DIFFICULTIES WITH ANGER AND AGGRESSION

Expressions of anger and aggression are not uniform. Not only will anger differ in its expression, but it will differ in its causation between individuals and within the same individual at various times. Aggression is multiply determined. Within the individual in question, the possibility of multiple expressions and multiple causation exists.

A range of behaviors can be called angry, from the noncompliant, resistive patient to the verbally explicit attacks of some patients to the explosive rage of the physically abusive patient. Each expression may have its neurologic, psychogenic, or sociogenic contributing factors. The initial understanding of the individual's expression of anger, its variants, and its contributing factors is essential if treatment resources are to be mobilized effectively. As a precursor to decision making, the clinician must realize that the manner in which he/she "understands" the patient's anger will influence the mobilization of therapeutic options that vary greatly in their applicability and appropriateness. The differential diagnosis must begin with a comprehensiveness which will result in the mobilization of therapy or therapies that will address the components of "this patient's" anger.

It is important during clinical analysis to include a review of and not just the most obvious expression of anger but all the variants that may be part of the patient's overall repertoire. The clinician must deal with the grades of anger within this individual's profile in order to defuse the entire fund of anger and not simply concentrate upon the most explosive anger. There is a matrix of possibilities within each patient (Table 23.1) that may occur exclusively, successively, or simultaneously.

Table 23.1: Range of Possible Manifestations of Anger

	Sociogenic	...........Psychogenic	...........Neurogenic
Pessimistic Angry Ideation			
Argumentative			
Oppositional Behavior			
Verbal Aggression			
Aggression Toward Objects			
Physical Aggression			

In the group of persons with brain injury, it frequently occurs that the expression of anger is influenced and contributed to by cognitive status. The manner in which cognitive status influences self-perceptions and perceptions of others becomes an important factor in understanding the variant of anger and aggression. The loss of executor functions and the loss of self-appraisal and self-monitoring that frequently result from brain injury set the stage for impaired interpersonal transactions and impaired social discourse which leads to interpersonal conflict. Therefore, in the understanding of behavioral expression, it is important to relate the person's cognitive status to the expression of anger. More importantly, the presence or absence of cognitive skill will frequently influence therapies mobilized in addressing the person's aggression.

Some anger is the product of a social transaction that has gone awry, and either member of the discourse could contribute to this feature. Characterizing the nature and limits of the person's anger and aggression helps in establishing the parameters of importance and significance. Furthermore, the efforts to describe the nature of the problem will help shed insight into the etiology and factors requiring attention. Impaired anger and aggression management may more properly be seen as an array of difficulties with differing combinations of factors driving the disorder.

It is important to assess how the type of anger expressed effects the individual and others. Although sounding simplistic, this exercise will quickly yield information regarding anger's influence on the individual's cognitive and motivational states and will help focus on how the anger influences social discourse and interpersonal transactions. Therapeutically, this simple inquiry will indicate what is to be done to the individual and what will need to be done to address the behaviors of others.

Angry/aggressive behaviors can be plotted along a continuum ranging from anger that is predominantly due to psychosocial factors, to intra-personal factors, and to expressions of anger that represent the loss of control and rage which may be more determined by neurogenic factors. The multifactorial features that contribute to anger are typically present in degrees with few etiologies being uni-variant. This becomes very important in our modeling of treatment.

All dys-control is not equal in importance or simply driven by one causation. Typically, it is the understanding of direction and multiple determination that will suggest a treatment approach tailored for the individual's needs. Needless to say, a prescriptive approach cannot be "cookbook" and requires versatility and uniqueness of understanding of time, place, and purpose for each person. The individuality of anger expression and the interface between neurologic, psychologic, and social factors driving anger expression must be acknowledged. In this way, treating anger dys-control does allow an insight into the multifactorial needs of treating personality and character changes. By understanding anger and personality within the context of an individual's neurology, psychology, and sociology, the client will be most served.

Beyond the individual techniques, it is the appreciation of anger (as of all personality traits) within the context of that individual's life that must be our starting point.

THE NEUROPSYCHOLOGY OF ANGER AND AGGRESSION

Physiological psychology has greatly contributed to the understanding of the biologic features of aggression and anger. Research in physiological psychology has revealed a number of brain sites that correlate with the presence or absence of aggressive behavior. In particular, the research differentiates unrestrained and uncontrolled expressions of anger and violence from predatory or stalking behaviors that lead to aggression. A variety of aggressive behaviors have been identified with differing circumstantial features and differing motivational components. Wilson (1975) has classified aggressive behaviors into several types based on their resulting outcomes:

1. Territorial aggression
2. Dominance aggression
3. Sexual aggression
4. Parental aggression
5. Predatory aggression
6. Anti-predatory aggression

Each of these types of aggressive behaviors has a purposeful end point. Not unlike the brain-injured individual, although not always knowingly, they, too, employ anger and aggression without the benefit of adequate management skills in order to effect a situation. Either purposefully or inadvertently, the expression of aggression by the injured person results in an altered end point and, thereby, dictates a change in circumstance. This purposeful nature is very important in our addressing and treating the behavior in question. There are a number of studies that indicate sites relevant to the expression of anger (Table 23.2).

There is also research that points out the role of neurotransmitters in the expression of anger. Although the relationship between these substances is complex, there have emerged findings that give some insight into the chemistry as well as the specific tracts associated with the expression of anger.

The absence of serotonin has been found to be one of the more consistent findings in aggression. Panksepp (1986) documents the role of serotonergic pathways and the expression of anger and aggression. The presence of serotonin appears to have an inhibiting affect on aggression. In particular, the presence of serotonin in prefrontal areas

Table 23.2: Brain Localization Studies Showing Sites Relevant to the Expression of Anger

SITE	AUTHOR	FINDINGS
Hypothalamus	Hess, 1928	Sham rage through stimulation
	Bard, 1928	Rage response after removal of all tissue above the hypothalamus in cats
Anteriormedial		
Nuclei of hypothalamus	Delgado, 1969	Affective attack response
Lateral nuclei		
hypothalamus		Predatory attack response
Amygdala	Vergnes, 1975, 1976	
	Tonkonogy 1991	
Cortical medial nuclei		Predatory attack
basolateral nuclei		Affective attack
Septum	Brady & Nauta, 1953	Lesions of septum lower threshold for rage response
Periaqueductal		Stimulation released affective attack
Grey Matter	Edwards & Flynn, 1972	
Ventromedial		Lesions eliminate affect attack but leaves predatory attack intact
Tegmentum	Adams, 1986	
Anterior		
Temporal Lobe	Garyfallos et al. 1981	"dys-control syndrome"
Frontal and Prefrontal		
Cortex	Heinrichs, 1989	Removes cortical inhibition over limbic structures

has a controlling effect. In contrast, the literature points out that with some reduced serotonin, there is an increase of aggressive behavior. There has also been evidence that persons who were aggressive toward themselves had reduced serotonin levels (Kruesi et al., 1992; Linnoila & Virkkunen, 1992).

In addition, elevated acetylcholine concentrations (Grossman et al., 1975) and dopamine levels (Eichelman, 1987) were also correlated with increased aggression. Increased levels of GABA were found to correlate with the reduction of aggression (Eichelman, 1987).

In humans, orbital frontal injuries have been associated with a "hypomanic" presentation with the noteworthy appearance of agitation and aggression. The so-called "releasing syndrome" is explained by the removal of cortical and, more specifically, frontal and prefrontal controls over limbic centers. This results in what researchers are describing as affect attack. Once expressed, the person returns to a quiescent state.

Frontal lobe injury has been amply associated with the loss of controls over emotionally charged behavior (Luria, 1983; Pribram, 1987; Mattson & Levin, 1990). Frontal lobe injury, which has a high incident rate among traumatic brain injury (TBI) patients, has yielded a variety of syndromes, with the dorso-lateral injuries frequently associated with a "releasing" and disinhibited profile of conduct inclusive of the expression of anger and aggression.

This array of emotionally charged behaviors accompanies specific cognitive alterations outlined by Hart and Jacobs (1993, pp. 2–4). These authors list four key factors as important in understanding the role of the frontal lobes in behavioral disturbance:

1. The frontal lobes decide what is worth attending to and what is worth doing.
2. The frontal lobes provide continuity and coherence of behavior across time.
3. The frontal lobes modulate affective and interpersonal behavior so that drives are satisfied within the constraints of the internal and external environment.
4. The frontal lobes monitor, evaluate, and adjust.

THE COGNITIVE AND SOCIAL PSYCHOLOGY OF ANGER AND AGGRESSION

Along with the identification of the menu of pathological states that could contribute to the expression of anger and aggression must go the understanding that these behaviors occur within a context.

In primitive man, when human behavior was assumed to have supernatural causes, the shaman of the Stone Age cave dwellers treated these behaviors via trephining or chipping away an area of the skull in order to, presumably, release the evil spirit residing within. The early Greeks and Romans practiced exorcism in order to rid the individual of the cause. This practice was revived during medieval times in which the body was made as unpleasant as possible so that the demon would leave.

The expression of aggression and anger is, to a large extent, controlled in society through the individual's adherence to codes of conduct and learned ways of expressing dissatisfaction and anger. Society relies on the rule-driven method of controlling aggressive behavior. However, under certain conditions, there are factors that lead the individual to violate these rules. It is at this point that the sociocentric features and the cognitive features that effect the expression of anger come into play.

For example, under ordinary conditions, the uninjured individual who is stressed or fatigued is more likely to be aggressive. Certainly, when threats or intimidation factors arise, the individual is likely to operate outside of the code of conduct typically controlling expressions of anger or aggression. Certainly, the individual who perceives the need to self-protect or to dominate the situation will likely violate the rules of conduct. In many cases, it is the person's perceptual and cognitive status that will determine their interpretation of a perceived threat or need to self-protect. Consequently, the rule of engagement will be determined by the person's perception and understanding of the circumstances.

Expressions of anger and aggression are modeled (Bandura, 1969) as well. In groups and communities, expressions of aggression have a contagious effect. The copying or mimicking of anger and aggression is routinely reported. To the degree that a consistent model of aggression is present in an environment or community, there is an inherent standard established giving "permission" or acceptance to that expression of aggression.

The individual who has sustained a brain injury to the cortical systems necessary for complex information processing and understanding frequently misinterprets others and has reduced skill to navigate conflict resolution and negotiation of outcomes. The relationship between faulty information processing and social misconduct is important. Recognition of the cognitive component in aggression, along with its social components, increases our options for effecting a change in conduct by addressing sites other than the purely neurologic systems of aggression in the brain.

The cognitive limitations associated with brain injury make social interpretation and social comprehension more challenging and more likely for mis-attribution. Furthermore, the loss of social transaction skills and the reduction in pragmatic language make social exchanges and social encounters more confounded and likely for misdirection.

Considering that the brain-injured individual enters a social realm with the added limitation of cognitive and emotional dys-control, it is not surprising that social discourse may be problematic. The loss of transactional skills in a social setting may be a major precipitant of the dys-control.

Added difficulties with self-appraisal and with self-monitoring make the brain-injured individual more vulnerable to social disarray. The loss of transactional skills along with a tendency for social mis-attribution can play a large part in setting the stage for the expression of anger and aggression that would otherwise be averted.

Varney and Menefee (1993) give an excellent overview of the relationship between the failure of psychosocial governance and the loss of executive functioning secondary to injury of the orbital frontal cortex. They point to the need for complex reasoning skills associated with the prefrontal in order to participate with others in social and productive settings. Without the cognitive skills, the adherence to social rules and the influence of social affiliations lose effect over governing daily conduct.

Social motives drive much of adult human behavior (Luria, 1983; Murray, 1938). Luria, in his recognition of higher cortical functions in man, realized the importance of executive functioning and the brain's role in establishing complex thought as it interfaces with motive, motivation, and ultimate control over conduct. The alteration to the brain brings with it the alteration in social motives, in particular, the motives of affiliation and power. With the disturbance to affiliation motives and with the disruption to the management of power motives, the individual loses the gratification of affiliations and also leaves uncovered the expression of power without the benefit of interpersonal input.

THERAPEUTIC INTERVENTION

Twentieth century society continues to struggle with how to treat severe disturbances of conduct among our members. Biological therapies have included insulin shock therapy as a physiological treatment for the unpredictable behaviors associated with schizophrenia. Electroconvulsive therapy (ECT) was introduced during the 1930s to treat a variety of behaviors, as was psychosurgery. The effectiveness of antipsychotic compounds on unpredictable or violent behavior cannot be overestimated, as described by Coleman (p. 622):

> *...It is difficult to convey the truly enormous influence they [medications] have had in altering the environment of the mental hospital. One of the authors, as part of his training, worked several months in the maximum security ward of one such hospital immediately prior to the introduction of this type of medication in 1955. The ward patients fulfilled the oft-heard stereotypes of individuals "gone mad." Bizarreness, nudity, wild screaming, and an ever present threat of violence pervaded the atmosphere. Fearfulness and a near-total preoccupation with the maintenance of control characterized the attitudes of staff. Such staff attitudes were not unrealistic in terms of the frequency of occurrence of serious physical assaults by patients, but they were hardly conducive to the development or maintenance of an effective therapeutic program.*
>
> *Then quite suddenly within a period of perhaps a month...all of this dramatically changed. The patients were receiving antipsychotic medication. The ward became a place in which one could seriously get to know one's patients on a personal level and perhaps even initiate programs of "milieu therapy."*

Psychosurgery with humans produced marked changes in persons with unremitting aggression or violent attacks. As early as the 1930s, prefrontal lobectomies and leukotomies were used to alter human aggression and agitation. Balasubramaniam and Kanaka (1976) and Richardson and Mitchell-Heggs (1973) report on the use of psychosurgery that selectively ablated areas of the brain including the amygdala, cingulate gyrus, hypothalamus, and other limbic sites as a means of "treating" aggressive responses in humans. Brown (1973) reports on stereotaxic surgery that eliminates violent episodes in patients who underwent bilateral amygdalotomy. Mark and Irvin's *Violence in the Brain* (1973) reviewed the significance of brain pathology to violent criminal acts and their impact on society.

We recognize the need to follow a scientific method in determining the employment of therapy or therapies that alter and improve the expression of anger and aggression. In addition, we recognize an array of resources that can be considered. In general we will discuss (1) the biologic therapies (primarily the use of medications), (2) the complementary employment of behavioral modification techniques, and (3) the social/ developmental approach to modifying aggressive behaviors.

PHARMACOLOGY OF AGGRESSION

Advances in the biochemistry of the brain have had a positive effect in the development of medications available to address the neuropathology of aggression. Silver, Yudofsky, and Hales (1994) in *Neuropsychiatry of Traumatic Brain Injury* present an excellent overview of the psychopharmacology of aggression. The authors are careful to point the differential approach to acute versus persistent aggression. Silver and Yudofsky correctly differentiate our historical method of non-specific and symptomatic treatment of aggression from our present ability to target specific neurotransmitter tracts and brain sites through our understanding of matching medications to specific neuronal networks related to the expression of anger and aggression

Several categories of medications have been employed to reduce or eliminate the expression of aggression. The anti-seizure medications and the anti-hypertensive medications are presented as excellent medications of choice for generic treatment of aggression due to neuronal or membrane destruction and receptor site malfunction. Other medication classes add increased power of influence either through poly-drug approaches or by selection due to specific accompanying symptoms along with the aggression.

Acute Aggression

Historically, the treatment of acute aggression was symptomatic in nature. By relying on the side effects of neuroleptic and anxiolytic medications, patients were sedated. This use, or (as Silver and Yudofsky present) this "misuse," has short-lived value and does not pass the cost/benefit analysis for maintaining an individual on this regime for a long time.

Due to the potential negative side effects ranging from suppression of cognition and arousal to the dangers of tardive dyskinesia, neuroleptic and anxiolytics find time-limited use. For example, Silver and Yudofsky (1994) point out that frequently the akinesia associated with neuroleptic is mis-attributed as "more agitation or aggression," and dosages are adjusted upward with a resulting "vicious circle." Furthermore, Silver and Yudofsky point out that there is some research evidence that injured motor neurons are effected adversely by such drugs as haloperidol. There does seem to be the need for risk-benefit analysis when using a dopamine antagonist when the individual displays clear motor system impairment.

Anxiolytic drugs with a primary effect of sedation are also questionable for long-term use. Benzodiazepines may have short-term effect by increasing the inhibitory transmitter GABA. However, the effects on cognition and reports of paradoxical effects on agitation and aggression argue against their use over the long term. Silver and Yudofsky (1994) recommend that antipsychotic and sedating medications be used only on a short-term basis, except with persons whose aggression is part of a psychotic thought disorder and impairment to reality testing.

There do exist other categories of medications with targeted effects that can be used to treat acute aggression. Amantadine has been used for dopamine agonist effects. Gualtieri (1989) reported use of amantadine during acute agitation during early stage recovery. Amantadine's effect on striatal and cortical dopamine systems is seen as the site of action in restoring the individual's control over aggression. Yudofsky (1994) points out there have been seizures following amantadine use in severe TBI and patients with poor arousal.

Clonodine, although very sedating and able to markedly lower blood pressure, is reported by Silver and Yudofsky (1994) as an option in managing acute aggression. Clonodine inhibits the activity of the brain site locus ceruleus and decreases adrenergic systems.

In addition, Yudofsky offers that Lorazapam has shown promise for managing acute episodes of aggression and offers a specific administration protocol for the use of Lorazapam. Propranolol, which will be discussed in its use with persistent states of aggression, can even be considered for acute aggression (Aiel, 1977).

Persistent Aggressive States

There are patients who take on a chronic state of aggressiveness beyond the Level IV stage of agitation. These patients will demonstrate a specific site of injury that correlates with the anatomical circuit of aggression. Patients with this profile will persist in their use of aggression and will no longer be considered in a transient state of agitated aggression. It is important to differentiate this patient from the emerging coma patient who is "passing through" a Los Amigos level IV stage. Clinically, we have seen patients admitted for care who have gone into a persistent state yet were still being seen as level IV. Whereas a level IV represents an emerging and transitional state, the persistent state of aggression will become an ongoing feature of the person's recovery.

Anti-Seizure Medications

Carbamazepine has become the medication of choice with patients whose aggressiveness may be related to a seizure focus. Furthermore, even without positive EEG findings, carbamazepine has been used to eliminate or lessen aggressive behavior. The site of action is considered to be the lessening of "kindling" response. The presence of subclinical "kindling" response in limbic and temporal lobe structures has been demonstrated to be related to the presence of rage and attack (Mark & Irvin, 1973). Although there has been clinical experience supporting the use of carbamazepine, there are cautions because of its medical side effects. Careful monitoring must include blood counts and liver function testing.

Valproic acid has also been used to regulate aggressive response in humans. This medication is also accompanied by a need for close medical monitoring. There are patients who have not tolerated carbamazepine that will benefit from valproic acid.

Lithium Carbonate

Lithium has long been used to manage the manic behaviors of patients with bi-polar disease. There is evidence that it may assist with the management of aggression in TBI (Moskowitz, 1991). Lithium's action in increasing serotonergic actions has been felt to explain its effectiveness. As reviewed by Yudofsky and Silver (1994), due to the brain-injured person's sensitivity to neurotoxin, the toxic side effects of lithium are important considerations in its use (Hornstein & Seliger 1989; Moskowitz & Altshuler, 1991).

Antidepressants

The antidepressants that are serotonin agonists have reportedly (Sobin et al., 1989) been effective in managing aggression in some patients. In particular, patients with agitation and mood lability in addition to their aggressiveness have benefitted from the serotonin agonist. Amitriptyline (Mysiw et al., 1988; Jackson et al., 1985), trazodone (Zubieta & Alessi, 1992), and fluoxitene (Sobin et al., 1989) have reported to be effective with aggression that accompanies emotional lability and mood alteration.

Anxiolytics

In aggression that is accompanied by high levels of anxiety and agitation, patients have responded to several anti-anxiety medications—in particular, buspirone (Gualtieri, 1991; Ratey et al., 1992). Because buspirone has caused agitation in some patients, Silver and Yudofsky (1994) recommend starting buspirone at lower dosages and gradually increasing every 3–5 days.

Clonazepam has also been used when aggression and agitation occur together. Although the findings are less specific to head injury and acquired brain injury, Freinhar and Alvarez (1986) reported control of aggression in elderly organic brain syndrome.

Anti-Hypertensive Medication

The use of beta blockers has been effective with persistent and episodic aggression. Beta blockers (e.g., propranolol or nadolol) may be particularly useful when once-a-day dosage is necessary due to compliance or medication adversity. Also, when the side effect of bradycardia occurs with the longer acting beta blockers such as propranolol, there are alternative medications such as pindolol. The evidence that beta blockers are effective with aggression comes without a clear explanation for mechanism of action. Both peripheral (Ratey et al., 1992) and central (Gengo et al., 1988) sites of action have been recognized.

These medications give the clinician the means to address essential disturbances to the central nervous system that underlie the expression of anger and aggression. The use of medication becomes a necessary complement to a comprehensive treatment of aggression when combined with neurobehavioral programming that addresses the behavioral aspects of aggression. Neither medications nor behavior programming can be viewed as a stand-alone approach to aggression, since aggression clearly has both neurogenic as well as a psychogenic driving mechanisms. The complementary relationship between the two factors of treatment extends to the need for compatible and complementary relationships between the treatment team members representing these two strong modes of addressing aggression in the brain injured (i.e., psychology and psychiatry).

NEUROBEHAVIORAL TREATMENT OF AGGRESSION

Since the founding of American behaviorism as the "second force" in psychology during the early 1900s, pioneers such as John B. Watson, E. Thorndike, and B.F. Skinner have advocated a strictly behavioral approach to the understanding of the organism. In opposition to the psychoanalytic technique of Sigmund Freud, American behaviorists did not assume the existence of unconscious structures as relevant to the study of the organism and focused upon information that was directly observable (i.e., behavior). Subsequently, decades of scientific study has provided us with a body of information that has proven useful in the modification of human behavior. A variety of behavioral strategies have been found to be effective in increasing or decreasing a target behavior, as summarized below.

Efforts to impose rules of learning on the expression of anger and aggression have taken some specific directions. With the realization that all anger is managed socially by having the individual adopt and employ rules of conduct, treatment of anger and aggression have similarities to the re-socialization of the individual facing recovery following brain injury. Although aversive conditioning approaches have a long history in the treatment of aggressive children and to some degree with adults (Bandura, 1969), the present trend is towards the use of positive reinforcement as a means of developing an increased repertoire of pro-social behaviors in order to reduce or eliminate aggressiveness. There is more emphasis on the instruction of acceptable alternatives and the development of the broader repertoire of behaviors in meeting need satisfaction.

We realize that during the acute expression of rage, where there is imminent danger to self or others, physical restraint and management may be necessary. Management of aggressive behavior is differentiated from behavioral treatment. Management is time- and situation-specific and speaks of imminent destructiveness. *Management* is akin to risk management with no inherent value beyond the immediate response to danger. *Treatment* has as its goal having the patient incorporate skills that can be generalized across time and place in order to ultimately self-manage anger and aggression. The attempt to develop and employ anger management skills and the attempt to incorporate these abilities in the person's overall recovery differentiates treatment from management. It is important to realize that although all members of a treatment team want to advance the patient's personal skills to manage anger, separate members of the team may have to differentially rely on management or treatment approaches. For example, nurses and therapists may have to rely on management strategies, while psychologists and psychiatrists focus on treatment. Simultaneously, within one care plan, there may be both management and treatment efforts employed.

BEHAVIORAL ANALYSIS

Treatment begins with a comprehensive understanding of the "anatomy" of the patient's aggression and anger. For all the reasons previously reviewed, the factors contributing to the aggressiveness must be articulated if a tailored approach is to be considered.

We would suggest a diagrammatic approach in addition to any plotting or frequency tabulations used. Multiple observations and exhaustive searches for antecedents and consequences of the behaviors in question should precede treatment intervention.

Although many data-gathering approaches may be employed (Jacobs, 1993), it is important that actuarial data be gathered in a fashion that will lead to solution of the individual's deficits.

We suggest a "tandem" data-gathering approach between a primary care giver and a support clinician serving as the observer, so as to capture the nature of the transactional disturbances. The primary care person will focus on task, while the observer takes the role of process observer. The nature of the transaction is captured, and the relationship between task demand and the care giver's approach is outlined so as to elucidate the formula of the transaction and the antecedents that may have triggered the episode. Also, the tandem transactional approach will allow for safety of the care giver. We have observed clinically that because the care giver frequently is so focused on completing the task, they naturally filter out "indicators" of an upcoming attack.

The observer is able to report changes and unnoticed behaviors in the patient so that the care giver is able to self-protect. Therefore, the tandem approach has built into it a risk management component.

This approach will have appeal to the allied therapists involved, letting them participate in data gathering while allowing them to remain involved with the goals they have set.

Within a task-specific situation, the information is then plotted along the curve. Observations longitudinally across time are also included or may be focused on exclusively without the more immediate transactional analysis available. In either situation, the collection of transactional and situational data becomes a task for all involved with the patient. This time of data collection is flexible but must be done if the anatomy of the aggression is to be completed. Multiple curves are plotted with the results being a frequency distribution of symptoms and times of onset and precursors (Figure 23.1).

With the attack (physical or verbal) at the bottom of the curve, the antecedents are plotted along the descending curve. Attempts to "back up" the antecedents as far in time as possible will be the challenge. Both environmental and external factors to the individual should be captured, but attempts to recognize internal states of the individual will also be necessary for a complete anatomy. In addition, and probably of more importance, the transactional factors between primary care giver and the brain-injured person should be captured. It is through the orchestration of the transaction that aggression will be prevented and treated. Therefore, it is essential that the transactional analysis be exhaustive. Any staff member who does "do well" with the patient should be observed so that the positive transactional symptoms can be captured. It will be within the context of the interpersonal transaction that the aggressive disorder will be modified. The dyad represents

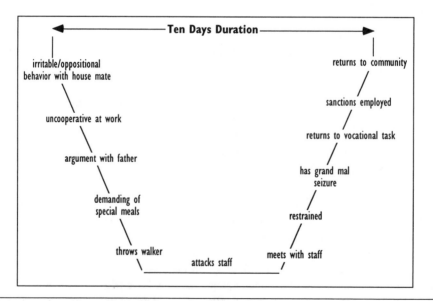

Figure 23.1: Display of aggression by a 23-year-old stroke victim showing an array of explosive difficulties including throwing objects, damage of property, and attacking individuals.

the most elementary context for social and interpersonal learning and rule acquisition. Within the context of this "anatomy" of an outburst, trigger factors—environmental and internal state factors—will begin to frame the direction for the specific approach to the individual's aggression. This approach also assures tailoring the approach to the individual, even though generic learning principals will be applied to the solution.

Each individual transaction also has meritorious information that must be captured. Using a transactional diagram (Figure 23.2), the specifics of task demand and trigger mechanism will be captured.

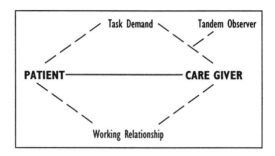

Figure 23.2: Task demand and trigger mechanism.

Once diagrammed, a selection of approaches can be considered. From the menu of possibilities, there is a range of techniques that can be employed. Management techniques could include restraints or the use of more modified approaches, such as therapeutic walks, to sensory re-directs (distraction of the patient) to "triangulation" of staff where two staff members repeatedly intercede to disrupt a third conflictive or inflamed transaction.

Behavior Techniques

Aggressive behavior can respond to the changing influences of behavior modification. Traditional approaches such as conditioning and reward schedules have been employed (Jacobs, 1993). Immediate changes in behavior have been accomplished by attempts to extinguish agitated and angry behaviors, and the approach is generally to focus on the aggression episode by episode. However, if aggression is taken as a specific example of a broader difficulty the individual has with self control and conforming to codes of conduct, then extinction or mere symptom reduction represents only a partial solution.

Skill Development

Because some aggressive episodes are the sequelae of impaired cognitive and executive functioning skills, skill development in these areas can offset the potential for aggression. Enhanced cognitive and self-managing skills indirectly improve competency and avoid the poor frustration tolerance that serves as a precursor to aggression and anger.

Training of social competency and, in particular, social discourse and interpersonal transaction skills greatly contributes to reducing unsuccessful social exchange that may set up the aggressive/angry outbursts.

Conditioning

Modification of aggressive responses begins with the efforts to condition an inhibitory response. In Harvey E. Jacob's text (1993), *Behavior Analysis Guidelines and Brain*

Injury Rehabilitation: People, Principles and Programs, the practitioner finds a new and refreshing use of well-founded behavioral principles. Jacobs (1993), in a sensitive and understanding fashion, is able to use behavioral principles without the loss of the personal identity of his patients (see strategies below). His attempt to treat the person through the application of behavioral principles bridges the gap between the humanist and the behaviorist.

STRATEGIES FOR INCREASING BEHAVIOR

- POSITIVE REINFORCEMENT: Presentation of a stimulus or event, contingent upon a response, that results in an increased probability of that response.
- SCHEDULES OF REINFORCEMENT: Delivery of a reinforcer based on time, specified rate of response, or both. Different schedules tend to have different effects on behavior. Schedules include the following:
  - *Continuous reinforcement*, in which each occurrence of the targeted response produces reinforcement.
  - *Fixed interval,* a schedule in which a fixed amount of time must elapse before a response produces reinforcement.
  - *Variable interval,* in which a variable amount of time, around some specified average, must elapse before a response produces reinforcement.
  - *Fixed ratio,* in which a fixed number of responses must occur before a response produces reinforcement.
  - *Variable ratio,* in which a variable number of responses, around some specified average, must occur before a response produces reinforcement.
  - *Differential reinforcement of low rates*, in which a specified amount of time must occur between each response in order to produce reinforcement.
  - *Differential reinforcement of high rates*, in which subsequent responses must occur within a specified amount of time in order to produce reinforcement.
- SHAPING: Differential reinforcement of successive approximations to some terminal behavior.
- TOKEN ECONOMY: A behavior modification system based on the exchange of generalized reinforcers.

STRATEGIES FOR DECREASING BEHAVIOR

- STIMULUS CHANGE: Alteration of stimuli in the prevailing environment, contingent upon a response, resulting in a decreased probability of that response.
- EXTINCTION: Withholding of reinforcement for a response that was previously reinforced, resulting in a decreased probability of that response.
- DIFFERENTIAL REINFORCEMENT: A procedure in which behavior to be eliminated is extinguished while alternative behavior is reinforced.
- TIME-OUT: A procedure that involves placing the person in a situation that will not allow him/her to come in contact with specific stimuli or consequences.
- PUNISHMENT: Presentation of a stimulus or event, contingent upon a response, that results in a decreased probability of that response.
- RESPONSE COST: Response-contingent removal of a positive reinforcer.

• OVERCORRECTION: Behavioral restitution following the occurrence of a specific behavior, resulting in a decreased probability of that behavior.

Behavioral techniques to treat aggression have been included in comprehensive behavior therapy manuals such as the one provided by Jacobs. He acknowledges that, when all other means of managing behavior have been unsuccessful, often the only alternative is the method of *Contingent Restraint*. This procedure involves physical restraint of an individual, contingent upon a response, that results in a decreased probability of that response. It is used when continuation of the targeted behavior is likely to result in physical harm to either the client or others. Use of this highly restrictive procedure depends upon properly trained staff and adequate professional supervision and should occur only under specific circumstances.

In general, effective behavior management programs depend upon rigorous training of staff, careful analysis of behaviors to be targeted, and consistency of application. Careful documentation and record-keeping are essential for the success of a systematic behavior plan.

This task has been somewhat accomplished by the behavior intensity reduction or deceleration activities. These would include attempts to extinguish the response or attempts to establish modeled behavior that represents a socially condoned manner of expression anger. Time outs or delays as antecedents to response could all be adopted. Through skill-training activities, the person copies or adopts an alternative expressive route.

Deceleration Techniques

There are those brain-injured persons who are aggressive and who lack the cognitive or mental status necessary to incorporate learned alternatives. They require a more simplified learning paradigm that focuses on diminishing the target behavior with the grander objective of pro-socialization left for a later time. Deceleration intervention is characterized by the early identification of a precursor to aggression and systematically redirecting the individual to alternative responses. This indirectly increases the individual's repertoire of behavior. The use of time outs, either self-directed or other-directed, falls into this category of approaches. The individual implements a inhibitory response at the earliest point of recognition. The individual and staff learn the antecedents to the aggression, and the patient is redirected to a time-limited time out. Other techniques include a use of modeling. The individual is to observe others' ability to cope with frustration or anger and then directed to model this performance. The use of modeling does fall into the more natural learning activities consistent with normal developmental tendencies. Extinction techniques are also employed with those having the cognitive status to realize the effect. The person would not be attended to during periods of agitation or anger (with the noted caveat that imminence of danger would not be ignored).

Behavioral Replacement and Repertoire Building

To truly increase behavioral repertoire and strength of response, a behavior replacement or behavior development process holds promise (Liberian & Wang, 1984). In this approach, the individual is taught to use alternative expressions of anger that are more socially sanctioned. The ability to increase assertiveness or correctly expressed opposition would fall in this category. However, the overall effort can be seen more broadly. Replacement and development of more pro-social behaviors can be developed to offset and stand in contrast to the aggressive behaviors. Crewe (1980) and Hollon (1973) used the reinforcement of positive behaviors and the extinction or non-response to angry/agitated behaviors with brain-injured patients. This approach known as Differential Reinforcement of Other behaviors (DRO) (Reeve, 1992) is a positive reinforcement strategy that stands in contrast to aversive methods of control. Theoretically, the development and attention to positive actions displace aggressive responses and strengthen the person's behavioral repertoire. With the increase of behavioral repertoire, the person is able to gain need satisfaction without the reliance on anger or aggression. With this approach, the staff will reinforce those behaviors that occur which are positive during the nonaggressive periods. The corollary effect is to extinguish aggressive or angry expressions. Within the scope of appropriate risk management, the non-response to aggressive acts would employ an extinguishing effect while promoting the pro-social choice.

Staff coordination and staff culture are very important in that all are to be dedicated to changing and expanding the repertoire of the person's behaviors. This stands in contrast to a staff that wants to just stop unacceptable aggressive behaviors.

Another related approach is that of Differential Reinforcement of Incompatible (DRI) behaviors. This approach focuses on building a repertoire of behaviors that targets and reinforces behaviors which are in opposition to the behavior to be eliminated. The staff would knowingly reinforce behaviors that are incompatible with aggression. They would reward the person during quiet times, or they would reinforce the person during friendly, calm, or appropriate social transactions. The staff would reinforce behaviors that meet need satisfaction through the expression of behaviors incompatible with aggression.

Protocols that rely on contingency systems are also appropriate as a more advanced approach. This approach requires the person's active participation, whereas the DRO and DRI schedules may be employed with a more passively involved patient. Through rewards, as in use of tokens or merits, the individual learns to inhibit unacceptable behaviors. This approach is commonly seen in token economies and can be modified to the reinforcement schedule desired. It is important to have a clear understanding of the person's need satisfaction profile so as to match contingencies to the individual case.

There are points of caution when employing contingency systems. With the brain-injured population, there has been some success, but the nature of the reward and token system needs consideration. The token system cannot be too abstract and must resemble, as much as possible, natural tokens. The more abstract tokens lose relevance with the person. Also, the agreed-upon reward has to be modified in light of the person's reduced self-appraisal skills and reduced cognition. A reward must be agreed upon that is realistic and risk manageable. Furthermore, the contingency schedule must not be so elaborate as to be defeated by the person's cognitive status.

The strategy to develop more socially acceptable behaviors will relate to our developmental strategies reviewed later. The increase of pro-social behaviors is the more encompassing solution to training the person to manage their own aggression. These substitution and replacement strategies need to be directed toward not only the targeted behavior but the precursors and pre-violence behaviors that tell of the upcoming aggression.

DEVELOPMENTAL AND PRO-SOCIALIZATION MODEL

As Gardner (1982) states,

Because excessive aggressiveness is a serious problem within our society, and perhaps across cultures, the roots of this behavior have been of particular interest to psychologists. While scholars claim that a tendency to aggressiveness is innate, and perhaps uncontrollable, many have a more optimistic view, feeling that aggression is neither necessary nor inevitable. The fact that aggressiveness is not noticeable in every individual and differs widely from one society to another at least holds open the possibility that it can be better understood and, possibly, better controlled.

The sociocultural approach to aggression has focused upon those forces that seem to either promote or prohibit aggressive behavior, particularly in children. In a seminal document, Sears, Maccoby, and Levin (1957) studied childrearing techniques and their effects upon behavior. They found that parents who were "permissive" (i.e., who tolerated aggressive acts in their children, yet who responded punitively when their tolerance was exceeded) tended to produce the most aggressive children. In contradiction to expectations, the more punitive the parent, the more aggressive the child. The combination of childrearing practices yielding the least aggressive children was low permissiveness and low punitiveness. Parents who are opposites in both their permissiveness and their punitiveness (Groups 2 and 3 in Table 23.3) have children who are similar in their aggressiveness.

Table 23.3: The Relationship between Punitiveness and Aggressiveness in Children (from Sears, MacCoby, & Levin, 1957)

	HIGH PUNITIVENESS	**LOW PUNITIVENESS**
HIGH PERMISSIVENESS	most aggressive aggressive children (Group 1)	moderately aggressive children (Group 2)
LOW PERMISSIVENESS	moderately aggressive children (Group 3)	least aggressive children (Group 4)

Further analysis of the data revealed that parents displayed other characteristics that appeared to contribute to aggressive behaviors in their children. These parents were highly anxious about childrearing, had low self-esteem, and were dissatisfied with their current situation. The parents disagreed about their methods of childrearing. In contrast, Becker (1964) described those parents whose children did not become aggressive. Their disciplinary techniques were love-oriented and featured much praise and punishing by withdrawal of love.

Although the dynamics of the parent-child situation are complex, there is much to be learned from these studies that is relevant for brain-injury rehabilitation. First, optimal rehabilitation (particularly for aggressive behavior) should take place within a specified culture or milieu. Secondly, the constant therapeutic influence of staff must recapitulate that of parents who produce nonaggressive children; staff must be seen as caring and warm, confident about their techniques, reasonably high in self-esteem, and satisfied with their work situation. Third, these values must be inculcated throughout the entire therapeutic community; the struggles of two parents to openly communicate their values and style of childrearing increase exponentially when there are dozens of staff persons. Frequent training, modeling of appropriate interactions, and review of staff roles in all episodes of aggressive behavior become hallmarks of the successful program. The cultural influences involved in successful rehabilitation are as important as those involved in successful childrearing (if equally elusive).

Over the last four years, the authors have investigated the treatment of aggressive patients in a less restrictive community re-entry program. At the outset, this approach intuitively would have benefit to the patient by providing opportunity to live and prosper in a non-institutional setting. Furthermore, the clinician would benefit from the ability to see this patient in "real life" settings and determine the ultimate recovery of the person in his/her ability to live in mainstream society. Family members would also prosper in their ability to see their loved one in a non-institutional setting and be able to enjoy their time with their family member outside of a confined environment.

In a practical sense, the question as to whether the aggressive patient can live outside of a restrictive environment was approached by employing many of the already reviewed techniques in combination. We were able to establish a treatment team that did successfully combine neuropsychiatric expertise with neuropsychologists, mental health professionals, and behavior modification experts. We were able to experience case-by-case examples of successful recovery of patients in some of the most important ways. Not only did these patients successfully meet the test of symptom reduction recovery, but these patients also were able to meet a more extensive goal of making a long-term difference in the outcomes with macro-systems of their life. These patients were not only able to reduce their aggression but improve their housing and family relationships, improve their productivity, reduce their attendant care needs and participate in larger social systems.

When we examined how we were able to accomplish these clinical successes, we recognized the role of a pro-socialization culture as a keystone to the treatment milieu. We have identified several features that we believe have made it possible for us to be successful with aggressive patients in the least restrictive environment.

First, we recognize the positive influence that community membership has on conduct. The open corrective feedback and open demonstration of behaviors in a community that responds in a corrective fashion cannot be underestimated. The emphasis on placing people in group activities and encouraging, even insisting upon, group membership and group participation has been important. Furthermore, the public display and its palliative effect on behavior seems to be a natural modifier.

Probably of most importance are the cultural characteristics of the staff and care givers within the treatment community. In review of the developmental literature regarding the nature of families and parents who promote the development of nonaggressive parents, we found many similarities among our staff members and these parenting models. Inherent in our model emerged the need for proper risk-assessment systems and corrective influences characteristic of each staff member.

Our alternative system of approach is to promote a truly "milieu" strategy and employ the socio-cultural approach to aggression in combination with the use of pharmacology and behavioral treatments. Based in developmental psychology, Sears, Maccoby, and Levin (1957), as stated previously, studied childrearing techniques and their relationship to the development of an aggressive off-spring. They found that parents who were "permissive" tended to produce aggressive children. The system surrounding the brain-injured person and the conduct and tolerances of the care givers thus takes on a new view. The systemic features of the care system that "grow" angry patients has been important in our work of managing aggressive behaviors in an open community setting. The inculturation of staff and the attitudes systemically expressed during the delivery of care become very important. The work of Sears et al. speaks of the need to train clear boundaries for acceptable behaviors within a given community.

The nature of the care giving system may have a palliative influence in the development of pro-social behaviors with the patients and their use of aggression. Least permissive/nonpunitive parents have least aggressive children. Contingencies and need for positive reinforcers may find clear applicability within this scope of thinking.

Other characteristics were also found to be related to the least aggressive patients. These patients were not unduly anxious about their roles with the staff. Staff persons had confidence in their skills and were satisfied with their roles with the patients. These two points speak to the need of a care team that is supported, prepared, and not anxious or doubtful of their roles. Sears et al. also found that parents with aggressive children expressed conflict over rearing practices. Within a care team, consensus of a coordination of approach should be supported by agreement in how the patient should be approached. Becker (1964) found that least aggressive children were raised by positive reinforcing parents with "love-oriented" disciplinary techniques.

Treating aggression within an open community may be possible by looking at the features of the care system as it replicates parenting features that contribute to the rearing of least aggressive children. Although the dynamics of the parent-child situation are complex and not unlike the patient-clinician relationship, there is much to be learned from these studies that focus on the features of those caring for the aggressive brain-injured patient. There can be value in a team approach which recapitulates that of parents who produce nonaggressive children; staff must be seen as caring and warm, confident about their techniques, reasonably high in self esteem, and satisfied with their work situation. These values must permeate the entire therapeutic community. Staff must be thoroughly trained, model appropriate interactions for patients, and review staff roles in all episodes of aggressive behavior.

We were left to conclude that our clinical success was due to the combined use of technology, medicine, psychology, and sociology (Table 23.4). We were able to combine the corrective influences of appropriate pharmacology with corrective forces of behavior modification, while enveloping all these strategies within a treatment milieu that is enculturated to promote a pro-socialization of the patient and to encourage that patient's group and community membership as the instrument to gain long-term need satisfaction.

Table 23.4: Complementary Relationship of Tripartite Model

Technical Domain	Neurology	Psychology	Sociology
Goal	Acute management with imminent danger	Restore complex cognitive skills	Group member skills
	Restore chemical integrity	Social discourse training	Role development
	Prepare individual as learner	Transactional cognitive remediation	Develop codes of conduct
		Emotional management skills	Social identity

Establishing the cultural, pro-socialization influences for nonaggression may be the hallmark of the successful program that will employ all the positive findings reviewed in pharmacology and behavior modification, in addition to the staff's conscious role of their own conduct's influence on patient aggression. Addressing aggression and all of the major personality alterations after brain injury is complex and requires resources (O'Shanick, 1994). Through the inclusive approach that we have employed, we have experienced its positive effects on patient care and on team building.

REFERENCES

Adam, D.B. (1986). Ventromedial tegmental lesions abolish offense without disturbing predation or defense. *Physiological &Behavior, 38,* 165–168.

Balasubramaniam, V., & Kanaka, T.S. (1976). Hypothalamotomy in the management of aggressive behavior. In T.P. Morley (Ed.), *Current controversies in neurosurgery.* Philadelphia: Saunders.

Bandura, A. (1969). *Principles of behavior modification.* New York: Holt, Rinehart and Winston.

Bard, P. (1928). A diencephalic mechanism for the expression of rage with special reference to the sympathetic nervous system. *American Journal of Physiology, 84,* 490–515.

Brady, J.V., & Naura, W.J.H. (1953). Subcortical mechanisms in emotional behavior: Affective changes following septal forebrain lesion in albino rat. *Journal of Comparative and Physiological Psychology, 46,* 339–346.

Brown, B.H. (1973). Further experience with multiple limbic targets for schizophrenia and aggression. In L. Laitinen & K.E. Livingston (Eds.), *Surgical approaches in psychiatry.* Baltimore: University Park Press.

Coleman, J.C., Butcher, J.N., & Carson, R.C. (1980). *Abnormal psychology and modern life* (6th ed.). New York: Scott, Foresman and Company.

Delgado, J.M.R. (1969). *Physical control of mind.* New York: Harper & Row.

Edwards, S.B., & Flynn, J.P. (1972). Corticospinal control of striking in centrally elicited attack behavior. *Brain Research, 41,* 51–65.

Eichelman, B. (1987). Neurochemical and psychopharmacologic aspects of aggressive behavior. In H.Y. Meltzer (Ed.), Psycholopharmacology: The third generation of progress (pp. 697–704). New York: Raven Press.

Fahy, T.J., Irving, M.H., & Millac, P. (1967, September 2). Severe head injuries: A six-year follow-up. *The Lancet,* 475–479.

Freihar, J.P., & Alvarez, W.A. (1986). Clonazepam treatment of organic brain syndromes in three elderly patients. *J. Clin. Psychiatry, 47,* 525–526.

Galluscio, E.H. (1990). *Biological psychology.* New York: Macmillan.

Gardner, H. (1982). *Developmental psychology* (2nd ed.). Boston: Little, Brown, & Co.

Garyfallos, G., Manos, N., & Adamopoulou, A. (1988). Psychopathology and personality characteristics of epileptic patients: Epilepsy, psychopathology and personality. *Acta Psychiatry Scand., 78,* 87–95.

Gengo, F.M., Fagan, S.C., de Padova, A., et al. (1988). The effect of B-blockers on mental performance in older hypertensive patients. *Arch. Intern. Med., 148,* 779–784.

Grossman, R., Beyer, C., Kelly, P., et al. (1975). Acetylcholine and related enzymes in human ventricular and subarachnoid fluids following brain injury. *Proceedings of the 5th Annual Meeting for Neuroscience, 76*(3), 506.

Gualtieri, C.T. (1991). Buspirone: neuropsychiatric effects. *Journal of Head Trauma Rehabilitation, 6,* 90–92.

———. Buspirone for the behavior problems of patients with organic brain disorders. *J. Clin. Psychopharmacology, 11,* 280–281.

Harlow, J. M. (1868). Recovery from the passage of an iron bar through the head. *Publ. Mass. Med. Soc., 2,* 327.

Heinrichs, R.W. (1989). Frontal cerebral lesions and violent incidents in chronic neuropsychiatric patients. *Biol. Psychiatry, 25,*174–178.

Hess, W.R. (1957). *The functional organization of the diencephalon.* New York: Grune and Stratton.

Hornstein, A., & Seliger, G. (1989). Cognitive side effects of lithium in closed head injury (letter). *J. Neuropsychiatry Clin. Neurosci., 1,* 446–447.

Jacobs, Harvey E. (1993). Behavior analysis guidelines and brain injury rehabilitation: People, principles, and programs. Gaithersburg, MD: Aspen Publishers.

Kendel, E.R., Schwartz, J.H., & Jessel, T.M. (1994). Principles of neural science (3rd ed.). Norwalk, CN: Appleton & Lange.

Kruesi, M.J.P., Hibbs, E.D., Zahn, T.P., et al. (1992). A 2-year prospective follow-up study of children and adolescents with disruptive behavior disorders: Prediction by cerebrospinal fluid 5-hydroxyindoleacetic acid, homovanillic acid, and autonomic measures. *Arch. Gen. Psychiatry, 49*, 429–435.

Levin, H.S., Benton, A.L., & Grossman, R.G. (1983). *Neurobehavioral consequences of closed head injury.* New York: Oxford University Press.

Lezak, M.D. (1978). Living with the characterologically altered brain-injured patient. *Journal of Clinical Psychiatry, 39*, 592–598.

Linnoila, V.M.I., & Virkkunen, M. (1992). Aggression, suicidality, and serotonin. *J. Clin. Psychiatry, 53* (Suppl. 10), 46–51.

Luria, A.R. (1966). *Higher cortical functions in man.* New York: Basic Books.

Moskowitz, A.S., & Altshuler, L. (1991). Increased sensitivity to lithium-induced neurotoxicity after stroke: A case report. *J. Clin. Psychopharmacology, 11*, 272–273.

Murray, H.A. (1938). *Explorations in personality.* New York: Oxford University Press.

Mysiw, W.J., Jackson, R.D., & Corrigan, J.D. (1988). Amitriptylin for post-traumatic agitation. *Am. J. Phys. Med. Rehabil., 67*, 29–33.

O'Shanick, G.J., & O'Shanick, A.M. (1994). Personality and intellectual changes. In J.M. Silver, S.C. Yudofsky, & R.E. Hales (Eds.), *Neuropsychiatry of traumatic brain injury.* Washington, DC: American Psychiatric Press.

Panksepp, J. (1986). The neurochemistry of behavior. *Annual Review of Psychology, 37*, 77–107.

Prigatano, G.P. (1986). *Neuropsychological rehabilitation after brain injury.* Baltimore, MD: The Johns Hopkins University Press.

Prigatano, G.P., & Schacter, D.L. (1991). *Awareness of deficit after brain injury.* Oxford, New York: Oxford University Press.

Ratey, J.J., Leveroni, C., Kilmer, D., et al. (1992). The effects of clozapine on severely aggressive psychiatric inpatients: A double-blind, placebo controlled study. *J. Clin. Psychiatry, 53*, 41–46.

———. (1993). The effects of clozapine on severely aggressive psychiatric inpatients in a state hospital. *J. Clin. Psychiatry, 54*, 219–223.

Reeve, J.M. (1992). *Understanding motivation and emotion.* New York: Harcourt Brace Jovanovich.

Rosenthal, M., Griffith, E., Bond, M., & Miller, J.D. (Eds.). (1983). *Rehabilitation of the brain injured adult.* Philadelphia: F.A. Davis.

Sears, R. R., Maccoby, E. E., & Levin, H. (1957). *Patterns of child rearing.* Evanston, IL: Row Peterson.

Silver, J.M., Yudofsky, R.H., & Hales, R.E. (1994). *Neuropsychiatry of traumatic brain injury.* Washington, DC: American Psychiatry Press.

Stuss, D.T., & Benson, D.F. (1986). *The frontal lobes.* New York: Raven Press.

Tonkonogy, T.M. (1991). Violence and temporal lobes lesion: Head CT and MRI data. *Journal of Neuropsychiatry and Clinical Neuroscience, 3*, 189–196.

Weigner, W.A., & Bear, D.M. (1988). An approach to the neurology of aggression. *Journal of Psychiatric Research, 22*, 85–98.

Wilson, E.O. (1975). *Sociobiology: The new synthesis* (Chaps. 11 and 13). Cambridge, MA: Harvard University Press.

Zubieta, J.K., & Alessi, N.E. (1992). Acute and chronic administration of trazodone in the treatment of disruptive behavior disorders in children. *J. Clin. Psychopharmacology, 12*, 346–351.

24 Training for Social Skills after Brain Injury

F. Machuca,[1] J.M. Martín Carrasco,[2] A. Martín González,[2] R. Rodríguez-Duarte,[1] and J. León-Carrión[1]

[1]Laboratorio de Neuropsicología Humana, Facultad de Psicología, Universidad de Seville, Seville, Spain
[2]Facultad de Psicología, Universidad Autónoma de Madrid, Spain

INTRODUCTION

The concept of social skills is not a new one, although applying it to patients surviving traumatic brain injury (TBI) is. One of the problems which most bothers the families and the rehabilitators of persons who have suffered brain injury is the problem of the patient having to return to daily life routines. From that moment on, the patient has to face demands that require efficient skills in social relations. It is no longer enough that the life of the patient be saved; now, all resources—medical, psychological, and social— have to be mustered with the aim of having patients live a normal life, even though this may not mean that they will be able to return to the life they had before the trauma. There is a concern, on the part of patients' relatives, that patients reach an adequate level of social activity. This interest is motivated by three fundamental factors: (1) by the young age of patients who suffer TBI, (2) by the increase in general quality of life and social welfare, and (3) by the technical and professional advances achieved. The rehabilitator's aim will center fundamentally on providing the patients with the skills necessary so that they can obtain the resources of their environment without being penalized for it and without an excessive use of energy. Not all patients are in a position to achieve this goal. Some of them had few social skills before the brain trauma occurred; others will have lost them or have seen them deteriorate after the trauma. Therefore, any type of integral treatment of persons with brain injury will have to take into account the proper moment to train the patient in social skills.

General neuropsychological rehabilitation should begin as soon as possible, and it would be convenient not to wait any longer than absolutely necessary after the patient has been discharged from the ICU to start the rehabilitation process.

It is not a case of reinserting patients back into society; it is a case of having patients return to social life in an effective manner, easily, and with the personal resources so that they can face, without additional costs, personal and social demands and needs. For some authors such as Ellis, Spivack, and Spettell (1994), Groswasser (1994), and Conder (1989), the return of patients to a work routine adapted to their capabilities is the best indicator of optimum results within the integral process of rehabilitation. The return to the work duties or study routine implies a recovery of cognitive capabilities, of the emotional state, and fundamentally of the patient's social skills. These authors have shown that the securing and keeping of an adequate work position is the most objective sign, among the patients themselves, of the success of the rehabilitation process. Nevertheless, one should not confuse the return to a work routine with the recovery of social skills.

According to León-Carrión (1994), enabling this type of patient to function has as its objective reaching the highest degree of personal and social autonomy and independence. This may be determined by three variables: the magnitude of the injury, the type of rehabilitation program, and the duration of time the latter was applied. Long periods of rehabilitation (4–5 months with minimal daily sessions of 5–6 hours) are adequate only for those patients who need them (i.e., for those who start out with a very low functioning level at the time of their admission in the rehabilitation program). Generally speaking, this type of program has better clinical results than less intense programs—2 to 3 hours per day—and for a shorter duration of time (less than 3 months). A greater intensity of the treatment increases the cognitive capacity of the subject. The main problem with long and intensive rehabilitation programs is their high costs (see Ellis, Spivack & Spettell, 1994).

The beginnings of training in social skills in psychology can be found in the work of Jack (1934) and Williams (1935). However, Wolpe (1958) was the first to use the concept of assertiveness in his book, *Psychotherapy by Reciprocal Inhibition*. Since then, many terms have been coined in attempting to define and conceptualize the list of capabilities that individuals call upon in their interactions with others. There are different names for the purpose of defining related concepts: personal competence, emotional freedom (Lazarus, 1971); personal effectiveness (Liebermann et al., 1975); social competence (Zeigler & Phillips, 1960); assertive behavior (Wolpe, 1958); and social skills. But the latter two are the ones most used in current psychology. The majority of patients who have suffered brain injury are involved in problems related to these types of skills.

Assertiveness and social skills have been, for some time, very closed concepts, and even today, they are used frequently and even indiscriminately. However, due to the confusion often created between assertiveness and aggressiveness, the term "social skills" has gained importance. The expression "assertiveness" has come to form part of those skills related to social skills, with the meaning of the collection of behaviors directed toward stressing protection or the development of personal rights and peculiarities and the control of related situations. The patients who are in the process of neuropsychological rehabilitation have to face situations such as defending their rights when the latter are in danger of being infringed; they have to learn to control their aggressiveness, which, in most cases, has a negative impact on social relationships.

With many of the current definitions of social skills, instrumental value appears as the relevant aspect. They are defined in this manner because of the help they provide in the adaptive order for the individual and for the benefits that can be obtained and preserved from their practice. Social skills are those kinds of behaviors that allow the subject to achieve what he/she needs and wishes without penalization. On the other hand, we should stress, from the general rehabilitation viewpoint of persons with brain damage, the importance of the role played by skillful social behavior in maintaining self-esteem. In neuropsychological rehabilitation, self-esteem plays a fundamental role since, for these patients, the better they are cognitively, the more they are aware of how poor their condition is after the trauma. This results in an emotional down, for which reason, if we set aside the rehabilitation of the emotional and affective aspects in the rehabilitation program, some of these patients may even engage in suicidal behavior (see Chapter 22).

CONCEPTUAL AND OPERATIONAL DEFINITIONS

For some authors, it is very difficult to try to present a concept of social skill. For Meichenbaum, Butler, and Grudson (1981), it is impossible to define socially skillful behavior because it is partially dependent on the situation in which it develops. Adopting this assumption, it is not difficult to imagine the problems generated in the attempt to find a clear definition and build a psychological model of social skills. Nevertheless, we can understand in a comprehensive manner that "the socially skillful behavior is that set of behaviors performed by an individual in an interpersonal context which expresses the feelings, attitudes, desires, opinions, or rights of this individual in a manner adequate to the situation in which he finds himself, while respecting the behaviors of the others, and which generally resolves the immediate problems of the situation while at the same time minimizing the probability of future problems" (Caballo, 1988) (i.e., effectively using the available resources in order to achieve the desired goal with the least possible penalization).

Socially skillful behavior, at times also known as "assertive behavior," is understood as the expression of interpersonal communication acquired in a learning process in which one considers the goal that the individual wishes to reach in the communication or interrelation situation. Adapting the characteristics given by Alberti (1977) to persons with brain damage, social skill

1. is a trait of behavior, not of the person.
2. is a trait specifically of the person and of the situation, not a universal characteristic.
3. must be considered within the cultural context of the individual, as well as in terms of other situational variables.
4. is based on the individual's ability to choose freely his course of action.
5. is a trait of effective social behavior, not a damaging one.

In the neuropsychological rehabilitation design, we should establish objectives that the patients must achieve. The aim is that brain injury patients achieve an assertive or socially skillful behavior such as the skill to

1. start, maintain, and finish a conversation.
2. express himself/herself negatively when it is pertinent to do so.
3. receive affirmatively criticism from other people.
4. withstand interruptions.
5. express and receive appreciation, love, praise, and affection.
6. receive fair treatment as a consumer.
7. ask others for favors.
8. defend one's own rights.

9. assume the responsibility to initiate action when responding to a personal desire or feeling.
10. act upon the physical and human environment in a manner that will achieve the adequate social reinforcement.
11. speak in public.
12. carry out a job interview.

With all these skills, the ability to communicate with others plays a fundamental role. It is very common that patients exhibit communication and speech problems (e.g., there are times they will not be able to speak and express what they want [motor aphasia] and other times they will not understand what they are being told [sensory aphasia]). This generally happens when the lesion occurs in the left side of the brain. In the course of interpersonal communication, a series of information transmission processes take place from one person to another or between more than two persons, during which one or several of the following functions take place—to inform, to order or instruct, to persuade, and to express or evoke.

Obviously in patients with brain damage, the effectiveness of the specific program in social skills training will depend on their cognitive functioning. This implies that the moment when patients have access to this type of program is conditioned by their progress in the other components of the program. It is important to stress this point because in the interpersonal communication process, the emotional and affective, cognitive, social, and contextual factors are implicated. In this process, due to the circumstances derived from the brain injury, a series of problems or "noises" could be produced that would prevent the messages of the communication from reaching the receptor in the same terms in which the transmitter wanted. One of the main communication obstacles is related to suspicion or paranoia, which usually appears as a sequela in this type of patient after brain injury. Some TBI patients are often very excitable because they think that the majority of things that take place around them do not take place naturally; they believe that there is someone who is manipulating them so that they function the way they do; they believe that everything has something to do with them. This makes living with these patients difficult because they always think that everything someone says or does has to do with them to the point that they see provocations where there are none. This type of perception seriously limits everything that is related to their social skills. Within the family, the patient may be understood and tolerated but probably such will not be the case with co-workers or with other people.

The most clear examples of distortive communication are those that take place during the so called "shared monologs" or "nonsense dialogs" in which at least two persons send each other messages without taking into account the information that each one of them is receiving from the other. The information that the source had the intention of sending does not always come through in the communication. In the communication game, a series of behaviors are carried out in order to have the message reach the other person. These behavior patterns may or may not be appropriate for either the person who sends the message or the person who receives the message.

The person is involved daily in multiple social interaction systems. In each one of them, he/she carries out roles adequate to and determined by socially established rules. The factors that intervene in the expression of social skills could be categorized as *cultural* (age, sex, social class, education), *individual* (attitudes, values, beliefs, interpersonal style, cognitive capability), *situational* (goals and purposes, social roles of the interacting parties, basic behavior repetoire, sequence of behavioral elements) and are ones that are consistent to the behavior.

We consider behavior effective when its consequence is the achievement of personal goals that are socially accepted and that maximize the reinforcement for all those subjects involved. Based on the above, we could point out four types of nonproductive behavior that would necessitate resorting to training in social skills and which should be avoided in the training of patients who have suffered brain injury:

1. *Inactivity*. Faced with a stimulus or situation which requires some sort of action, the individual remains still. At times, the person does things that have little or nothing to do with the solution to the situation, or behaviors are not an adequate response to the initial stimulus. Some patients, at certain moments of recovery, become apathetic, indifferent, and depressive. This happens mainly with those patients who have suffered injury to the right orbito-frontal zone, in the left frontal lobe, or in the basal ganglia (León-Carrión, 1994).

2. *Overadaptation*. This happens in situations when the person does not act in accordance with his/her own goals but rather in accordance with what he/she thinks are the goals and wishes of others.

3. *Anxiety*. This occurs when the behavior patterns consist of stereotyped, repetitive, or uncontrolled activities that have nothing to do with solving the problem or controlling the aim of the situation. It is possible that anxiety is a very frequent state observed in all those patients who have suffered from TBI. This usually happens once they start to recover their cognitive capabilities; at times, these patients behave as if manifesting the disorders of a post-stress situation. This state of anxiety could cause them to avoid things and situations or cause them a restlessness that keeps them tense most of the time (León-Carrión, 1994).

4. *Aggressiveness*. Violent behavior may follow the anxiety phase. In this sense, the stored and unchanneled energy from the previous phases is commonly discharged through some sort of aggressive act. Some patients become irritable, irascible, and aggressive. This is observed especially among those patients with injury in the temporal lobe, especially in the frontal one. They have a low tolerance for frustration, and when confronted with any type of obstacle, they respond with violent or poorly structured behavior. This also usually happens when the cognitive functioning or the patient's intellectual state is also deteriorated. Suspiciousness, paranoid ideation, anxiety, or a state of agitation influence in equal manner this aggressiveness (see Chapter 23). In this case, we try to bring together the affective component with the cognitive one. Ellis (1975) maintains that, frequently, the more rationally people think, the greater are the chances that they will act assertively. We could say that the ideology of assertive behavior bases itself in a collection of rational, realistic, and logical beliefs, which support or have as their basis a set of basic personal rights that serve to avoid being manipulated by others. But it is not easy for a person who has survived TBI to be rational, realistic, and logical, although it is not impossible either.

Other behavioral aspects of social skills should be noted. We have indicated that communication becomes evident through people's behavior. Within this behavior, we include both verbal and nonverbal behavior. We use verbal behavior to express ideas, make requests, inform, express feelings, reason about things, ask questions, etc. In this sense, we must not forget the possible obstacles or noises that might appear during the transmission of a verbal message. The nonverbal behavior in communication includes other dimensions: facial expression, gaze, posture, gestures, the spacial proximity between the interlocutors, physical contact, the tone, volume and speed of speech, personal appearance, etc. Some authors state that in communication, over 50% of the information reaches the receptor at a nonverbal level and, to a greater extent, at a visual level. All these aspects have to be considered in the training of persons with brain injury. Verbal, nonverbal, and visual behavior must be reinforced with these patients.

TRAINING IN SPECIFIC SOCIAL SKILLS

The sub-program in social skills training for patients surviving brain injury that follows an integrated neuropsychological rehabilitation program consists of, in its total development, the following four elements:

1. *A training process in social skills for specific behaviors.* These have to be integrated in the behavioral repertory of the person according to the "Theory of Social Learning," which explains the learning processes through direct observation, instructions, modeling, role-playing, feedback, and reinforcement. As a starting point, we will refer to the influence of vicarious learning in our behavior: the observer acquires a behavior which he/she had not exhibited before as a result of his/her being exposed to a model. The rehabilitator should adapt as much as possible to the characteristics of the patient with whom he/she is going to work. The results that the model may obtain from the behavior he/she projects may function vicariously for the observer, increasing the probability that the patient will produce a similar behavior.

   The acquisition of social skills would also take place by means of direct teaching or through verbal instructions, during which the subject acquires reinforcements, and cognitive expectations intervene as a consequence of the reinforcements or of the self-effectiveness. Role-playing in different situations could cause the effect of generalizing the skills acquired by means of the previously described mechanisms. This entire process of acquisition/generalization of behavior goes along with the development of reactive organic systems and with the cognitive capabilities of the individual. Basically, the inappropriate execution or nonexecution of social adaptive behavior could be explained by personal, behavioral, and situational factors. In these patients, the explanation could rather be found in the lack of cognitive skills to enable them to encode and decode adequately all the relevant information that comes into play in any interaction, be it due to psychological disorders, which raise the level of anxiety and cause perceptual errors or slants, or to coma, or to deterioration of the motor order.

2. *An anxiety reduction process in socially problematic situations.* Normally a decrease in anxiety is achieved in an indirect manner (i.e., by carrying out the more adaptive behavior that supposedly is incompatible with the anxiety response). If the anxiety level is very high, a progressive relaxation technique could be used that would achieve a desensitization to the problem situation. For those patients who remain tense most of the day, it is appropriate that the family try to create a peaceful and quiet environment. At times, it is very relaxing and calming for patients to speak about those topics that will reduce their anguish without being repetitive. We must avoid having patients take advantage of the family's availability and spend all their time in an obsessive manner asking about the same

things. In addition to the relaxation sessions, relaxing baths and soft music are helpful for survivors of TBI.

3. *A cognitive restructuring process for the modification of values, beliefs, manner of thinking, and attitudes.* Frequently cognitive restructuring is carried out in an indirect manner in the same way as with anxiety; however, with this type of patient, the rehabilitation of cognitive functions becomes a priority goal. The most adequate rehabilitation in TBI is the one that is integrated in which we are simultaneously working on the cognitive, behavioral, and emotional deficits of the patient, always starting the rehabilitation process from those functions that are in the best shape. As subjects improve in their cognitive rehabilitation, more beneficial social behaviors and skills will be added to their psychological activity, which consequently will strengthen new cognitive processes and stabilize emotional difficulties.

4. *A training process for problem solving.* Research has been done on the development of the ability to solve problems. Much of it claims that practice in problem solving causes changes in the organization of the cognitive processes at different levels of complexity (Anderson, 1983). These changes seem to indicate modifications in the use of working memory during the problem-solving process. Caralson, Khos, and Yaure (1990) studied the ability to solve problems at three different organizational levels: strategy, sub-objectives, and operators at the same time that they investigated time storage, the manipulation of information, and the coordination of multiple representations. Their studies demonstrated the following:

    a. The different measures of problem solving show that there is a quick initial improvement of skills, but that there is relatively small benefit with continued practice. This suggests that learning occurs both at the strategy level as well as at the operative level.

    b. The effects of practice can be noticed especially in the inference that is made and in the selection of operations to minimize the cost of the process.

    c. Practice reduces the interference in the passive storage chores more than the interference of chores that require an active manipulation of information. The cost of integrating the exposed and integrated information in solving problems declines with practice but remains essential even with high practice levels.

    d. Transfer to new circuits after a moderate amount of practice is important but not perfect, since there is a distinction between the learning that produces speed and the strategic restructuring in order to achieve the goals desired.

One could say that the acquisition of skills for the solution of problems is a process that develops through experience and practical activity. These are the two factors that are going to condition the entire process including, obviously, in the experience and practical activity, cultural and contextual aspects.

Luria (1969) indicated that the very mild frontal syndrome can provide an idea of the importance of the frontal lobe in the solving of problems. Generally speaking, such people are characterized by:

1. A disintegration of the systematic program used to solve problems. They carry out the operation in an isolated and uncontrolled manner and from fragments that are also isolated and separated from their contexts.
2. They are unable to inhibit fragmentary and premature reactions. They exhibit uncontrolled responses at different stages of the problem, and the analysis and synthesis of the problem, which constitute the orientation basis for any type of intellectual activity, disappear.
3. They exhibit a current of inertia and lack of activity.

An interesting study conducted by Cox and Ostby (1989) on social problem-solving skills in survivors of a brain injury shows that the skills in resolving social problems are correlated with categorization, sequencing, neural control, and intelligence, as well as with behavioral security and communication measures. Since not all TBI patients exhibit the same types of deficits, Table 24.1 shows a series of behavioral characteristics found in different frontal syndromes that will have a negative influence on the social habits of these patients and which, as a function of them, will greatly influence the rehabilitation process (see also Chapter 15).

Table 24.1: Essential Behavioral Characteristics of Frontal Syndromes (from León-Carrión, 1995)

LESION	BEHAVIORAL CHARACTERISTICS
Frontal orbital syndrome	a. Disinhibition b. Pseudopsychopathic or manic type syndrome c. Affective disorders
Frontal dorso-lateral syndrome (unilateral or bilateral)	a. Apathy b. Pseudodepression c. Dysphasia (left hemisphere lesion) d. Aprosody (right hemisphere lesion)
Frontomedial syndrome	a. Behavioral initation deficits b. Difficulties starting or becoming active in any type of physical activity c. Apathy, akinesia, mutism
Frontoparietal syndrome	a. De-automatizacion of movements b. Motor deficits c. Sensory deficits
Frontotemporal syndrome	a. Aphasias b. Deficits in understanding words c. Serious verbal deficits d. Motor deficits
Frontodiencephalic syndrome	a. Serious awareness disorders b. Mnemonic deficits c. Time-space disorientation

To conclude, with social skills training, patients should try to obtain the following personal resources:
1. The development of a system of beliefs that will result in their respecting the rights of others as well as their own.
2. The ability to distinguish assertive, passive, and aggressive behavior.
3. The cognitive restructuring of the manner of thinking in concrete situations.
4. The practice of assertive responses.

THE DESIGN OF THE TRAINING PROGRAM IN SOCIAL SKILLS IN PATIENTS WITH TBI

As is the case at the beginning of the training sessions, it is indispensable to evaluate in which social skills areas it is necessary to intervene or in which of them the subject finds the most difficulty resolving. Once these situations have been discovered, training may continue so that patients may anticipate and discriminate problematic social situations in order to optimize decisions regarding how and when to apply the learned skills. This training consists of discussing the nature of the situations (implicit norms, roles to carry out, verbal codes to be used, and appropriate tone of voice for the conversation to be held) and the structure of the goal the subject is after. It is recommended that the social skills program not be done in isolation, and, therefore, should be integrated into a general neuropsychological rehabilitation program.

General considerations in the training of patients are as follows:

1. The training should focus on patients' individual strengths so as to compensate deficits and avoid weaknesses.
2. The training should focus on the tasks as well as on the learning process.
3. The training may include strategies based on computers and tutors.
4. The frequency of sessions should be sufficient so that there is not a detriment in the execution from session to session. It is advisable that at least three sessions per week be carried out, to include daily exercises with relatives.
5. Priority should be given to those skills necessary in order to be able to give and receive social support.
6. The most effective training is that which is accompanied by cognitive and affective techniques.
7. The training carries with it a decrease of anxiety and the development of the cognitive skills.

Fundamentally, the rehabilitation is based on those social aspects in which the individual performs best or which are least deteriorated, so that from that point, we may compensate those deficits associated with the brain injury the patient has suffered.

PROCEDURE PHASES OF THE NEUROPSYCHOLOGICAL REHABILITATION PROGRAM IN SOCIAL SKILLS

Before proceeding to the phase in the program of the rehabilitation of social skills, other program phases should be completed that facilitate some minimal aspects or requirements in order to be able to have access and be successful in the rehabilitation program in social skills.

Phase I: Evaluation of Social Competence

Due to the characteristics of patients with TBI, neuropsychologists are going to find, when they reach the rehabilitation of social skills phase, persons who present multiple deficits at the psychophysiologic level, as well as at the cognitive and behavioral levels. These considerations have a priority role in rehabilitation and at the time of facing social relations. Therefore, the neuropsychological status of the patient must be known and evaluated.

1. *Psychophysiological Aspects:* It is important to keep in mind the following three fundamental aspects in order to begin planning adequate rehabilitation.

   a. *Level of Activation.* It is necessary that subjects be able to keep themselves awake and with an adequate level of awareness—patients should be aware of where they are, who they are with, and what the situation is. If they do not have these capabilities, it will be difficult to develop a socially acceptable behavior.

   b. *Sphincter Control.* Although this could be solved with the use of diapers (which would gather the urine and feces), it would not be the most adequate solution when trying to hold meetings with friends, especially if patients cannot control their anal sphincter. This could affect patients negatively, since part of the group could reject them, which, in turn, could lead to social isolation.

   c. *Sensory-Motor Aspects.* Patients should have at least some possibility of controlling their gaze, some of their gestures, the capability of keeping their body in a stable manner, the capability of receiving minimal visual and/or audio information, etc.

2. *Cognitive Aspects.* In this section, the ability to understand and communicate plays a fundamental role. If subjects are unable to communicate or to understand that which is being communicated to them, they will have difficulty achieving a socially effective relation.

   a. *Attention.* All psychological activity and human behavior needs and consumes different amounts of attention; therefore, when they are deteriorated, the remaining functions will also be affected. There are different levels of attention and concentration that may produce different types of deficits. Patients may have problems focusing attention (e.g., when you ask them to look at you, and they are unable to do so). It is possible that patients are able to do what you ask and that they may be able look you in the face but may be unable to keep their attention focused because they have a problem of sustained attention. It may be that patients can do the above requirement well but may be distracted easily. They are able to fix their attention but become distracted with any irrelevant thing; this is known as a problem of *selective attention.* Perhaps the problem is just the opposite—they are unable to change easily from one attention focus to another one; this is a problem of *attention flexibility.* Finally, perhaps the only problem patients have is that they are unable to maintain their attention on more than one thing at a time (i.e., they are unable to do two things at once). All these deficits are relevant and interfere with daily life (León-Carrión, 1995).

   b. *Memory.* Memory plays a fundamental role in the acquisition and development of social skills because of its role in facilitating patients' recognition of people and things they deal with daily. In order to perform socially, subjects must be able to recognize routes and places, for example, in order to return home. Therefore, in order to be able to start a neuropsychological rehabilitation program, patients must have begun to recover their working memory and space and time memory and have the capability of consolidation (see Chapter 20).

c. *Language.* Patients must have some measure of communication ability at some level. It does not matter if they have some type of motor aphasia (i.e., inability to speak), if they are able to communicate by other means—writing, gestures, etc. This is not the case with sensory aphasia (Wernicke's); if patients cannot understand what they are being told, it will be very difficult for them to maintain even the most basic level of communication. It requires that they have already recovered their mental capabilities and that they are able to understand and reason at a certain level. The evaluation of the communication deficits of patients with brain injury has usually been based on informal clinical exploration, but, recently, an evaluation scale for communication skills has been developed based on a behavior model. The traditional manner of evaluating aphasia (in the standard manner) excludes many of the natural elements of communication such as speech, gestures, gaze, etc. By contrast, the new speech evaluation scale for adults with brain injury evaluates separately six relevant items of communication for this type of patient: understandability, fixed gaze, formation of sentences, holding a topic, narrative coherence, and initiation of conversations, all of which provide relevant information for the treatment (Ehrlich & Barry, 1989).

d. *Formation of Concepts and Executive Functions.* After suffering from brain injury, it is very probable that patients have problems with reasoning and in resolving effectively situations that are somewhat complex. It is our experience that this is a very common finding. It has to do with patients having problems adequately handling the information that reaches them from their surroundings. They are going to have difficulties in understanding and adequately integrating the demands of daily living. In order to be able to resolve a problem, they need a good capability of analysis, synthesis, and organization of information in order to be able to give an adequate response. If they are not sufficiently recovered in their cognitive capabilities, the most important step is the training in neurocognitive rehabilitation, and although the program of social re-entry will be a part of the program, it will not be an independent program.

3. *Behavioral aspects.* One of the most serious problems patients have, and which makes it difficult for them to lead a more or less independent social life, is the one related to the type of behavior they exhibit (especially when they exhibit difficulty in controlling impulses, which is quite normal with this type of patient). It means that patients are not able to control irritability or anger, or they may even become aggressive for no reason at all. Their inability to control sexual impulse will also be an obstacle for social re-entry. If patients are always trying, commenting, or gesticulating sexually, those around them will become extremely uncomfortable.

Phase II: Individual, Idiosyncratic, and Contextual Design of the Rehabilitation Program in Social Skills

In this second phase, a series of individual, concrete, and specific goals are established for patients so that they will serve to generate a rehabilitation plan that will make it possible to reach the individual goals previously defined. The choice of these goals is one of the most important aspects that the rehabilitator must watch, since it is on this that the later subjective perception by the patient and relatives of the success or failure of the rehabilitation program of the social skills will depend.

The design of these objectives must be done by previously obtaining a good knowledge of the premorbid social functioning of the subject to avoid setting up the recovery of habits that the patient did not have before the accident. It is very important to know the environment in which the patient relates at a family level, among friends, on the job, etc. so that the rehabilitation of social skills are adequate to his/her real needs.

Three variables are significant in the elaboration and design of the goals to achieve an adequate social re-entry—age, social class, and marital status of the patient. Younger patients have a greater facility for change, forgetting, and restructuring their social relations than middle-aged patients, when re-entry in social life will be conditioned on characteristics of the patient's previous social life (i.e. was he/she someone who would go out with friends or enjoy fun activities outside the home before the accident?). When the injured person is very old, the possibility of his/her again having a social life is minimal.

The social class of the patient prior to the accident must also be considered. According to León-Carrión (1994), the greater the educational level and/or economic level of patients, the better the recovery results. The influence of marital status in the patient's rehabilitation is important. Married patients have some sort of social life, even if only in a family environment. Single patients need more contact with other people, and going outside of their regular environment is not only socially beneficial but also advisable from the cognitive point of view. These patients are especially indicated to participate in a program of rehabilitation of social skills.

In addition to individual patient goals, there is a series of general goals that should be considered when designing the rehabilitation program. With the goal of achieving assertive behavior in patients with brain injury, the training must also improve or/and re-establish human dignity as follows (based mainly on Jacubowsky and Lacks [1975]):

1.   Maintaining their dignity and self-respect by behaving in a skillful or assertive manner without violating the rights of others.
2.   Being treated with respect and dignity.
3.   Being able to reject requests without feeling guilty.
4.   Being able to experiment and express personal feelings.
5.   Being able to stop and think before acting.
6.   Being able to change one's mind.
7.   Being able to ask for whatever they want (while at the same time being aware that another person has the right to say no).
8.   Choosing to do less than is humanly possible.
9.   Having the option of deciding what to do with their own body, time, and property.
10.   Being able to ask for information.
11.   Having the right to make mistakes.

12. Being able to feel good about themselves.
13. Being able to have their own needs and to recognize that those needs are as important as the needs of others.
14. Having opinions and voicing them.
15. Having the right to get that for which they have paid.
16. Having the right to choose to not behave in an assertive manner.
17. Having the right to have personal rights and to defend them.
18. Being able to be heard and taken seriously.
19. Being able to be alone when choosing to do so.
20. Having the right to do anything they want as long as it does not violate the rights of others.

As a final goal, the rehabilitator should see that the responsibility shifts gradually from the relative or caretaker to the patient until he/she is able, independently, to lead a normal social life.

Phase III: Program Implementation

For each area of skill to be trained, the following series of steps could be used:

- **Step 1—Instructions.** The rehabilitators, when beginning each area of training, will review the behavioral-cognitive components covered in previous sessions and offer a perspective in which the different behaviors integrate themselves and in which the different behaviors have to be practiced simultaneously. After establishing this bridge between sessions, they should describe to the patient the component running through the session which they are going to work on next, showing possible examples in which this component is part of an interaction. The cognitive component underlying the behavioral exercises must be clearly stated and integrated by the patient. Similarly, the affective component associated with the training exercises of each skill must be worked through by the rehabilitator with the patient. The discussion of the benefits of the illustration of the training chores will ease the internalizing of their value and will serve as an initial step to what is called "self-taught training," during which the subject verbalizes an instruction before carrying out the skill behavior. These self-instructions should be carried out after the display of the model.

- **Step 2—Modeling.** The model displays the entire behavior, with all its components, centering the patient's attention on one component during each session. The effectiveness of the modeling is greater when the patient is offered different types of models and modeling, because it maintains the observer's attention and because it offers several examples of the behavioral component in different social situations, which facilitates the generalization of the behavior. However, in patients with brain injury, focus should be on the exposure to specific behavior models, not on a varied selection that might confuse patients rather than benefit them or that might delay or impede their progress in the training process. The model may be presented live or in a hidden fashion. In the hidden model, intimate scenes might be used, since subjects imagine a model exhibiting those behaviors that they would like to exhibit. In addition, it does not require previous preparation; however, this carries greater risks of being used in an inappropriate manner. While it is a very useful type of modeling for achieving subjects' disinhibition prior to the situation which has to be dealt with, it does not guarantee the acquisition of the behavior to which they were exposed. In patients with brain injury, hidden modeling is not advisable due to the neurocognitive deficits they present. Live modeling may be carried out by the therapist during the session and offers greater possibilities of control over the model. To make the encoding of behaviors easier, the behavior may be displayed repeatedly. It requires less effort on the part of the patient, and it is possible for the model and the observer to carry out the behavior simultaneously, with the model acting as the guide of the behavior.

- **Step 3—Role-playing.** This is used both in the evaluation phase and in the training phase. Unlike with the evaluation moment, during training, those behaviors and situations are role-played that have shown themselves to be problematic during the evaluation, starting with those that are least affected and progressing toward those that exhibit the greatest deficits. Additionally, during the training, patients do not behave as they would normally but must follow closely the instructions given by the trainer. Patients must receive information on how to perform the role-playing and whether they are getting close to the proposed model. Feedback is important, as well as the reinforcement patients receive from the rehabilitator, who will inform them how well they performed the component that they were role-playing, as well as the other components that may have been role-played before and which were necessary to apply in the role-playing being carried out at the moment. There are two types of role-playing—manifest and hidden. In the hidden role-play, subjects imagine themselves exhibiting the behavior. In the manifest role-play, patients have to adjust their role-playing to the instructions given by the trainer. Hidden processes are not the best for patients with brain injury.

- **Step 4—Shaping.** This is performed fundamentally through a feedback process during which adequate behaviors are reinforced. In this process, patients are offered the behaviors that they exhibited during the model imitation phase. The therapist reviews the execution, making the necessary comments aimed at retaining the adequate behaviors and at eliminating the inadequate ones. This system allows for the possibility of reviewing the displayed behaviors many times and isolating different components each time. For this reason, it is very effective in the training of complex nonverbal behaviors.

   Feedback should be started by mentioning some positive aspect of the display, noting some change in relation to the previous role-playing, taking advantage of the moments when the component being practiced appears, even though its frequency may be low, and the patient's attempts in displaying the behavior may not have been successful. Once the subject has been reinforced positively, the therapist comments on the components that are still wrong, trying to find reasons why an inadequate behavior has appeared or the desired behavior has not appeared. This all should be accompanied by new directions that indicate how to change the behavior and further practice by role-playing.

   Reinforcement takes on a special importance in this phase, although in the therapist-patient relationship, there is a continuous reinforcement process. The reinforcement is aimed at motivating patients to improve their behaviors and to increase the number of their correct responses. They must be positive reinforcements since they greatly improve the internalizing of the behavior and, consequently, external control gradually becomes unnecessary. Negative reinforcements carry emotional side effects and are less informative.

If the review of the execution of the behavior is carried out in a group (with friends, with relatives that participate in the training), it must be controlled by the therapist. A certain amount of training of the group would be beneficial in the area of the criticism, so that the comments they may make may be beneficial.

With the final step, the aim, on the one hand, is that patients maintain the skills learned through time with the aid of an intermittent reinforcement program. On the other hand, the aim is also that what has been learned during the sessions be placed into practice in real life environments, in different situations, and before different people. Finally, it is desirable that the acquisition of the trained skills ease the acquisition of new behaviors.

In order to achieve these objectives, patients must grasp the general principle of each component during the sessions and create their own examples of real situations in which the rehearsed component has to be applied. Subjects must not simply imitate the model but rather apply the new component to different situations of daily life. This can be achieved by modifying the interlocutor's comments in the role-playing and by changing the descriptions of the scenes used during the training sessions, as well as by making sure that the interlocutor for each session is not always the same person.

It is advisable that, in the behavior training, those behaviors which will maximize success and minimize failures be reinforced.

If patients do not have many opportunities in their daily lives to practice the acquired skills or if, in the training follow-up stage, problems should be noted with the performance of behaviors, it is important that new training sessions of the components having problems be carried out.

- **Step 5—Generalization.** The use of reinforcement is especially important in the generalization process. The group must reinforce patients when they inform them that they have used trained behaviors in real life situations. At this stage, it is advisable to include other people from patients' real life environment so that they may serve as sources of information and reinforcement for patients.

CONCLUSIONS

The possibility of the patient being able to return to a social life and being able to go out on the street is conditioned on several factors. Patients must have at least minimal skills to relate to others; if that is not the case, they will have to first undergo a program of neuropsychological rehabilitation that will allow them to reach an adequate level in order to be able to have access to an attempt to restore their social lives.

There are several factors that are impediments for brain-injured patients' social re-entry. First, physical control habits and sphincter control are important, along with having the capability of communicating at some level; it is essential that such patients have recovered mental capabilities (León-Carrión, 1994).

REFERENCES

Alberti, R.E. (1977). Assertive behavior training: Definitions, overview contributions. In R.E. Alberti (Ed.), *Assertiveness: Innovations, applications, issues*. San Luis Obispo: Impact.

Anderson, J.R. (1983). A spreading activation theory of memory. *Journal of Verbal Learning and Verbal Behavior, 22,* 261–265..

Caballo, V.E. (1988). *Teoría, evaluación y entrenamiento de las habilidades sociales.* Valencia: Promolibro.

Caralson, R.A., Khos, B.H., Yaure, R.G., & Schneider, W. (1990). Acquisition of a problem-solving skill: Levels of organization and use of working memory. *Journal of Experimental Psychology: General, 119,* 193–214.

Conder, R.L. (1989). Recommendations for clinical and research evaluation of vocational re-entry programmes for survivors of traumatic brain injury. *Brain Injury, 3,* 1–4.

Cox, D.R., & Ostby, S.S. (1989). Head injury and social problem solving skills. *Journal of Clinical and Experimental Neuropsychology, 11*(1), 59.

Ehrilch, J., & Barry, P. (1989). Rating communication behaviors in the head-injured adult. *Brain injury, 3,* 193–198.

Ellis, A. (1990). *Manual de terapia racional-emotiva.* Bilbao: Desclee de Brouwer.

Ellis, A., & Harper, R.A. (1975). *A new guide to rational living.* North Hollywood: Wilshire.

Ellis, D.W., Spivack, G., & Spettell, C.M. (1994). Rehabilitation treatment variables that affect outcome after brain injury. In A.-L. Christensen & B. Uzzell (Eds.), *Brain injury and neuropsychological rehabilitation: International perspectives.* Hillsdale: Lawrence Erlbaum Associates.

Grosswasser, Z. (1994). Rehabilitating psychosocial functioning. In A.-L. Christensen & B. Uzzell (Eds.), *Brain injury and neuropsychological rehabilitation: International perspectives.* Hillsdale: Lawrence Erlbaum Associates.

Jack, L.M. (1934). *An experimental study of ascendant behavior in preschool children.* Iowa City: University of Iowa Studies in Child Welfare.

Jacubowsky, P.A., & Lacks, P.B. (1975). Assessment procedures on assertion training. *The Counseling Psychologist, 5,* 84–90.

Lazarus, A.A. (1971). *Behavior therapy and beyond.* New York: McGraw-Hill.

León-Carrión, J. (1994). *Daño cerebral: Guía para familiares y cuidadores.* Madrid: Ed. Siglo XXI.

———. (1995). *Manual de neuropsicología humana.* Madrid: Ed. Siglo XXI.

Liebermann, R.P., King, L.W., De Risi, W.J., & McCann, M. (1975). *Personal effectiveness.* Champlain: J.L. Research Press.

Luria, A.R. (1969). Frontal lobe syndromes. In P.J. Vinken & J.W. Bruyn (Comps.). *Handbook of clinical neurology* (Vol. 2). Amsterdam: Elsevier.

Meichenbaum, D., Butler, L., and Gruson, L. (1981). Toward a conceptual model of social competence. In J. Wine & M. Smye (Eds.), *Social competence.* New York: Guilford Press.

More, A.D., Stambrook, M., & Peters, L. (1989). Copping strategies and adjustment after closed-head injury: A cluster analytical approach. *Brain Injury, 3,* 171–175.

Weheman, P., Kreutzer, J., West, M., Sherron, P., Diambra, J., Fry, R., Groah, C., Sale, P., & Killam, S. (1989). Employment outcomes of persons following traumatic brain injury: Pre-injury, post-injury, and supported employment. *Brain Injury, 3,* 397–412.

Williams, H.M. (1935). A factor analysis of Berne's social behavior in young children. *Journal of Experimental Education, 4,* 142–146.

Wolpe, J. (1958). *Psicoterapia por inhibición recíproca.* Bilbao: Desclee de Brouwer.

Ziegler, E., & Phillips, L. (1960). Social effectiveness and symptomatic behaviors. *Journal of Abnormal and Social Psychology, 61,* 231–238.

25 Rehabilitation for Employment and Leisure Activities

Tom Teasdale and L. Siert

Department of Psychology, Center for Rehabilitation of Brain Injury
University of Copenhagen, Denmark

INTRODUCTION

Neuropsychological rehabilitation following brain injury requires a dual focus on what can be called the *molecular* and *molar* aspects of the injury. The molecular aspects comprise the evaluation, restoration, and, perhaps, circumvention of identified deficits of, in particular, cognitive functioning. The preceding chapters of this book bear testimony to the intensive research and clinical efforts that have traditionally been directed towards the specific cognitive deficits of attention, memory, perception, language, etc. At the same time, however, it is important to recognize that brain injury, through a variety of routes, including but not exclusively comprising cognitive deficits, impacts considerably on daily life and that this impact needs also to be addressed directly in a "molar" or global fashion. It is, in our view, not enough to attempt to remediate identified cognitive deficits in isolation with the hope that the patient's daily life will thereafter restore itself.

For adults of working age, it is a very common and critical disruption to daily life that the capacity to satisfactorily perform a job is seriously reduced. Although this might appear to result in more time to engage in leisure-time activities, hobbies, sports, voluntary work, etc., rehabilitation professionals are all too aware that these activities are typically reduced following a brain injury, rather than increased. The reasons for these two related problems in employment and leisure, and proposed solutions to them, have much in common, but they are not fully overlapping. The present chapter will consider each separately.

REHABILITATION FOR EMPLOYMENT

Traumatic brain injury (TBI) occurs most commonly to young adults at or near the beginning of their working lives, and other forms of acute onset injury (e.g., stroke and cerebral infections) can also occur with an adult at any point in a lifelong working career. Very severe injuries, of course, will, all too often, result in chronic physical disability, even vegetative state, in which return to employment will be impossible. Even for less severe cases, however, loss of employment is common. For example, in a classic study in Britain, Brooks et al. (1987) found that less than 30% of a sample of head-injured adults were employed when followed up as much as seven years after injury. In a similar study in the United States, McMordie et al. (1990) found less than 20% of brain-injured patients in competitive employment.

There is, however, an increasing optimism, encouraged by positive results from a steadily increasing number of post-acute rehabilitation centers, with regard to the moderate-to-severe levels of injury, in which hope of return to employment would earlier have been abandoned.

There are two typical courses in the emergence of difficulties in post-injury employment. One course is that following the acute treatment of the injury, it is recognized that a return to earlier employment will be impossible. This is most apparent where the patient, perhaps as a result of a stroke, has been left with a severe aphasia and/or with motor dysfunctions such as a hemiplegia. A job requiring good communication skills would be impossible for the former, and a job requiring unhampered mobility would be impossible for the latter. Such patients may be referred directly to post-acute rehabilitation since it is immediately evident that they will require retraining if they are to achieve any form of return to employment.

The second route that is often encountered in rehabilitation settings occurs in cases where patients attempt to return to their employment and fail in this attempt. Brain injuries that do not leave the patient with a physical or speech disability can result, as documented in other chapters, in a variety of deficits which are less immediately manifest (e.g., concentration and memory difficulties). To these can be added the wide range of characteristics particularly associated with frontal lobe injuries including organization and planning, social regulation, and impulse control, often called the *dysexecutive syndrome* (Baddeley & Wilson, 1988), and other personality changes. In such cases, the nature of the deficits may only become apparent after patients have returned to their former employment. The confrontation with the demands of the job often reveals the first clear sign to the patients, or perhaps more likely to their colleagues and employer, that the demands can no longer be met. Dismissal may follow, although in some enlightened conditions, leave of absence, especially in order to undergo a post-acute rehabilitation program, may be granted.

Factors effecting return to employment have been the object of several reported studies of brain-injured patients. Grosswasser (1994) followed up over 300 patients at the Loewenstein Rehabilitation Hospital, dividing them into "good recovery," defined as return to competitive employment or to regular education, and "poor recovery." Age was not a major factor, but hemiparesis and cognitive and language deficits were, together with behavioral disturbances. Uzzell et al. (1987) followed over 50 TBI patients with a wide range of degrees of severity of injury as estimated from the Glasgow Coma Scale (GCS) within six hours of the injury. She found a strong relationship between return to employment and degree of severity, with over half the patients with a GCS > 8 returning to employment but less than 25% of patients with a GCS = < 8 doing so. In a recent study of almost 100 patients, Ponsford et al. (1995) found four variables to be predictive of post-injury employment status: age, GCS, duration of Post-Traumatic Amnesia (PTA), and a global value derived from a disability rating scale.

Godfrey et al. (1993) also found age and duration of PTA to be significant predictors, as were a number of neuropsychological tests, notably Ravens Progressive Matrices and the Paced Serial Addition Task (PASAT). Ruff et al. (1993) examined the predictive value of neuropsychological tests and questionnaire-derived scores. They found that, in addition to age and coma duration, a number of Wechsler Adult Intelligence Scale subtests (notably vocabulary) and a Depression score from the Katz Adjustment Scale questionnaire were related to post-injury employment status. The importance of emotional and personality factors was also emphasized by a study of Lubusco et al. (1994), who found that return to employment in a group of TBI patients was predicted by a relatively higher external "locus of control" and by a lower score on the Beck's Depression scale.

With the exception of Grosswasser's study, age has rather consistently been found to be a major factor. In general, older patients return less often to their former employment than younger ones. Some of this effect may be attributable to the generally slower and less complete recovery with increasing age that characterizes most forms of illness, but there is no doubt that societal and individual expectations also play a role. A head-injured patient of age 50 will often be more encouraged, and more willing, to accept a disability pension than a patient of half that age.

Given, however, that patients of working age have been referred to neuropsychological rehabilitation in the hope of their being able to return to some form of employment, how may this best be achieved? We would argue that it is best achieved in three stages: (1) assessment, (2) intensive rehabilitation, and (3) follow-up in the work environment.

Assessment

This topic has been dealt with in detail in previous chapters, but some points of specific relevance to employment need to be emphasized in the present context. The first requirement is a full assessment of patients' abilities and disabilities. This must include neuropsychological as well as physical assessment. To begin with the latter, it is necessary to know not only what direct motor and sensory deficits might have resulted from the injury, but also the general physical condition of the patient. Following injury, many patients become less physically active, leading highly sedentary lives resulting in poor physical condition. It is also important to know whether there have been other medical sequelae of the injury. Post-injury epilepsy or hemianopsia, for example, would rule out forms of employment involving driving.

Neuropsychological assessment should include the usual range of cognitive abilities, and therapists should note not only dysfunctions but also spared, intact functions since the latter will form the foundation of the patient's employability. An evaluation of personality and social characteristics is no less important. Some brain-injured patients may become profoundly depressed following the realization that they no longer have capacities that they previously took for granted. Other patients, often those examined closest in time to their injury, may be unaware of or unable to confront the fact that they have suffered any loss of capacity at all.

A third psychological aspect to be explored is the patient's expectation with regard to return to employment. This issue can be complex and may vary widely from patient to patient, even given the same apparent type and degree of injury. It is often, but not always, the case that the patient will have a strong wish to return to employment. This is hardly surprising given not only economic considerations concerning income but also the central role that a job has in most cultures for the adult's sense of personal identity and for their social relationships. It should here be added that the return to employment will also often be a major concern for the patient's close family, be they parents or spouse, and not the least, for the agency financing rehabilitation efforts, whether through state social services or private insurance plans. It may seem a severe criterion, but the success or failure of rehabilitation programs often tends to be gauged in terms of their ability to achieve a return to employment for their patients.

Intensive Rehabilitation

There is a converging view, found both in Europe and North America, that moderate-to-severe brain injury requires a period of focused, concentrated rehabilitation in the post-acute phase, following stabilization of the medical condition. Models for this form of rehabilitation are provided by Ben-Yishay (1993) and Prigatano (1989) in the United States, as well as by Christensen in Europe (1995). With specific regard to return to employment, it may be stated generally that such rehabilitation should set a number of specific targets and work with specific strategies.

One primary and general target is to give patients an insight into the nature of their problems, be they cognitive, emotional, behavioral, personality, or social. The corresponding strategy here is feedback to the patient. As indicated above, patients may be unaware of the nature of their deficits. The importance of attaining insight through feedback must be stressed for two reasons. First, the patient will not be able to improve without a realization of where improvement is desirable. Secondly, and no less importantly, the patient must be given the ability to use compensatory strategies for dysfunctions for which no great degree of direct amelioration may be possible. This will happen in the physical field, where, for instance, sensory or fine motor skills may never return fully but also in the field of psychological characteristics. Current evidence is not generally encouraging with regard to the degree to which, for instance, good memory functioning can be restored (Wilson, 1992), and, therefore, rehabilitation needs to concentrate on the use of alternative strategies (e.g., the use of diary techniques, written shopping lists, electronic organizers, etc. [Lynch, 1995]).

The use of computer training procedures is increasing in rehabilitation settings (Lynch, 1992) and, therefore, deserves a special mention. While such procedures can be of use in revealing deficits to the patient and while many patients are quite positively motivated towards interactive computer programs, evidence of their efficacy is as yet sparse. There is, moreover, a danger that valuable time in the rehabilitation setting may be lost engaging in what may be no more than "placebo" activities. Unsupervised interaction with a computer cannot, in our opinion, be a substitute for interaction with, and under the guidance of, a therapist. According to Ruff et al. (1994), the computer *per se* is not the answer; it is rather *how* the computer technology is introduced to effectively assist the patient and the practitioner. In some instances, however, a case may be made for the use of such programs, perhaps particularly language training programs for aphasics, in the home environment as an adjunct to the rehabilitation program.

As pointed out elsewhere in this volume, social interaction should form an essential part of a rehabilitation program. Successful return to employment, particularly in those jobs involving contact with the general public, is as often hindered as much by loss of social skills as by loss of cognitive ones. The use of video-recordings of role-playing situations can be a vivid means for the therapist to provide patients with feedback regarding their own social skills or lack thereof.

As a further example of structured social interaction of particular relevance to developing a return to employment, we can here cite the "morning meeting," which begins each day of the Copenhagen rehabilitation program. This is described in detail in Chapter 4 from which it will be seen that the meeting effectively simulates much of the interpersonal interaction and socially delegated responsibilities that characterize activities in many workplaces.

Another important aspect of rehabilitation during this intensive phase is what may be characterized as specific job-relevant training. At some early phase in the process, a target with regard to subsequent employment should be set wherever possible. From this goal will follow automatically a specification of the job-relevant skills required. These skills can be as varied as the job market itself and can, therefore, best be illustrated by individual case examples from our clinical experience.

- A former translator working with a bureau was trained to use the most recent version of the word-processor that had been introduced at his place of work during his lengthy absence following a stroke. In this way, he was able to return to his bureau already familiar with the most basic tool used there. Additionally, he was given exercises in translation from Spanish to Danish resembling those undertaken by his bureau, and his success at this was monitored closely.

- A small group of patients, who had worked in the financial sector, was given the task of following newspaper-published developments in interest rates, investment stocks and shares, and exchange rates during the period of their rehabilitation. A motivating competitive element was introduced into this task by each member of the group fictitiously "investing" the same sum at the beginning of the program (as did the therapist) and aiming, thereafter, to maximize "profit" throughout the period of the program. The group plotted the rise or fall of their respective fortunes graphically each week.

- A former guitar teacher gave "lessons" to a moderately skilled guitar-playing psychologist during the course of rehabilitation. In this way, she improved not only her own virtuosity but also was required to concentrate on her pedagogical skills in planning lessons, communicating instructions, and observing and giving feedback on the performance of her "pupil." Concurrently and importantly, the psychologist was able to give her feedback, through reviews submitted to her primary therapist, on her own performance as a teacher.

- It was planned that a right-hemisphere stroke patient should, after rehabilitation, join her brother in his antique business, despite her having little prior experience. Part of her time during rehabilitation was, therefore, employed in her reading, discussing, and summarizing relevant literature, especially on the subject of mirrors in which her brother specialized.

- A severely aphasic man with right-sided hemiparesis was trained to use the numeric keypad of a personal computer to key in numeric data. This was done in preparation for a return to the computer division at his former employment, where he had been offered part-time work entering numeric codes from sales representatives' order forms.

Specific job-related skill-training is thus highly desirable and generally attainable given a versatile and imaginative staff of therapists. A particular problem arises for young brain-injured patients, namely those who, at the time of injury, were not in employment but were still at school or pursuing a higher education. In some cases, the interruption of schooling may have left them without the attainment of basic skills in, for instance, language and mathematics. Where this has happened, it is important to incorporate into the rehabilitation program some special education teaching in order that such skills, usually fundamental to any form of employment, can be improved. The issue of brain injury in children is dealt with in detail in Chapter 27. In the case of patients injured while pursuing higher education, careful consideration will need to be given as to whether or not the continuance of that education is a realistic goal following the rehabilitation program.

Although an appraisal of the potential for a return to employment should be made at the beginning of the intensive phase of a rehabilitation program and modified as appropriate throughout its course, it is towards the end of the program that the issue becomes critical. It may be particularly important for motivation that the patient should have a clearly defined and established continuation when the program ceases. If this does not happen, then the patient can become discouraged, with a tendency to fall back into despair and lethargy, and, in this way, the benefits of the program will be quickly dissipated. Occasionally, one may observe overdependent behavior in which the patient is reluctant to leave the reassuring and supportive environment that the rehabilitation center has provided. Continuity with a working environment is therefore important. The case for a careful integration of involved parties in the rehabilitation process (e.g., medical, educational, employment, and social services, possibly under the coordination of a case manager) has been well made by MacMillan et al. (1988), among others.

Follow-Up

Ideally, thus, even during the course of the rehabilitation program, a precise plan will have been arranged for the return to employment. This plan will have addressed at least three issues: (1) where the patient will work, (2) how much and at what level he/she will work, and (3) how he/she will be reimbursed. In all cases, it should be stressed that a close coordination between the rehabilitation center and the place of employment is highly desirable, both before and after the transfer. It has often been pointed out that there has been a strong tendency for brain-injured patients to get "lost in the cracks" between services, and, in a sense, "follow-through" would be a better term than "follow-up."

With regard to where the patient will work, the most natural starting point would be his/her former workplace. It is our general experience that previous employers are favorably disposed towards the re-employment of their now brain-injured workers. This derives from laudable socially responsible attitudes regarding the reintegration of handicapped people. Furthermore, in some cases, the patient, particularly one for whom a relatively short time has elapsed since injury, may have a legal entitlement to return to his/her former job.

At the same time, there can be particular difficulties for the patient returning to a former workplace. There may be an implicit expectation that he/she can return to all former duties and tasks, and a gradual frustration and irritation on the part of colleagues and employers may occur if it becomes evident that the brain-injured patient cannot fully meet all these demands. In this way, much of the initial good may gradually evaporate, and the patient could ultimately experience a confidence-destroying fiasco, ending in abandonment of the employment. Such an experience would also make it the more difficult for the patient to commence another attempt later, however much more manageable.

It may, therefore, be advisable to consider the possibility that an alternative place of employment could be a better solution. Finding such employment may, however, not be a simple matter. In many developed economies, there are chronic high levels of unemployment that work against the employment prospects of all handicapped persons. Our experience in Denmark has been that social service departments have often been helpful in mediating job opportunities. In other cases, such opportunities arise somewhat serendipitously, as, for instance, through the patient's own social, business, or family connections.

Whatever place of work is determined, however, the issue of the nature of the work must also be considered carefully. Most brain-injured people will, even after rehabilitation, not, at least immediately, have a full working capacity. It is, therefore, strongly advisable to introduce a graduated workload in which both the length of the working day and the nature of the tasks and responsibilities involved are initially set safely within the patient's capacity. Only as the patient workload demonstrates management of the workload should an increase be phased in. As stated above, it is important that the patient should not experience failure through being overburdened at the outset, since this could lead to abandoning the employment altogether.

The question of remuneration is likewise important. Social legislation varies from country to country, but it will probably be widely true, as it is in Denmark, that a range of options exists whereby employment can be state-subsidized, either permanently or for a trial period. These options should be thoroughly explored since they can greatly increase the willingness of employers to hire brain-injured people. In relation to state support of employment, the converse issue of disability pensions must also be considered. For what, in our experience, has been a minority of patients, the prospect of a receiving a disability pension is not always unattractive. This may particularly happen where state or private schemes would provide an income approaching the pre-injury salary. Even here, it may be important not to support the patient in this wish too readily for two reasons. In part, the therapist generally has a broader obligation to make an independent assessment of the working capacity of the patient, and, thereby, his/her ability to again become an economically productive member of society, and, in part, the therapist needs to be aware that abandoning at too early a stage any plans for a return to employment leaves the patient with a long-term reduced quality of life, regardless of that person's current perception of how his/her life would be "free" from a daily routine of going to work.

Some brain-injured people prefer to return to an employment without revealing the nature of their injury to their employers or colleagues. This is fully understandable and may perhaps be possible in cases where the sequelae are few and slight or where recovery has been complete. But more typically, the injury and its consequences cannot, at least in the long run, remain hidden. Certainly in such cases, it is advisable for professional therapists to involve themselves actively in the process of the patient's returning to employment. This can take the form of assessing the job situation into which the patient will return and planning a graduated shouldering of tasks as outlined above.

While thorough and individually tailored preparation for employment in an intensive rehabilitation setting and close monitoring in the work environment in follow-up thereafter undoubtedly can contribute much to successful long-term return to employment, newer initiatives are focusing upon direct interventions in the work environment itself. Kreutzer, Wehman, and colleagues ((Wehman, Kreutzer, Stonnington, & Wood, 1988; Wehman, Sherron, Kregel, Kreutzer, Tran, & Cifu, 1993) have strongly advocated this model in which employment "specialists," alongside "clients" at the workplace, are able to help patients to "overcome their inability to generalize or retain skills and other major social, behavioral, and physical problems which have traditionally hindered their ability to maintain employment" (Wehman, Revell, Kregel, Kreutzer, Callahan, & Banks, 1991). Prior to placement, the client is matched to the available job on the basis of an assessment of his/her skills, both cognitive and social, and preferences. Advocacy of the scheme with potential employers is also a major element. Interventions, such as work and social-skills training, are also provided at the place of employment. The employment specialist will also help the client with issues of transportation, accommodation, and public benefits and, where necessary, familial and social relationships. In the initial phases, the specialist may accompany the client continuously, and this will gradually decline as the client's skills and capabilities and his/her integration into the workplace increase. Periodic contact is, however, maintained with both the client and the employer.

As another somewhat different example of what can be done in this manner, we shall here outline a recently introduced project with which we are involved and which is not, at the time of writing, described elsewhere. Our center has begun a joint project with the social services department of one of the counties to the north of Copenhagen. The essence of the project involves enlisting the services of a support person to assist the brain-injured patient at the workplace itself. This person should be someone already employed at the workplace and, therefore, fully acquainted with its organization and demands, and likewise acquainted with the other members of staff whom the patient will encounter and alongside whom he/she will have to work. The support person will typically work in close proximity to the brain-injured person and can be called upon by the latter as needed to assist with whatever task he/she has in hand. The employer is reimbursed (through a project fund provided by the Ministry of Social Services) for the salary of the support person for the number of hours during which they are functioning in that role. Thus, the employer does not sustain any economic loss while participating in the scheme. The number of hours is agreed upon contractually prior to the implementation of the scheme and is reviewed periodically. It varies considerably from case to case, depending on the number of hours the brain-injured person works and upon their need for help.

In addition to the on-site support person, the project involves a collaboration between a coordination group of three relevant professionals—a social worker from the county in question, a handicap consultant from the Danish employment exchange, and a neuropsychologist (L.S.). The broad range of expertise constituted in this group is regarded as essential for the success of the project. The social worker has responsibilities for providing general information concerning the project to local authorities, general practitioners, and other potentially interested parties. He/she also has direct responsibilities for practical negotiations and administration. The handicap consultant has the responsibility of finding suitable places of work and initiating contact with these in cases where the brain-injured person does not have the possibility of returning to his/her former workplace. The neuropsychologist has responsibilities for the initial visit to the place of work to explain the nature of the brain-injured person's strengths and weaknesses to the future employer. Following this meeting and the selection of a suitable support person, the neuropsychologist is also responsible for the initial training of the support person in general aspects of the consequences of brain-injury and the specific problems that can arise for the brain-injured person in question. He/she is likewise responsible for follow-up and supervision of the support person and other close colleagues in the workplace. This involves visiting the workplace at least once a month and perhaps more frequently when required. It is also important to emphasize the quality of the direct contact between the neuropsychologist and the brain-injured person in providing support for the latter.

The coordination group meets at least once monthly to monitor the cases currently engaged in the project and to consider new referrals. These referrals can be made from various sources, including the Center for Rehabilitation of Brain Injury's own patients, upon completion of the intensive day-program. In all cases, medical, social, and employment records are evaluated, and the patient is invited to an assessment session that includes neuropsychological testing (by L.S.) unless this has recently been undertaken elsewhere. When a positive decision is made, a specific plan is drawn up with the cooperation of the employer, the selected support person, and the brain-injured person.

Experience hitherto with the project (about 25 cases) has been very largely satisfactory and has underlined the importance of providing information to all parties involved and encouraging motivation from all parties. It has shown the advisability of openness in the placement, such that other employees are aware of the arrangement and are made aware that the brain-injured colleague is not to be treated as if he/she were ill but simply as someone in need of help, at least initially, to learn (or relearn) to cope with the demands of the job. Similarly, it has confirmed the benefit of the on-site support person in assisting with this coping. The project, which has been initially funded for a four-year period, is overseen by an external evaluation delegated by the Ministry of Social Services. Should the project be successful, it is expected to lead to a change in Danish social legislation such that a brain-injured person will be entitled to the state support necessary to finance the implementation of a support person arrangement at an appropriate place of employment.

A frequently asked question is: How successful is rehabilitation in securing a return to employment? This issue has been plagued by the difficulty of comparisons between published reports using different patient samples. Nonetheless, against a background of earlier reports of return to employment at rates of 30% or less ((Brooks, McKinlay, Symington, Beattie, & Campsie, 1987; McMordie, Barker, & Paolo, 1990), more positive reports suggesting rates of 60% or more from several post-acute rehabilitation centers (Cope, 1994), including our own (Christensen, Pinner, Moller Pedersen, Teasdale, & Trexler, 1992), are encouraging.

Despite this prima facie evidence and widespread clinical experience, the viewpoint is still sometimes that the better rates might have occurred "spontaneously" (i.e., without the time, effort, and expense of the post-acute rehabilitative interventions). For this reason, a recently published report by Prigatano et al. (1995) is particularly important. In their study, 38 brain-injured patients who had undergone a post-acute rehabilitation program (similar to the Copenhagen program) were compared with 38 matched control patients who had not undergone the program. For both groups, the follow-up time post-injury averaged about three years. In the rehabilitation group, 63% were working full-time or part-time, and fewer than 3% were deemed unable to work. Among the control patients, the corresponding figures were 46%, and 36% were deemed unable to work. It is also of interest to note that among the rehabilitation group, a productive outcome was strongly related to therapists' ratings of the quality of alliance with the patients, again emphasizing the point made earlier of the importance of establishing a good therapeutic relationship with the patient in the rehabilitation program.

REHABILITATION FOR LEISURE ACTIVITIES

Since brain injury can so often result in loss of employment in more severe cases or reduced employment in others, perhaps even in spite of rehabilitation efforts, it is important to address the issue of how patients spend their leisure time. This is not only because reduced employment necessarily creates more free time in which to engage in leisure activities but also, more centrally, because the restoration of personal identity, a fulfilling lifestyle, and social relationships can all be fostered by promoting worthwhile activities. For the brain-injured adult who is in a marital relationship, the sedentary, unproductive, and socially isolated lifestyle that may follow places considerable strains on the relationship itself. For the brain-injured patient who is not in such a relationship, the same lifestyle considerably reduces the prospects of ever entering one.

The difficulty of promoting leisure activities in brain-injured patients may sometimes be compounded by the fact that inactivity has been a partial contributing factor in the injury itself. This occurs in some stroke patients, where lack of physical activity is a known risk factor (Lindenstrom, Boysen, & Nyboe, 1993). This needs, however, to be seen against the increased risk of head injury associated with some forms of sporting activity (Engberg, 1995) and, in some countries more than others, with cycling (Thompson, Rivara, & Thompson, 1989).

As noted by Brooks (1992), the consequences of brain injury for leisure activities have been much less widely studied than the consequences for employment. The extant literature, however, clearly indicates that leisure activities decrease both quantitatively and qualitatively following a brain injury. In an early study, Oddy et al. (1978) followed up 50 young adults six months after a severe closed head injury. They found that leisure activities were reported as being among the most affected areas of the patients' lives. In a seven-year follow-up of the same patient group, Oddy et al. (1985) noted, however, some improvement in this respect, although this was mainly confined to the less severely injured. The chronic nature of these effects was also underlined by Klonoff et al. (1986), who demonstrated reduced leisure activities, and particularly social activities, in a similar group of brain-injured patients 2–4 years post-injury. Ponsford et al. (1995) found that only 10% of their head-injured sample were able to engage independently in all of their pre-injury recreational activities and interests. Hall et al. (1994) found lack of leisure activities (and lack of social contacts) to be among the most common complaints regarding brain-injured patients made by their close relatives up to two years post-injury. Reviewing the literature, Morton and Wehman (1995) noted the frequency of passive and essentially solitary leisure activities indulged at home such as watching television and listening to music.

In a comparatively rare controlled study of the effect of rehabilitation on leisure activities in a brain-injured group, Jongbloed and Morgan (1991) found no statistically significant differences between the experimental and control groups in activity involvement or satisfaction with that involvement. They note, however, that their intervention—involving only five home visits by occupational therapists—may have been too little to have any substantial effect. We have been able to report rather more success from our rehabilitation day-program. In a follow-up of 67 patients at one and three years following the program, the proportion of patients engaging in leisure activities that brought them out of their homes and into the company of others has risen to levels equaling those pre-injury (Lambert & Willett, 1993; Hassett, Jr., Doolittle, Molloy, & Lalka, 1987).

To an even greater extent than for the rehabilitation for employment, the potential for rehabilitation of leisure-time activities is highly differentiated since it will depend very much on the individual case. In some instances, it will involve encouraging taking up and pursuing further an interest that the patient already had. In other instances, this may be impossible, in particular, because of physical handicaps. Some clinical examples may illustrate something of what may be achieved.

- A TBI patient proved during rehabilitation to be unexpectedly knowledgeable about birds. Although the patient had never specifically cultivated this interest, the extent of his knowledge was revealed to him by demonstrating his ability to recognize and name bird species from both their appearance and from their song. This awoke a motivation, and he was encouraged to pursue the interest further by engaging in regular nature walks, reading on the topic, and by joining an ornithological society.
- A stroke patient had formerly been a busy company manager with little time for leisure activities. The aphasia that resulted from his stroke left his appreciation of music unaffected, and he became a frequent concert-goer and took evening class courses in music history.
- A frontal-lobe injured patient with intact verbal and memory skills but unable to return to her former strenuous work, indulged a life-long ambition to join an amateur dramatic society, helping with the stage management and making small appearances in productions.

The importance of these examples lies in the fact that they involve social activities. Although pastimes that are less inherently social such as, perhaps, stamp and coin-collecting or painting, can be of considerable value for the brain-injured patient no longer able to work, the risk of home-bound social isolation should be recognized and preferably countered in some other ways. At various times, our center has fostered activity groups for former patients. In one case, an evening chess club led to the long-term pursuance of chess playing at home between several members of the group. In another case, a class in 12-meter boat sailing (a skill that can be managed solo even in the presence of hemiparesis) was successful in teaching several former patients both the theoretical and practical skills involved and lead to this becoming an enjoyed sporting activity for them.

The influence of rehabilitation on leisure time activities has not been widely reported. At our own center, however, we found that at one and three years post-rehabilitation, the amount of time reportedly engaged in social activities outside the home had reached levels equal to those prior to injury, despite having dropped markedly between the time of injury and entry into the program (Teasdale & Christensen, 1994). Importantly, there was no decline during the period between one and three years post rehabilitation, suggesting that levels of social activity were being maintained rather than, as one might have feared, declining with increasing time after the boosting effect of the program itself.

In addition to evening- and day-class courses specifically designed as time-limited measures to propel brain-injured patients towards subsequent independent activities, there may also be a need, especially among the more severely injured, for a much longer term support system. Harvey Jacobs et al. (1990) described this as "lifelong living programming." Mathews (1990) describes non-residential independent living centers in which disabled people, including those with brain injury, are able to engage in collective social activities and be of mutual help in areas such as housing, skills training, advocacy, peer counselling, attendant services, and transportation. Strong emphasis is placed on consumer control rather than on external, non-handicapped administration. Mathews notes, however, that such centers are less frequently attended by brain-injured patients than by other "handicapped" groups such as psychiatric patients and the mentally retarded. It could well be the case that brain-injured patients do not generally mix well other with such groups, and that it might be better, where possible, to provide facilities for them as a distinct group.

Jacobs (1995) has himself recently described a number of "clubhouse" models along these lines that are either operating or under development. The clubhouses are peer-directed and are non-medical in orientation. Thus, those attending are not patients but members. The limited professional staff support rather than direct the program. Jacobs notes that most of the people referred to the clubhouses are more severely disabled than the norm but that excellent outcomes, in terms of independent living, can be attained.

As a new initiative, a similar program is currently being piloted in Copenhagen. A small day-and-evening center, financed indirectly by the Ministry of Education, has opened offering a range of activities including courses in cognitive training under the guidance of qualified staff as well as small discussion groups and such informal social interactions as common lunches. Additionally, there are courses in creative activities such as guitar-playing, drawing, and painting. In the next phase of development, the center will have a weekly open-house day for more general meetings and social activities.

In conclusion, one other form of "leisure" activity should be mentioned. One of the most constructive ways in which brain-injured people, together with their close relatives, could occupy themselves is through active participation in support groups (Miller, 1992; DiCesare, Parente, & Anderson Parente, 1990). In addition to channelling communication and interaction between brain-injured people, support groups, particularly when organized as national associations, can provide valuable focus in the political and societal fields by increasing public awareness of the brain injury problem in order to reduce the extent to which it is a "silent epidemic." These issues are dealt with in Chapters 24 and 26.

REFERENCES

Baddeley, A., & Wilson, B. (1988). Frontal amnesia and the dysexecutive syndrome. Special Issue: Single-case studies in amnesia. Theoretical advances. *Brain and Cognition, 7,* 212–230.

Ben Yishay, Y., & Diller, L. (1993). Cognitive remediation in traumatic brain injury: Update and issues. *Archives of Physical Medicine and Rehabilitation, 74,* 204–213.

Brooks, N. (1992). Psychosocial assessment after traumatic brain injury. *Scandinavian Journal of Rehabilitation Medicine, 26* (Suppl.), 126–131.

Brooks, N., McKinlay, W., Symington, C., Beattie, A., & Campsie, L. (1987). Return to work within the first seven years of severe head injury. *Brain Injury, 1,* 5–19.

Christensen, A., & Teasdale, T.W. (1995). A clinically and neuropsychologically led post-acute rehabilitation program. In M.A. Chamberlain, V. Neumann, & A. Tennant (Eds.), *Traumatic brain injury rehabilitation: Services, treatments and outcome* (pp. 88–98). London: Chapman & Hall.

Christensen, A.-L., Pinner, E.M., Moller Pedersen, P., Teasdale, T.W., & Trexler, L.E. (1992). Psychosocial outcome following individualized neuropsychological rehabilitation of brain damage. *Acta Neurologica Scandinavica, 85,* 32–38.

Cope, D.N. (1994). Traumatic brain-injury rehabilitation outcome studies in the unites states. In A. Christensen & B.P. Uzzell (Eds.), *Brain injury and neuropsychological rehabilitation: International perspectives.* (pp. 201–220). Hillsdale: Lawrence Erlbaum.

DiCesare, A., Parente, R., & Anderson Parente, J.K. (1990). Personality change after traumatic brain injury: Problems and solutions. *Cognitive Rehabilitation, 8,* 14–18.

Engberg, A. (1995). Severe traumatic brain injury: Epidemiology, external causes, prevention, and rehabilitation of mental and physical sequelae. *Acta Neurologica Scandinavica, 92,* 164 (Suppl.).

Godfrey, H.P., Bishara, S.N., Partridge, F.M., & Knight, R.G. (1993). Neuropsychological impairment and return to work following severe closed head injury: Implications for clinical management. *New Zealand Medical Journal, 106,* 301–303.

Grosswasser, Z. (1994). Rehabilitating psychosocial functioning. In A. Christensen & B.P. Uzzell (Eds.), *Brain injury and neuropsychological rehabilitation: International perspectives* (pp. 187–200). Hillsdale: Lawrence Erlbaum.

Hall, K.M., Karzmark, P., Stevens, M., Englander, J., O'Hare, P., & Wright, J. (1994). Family stressors in traumatic brain injury: A two-year follow-up. *Archives of Physical Medicine and Rehabilitation, 75,* 876–884.

Hassett, Jr., J.M., Doolittle, T., Molloy, M., & Lalka, D. (1987). Hypersensitivity reaction to anticonvulsants following head injury. *New York State Journal of Med, 87,* 571–573.

Jacobs, H.E. (1995). The clubhouse model for social integration. Paper presented at the First World Congress on Brain Injury, Copenhagen, Denmark.

Jacobs, H.E., Blatnick, M., & Sandhorst, J.V. (1990). What is life-long living, and how does it relate to quality of life? *Journal of Head Trauma Rehabilitation, 5,* 1–8.

Jongbloed, L., & Morgan, D. (1991). An investigation of involvement in leisure activities after a stroke. *American Journal of Occupational Therapy, 45,* 420–427.

Klonoff, P.S., Snow, W.G., & Costa, L.D. (1986). Quality of life in patients 2 to 4 years after closed head injury. *Neurosurgery, 19,* 735–743.

Lambert, S.M., & Willett, K. (1993). Transfer of multiply-injured patients for neurosurgical opinion: A study of the adequacy of assessment and resuscitation. *Injury, 24,* 333–336.

Lindenstrom, E., Boysen, G., & Nyboe, J. (1993). Lifestyle factors and risk of cerebrovascular disease in women: The Copenhagen City Heart Study. *Stroke, 24,* 1468–1472.

Lubusko, A.A., Moore, A.D., Stambrook, M., & Gill, D.D. (1994). Cognitive beliefs following severe traumatic brain injury: Association with post-injury employment status. *Brain Injury, 8,* 65–70.

Lynch, W.J. (1992). Ecological validity of cognitive rehabilitation software. *Journal of Head Trauma Rehabilitation, 7,* 36–45.

_____. (1995). You must remember this: Assistive devices for memory impairment. *Journal of Head Trauma Rehabilitation, 10,* 94–97.

Mathews, R.M. (1990). Independent living as a life-long community service. *Journal of Head Trauma Rehabilitation, 5,* 23–30.

McMillan, T.M., Greenwood, R.J., Morris, J.R., & Brooks, D.N. (1988). An introduction to the concept of head injury case management with respect to the need for service provision. *Clinical Rehabilitation, 2,* 319–322.

McMordie, W.R., Barker, S.L., & Paolo, T.M. (1990). Return to work (RTW) after head injury. *Brain Injury, 4,* 57–69.

Miller, L. (1992). When the best help is self-help: or, Everything you always wanted to know about brain injury support groups. *Journal of Cognitive Rehabilitation, 10,* 14–17.

Morton, M.V., & Wehman, P. (1995). Psychosocial and emotional sequelae of individuals with traumatic brain injury: A literature review and recommendations. *Brain Injury, 9,* 81–92.

Oddy, M., Humphrey, M., & Uttley, D. (1978). Subjective impairment and social recovery after closed head injury. *Journal of Neurology, Neurosurgery and Psychiatry, 41,* 611–616.

Oddy, M., Coughlan, T., Tyerman, A., & Jenkins, D. (1985). Social adjustment after closed head injury: A further follow-up seven years after injury. *Journal of Neurology, Neurosurgery and Psychiatry, 48,* 564–568.

Ponsford, J.L., Olver, J.H., Curran, C., & Ng, K. (1995). Prediction of employment status 2 years after traumatic brain injury. *Brain Injury, 9,* 11–20.

Prigatano, G.P. (1989). Bring it up in milieu: Toward effective traumatic brain injury rehabilitation interaction. Special Issue: Traumatic brain injury rehabilitation. *Rehabilitation Psychology, 34,* 135–144.

Prigatano, G., Klonoff, P.S., O'Brien, K.P., Altman, I.M., Amin, K., Chiapello, D., Shepherd, J., Cunningham, M., & Mora, M. (1995). Productivity after a neuropsychologically oriented milieu rehabilitation. *Journal of Head Trauma Rehabilitation, 9,* 91–102.

Ruff, R.M., Mahaffey, R., Engel, J., Farrow, C., Cox, D., & Karzmark, P. (1994). Efficacy study of THINKable in the attention and memory retraining of traumatically head-injured patients. *Brain Injury, 8,* 3–14.

Ruff, R.M., Marshall, L.F., Crouch, J., Klauber, M.R., Levin, H.S., Barth, J., Kreutzer, J., Blunt, B.A., Foulkes, M.A., Eisenberg, H.M., et al. (1993). Predictors of outcome following severe head trauma: Follow-up data from the Traumatic Coma Data Bank (see comments). *Brain Injury, 7,* 101–111.

Teasdale, T.W., & Christensen, A. (1994). Psychosocial outcome in Denmark. In A. Christensen & B.P. Uzzell (Eds.), *Brain injury and neuropsychological rehabilitation: International perspectives.* (pp. 235–244). Hillsdale: Lawrence Erlbaum.

Thompson, R.S., Rivara, F.P., & Thompson, D.C. (1989). A case-control study of the effectiveness of bicycle safety helmets. *New England Journal of Medicine, 320,* 1361–1367.

Uzzell, B.P., Langfitt, T.W., & Dolinskas, C.A. (1987). Influence of injury severity on quality of survival after head injury. *Surgical Neurology, 27,* 419–429.

Wehman, P.H., Kreutzer, J.S., Stonnington, H.H., & Wood, W. (1988). Supported employment for persons with traumatic brain injury: A preliminary report. *Journal of Head Trauma Rehabilitation, 3,* 82–93.

Wehman, P.H., Revell, G., Kregel, J., Kreutzer, J.S., Callahan, C., & Banks, D. (1991). Supported employment: An alternative model for vocational rehabilitation of persons with severe neurologic, psychiatric, or physical disability. *Archives of Physical Medicine and Rehabilitation, 72,* 101–105.

Wehman, P.H., Sherron, P., Kregel, J., Kreutzer, J., Tran, S., & Cifu, D. (1993). Return to work for persons following severe traumatic brain injury: Supported employment outcomes after five years. *American Journal of Physical Medicine and Rehabilitation, 72,* 355–363.

Wilson, B.A. (1992). Recovery and compensatory strategies in head injured memory impaired people several years after insult. *Journal of Neurology, Neurosurgery and Psychiatry, 55,* 177–180.

26 Community Inclusion: The Ultimate Goal of Rehabilitation

Al Condeluci

United Cerebral Palsy
Pittsburgh, PA

INTRODUCTION

The ultimate goal of all rehabilitation efforts is the successful return of disabled individuals to their communities. Although rehabilitation may have many dimensions and aspects, all disciplines consider their efforts successful if individuals are reunited with family and experience meaningful realities within their communities. Indeed, all functions of daily living activities are pointless unless there exists a viable setting in which people can use their renewed skills.

To this end, most rehabilitation practices focus attention and energy on the mastery of community skills, be they physical, cognitive, emotional, sensory, or technical. Success ultimately is the ability to use gains developed in rehabilitation in real community settings. Thus, the focus of most rehabilitation disciplines has been to assess the deficit, determine needs, establish strategies, activate the best strategy, and then evaluate the results. The goal is to redevelop skills or create compensatory skill approaches necessary in the discipline for community success.

In spite of the noble goals and the best intentions of professionals in the field, successful community placements for people with acquired brain injuries leaves much to be desired. The majority of people with disabilities, especially those with severe acquired brain injuries, are not successfully included in the community. In fact, the plethora of long-term community "programs" for people with head injuries has not only created a new industry in rehabilitation but has signaled the clear inability to successfully return individuals to the generic community. Rather than have people with injuries return to their communities, thousands of individuals are being "cared for" in group homes, long-term care facilities, and other separate environments.

To better understand this phenomena, there are a number of ways outcomes can be evaluated in determining community inclusion success. One approach is to look at four critical outcome dimensions and gauge overall realities in each of these areas. Reviews of each area are telling. The dimensions are

1. Where one ends up living.
2. Meaningful community activities.
3. Opportunities for intimacy.
4. Opportunities to rejuvenate.

Where One Ends Up Living

There is no question that housing outcomes after rehabilitation for people with acquired brain injuries are dismal. Most people end up with family members, even though many patients would prefer to be on their own or back with spouses. In a review of 40 people with brain injuries in the greater Buffalo (NY) area (Condeluci & Swales, 1990), 32 people (85%) were living at home primarily with parents. However, these people reported that they were not happy being with their parents or parental-like spouse. Similarly, other studies of people with disabilities who live at home show similar concerns or dissatisfaction. Accessible, affordable, and safe housing is virtually nonexistent for people with disabilities in most areas of North America. In fact, as the housing market continues to shift and rents rise, more and more people are forced to consider less and less desirable settings and locations.

For individuals with brain injuries of a more significant severity, the housing options are even worse. Families are often not able to care for their son/daughter/spouse and must place them in institutional settings. Far too many people with disabilities find themselves in group homes, intermediate care facilities, or long-term care homes designed for the frail elderly.

Meaningful Day Activities

This area refers to work or community options that society would consider meaningful and appropriate for adults, and the realities for people with disabilities is equally tragic. A 1992 Harris poll survey in the United States that explored disability issues found serious deficiencies in the area of employment. Eight-six percent of individuals polled in this large national sample were found to be unemployed or seriously underemployed in America. Those who were employed made significantly less than their non-disabled peers.

Beyond all this, anecdotal reviews of any community gathering venues in America will find a stark absence of people with disabilities. Consider any group or association that you belong to and consider the representation of disability in these groups. How many people with disabilities do you routinely see in your everyday experience? When posed at professional conferences or seminars, the answer to this question is often "none" or "very few."

Beyond these more tangible observations, many individuals with significant disabilities report that even when they are able to engage in a meaningful activity, they are often avoided by their peers. They might be "in" the setting but do not feel "of" the setting.

Opportunities for Intimacy

We know that the divorce and separation rate in Western society today is high. Some estimates put it as high as 50%. Many people have difficulties with intimacy. Still, for people with disabilities, the divorce and separation rate is even higher. Perhaps more devastating is that beyond these intimacy breakups, friendships and support networks also fade away after injury. Personal testimonies from individuals with disabilities and their families continue to confirm the loneliness and isolation often felt.

Indeed, survivor perspectives on their own outcomes confirm the importance of intimacy and relationships (Condeluci, Ferris, & Bogdan, 1992). In three distinct studies, the critical area relating to social and personal connections were rated as very important by people with acquired brain injuries.

More anecdotal feedback continues to confirm the frustration with meeting people and forming lasting, long-term relationships. At the United Cerebral Palsey Center for Personal Development, a community-based setting for people to discuss personal issues in Pittsburgh, PA, one of the most requested topics over the center's 22-year history is the Relationship and Intimacy class. It is an area of interest and need for us all.

Opportunities to Rejuvenate

When looking at the opportunity for people with disabilities to experience recreation, three important variables must be in place. One is the money individuals must have to purchase recreation activities. Even popcorn and a video at home costs money. But most people with disabilities are economically disadvantaged, locked out of jobs and opportunities. Second, individuals must have friends with which to share recreational activities. If friends fade or disappear after disabilities, as most individuals and families report, people will be limited in this area. Finally, individuals must be able to get to and into the place of recreation. Again, transportation and access, even with the advances in America brought on by the Americans With Disabilities Act (ADA, PL101-336), is difficult in most communities today.

Thus, regardless of rehabilitation activities after an injury of disability, people with severe manifestations are largely isolated and excluded from the very things that most of us would consider basic to community inclusion.

This chapter is an exploration and overview of the notion of community. If rehabilitation is to help people set the goal of community inclusion, it is imperative that we better understand the nature of community and, more importantly, find better ways to address this challenge.

A PARADIGM SHIFT

Most rehabilitation efforts for persons with acquired brain injuries are derived from a medical model (NHIF Directory, 1994). This approach is appropriate when the major goal of rehabilitation is to save the person's life or stabilize their vital functions. Indeed, with acquired brain injury advances in medical and early rehabilitation interventions, more people are saved today than ever before. As people continue in the rehabilitation process, however, the goals and challenges begin to shift. After the primary efforts of stabilization have occurred, the focus begins to move from internal to external issues. At some point in the equation, the individual, their family, and the professionals around them begin to think about discharge and community re-entry.

With this shift in mind, professionals in rehabilitation need to understand that a focused body of practice is developing in the area of community inclusion (Taylor, Racino, Knoll, & Lutfiyya, 1987). Researchers and practitioners are recognizing that traditional and medical models need to give way to newer foundations (Zola, 1986). It is becoming commonly accepted in the disability movement that community success and support systems around people with disabilities must take on a broader empowerment focus with an emphasis on interdependence and partnerships (DeJong, 1983; Condeluci, 1991).

This common theme that underscores the interdependent model builds from a community base and is fueled by the notions of capacities and valorization (Wolfensberger, 1992; Condeluci, 1995). The major convictions that underlie this newer model are

- Consumer choice and participation.
- Age appropriateness.
- Right to choose.
- An accepting and respectful environment.

In traditional approaches with acquired brain injuries, patients and their families have little opportunity to participate in decisions. Certainly, they are informed and consulted, but the medical model clearly positions the professional as the expert with much greater capacity to make the best decision. Further, the medical treatment model often offsets and congregates individuals with disabilities in facilities and settings that create a variety of community stigmas. Most community members know the settings in their town where the "handicapped" go for treatment. Indeed, when people are congregated, isolated, sheltered, or segregated, negative dynamics occur (Biklen & Knoll, 1987) including

- labels and stereotypes,
- lack of privacy and control,
- association with others perceived as less valuable,
- lower standards, and
- promotion of dependency.

These dynamics create powerful and often devaluing images of persons with disabilities. They cast a deep stigma in the community's eye that is difficult to erase (Goffman, 1963; Shapiro, 1993). This stigma and negative image follows people with brain injuries as they attempt to re-enter communities. Further, given the deep-rooted dimensions of the medical model, there is a propensity for individuals with disabilities to perceive themselves within the confines of the stereotype. Not only does society see them this way, but they begin to believe that they are sick and incapable (Illich, 1976).

A better understanding of the medical model occurs by comparing it with the community-based, interdependent model (Table 26.1) (Condeluci, 1991).

Table 26.1: Medical Model Compared to Community-Based Model

ISSUE	MEDICAL MODEL	INTERDEPENDENT MODEL
PROBLEM	A damaged brain	Lack of supports
LOCUS	In person	In community
FOCUS	Deficits	Capacities
SOLUTIONS	Classify	Develop supports
	Congregate fix	include power
IN CHARGE	Expert	Individual/Family
OUTCOME	Fix/Accept	Relationships

As this comparison demonstrates, a community-based perspective must shift within the paradigm of treatment from a microscopic perspective of the person or their brain injury as the problem to a more systematic approach with the interdependent model that looks to existing capacities and ways that people can be included and involved. This is not an easy shift for society to make.

In most cultures, differences in people cause exclusions (Condeluci, 1995). Communities often separate people out, both formally and informally, in ways that create stigma and misunderstanding. In any generation, vivid evidence can be found to use differences to discriminate, devalue, or exclude. Civil rights literature in the United States chronicles the phenomena of segregation, devaluation, and oppression that played out in hatred, anger, and death (Branch, 1988; Garrow, 1986). To some extent, some would argue, these manifestations continue today.

These observations have implications for brain injury rehabilitation. When the focus of attention is on what is "wrong" with people or what makes them different, this energy has powerful reaches into the community. The natural result is that typical community members feel no relationship to the "different" person and keep away. More tragically, given the propensity of "special programs," the community abdicates its responsibility to the injured person, yielding to the professional community to "take care" of the injured individual, not only in the acute phase, but for the long term.

A reexamination of current practices should offer a real challenge to acquired brain injury service systems and professionals today. If the medical model produces a deficit approach, then it would follow that these programs are creating even greater gaps with the community. The longer this model prevails, especially after stabilization, the more we will condition the community to keep arms length from people with disabilities.

The interdependent model, however, challenges this assumption. It starts to reframe the basic questions and suggests a focus on the culture and environment. It assumes that the person with the disability can and should take a lead role. It suggests that the target for change is not the individual but the culture at large (i.e., similarities are far greater).

To encourage an interdependent model, however, requires that we know, understand, and can relate to culture and communities. This is where current acquired brain injury rehabilitation has fallen short. Most acquired brain injury rehabilitation efforts attempt to change the person to some extent, even those programs that specialize in community re-entry. When we can no longer dramatically change the person who still manifests challenging behaviors, then the traditional solution is to create segregated, assisted living, or work communities. What has resulted is the growing development of retreats, ranches, farms, group homes, workshops, and other separated residential or activity milieus for long-term support.

Before we relegate these more challenging individuals to separate environments, we can and must do more within our existing environments. We need to test, adjust, and create alternative solutions in an effort to promote more viable community outcomes. To institutionalize one person because we did not try an alternative community approach is not only a tragedy but a travesty in rehabilitation.

UNDERSTANDING COMMUNITY AND CULTURE

"Community" is a concept that is vital to most paradigms today. Industry, education, politics, religion, medicine, and other disciplines speak to the essential inclusion of community into their perspectives. There are a number of ways to look at community, but first we must become familiar with the following definitions:

- *American Heritage Dictionary* (3rd ed., 1992): "A group of people living in the same locality and under the same government. A group of people having common interests with sharing, participation and fellowship."
- *Webster's Dictionary* (Complete Unabridged, 1985): "Community is a unified body of individuals. People with common interests living in a particular area. The area itself. The interacting population of various kinds of individuals. A group of people with common characteristics living together within a large society."
- *The Neighborhood Organizer's Handbook* (Warren & Warren, 1979): "The community of a place—the proximate neighborhood setting is a vital part of growing up, of raising families, of meeting many of the changes and stresses of urban life."
- *Rural Sociology* (Hillary, 1955): "Community is a group integrated through a system of spatially contingent, interdependent biotic, cultural, and social relations and structure which have evolved in the process of mutual adjustments to environmental situations."
- *Beyond Community Services* (McKnight, 1988): "Communities are collective associations. In a sense, they are more different than friendship...it is groups of people who work together in a face-to-face basis and are engaged in public rather than private life."
- *Community Structure and Analysis* (Sussman, 1959): "Community is a human population living in a given geographical area which has interdependence and often specialization of function and which shares a common culture."
- *Quest For Community* (Nisbit, 1972): "Community thrives on self-help, either corporate or individual, in everything that removes a group from the performance on an involvement in its own government can hardly help but weaken the sense of community. People do not come together in significant and lasting associations merely to be together; they come together to do something that can not easily be done in individual isolation."
- *Discovering Community* (O'Brien, 1986): "We can promote a sense of community if we develop the competence to overcome our habits of segregation, professionalization, and bureaucratization on even the smallest scale. Discovering community means testing the everyday assumptions of the service world through the actions of reflections."
- *The Gift of Hospitality* (O'Connell, 1988): "Community is no different for people with disabilities than for any of the rest of us. It is the free space where people think for themselves, dream their dreams, and come together to create and celebrate their community humanity."

In a broader sense, community relates to vital human interaction. It is when people come together for a common purpose. Community recognizes a need for privacy but equally allows for a fluid flow of integration and interchange. Given this dimension of communality, it is easy to pervert the nature of community by suggesting that people of common identity *should* all live together. This approach has been followed when groups of people such as those who are disabled have been segregated into common environments. Some experts in brain injury rehabilitation have argued that such common settings for people with acquired brain injuries might be the best long-term solution. This perspective needs to be understood as a perversion of the community definition. A key factor in community is the freedom to choose. There is a fundamental difference between choosing to be with people of common bond, such as ethnic or religious similarity, and being relegated to such settings by others who think it is best.

An easy way to understand the real nature of community is to compare it to structured human service settings such as sheltered workshops or group homes. McKnight (1988) suggests that one of the differences between human service settings and natural communities is that human services operate on *control* while communities operate on *consent*.

There is no question that organized human service settings are structured and controlled. They operate from a command paradigm where a single leader makes a decision, and there often is little debate. I have visited countless human service long-term support settings, even those purporting to be "community-based," that required me to sign in and had a bevy of policies and procedures that drove the system. On the other hand, most community settings are more informal. Although there may be manifestations of structure with formal and informal rules and regulations, the focus of action is, for the most part, driven by consent.

Second, human services are slow and deliberate while communities respond quickly. As structured systems, human service entities follow procedure and the chain of command. Often, any ideas, even those that might require immediate response, must go through a tedious process before they are accepted. I have experienced systems that dictate that ideas must be framed with "white papers" that define and defend their efficacy, then be subjected to a committee review before they will be considered for implementation. Conversely, when something needs to happen in community setting, there is no need for "white papers." People gear up and take on what needs to be done. This spirit of quick response, however, seems to have been perverted by specialization (Illich, 1976); that is, as communities become more and more organized, specialization grows and begins to stunt quick actions by deferring to the "experts" (Horton, 1990).

Third, human services require channeled solutions while communities inspire creative reactions. There is no question that creativity can be stunted by the tedious process of approval and sanctioning. As an idea gets deliberated, it is often distilled. The net result is often a softer and often less efficient version of the idea. With communities, however, ideas are usually quickly embraced and carried out.

The difference between assisted settings, such as those set up for people with acquired brain injuries and the community at large is (Table 26.2) further elaborated by O'Connell (1988).

Table 26.2: Comparison of Assisted Settings and Community Settings

ASSISTED SETTINGS	COMMUNITY
People are known by what's wrong, their label, or their condition.	People are known as individuals.
People are incomplete, need to be changed or fixed.	People are as they are with opportunity to be.
Relationships are unequal—workers do for the client.	Relationships are reciprocal.
People are broken into parts, separated into groups.	People are accepted as whole and viewed as a part of whole society.
Problems are solved by consulting authorities, policies, procedures.	People seek answers from their own experience and the wisdom of others.
There is no room to acknowledge mistakes and uncertainty.	People can make honest efforts and acknowledge honest mistakes and fear.
All problems have national solutions.	There is room for confusion, mystery, and recognition that some things are beyond human control.

Clearly, assisted settings, as are typical in long-term arrangements for people with brain injuries, follow an assisted living script. In most cases, they are influenced by the medical model perspective. By using an interdependent model and coming to understand one about community, perhaps the goals of inclusion and re-entry might be more enhanced.

To understand community, there are other dimensions to be considered. Mial suggested five ways to examine the concept of community (1960) as follows:

1. As a geographic area.
2. As a legal unit of government.
3. As a set of attitudes, beliefs, and loyalties.
4. As a collection of neighborhoods.
5. As a network of associations.

Although the term "community" can have broader implications such as in describing a collection of people (i.e., disability community), it can also be used in other descriptive formats.

Another analysis of community (Warren & Warren, 1979) identifies six distinct functions of community as follows:

1. As a **SOCIABILITY ARENA**. This refers to the social relationships that can grow from community.
2. As an **INTERPERSONAL INFLUENCE CENTER.** This refers to the interpersonal supports that people share when in distress.
3. For **MUTUAL AID.** This level deals with the banding together that can happen when disasters occur.
4. As an **ORGANIZATIONAL BASE.** At this level, associations occur around points of mutual interest.
5. As a **REFERENCE GROUP.** This dimension suggests an identification often associated with pride or location.
6. As a **STATUS ARENA**. This final category serves to allow neighbors to gauge or parade their status in the community.

These functions offer some sense of the purpose that communities serve. All or some of these six functions come into play when people gather together in some common proximity. Beyond this, Warren and Warren also focus on the formal dimensions of community as follows:

1. **INTEGRAL**. Here the community is closely linked and woven together. Players have a deep and common bond.
2. **PAROCHIAL**. At this level, the community is bonded together, but some of the close linkages may be missing.
3. **DIFFUSE**. This third level finds a community that has a common identity, but is missing some of the close interactions.
4. **STEPPING STONE**. This community type allows for interactions and linkages but is often missing identity.
5. **TRANSITORY**. These settings offer occasional linkages between players but are missing the depth of identity.
6. **ANOMIC**. This final category finds almost no commonality between players. People keep to themselves and have little, if any, reliance on each other.

These formal dimensions of community are helpful in considering the challenge of incorporating an interdependent paradigm. If the goal of rehabilitation is to ultimately assist people as they form relationships between family, neighbors, and former friends, we must understand community territory and dimensions. Quite clearly, the typography identified by Warren and Warren shows a cascading interpersonal flow of community. This kind of understanding ought to be factored into the rehabilitation process when we attempt to facilitate the community placement process.

A final point in the examination of community rests with an acknowledgment of culture. Often the concepts of community and culture are blended, yet they do have distinct elements. Culture is a network of people bound together by some common cause or interest (Condeluci, 1995). This broader definition can relate to groups of people that are also defined in the context of community (e.g., a church community is indeed a culture, but a neighborhood, although people share space, may not hold all the variables of culture).

Cultures are distinguished by common rituals, rules, boundaries, and jargon. They have either formal or informal leaders, and membership is held constant by at least one prevailing theme that everyone holds dear. New members often have to prove themselves before they are invited to join or become accepted into the culture. Indeed, in most all cultures, before newcomers get fully sanctioned within the culture, they usually are escorted by an accepted or respected member. These people who reach across the boundaries of the culture are called "gatekeepers."

This notion of the gatekeeper is a potentially helpful one for rehabilitators to understand. For people to truly be included into a culture requires that insiders approve. Regardless of the physical or functional gains that rehabilitation can help with, these things are useless in the goal of inclusion if a gatekeeper is not available to guide people in. Most people reading this chapter probably have had personal experience with gatekeepers. Some have served as gatekeepers, and others have become sanctioned themselves because of them. All of us have experienced the relevance of this phenomena of becoming valued within the context of culture.

Some types of cultures that might have relevance in the process of rehabilitation include

1. Family culture.
2. Spiritual culture.
3. Work culture.
4. Age culture.
5. Neighborhood culture.
6. Ethnic culture.
7. Sex or sexual orientation culture.
8. Common interest culture.

All of these areas are clear cultures, and many are types of communities as well. Each category has its clear boundaries and points of common interest. These areas also can play a critical role in the inclusion of people with brain injuries. The more that support people understand the elements that influence these cultures, the easier it might be to find gatekeepers and guides that can escort the estranged individual back into the culture. The important element, however, is that the individual with a disability has, or subscribes to, the commonality that bands the culture together.

IMPLICATIONS FOR REHABILITATION AND ACQUIRED BRAIN INJURY

One way to implement a holistic approach is to orchestrate a circle of community support around the person. This circle consists of a variety of players—some are professionals and others are from the community—who talk with and commit to a plan for the person with the brain injury. This gathering is not a staffing in the traditional sense, but a brainstorming session where those around the individual with a disability, be they in a home, work, or community setting, can speak to or commit to a part of a community inclusion plan. The only goal of the circle gathering should be to promote and keep the individual with a disability involved within the community.

This circle of support concept has worked successfully in a variety of settings (O'Brien & Lyle, 1987). In many of these contexts are neighbors, friends, associates, family members, or professionals, all ready and willing to see the individual with a disability return to the community.

This circle-of-friends approach can work well with people with a brain injury as they attempt to re-enter clubs, groups, associations, work, the church, or any other type of cultural gathering. Indeed, when a valued member of a group joins the circle of friends, they can also serve as a gatekeeper who can guide the individual with a disability back into the group. When other members of the group see the gatekeeper with the disabled individual, the natural reaction is to welcome the person back to the group. In a way, the value attributed to the gatekeeper gets transferred to the individual with a disability, making their acceptance and inclusion that much easier. This process is called "cultural diffusion."

This shift in value from one person to another follows a concept called "Valued Image Juxtaposition" (Wolfensberger, 1971) (i.e., when a person who already holds value in a cultural setting is juxtaposed with an individual who has no value to the group or might be devalued by society). In general, their value will rise with the group. Conversely, when a person who is devalued by society is juxtaposed with another who is equally devalued, the net effect will be a continuation of devaluation for both people. In either example, it is important to know that value spreads between people either up or down the scale.

SHIFTING ROLES FOR REHABILITATION

Given a sensitivity to community, culture, and the interdependent paradigm, a number of new roles emerge to support people with acquired brain injuries. These roles build from the basic notion of inclusion and offer some community possibilities as follows:

- *Community Case Manager.* This role is key for basic management of community issues. In many situations, the case manager has solid history with the survivor. This person can play a primary role in balancing the myriad of issues that emerge when people return to the community.
- *Personal Attendant.* These support people provide direct physical and/or cognitive supports for the individual with a brain injury. As the first person to interrelate with the survivor each morning, the personal attendant can help set a

positive tone. Fears, concerns, and anxieties can be discussed before the survivor sets out for the day.

- *Bridgebuilder.* This newer role has been found to be extremely helpful to individuals with disabilities who return to community (Mount, Beeman, & Ducharme, 1988). The bridgebuilder ensures that the person with an acquired brain injury is a viable player in the community. They are concerned about linking the individual to typical and natural relationships. The community bridgebuilder attempts to find an interest or link for the individual to their neighborhood. These interests, such as a hobby or avocation, function as a "ticket" to commonality. All people have tickets to commonality, and the bridgebuilder finds and then uses these gifts to connect people.

- *The Family.* As simple as it may seem, community success in brain injury rehabilitation is critically tied to family intervention and support. Community rehabilitators know all too well that the inclusion plans that really succeed are the ones that are supported by families. Indeed, if the family is against the community plans, the potential for success will be greatly compromised. As with the personal attendant, the family can hold the key to attitude, motivation, and consequently, success. Family energy is powerful and needs to be drawn into a holistic approach.

CULTURING COMMUNITY

Often, when the topic of community comes up in rehabilitation discussions, the inference is that of community education. Most people think that to consider community is to assure that the community comes to understand disability, and through this understanding, comes to be more inclusive. In reality, the notion of harnessing community in the rehabilitation process is very different from the concept of community education.

Community education is a deliberate and focused attempt to promote a particular thesis to a particular group of people. The educator has a plan and often compliments his/her approach with books, pamphlets, materials, etc. The goal is to get the audience to appreciate the new concept and then to take some action. It implies that the teacher knows more than the audience, and the goal of teaching is to transmit this new information to the group.

Culturation, on the other hand, is a much more informal process. It is the insidious transmission of information, usually between peers. It is about presence, patterns, and observable cues that are couched in the environment and language of the members of the culture. It is about informal leadership patterns, valued roles, and influential cultural features that lead the way to appreciation and understanding.

Often, community education is antiseptic and downward (i.e., the teacher packages the information, introduces it to the audience, then tests or hopes that the audience will retain the information and use it as it was intended). With culturation, the process is different. It is not clear who influences the process and exactly when the information might play out. As something new, such as a person or a new idea, is introduced to the culture, it is done so in a softer way. People just come to know through presence and constancy.

To a certain extent, culturation is a process that anchors because it stands the test of time. Community education, on the other hand, can be manipulated or perverted in a way that it may not make a real impact on the audience. If we want a community to be more inclusive of people with acquired brain injuries, is it better to call a town meeting and teach the neighbors about disability, or do we find some valued neighbors and introduce them to a neighbor with an acquired brain injury and hope the connection and presence of the person with the disability makes an impact?

This is not to suggest that culturation is a panacea, an easy answer to the community inclusion challenge. It does have some clear drawbacks. One is its slow pace and tedious approach. Culturation requires a constant presence which takes time. Another challenge is that many variables of the community are uncontrollable. This means that the community builder must accept the uncertainty that goes with the culturation. Regardless, when thinking about the challenge of inclusion, culturation offers a solid alternative for the rehabilitation professional.

CONCLUSION

Understanding community and culture are critical to enhancing the long-term re-entry success for people with acquired brain injuries. Historically, these individuals have been treated from a medical model, yet if we are to truly be successful, we must create a bridge and dialogue between the medical and interdependent paradigms. Professionals in rehabilitation must come to understand the viability of interdependence, community, and culturation and include these principles in their work.

We know that people with acquired brain injuries want to belong to community. We also know that the traditional approaches have not produced the outcomes we would like to see. By adopting an interdependent perspective and using a culturation approach, we may be able to enhance opportunities for people to become reintegrated into their respective lives.

Know, however, that this will not be easy. The medical model has cast deep roots, and most rehabilitators are comfortable with a treatment-based model. Still, we must be open. If we have not enjoyed the outcomes by which people with acquired brain injuries are easily incorporated into their previous neighborhoods and groups, then change must occur.

Life is a tight ecological web with links up and down the scale. Our micro worlds— our abilities, personality, and character—are uniquely related to our macro world— family, friends, community, and greater society. One cannot be considered without the other. Considering the ideas explored in this chapter does just that, blending the personal with the societal. To do anything less is to continue to keep people apart. We can, and we must do more.

REFERENCES

Biklen, D., & Knoll, J. (1987). The disabled minority. In S. Taylor, D. Biklen, & J. Knoll (Eds.), *Community integration for people with severe disabilities.* New York: Teachers' College Press.

Branch, T. (1989). *Parting the waters.* New York: Simon & Schuster.

Condeluci, A. (1991). *Interdependence.* Winter Park, FL: GR Press.

———. (1995). *Interdependence* (2nd ed). Delray Beach, FL: St. Lucie Press.

———. (1995). *Beyond difference.* Delray Beach: St. Lucie Press.

Condeluci, A., Ferris, L., & Bogdan, A. (1992). The survivor perspective. *Journal of Head Trauma Rehabilitation, 7*(4), 37–45.

Condeluci, A., & Swales, P. (1990). *From no one to someone.* Buffalo, NY: Headway for Brain Injured.

Garrow, D. (1986). *Bearing the cross.* New York: Morrow and Co.

Goffman, E. (1960). *Stigma.* New Jersey: Prentice Hall.

Harris Survey. (1992). *Disabled American's self perception: Bringing disabled Americans into the mainstream.* Washington, DC: Federal Register.

Hillary, G. (1955). The community. *Rural Sociology, 20,* 52–68.

Horton, M. (1990). *The long haul.* New York: Doubleday.

Illich, I. (1976). *Medical nemesis.* New York: Pantheon.

McKnight, J. (1988). *Beyond community services.* Evanston, IL: Northwestern Center For Urban Affairs.

Mial, D. (1960). *Our communities.* New York: NYU Press.

Mount, B., Beeman, P., & Ducharme, G. (1988). *What we are learning about bridgebuilding.* Manchester, CT: Communities, Inc.

NHIF. (1944). *Directory of services.* Washington, DC: NHIF.

Nisbit, R. (1972). *Quest for community.* New York: Oxford University Press.

O'Brien, J. (1988). *Discovering community.* Decatur, GA: Responsive Systems Association.

O'Brien, J., & Lyle, C. (1987). *Framework for accomplishment.* Decatur, GA: Responsive Systems Association.

O'Connell, M. (1988). *The gift of hospitality.* Evanston, IL: Northwest Center for Urban Policy.

Shapiro, J. (1993). *No pity.* New York: Times Books.

Sussman, M. (1959). *Community structure and analysis.* NY: Thomas Crowell Co.

Taylor, S., Racino, J., Knoll, J., & Luftiyya, Z. (1987). Down Home. In S. Taylor, D. Biklen, & J. Knoll (Eds.), *Community integration for people with severe disabilities.* New York: Teachers' College Press.

Warren, R., & Warren, D. (1979). *The neighborhood organizer's handbook.* Notre Dame, IN: Notre Dame Press.

Wolfensberger, W. (1971). *Normalization.* Toronto, ON: NIMR.

———. (1992). *A brief introduction to social role valorization as a high-order concept for structuring human services* (Rev. ed.). Syracuse, NY: Training Institute for Human Service Planning, Leadership and Change Agentry.

PART V:

SPECIAL TOPICS

27 Traumatic Brain Injury in Children: Neuropsychological, Behavioral, and Educational Issues

Ronald C. Savage,[1] Dennis C. Russo,[1,2] and Rita Gardner[1]

[1]The May Institute, Randolph, MA
[2]Department of Psychiatry, Harvard Medical School, Boston, MA

INTRODUCTION

Throughout the world, injury and disease disrupt the lives of many of our children and youth. Injury, in general, is the leading cause of disability among children between birth and age 19 (Savage, 1993). Traumatic brain injury (TBI) is the largest killer and disabler of children and adolescents of all types of injury (IBIA, 1995; NHIF, 1992; Baker, O'Neill, & Karpf, 1984). The number of children and adolescents sustaining brain injuries is staggering. Epidemiologic estimates in several countries indicate 220 to 300/100,000 youths under the age of 15 will sustain a brain injury each year (Annegers, Grabow, Kurland et al., 1980; IBIA, 1995). Infants and toddlers who sustain injuries from abuse are not often recorded in our head trauma registries, yet it is estimated that two-thirds of these children suffer head trauma (NHIF, 1992). For teenagers, due to their active lifestyles, these estimates can increase to 600/100,000 in youths between the ages of 15 and 20 years (NHIF, 1992; Klauber, Barrett-Conner, Marshall, & Laws, 1991). With regard to TBI, over 1 million children in the United States are injured annually, with 165,000 of them requiring hospitalization. Sixteen to twenty-thousand of those children experience severe, life-long sequelae as a result of their injury (NHIF, 1992).

The National Pediatric Trauma Registry (NPTR, 1993) has, since 1985, gathered data on the causes, circumstances, and consequences of injuries to 28,692 children who were admitted to 61 children's hospitals or trauma centers in the United States. As recorded by the Registry, TBI in children was caused by motor vehicle accidents, falls, pedestrian injuries, near drownings, other trauma, gunshot wounds, and physical abuse. TBI was the most frequent injury diagnosis (28%), followed by fractures to the bones of extremities and torso and open wounds. The presence of TBI was associated with a three-fold increase in the likelihood of four or more functional limitations (i.e., vision, hearing, speech, self-feeding, bathing, dressing, walking, cognition, and behavior).

Advances in emergency medical treatment and technologically innovative care during the critical, acute recovery phase have improved the odds of surviving a TBI while increasing the need for TBI rehabilitation programming and long-term services. The burden of responsibility for the care of TBI survivors rests with medical specialists, allied rehabilitation therapists, primary care physicians, educators, and families. Each has a role in caring for the child or adolescent survivor that requires a knowledge of the brain behavior relationship associated with the injury, sensitivity to the individual's awareness of the injury, the child's developmental needs, and comprehensive educational planning. This chapter will focus on the cognitive, psychological, and educational issues facing professionals dealing with school-age students who have experienced TBI.

Once the student's acute medical condition is stabilized after a TBI, his/her cognitive and behavioral functioning should be determined. Disruption in general cognitive functioning can originate from inaccuracies in the sensory input or reception and storage of environmental information or be traced to inaccuracies and disruption in the organization and output (expression) of information produced by the students themselves. The observed impact of an injury can result from physical injuries separate from the brain injury (e.g., a broken hip), be an expression of the brain injury itself (e.g., ataxia), or a reaction to the deficits associated with the both types of injuries (e.g., irritability). Thus, the degree of brain damage can be observed in the behavioral and cognitive deficits associated with a particular part of the brain and the extent to which a disruption in communication from one area of the brain to another occurs. For example, damage to the mid-brain, including the limbic system, may result in underarousal or overarousal and may manifest itself as lethargy and depression (e.g., basal ganglia damage) or agitation (e.g., damage to the reticular activating system). Plasticity and compensation in the areas of the brain that are damaged, in addition to the extent of injury, account for the temporary or long-term nature of the behavioral and cognitive deficits noted.

Higher order cognitive functioning is centered in the cortex, the "thinking" part of the brain. Anatomically, the area from the sensory strip posterior, including the parietal, temporal, and occipital lobes can be thought of as the sensory input area of the brain. Damage to the occipital lobe can affect visual input and visual perception even though the eyes themselves are not damaged. Lesions in the parietal lobes can affect tactile input, and damage to the temporal lobes can affect auditory input of information and memory. The output region of the brain is from the motor strip anterior (the frontal lobes). Despite intact sensory input, if this area of the brain is damaged, the student may have difficulty in effectively using the information received. Hemispheric differences are also present in the brain. Injury to either hemisphere, coup-contracoup injuries, shearing injuries, or damage to the corpus callosum can severely effect the ability of the brain to receive, process, store, and use information. The most common cognitive complaints following a brain injury are difficulty in learning, decreased memory and concentration, decreased intelligence, and slowing of cognitive processes (Klonoff, Clark, & Klonoff, 1993). Unfortunately, even mild TBI can have a long-term impact on the student's cognitive functioning (Klonoff et al., 1993; Eichelberger & Ball, 1991; Savage, 1987), and these deficits are often diagnostic when neurologic data (e.g., CAT, MRI) are equivocal. Processing difficulties, memory storage and retrieval deficits, and other higher level cognitive skills can be assessed through neuropsychological testing and integrated with other neurologic data.

NEUROPSYCHOLOGICAL ASSESSMENT

The neurological data obtained from CT and MRI scans is invaluable in isolating the specific structural areas of the student's brain that have suffered damage, assuming the injury is not mild (Zasler, 1993). But the relationship of the damage to functional ability is ascertained through neuropsychological assessment. The neuropsychological examination varies in format—tests chosen and order of presentation or protocol—based on the referral question but, in general, evaluates the student's cognitive abilities, visual/perceptual/motor abilities, and psychological functioning. Information from the neuropsychological evaluation is used to establish the student's base level of functioning, which can then be used to develop rehabilitation programming and to monitor progress during the recovery period. The latter is especially important during childhood because the brain continues to develop and/or organize independent of the injury throughout this period (Allison, 1992; Lehr & Savage, 1990; Savage, 1987). Without ongoing assessment, additional "hidden" deficits may appear when the student fails to reach a developmental milestone or obtain certain concepts.

The psychological tests available for the neuropsychological assessment of children with TBI are numerous (see Begali, 1992). Franzen and Berg (1989) and Spreen and Strauss (1991) also describe many of the fixed batteries and individual psychological tests available to the neuropsychologist. The domains covered by these assessments include general cognitive abilities (including academic achievement), sensory perceptual, visual/perceptual/motor, attention, concentration, memory, executive processing, behavioral, and psychosocial functioning.

Assessment of cognitive abilities includes determining if past academic functioning and remote memory for personal information are intact and to what degree the student has the ability to learn new information. Both types of learning play an important prognostic role in the assessment of cognitive function. It has been the experience of clinicians and teachers that total amnesia, except for the accident events, is rare among students with brain injury. Rather, there is an "islands of knowledge" phenomenon where gaps in information and skills surround fragments of memory. In addition, skills learned immediately prior to the injury are more likely disrupted than overlearned concepts (Levin, Culhane, & Hartman, 1991). For instance, initially on return to school after a TBI, some students may appear academically intact, especially if they were above average prior to their accident (Savage & Wolcott, 1988). These students may "coast" on their old learning, only to have their performance drop below grade level as new information must be assimilated (Klonoff et al., 1993).

The value of neuropsychological assessment to the care of a student with TBI becomes clearer when difficulties in each domain are highlighted. In regard to academic achievement, previous school records are compared with current academic performance, and gaps in recall of information are noted. If such gaps are present, the evaluation will determine if the student is having difficulty in the recall of information, a slowness in processing directions, or interference from other deficits such as fine motor difficulties during a task (e.g., arithmetic calculations). The results of standardized assessments of academic achievement can be validated in the classroom through discussion with the student's teacher and the examination of regular academic work (e.g., mathematics worksheets).

Probably the most critical factor involved in an student's adaptation to daily activities and certainly school performance is the level of their executive functioning. In this domain, neuropsychological assessment is expanding to include a wider range of quali-tative and quantitative measures (Lezak, 1993) so that the subtle but significant difficul-ties encountered can be diagnosed. Injury to the frontal lobe and temporal horn due to the sharp projections of the skull (e.g., the sphenoid processes, posterior to the orbits) is common in students who receive TBIs. Executive functioning is associated with frontal lobe integrity and includes the ability to monitor and regulate one's behavior, the ability to profit from feedback (including mistakes), the ability to maintain and switch sets (cognitive flexibility), the inhibition of impulses, and the lack of perseveration in re-sponses. Deficits in these areas can be devastating.

BEHAVIORAL ASSESSMENT

Neuropsychological assessment often takes place in-vacuo (i.e., the tests themselves are designed to measure primary neuropsychological functions). Testing is, therefore, conducted in sterile surroundings, with stimulation carefully controlled, in order to tease out the particular mosaic of deficits present in a particular student. Such static testing needs to be supplemented with more dynamic, in-vivo behavioral assessment. While the mapping of dysfunction is critical to the design of educational and rehabilitative pro-grams, it is behavior in context that proves to be the major stumbling block of children with brain injuries.

Indeed, initial deficit that is the direct result of trauma is elaborated through the history of the child's contacts with his world. TBI is a chronic impairment, and education efforts need to be focused on long-term behavioral issues as well as short-term medical-restorative rehabilitation. Viewing the problematic behavior of children with TBI from a behavioral perspective, one can see that it is the normal outcome of the injury and requires aggressive intervention (Russo & Navalta, 1995).

Over time, cognitive handicaps become associated with success or failure, secondary gain, or escape from demands, and these "learned" elaborations may be primary prob-lems, even early in the recovery process from brain injury. Such cognitive deficits influence complex learning. This type of learning is frequently seen in understanding the meaning of other's behavior, in the development of social relationships, and in the control of one's environments. Such social situations are conditional, as opposed to neuropsycho-logical tests which are more linear in construction. The behavior analysis must be designed to understand the child's behavior in the context of daily living: how a child becomes frustrated and aggressive in reaction to verbally presented instructions due to auditory sequencing issues; how unsuccessful social interaction produces withdrawl and depression; or how impulsivity places a child at risk for further injury. It is not sufficient to merely identify these tendencies in neuropsychological assessment in the rehabilitation or hospital setting. The specific ways they manifest themselves in the real world must be studied as well in order to formulate an adequate plan for their remediation. The home and school, and interactions with peers and families, therefore, become the testing suite for behavioral assessment.

Fortunately, there exists a wide array of techniques for the functional assessment of behavior that have been developed for use with other populations. Behavior management strategies (Cohen, 1986), research-based educational programming (Ewing-Cobbs et al., 1986), and functionally based assessment (Haley, Hallenborg, & Gans, 1989) are crucial factors in re-entry into the school setting, a process that has been recognized as a critical phase in recovery for children with TBI (Carney & Gerring, 1990). Behavioral programs for children with brain injury are well developed (Deaton, 1987), and their value in teaching academic skills is documented (Glang, Singer, Cooley, & Tish, 1992).

Inclusive in the functional analysis process must be an analysis of the communication environment and communication abilities of the injured child. There is a growing body of literature that establishes the need for behavioral assessment to include the communicative nature of behavior. This assessment allows for the development of communication-based, alternative strategies (Bird, Dorez, Moniz, & Robinson, 1989; Durand, 1990; Reichle & Wacker, 1993). In establishing mechanisms that ensure a child's individual functional communication ability, the family communication system and the school environment are critical to reestablish positive living relationships (Ylvisaker, Feeney, & Urbanczyk, 1993). After a TBI is incurred, communication systems may be significantly altered, and collaboration with the speech-language pathologists and behavior analysts will facilitate in an integrated intervention system to facilitate a child's behavioral progress (Ylvisaker & Feeney, 1994).

While children with TBI are significantly different in the etiology and causation of their behavior than noninjured peers or other populations such as children with retardation, autism, or birth-related, cognitive defects, the general approach of behavioral functional analysis is useful with this population.

What is clearly necessary is an integration of behavioral assessment with neurospychological assessment (i.e., how impairment and subsequent disability become a handicap to the child). Too often, studies in the literature of behavioral treatment have focused primarily on the typography rather than its function (Burke & Lewis, 1986; Wood, 1988; Zencius, Wesolwski, & Burke, 1989).

Precursors to behavioral treatment require an understanding of the specific history of disease or trauma, a clear neurological diagnosis, an evaluation of the "epoch" of recovery, and an evaluation of the patient's neuropsychological limitations and strengths. These antecedents to behavioral analysis allow the educational assessor to identify areas of deficit that are neurologically motivated, to create plans for "compensatory strategies" to assist in learning, and to prevent behavioral efforts from being aimed at areas for which little hope of modification exists.

A behavioral analysis is then conducted for the particular behavior involved. The behavior is, first, operationally defined, a method for its measurement is developed, and a base rate is obtained. A functional assessment then evaluates when and why the behavior occurs. The assessment tests hypotheses such as "the behavior functions to produce attention for the child," "the behavior functions to reduce demand or allow escape or avoidance," or "the behavior is self-stimulatory in nature." A given behavior may exhibit any or all of these functions. Additionally, with a brain injury, children may exhibit neurologically motivated behaviors such as impulsive behavior, aggression, hyperactivity, hypersexuality, lack of memory, or poor attention. An understanding of or hypothesis about the causation of behavior allows intelligent treatment to be conducted both to reduce problem behaviors and to increase positive behaviors. Likewise, functional assessment provides valuable clues as to the most appropriate locus of treatment. Treatment in such conditions may focus on antecedents, on consequences, or on the training of alternative behaviors.

In summary, behavioral treatment needs to be based on an understanding of the context of behavior, the characteristics of the learner, the type of behavioral difficulty, and the motivation and causation of behavior in order for effective educational to occur.

RETURNING TO SCHOOL

Returning to school and home is a primary goal for students after a TBI (Savage & Wolcott, 1988; Ylvisaker, 1991; Begali, 1992; Blosser & DePompei, 1994). It may also be a very challenging time for the student, the family, the child's friends, and the school. Carefully coordinated planning is necessary to create a successful school re-entry for these students, a process that begins shortly after the injured student is medically stable and may continue for several years after returning to school.

Too often children are discharged from acute medical facilities without receiving adequate recommendations for rehabilitation or education. Children may actually be more vulnerable to the effects of brain injury when compared with adults (Isaacson, 1975), even though hypotheses such as greater plasticity of the brain during childhood (Rosner, 1974) suggest that children's recovery after brain injury is superior to that of adults. Inaccurate professional perceptions of the impact of brain injury on children (Hart & Faust, 1988) may lead to incorrect treatment or in not providing treatment at all. It is, unfortunately, the case that their relatively good physical recovery becomes the focus of the acute care team, and specific education and recommendations for return to the community are not often forthcoming (Lash, Russo, Navalta, & Baryza, in press). During the first several years after discharge, children's behavior may deteriorate with new behavioral disorders, learning problems, and social difficulties arising (Russo & Navalta, 1995; Rutter, Chadwick, Shaffer, & Brown, 1980).

The return to school can, therefore, be devastating if the healthcare facility (hospital or rehabilitation center) and the student's home school do not interact as soon as possible and as often as possible (Carter & Savage, 1988; Ylvisaker et al., 1991; Begali, 1992; Mira et al., 1992; Lash, 1992). Hence, as soon as a child or an adolescent is admitted to a healthcare facility, the school re-entry and transition process needs to start. Healthcare professionals need to immediately inform the school that they are presently caring for one of their students. They should then arrange to have the family and/or the attending physician formally request that the school come in and evaluate the child.

This evaluation is the important first step in initiating the special education process and services the student may need. Unfortunately, many students are not referred to the school system for evaluation and are merely discharged back to school with little, if any, support services in place (Savage, 1991). While brain injury creates new deficits, it also affects the performance of previously learned skills as well. Other premorbid factors such as substance abuse, psychiatric history, and dysfunctional families (Rivara et al., 1993) are also likely to affect school re-entry and lead to increased post-traumatic behavior disorders.

This underscores the role of the healthcare providers as advocates for their student-patient. If a physician, for example, acts promptly and immediately refers the student for a special education evaluation, the school-based special educators or psychologists can then visit the student in the healthcare facility prior to discharge and decide what kinds of services the student and family will need and how to best coordinate these services with the healthcare facility and the school. (Savage, 1991; Ylvisaker et al., 1991). Developing communication protocols between healthcare facilities, school systems, and families will help eliminate the "cracks" between systems to which all too many students and their families fall victim.

Just as there are great differences in the needs of students returning to school after TBI, so also are there substantial differences in the experience, knowledge, and skill of school staff, in the systems available to serve complex students in community schools, and in the degree of flexibility that teachers, administrators, and others bring to educational decision making for students with disability. Most educational systems do not have the training or funds required to meet the needs of children with TBI (Cooley & Singer, 1991). Increasing efforts to educate professionals regarding brain injury are, however, occurring (Blosser & DePompei, 1991).

There is wide disparity in the ability of educational systems to serve the child with brain injury. Many schools need little more than an update from the hospital about the student's current level of performance. Others require serious staff training and improved systems for flexible educational planning. Healthcare professionals may be helpful in orienting school staff to critical issues in TBI, just as school staff can help hospital professionals make their assessments and interventions more relevant to the student's educational needs.

Once the school has determined that the student is in need of special education services and has appropriately identified the student as a student with TBI, then the school can begin to develop an individual education plan (IEP). The IEP can serve as the contract between the student's family and the school system regarding the kinds and extent of services the student needs (Carter & Savage, 1988; Ylvisaker et al., 1991). In the case of those students whose TBIs are mild, comprehensive special education programming may not be immediately necessary. Those students may only need to be monitored or have their schedules modified for a period of time to insure that any neurologic sequela has resolved. During this time, the school nurse, classroom teachers, and family can then alert the student's physician and/or neuropsychologist to any persistent problems the student may experience.

In the case of students with more severe injuries, the initial IEP should be a "joint venture" among the healthcare facility, the school, and the family. This initial IEP can reflect the neuromotor, cognitive, and psychosocial needs of the student from a functionally based and process-centered approach that will enable students to become increasingly more involved in their school, family, and community as they continue to recover.

For example, consider a student with a TBI who is back in school but is experiencing difficulty remembering historical dates and facts in social studies class. This student may need a work area in the classroom restructured to enhance attention and concentration and to use specific memory strategies to help store and retrieve information. Such therapeutic interventions that worked well in the rehabilitation setting can be carried over into the school setting and shared with the family so that they can be continued at home. When early collaborative planning starts in the rehabilitation setting and is extended into the school, it helps merge the healthcare and school systems with the family in a unified, ongoing program. Again, with the IEP, everyone can negotiate and agree to service delivery models that are in the best interests of the student.

PLANNING THE ACADEMIC PROGRAM

Healthcare facilities and school systems that have "connected" their services have also learned that "school re-entry" is not a one-time event in the student's life. Returning to school is a series of transitions from the moment the student is injured until he graduates from school and beyond. When changes in behavior or performance are observed, teachers, possibly in consultation with the school psychologist, counselor, or special educator, must decide what accommodations will be necessary and effective and how long they should be in place. The goal is to help the student avoid academic and social failure during the period of time that he/she is recovering from the injury, while simultaneously not creating dependence on accommodations. The following are illustrations of frequently used accommodations:

1. Reduced assignments.
2. Increased time to complete assignments or tests or to respond in class.
3. An assignment book to keep track of assignments and a meeting with the teacher at the end of the day to ensure that the student knows what homework to do.
4. Rest periods during the day.
5. Clear orientation to tasks, with outlines for large tasks and study guides.
6. Explanation to peers of the short-term consequences of TBI, along with counseling of peers to ensure their understanding of impulsive or otherwise socially awkward behavior.

Hence, classrooms, curricula, and teacher responsibilities may need to be reconfigured to deal with these cognitive and psychological needs so learning can occur. For example, counseling supports may need to be set up to help the student discuss personal feelings and learn ways to accommodate socially, and additional family/community services may need to be increased to insure long-term success. Or the student may need to "check in" with the special educator each morning to make sure he/she has the right materials, books, etc. for classes that day. Later the student may need to "check out" with the teacher regarding homework, upcoming tests, and any special assignments. The student may need additional speech, physical, and/or occupational therapies integrated into their academic schedule through the IEP rather than pulling the student out of school for traditional outpatient services. Classroom teachers may need to modify the academic work load by providing study guides, giving additional time for assignments, or using specific cognitive and behavioral strategies to enable the student to learn better.

Unfortunately, academic, behavioral, and social consequences of the injury often evolve in unpredictable and, possibly, negative ways over months and years following the injury (Rutter, 1982). For example, a preschooler with severe injury may experience apparently good recovery in the early months and years after the injury. However, because the injury may interfere with the neurologic maturation necessary for the next major developmental transition, he/she may have great difficulty with the cognitive and behavioral demands of the early grades. Furthermore, transitions within school (e.g., from grade school to middle school and from middle school to high school), may reveal consequences of earlier injury because of the ever increasing demands for behavioral self-regulation, emotional and cognitive maturity, and efficiency of information processing. As the child attempts to negotiate social and academic challenges normally facilitated by maturation of parts of the brain that have been injured, new and possibly unpredicted obstacles may arise (Eslinger, Grattan, Damasio, & Damasio, 1992; Fletcher, Miner, & Ewing-Cobbs, 1987; Grattan & Eslinger, 1991; Mateer & Williams, 1991). Therefore, when medical and educational professionals speak about the return to school, they must attempt to visualize the needs of the child over the course of an entire school career and beyond.

It is useful to look at school as a series of developmental experiences including the preschool years, beginning school years, middle school years, and later school years, and compare those stages with neurologic development. In the preschool years, children experience tremendous growth in all areas, especially cognition, communication, and movement. They are increasingly involved in the larger social world as well. Although much of this development occurs within the family context, preschool-age children are also involved in many early school experiences. For a preschool-age child with TBI, effective school "entry" (rather than re-entry) requires teachers to introduce, monitor, and adjust learning and social demands so that the child does not become frustrated. The child's increasing ability to regulate attention, acquire increasingly abstract concepts at a normal rate, master the language, achieve motor development milestones, and learn how to interact effectively with peers and adults will be significant benchmarks of how well he/she is recovering and continuing to develop.

In the elementary and middle school years, children's brains continue to develop rapidly (Lehr & Savage, 1992). Many neurological connections are made, and children are immersed in systems of academic learning. Socially, children are expected to function in an increasingly independent manner, work within groups with peers and other adults, and regulate their behavior to conform to social standards. Children with TBI often struggle with increasingly heavy cognitive and academic challenges and the demand for flexibility posed by changing classroom settings and interactions with more than one teacher (especially if special education services are involved). Physical activities require increasingly thoughtful safety and social judgment. Of equal or greater importance, the psychosocial demands of emerging adolescence add to the uncomfortable feeling of "difference" and to the desire to do whatever is necessary to be like one's friends. Although students with TBI may not be aware of or in control of behavioral changes, they predictably react emotionally to academic overload and feelings of rejection both by peers and family members.

As children move into adolescence and the beginnings of adulthood, they are confronted with ever increasing academic curricula, as many as 8–10 teachers to work with, and a host of physiological and psychological changes. Issues of physical maturation and attractiveness, sexuality, self-identity, independence, confidence, and self-worth figure prominently in their evolving lives. Adolescents are "on the go," driving cars, going out on dates. Adolescents with TBI may experience great difficulty in any of these areas at a time when they also need to be able to think logically, make adult-like decisions, process vast amounts of information, and solve complex problems. This period of development can leave many adolescents with TBI "standing in the dust" of their peers and create insurmountable feelings regarding their losses, inabilities, and hope for a future outside of school. Such losses can trigger anger, depression, and inappropriate behaviors and lead to substance abuse and suicidal thoughts (Lehr, 1990; Lehr & Savage, 1992).

This developmental perspective mandates a long-term orientation to recovery and ongoing development after brain injury and to the complications that may surface over time. Needs must be projected and identified over a series of school transitions that match the milestones of cognitive, psychosocial, and motor development. Classrooms, curricula, and teacher assignments may need to be reconfigured periodically to meet changing learning needs. Counseling may be needed to help students discuss their feelings and learn ways to accommodate socially. Family/community services may be needed to ensure long-term success.

Often neglected is the issue of post-school experiences (Wolcott & Lash, 1993). The cooperative planning of where individuals may work, where they may live, and how they will be included in the community needs to begin in the early student years. The involvement of vocational rehabilitation services and independent living centers in post-secondary education experiences are part of the overall series of transitions as well (Savage, 1987). Many young adults with TBIs end up living closet lives at home after they have "graduated" from school. As healthcare centers recognize the need to connect their services with the school, so do schools need to connect their services with the outside world. Schools can provide very supportive community-like environments for the student to succeed, but post-school experiences, if not planned for, can become a nightmare. Collaboration with area vocational services, independent living centers, community-based advocacy agencies, and other support systems needs to occur in the student's educational program prior to graduation in order to establish a coordinated transition plan from school to community.

Again, it is the Individual Education Plan (IEP) for a child with a TBI that guides both the short- and long-term services. In stark contrast to children with developmental disabilities, the needs of a child with a traumatic injury may vary significantly over time. A child with TBI has very unique educational needs (Savage, Lash, Bennett, & Navalta, 1995) that change as their medical condition changes. Thus, the needs of children with brain injuries are continually changing and evolving and as part of the planning process, there must be a clear focus on what will be the next step in the continuum of care as the recovery process occurs. This recovery is individual to each child, and the design of care must reflect that individuality. For example, a child who needs a specialized placement due to behavior discontrol and requires significant supervision and behavioral intervention may not need the same level of service even 12 months post-injury. A student who transitions to public school may need tutorial teachers who are specially trained in brain injury and developing educational programs that reflect the unique nature of the student's injury.

What is clear is that with the Individual Education Plan, professionals and families need to work on developing a continuum of care that provides whatever services their child requires to foster educational progress. During these transitions, communication with the local school system is imperative (DePompei & Blosser, 1995). Students with TBI often are most appropriately served in the general classroom (Carter & Savage, 1985), yet they may require a series of transitions between less restrictive environments in order to be successful in the general classroom.

ACQUIRED BRAIN INJURY

While discussion in this chapter has focused on children with TBI, a huge number of children exist with acquired brain injuries secondary to disease. Children who are the victims of diabetic coma, stroke, a-v malformation, encephalitis, meningitis, cognitive dysfunction secondary to toxic exposure (lead, cocaine, alcohol), diseases that alter cognitive function (kidney failure, brain tumors), or those for whom medical treatment has caused iatrogenic cognitive outcomes often present with similar neurobehavioral difficulties and require carefully focused educational intervention of the type we have outlined here. The methods of assessment for this population are similar and, in many cases, identical to children with TBI, and there is little value in making a distinction between children with acquired neurological disorders for this reason.

CONCLUSION

Children and adolescents with brain injuries and their families often face long-term struggles and challenges. As the general public better recognizes these needs and develops systems among hospital, schools, and communities, improved services will result. Earlier referral by the healthcare providers and the collaborative development of individual education plans will enable professionals to blend their services and provide families with systems to insure service delivery for their children.

ENDNOTES

1. Preparation of this chapter is supported in part by Award #H133B00344 from the National Institute on Disability and Rehabilitation Research, U.S. Department of Education.

REFERENCES

Adolph, K., Eppler, M., & Gibson, E. (1993). Development of perception of affordances. In C. Rover-Collier & L.P. Lipsitt (Eds.), *Advances in infancy research 8*. Norwood, NJ: Ablex Publishing Corporation.

Ainsworth, M.D.S. (1989). Attachments beyond infancy. *American Psychologist, 44,* 709.

Allison, M. (1992, Oct/Nov). The effects of neurologic injury on the maturing brain. *Headlines,* 2.

Annegers, J.F. (1983). The epidemiology of head trauma in children. In K. Shapiro (Ed.), *Pediatric head trauma*. Mount Kisco, NY: Futura Publishing Company.

Annegers, J.F., Grabow, J.D., Kurland, L.T., & Laws, E.R. (1980). The incidence, causes and secular trends of head trauma in Olmsted County, Minnesota 1935–1974. *Neurology, 30,* 912.

Baker, S.P., O'Neill, B., & Karpf, R. (1984). *The injury fact book*. Lexington, MA: Lexington Books.

Begali, V. (1992). *Head injury in children and students: A resource and review for schools and allied health professionals* (2nd ed.). Brandon, VT: Clinical Psychology Press.

Berrol, S. (1992). Terminology of post-concussion syndrome. *Physical Medicine and Rehabil.: State of the Art Reviews, 6,* 1.

Bird, F., Dores, P.A., Moniz, D., & Robinson, J. (1989). Reducing severe aggressive and self-injurious behaviors with functional communication training: Direct, collateral, and generalized results. *American Journal of Mental Retardation, 94,* 37–48.

Blosser, J. L., & DePompei, R. (1991). Preparing educational professionals for meeting the needs of students with traumatic brain injury. *Journal of Head Trauma Rehabilitation, 6,* 73–82.

Bowlby, J. (1988). Developmental psychiatry comes of age. *Am. J. Psychiatry, 145,* 1.

Burke, W.H., & Lewis, F. (1986). Management of maladaptive social behavior in a brain injured adult. *International J. of Rehabil. Res., 9,* 335–342.

Carney, J., & Gerring, J. (1990). Return to school following severe closed head injury: A critical phase in pediatric rehabilitation. *Pediatrician, 17,* 222–229.

Carter, R.R., & Savage, R.C. (1988). Transitioning pediatric patients into educational systems: Guidelines for professionals. *Cognitive Rehabil. 6,* 10.

Casey, R., Ludwig, S., & McCormick, M.C. (198). Minor head trauma in children: An intervention to decrease functional morbidity. *Pediatrics, 80,* 159.

Cohen, S. B. (1986). Educational reintegration and programming for children with head injuries. *Journal of Head Trauma Rehabilitation, 1,* 22–29.

Cooley, E., & Singer, G. (1991). On serving students with head injuries: Are we reinventing a wheel that doesn't roll? *Journal of Head Trauma Rehabilitation, 6,* 47–55.

Deaton, A. V. (1987). Behavioral change strategies for children and adolescents with severe brain injury. *Journal of Learning Disabilities, 20,* 581–589.

DePompei, R., & Blosser, J. (1995, Spring). Transition planning from hospital to special education placement in school. *TBI Challenge,* 3–2.

Dikman, S., Machamer, J., & Temkin, N. (1993). Psychosocial outcome in patients with moderate to severe head injury: Two-year follow-up. *Brain Injury, 7,* 113.

Durand, V.M. (1990). *Severe behavior problems: A functional communication training approach*. New York: Guilford.

Eichelberger, M., & Ball, J. (1991). EMSC: Focus on the traumatically brain injured child. Washington, DC: Children's National Medical Center, Department of Pediatrics.

Eslinger, P., Grattan, L., Damasio, H., & Damasio, A. (1992). Developmental consequences of childhood frontal lobe damage. *Archives of Neurology, 49,* 764.

Evans, R.W., & Ruff, R.M. (1992). Outcome and value: A perspective on rehabilitation outcomes achieved in acquired brain injury. *Journal of Head Trauma Rehabilitation, 7,* 24.

Ewing-Cobbs, L., Fletcher, J. M., & Levin, H. S. (1986). Neurobehavioral sequelae following head injury in children: Educational implications. *Journal of Head Trauma Rehabilitation, 1,* 57–65.

Franzen, M., & Berg, R. (1989). *Screening for brain impairment.* New York: Springer Vaerlag.

Gibson, J.J. (1989). The ecological approach to visual perception. Boston, MA: Houghton Mifflin.

Glang, A., Singer, G., Cooley, E., & Tish, N. (1992). Tailoring direct instruction techniques for use with elementary students with brain injury. *Journal of Head Trauma Rehabilitation, 7,* 93–108.

Haley, S.M., Hallenborg, S.C., & Gans, B.M. (1989). Functional assessment in young children with neurological impairment. *Topics in Early Childhood Special Education, 9,* 106–126.

Harrington, D., Malec, J., Cicerone, K., & Katz, H. (1993). Current perceptions of rehabilitation professionals towards mild traumatic brain injury. *Arch. Phys. Med. Rehabil., 74,* 579.

Hart, K.J., & Faust, D. (1988). Prediction of the effects of mild head injury: A message about the Kennard Principle. *Journal of Clinical Psychology, 44,* 780–782.

Heaton, R. (1981). Wisconsin Card Sorting Test. Odessa, FL: Psychological Corporation.

Hofmann, A. (1992). Managing students and their parents: Avoiding pitfalls and traps. *Student Medicine: State of the Art Reviews, 3,* 1.

Individuals with Disabilities Education Act (IDEA). (1991). United States Department of Education. Washington DC: Office of Special Education and Rehabilitative Services.

International Brain Injury Association. (1994). *Facts about traumatic brain injury.* Washington, DC.

Isaacson, R.L. (1975). The myth of recovery from early brain damage. In N. Ellis (Ed.), *Aberrant development in infancy.* London: John Wiley & Sons.

Jaffe, K., Fay, G., Polisau, N., Martin, K., Shurtleff, H., Rivara, J., & Winn, H. (1993). Severity of pediatric traumatic brain injury and neurobehaviorial recovery at one year—A cohort study. *Arch. Phys. Med. Rehabil., 74,* 587.

Jenkins, E., & Bell, C. (1992). Student violence can't be curbed. *Student Medicine: State of the Art Reviews, 3,* 71.

Kalsbeek, W.D., McLaurin, R.L., Harris, B.S., & Miller, J.D. (1980). The National Head and Spinal Cord Survey: Major findings. *J. Neurosurg., 53,* 519.

Kay, T. (1986). The unseen injury: Minor head trauma. Washington, DC: National Head Injury Foundation.

———. (1993). Neuropsychological treatment of mild traumatic brain injury. *Journal of Head Trauma Rehabilitation, 8,* 74.

Kay, T., et al. (1993). Definition of mild traumatic brain injury. *Journal of Head Trauma Rehabilitation, 8,* 86.

Klauber, M.R., Barrett-Connor, E., Marshall, L.F., Bowers, S.A. (1981). The epidemiology of head injury. *Am. J. Epidemiol., 113,* 500.

Klonoff, H., Clark, C., & Klonoff, P.S. (1993). Long-term outcome of head injuries: A 23-year follow up study of children with head injuries. *J. Neurol. Neurosurg. Psychiatry, 56,* 410.

Klonoff, P.S., Lage, G.A., Chiapello, & D.A. (1993). Varieties of the catastrophic reaction to brain injury: A self psychology perspective. *Bulletin Menniger Clinic, 57,* 227.

Kraus, J.F., Black, M.A., Hessol, N., Ley, P., Rokow, W., Sullivan, C., Bowers, S., Knowlton, S., & Marshall, L. (1984). The incidence of acute brain injury and serious impairment in a defined population. *Am. J. Epidemiol., 119,* 19.

Lash, M. (1992). *When your child goes to school after an injury.* Boston: Tufts University.

Lash, M., Russo, D. C., Navalta, C. P., & Baryza, M. J. (1994). Families of children with traumatic injuries identify needs for research and training. *Neurorehabilitation* (submitted for publication).

Lehr, E., Savage, R.C. (1990). Community and school integration from a developmental perspective. In J. Kreutzer (Ed.), *Community integration following traumatic brain injury.* Baltimore: Paul Brookes Publishing Company.

Levin, H., Culhane, K., Hartman, J., Edankovich, K., et al. (1991). Developmental changes in performance on tests of purported frontal lobe functioning. *Developmental Neuropsychology, 7,* 377.

Levine, M.J., VanHorn, K.R., & Curtis, A.B. (1993). Development models of social cognition in assessing psychosocial adjustments in head injury. *Brain Injury, 7,* 153.

Lezak, M.D. (1993). Newer contributions to the neuropsychological assessment of executive functions. *Journal of Head Trauma Rehabilitation, 8,* 24.

Loveland, K.A. (1991). Social affordances and interaction II: Autism and the affordances of the human environment. *Ecological Psychology 3,* 99.

Mateer, C. (1992). Systems of care for post concussive syndrome. *Physical Medicine and Rehabilitation: State of the Art Reviews, 6,* 143.

McHugh, P.R. (1987). William Osler and the new psychiatry. *Annals of Internal Medicine, 107,* 914.

Mira, M.P., Tucker, B.F., & Tyler, J.S. (1992). Traumatic brain injury in children and students: A sourcebook for teachers and other school personnel. Austin, TX: PRO-ED Publishing.

National Head Injury Foundation. (1992). *Pediatric head injury.* Washington, DC: National Head Injury Foundation.

National Pediatric Trauma Registry. (1993). *Summary of findings.* Boston, MA: Research and Training Center on Childhood Trauma.

Neisser, U. (1988). Five kinds of self-knowledge. *Philosophical Psychology, 1,* 35.

Nowicki, S., & Duke, M. (1992). *Helping the child who doesn't fit in.* Atlanta: Peachtree Publishing.

Offer. D., & Schonert-Reichl, K. (1992). Debunking the myths of adolescence: findings from recent research. *J. Am. Academy of Child & Student Psychiatry, 31,* 100.

Ommaya, A.K., & Gennarelli, T.A. (1974). Cerebral concussion and traumatic unconsciousness: Correlation of experimental and clinical observations on blunt head injuries. *Brain, 97,* 633.

Price, B., Doffnre, K., Stowe, R., & Mesulum, M. (1990). The compartmental learning disabilities of early frontal lobe damage. *Brain, 113,* 1383.

Reichle, J., & Wacker, D.P. (Eds.). (1993). Communicative alternatives to challenging behavior. Baltimore, MD: Paul H. Brookes.

Rivara, J. B., Jaffe, K. M., Fay, G. C., Polissar, N. L. Martin, K. M., Shurtleff, H. A., & Liao, S. (1993). Family functioning and injury severity as predictors of child functioning one year following traumatic brain injury. *Archives of Physical Medicine and Rehabilitation, 74,* 1047–1055.

Rogers, C.R. (1961). *On becoming a person.* Boston, MA: Houghton Mifflin.

Ruff, R.M., Marshall, L.F., Crouch, J., Klauber, M.R., Levin, H.S., Barth, J.T., Kreutzer, J., Blunt, B.A., Foulkes, M.A., Eisenberg, H.M., Jane, J.A., & Marmarou, A. (1993). Predictors of outcome following severe head trauma: Follow-up data from the Traumatic Coma Data Bank. *Brain Injury, 7,* 101.

Russo, D.C., & Navalta, C.P. (1995). Some new dimensions of behaviour analysis and therapy. In H. van Bilsen, P.C. Kendall, & J.H. Slavenburg (Eds.), *Behavioral approaches for children and adolescents: Challenges for the next century.* New York: Plenum Publishing.

Rutter, M., Chadwick, O., Shaffer, D., & Brown, G. (1980). A prospective study of children with head injuries: I. Design and methods. *Psychol. Medicine, 10,* 633–645.

Savage, R.C. (1987). Educational issues for the head injured student and young adult. *Journal of Head Trauma Rehabilitation,2,* 1.

———. (1991). Identification, classification, and placement issues for students with traumatic brain injuries. *Journal of Head Trauma Rehabilitation, 6,* 1.

———. (1993, Summer). Children with traumatic brain injury. *TBI Challenge,* 4–5.

Savage, R.C., & Wolcott, G.F. (1988). An educator's manual: What teachers need to know about students with traumatic brain injuries. Washington, DC: National Head Injury Foundation, Inc.

Savage, R.C., Lash, M., Bennett, K., & Navalta. (1995, Spring). Special education for students with brain injury. *TBI Challenge,* 3–7.

Schwartz, M., Mayer, N., Fitzpatrick DeSalme, E., & Montgomery, M. (1993). Cognitive theory and the study of everyday action disorders after brain damage. *Journal of Head Trauma Rehabilitation, 8,* 59.

Shapiro, K. (Ed.). (1983). *Pediatric head trauma.* Mount Kisco, NY: Futura Publishing Company.

Smith, C.R. (1983). *Learning disabilities: The interaction of learner, task, and setting.* Boston/Toronto: Little, Brown and Company.

Spreen, O., & Strauss, E. (1991). *A compendium of neuropsychological tests.* New York: Oxford University Press.

Teasdale, G., & Jennett, B. (1974). Assessment of coma and impaired consciousness: A practical scale. *The Lancet, 2*, 81.

Valenti, S.S., & Good, J.M.M. (1991). Social affordances and interaction: I: Introduction. *Ecological Psychology, 3*, 77.

van Acker, R., & Valenti, S.S. (1989). Perception of social affordances by children with mild handicapping conditions: Implications for social skills research and training. *Ecological Psychology, 1*, 383.

Varney, N., & Menefee, L. (1993). Psychosocial and executive deficits following closed head injury: Implications for orbital frontal cortex. *Journal of Head Trauma Rehabilitation, 8*, 32.

Wolcott, G.F., & Lash, M. (1992). *Educating children with traumatic brain injuries.* Weston, MA: Wolcott and Associates.

Wood, R. (1988). Management of behavior disorders in a day treatment setting. *Journal of Head Trauma Rehabilitation, 3*, 53–61.

Yivisaker, M., Feeney, T.J., & Urbanczyk, B. (1993). A social-environmental approach to communication and behavior after traumatic brain injury. *Seminars in Speech and Language, 14*, 74–87.

Ylvisaker, M., Hartwick, P., & Stevens, M. (1991). School re-entry following head injury: Managing the transition from hospital to school. *Journal of Head Trauma Rehabilitation, 6*, 10.

Zasler, N. (1993). Mild traumatic brain injury: Medical assessment and intervention. *Journal of Head Trauma Rehabilitation, 8*, 13.

Zencius, A., Wesolowski, M., & Burke, W. (1989). Comparing motivational systems with two noncompliant head injured adolescents. *Brain Injury, 3*, 67–71.

28 Rehabilitating Brain Damage in Hispanics

Marcel O. Pontón,[1,2] José Gonzalez,[2] and Marisa Mares[3]

[1]Harbor UCLA Medical Center, CA
[2]Neuropsychiatric Institute, Department of Psychiatry and Biobehavioral Sciences,
    UCLA School of Medicine, CA
[3.]Cal State, Dominguez Hills, CA

INTRODUCTION

Why include a chapter on the treatment of head-injured Hispanic patients in this book? Do they have a different recovery course? Do they experience unique issues in their rehabilitation not discussed in the literature thus far? Are there cultural issues that impact the therapeutic process that require specific attention? The answer to these questions is a resounding "perhaps." A more honest answer is "we don't know." Much like the paucity of neuropsychological research with this population (Pontón et al., 1996), the literature yields no results on psychotherapy with head-injured Hispanic patients.

This chapter presents a clinical approach to the psychotherapeutic management of Hispanic patients who have suffered a head injury. Rather than discussing overall frameworks (Prigatano, 1986), stages of recovery (Lezak, 1988) or a general understanding of the role of therapy with brain-injured patients (Cicerone, 1989, 1991), this chapter will focus on specific techniques to use with the Latino population.

At the outset, several caveats should be laid out. First, the techniques and approaches discussed here assume that the neuropsychologist can communicate directly with the patient in his/her native language. Second, the chapter deals with Hispanic patients in a U.S. context. Third, it assumes that patients were involved in some form of gainful employment prior to their injury and, therefore, have access to certain insurance benefits for their treatment. However, the issues involved in rehabilitation are faced by survivors of head injury regardless of their employability status.

The emphasis of this chapter is clinical. It offers certain guidelines and suggestions for providing psychotherapy to this population using a functionally eclectic model that is partial to cognitive behavioral approaches. Each of the techniques discussed is described in terms of its purpose, implementation, and limitations. Wherever applicable, tables and resources are discussed to aid the clinician in treatment planning. The four techniques discussed here are neither novel nor unique. They are well grounded in the psychotherapeutic literature. However, they are clearly geared towards the Latino population and are articulated in the context of the first author's clinical experience with this population. We discuss the techniques of *symptom validation, journaling, structuring, and reframing.* The last technique is divided into three different applications. Case studies illustrate the application of the techniques in clinical practice.

SYMPTOM VALIDATION

> *Andamos entre sombras, equivocando puertas,*
> *recorriendo un oscuro país desconocido,*
> *creyendo que son falsas las cosas que son ciertas*
> *o dando por seguras las cosas que no han sido*
>
> —Miguel Angel Buesa

Complaints of physical, emotional, and neurocognitive dysfunction are abundant during rehabilitation (León-Carrión, 1994; Parker, 1990; Gainotti, 1993; McAllister, 1994). Patients with unsophisticated coping mechanisms tend to overinterpret their symptoms in an exaggerated and unrealistic manner (Cicerone, 1991). Sensations of pain, discomfort, dizziness, or somatosensory sequelae are reported constantly as confirming the patient's subjective perception of severe and generalized dysfunction (Mittenberg & Burton, 1994; Bohnen et al., 1994). The subjective experience of these symptoms may, in turn, fuel the patient's level of anxiety and depression, creating a vicious cycle of despair (Cole, 1992). Complicating matters is the common experience that the physician, neuropsychologist, therapist, or nurse evaluating the patient will not be able to corroborate the symptoms objectively and may, therefore, respond by ignoring the patient's complaints. Moreover, such presentation is sometimes seen by clinicians as "whining," "attention-seeking behavior," or, most commonly, as malingering.

The clinician may be correct in interpreting the severity of the symptoms presented by the patient as exaggerated. However, rapport and ultimately therapeutic progress will not be advanced if the patient's concerns are ignored (Whitehouse, 1994). AA, a 30-year-old man with a severe head injury and multiple trauma after falling 20 feet on a construction site, had a typical reaction:

> *The doctors here do not pay attention to me. They think I'm lying. I keep telling them over and over about my problems, and they shrug me off. They never tell me what is wrong with me; they don't answer my questions, and they don't even do anything for me. The [physiatrist] saw me for five minutes and that's it. I need a pill or something. I'm not going anywhere until all of my problems are resolved.*

This complaint is typically heard from monolingual or bilingual Hispanic patients. It reflects frustration, anger, and ultimately, it can evolve into lack of cooperation with treatment. Many Latino patients regard the ignoring of their symptoms by clinicians and staff as insulting. It is at this stage when many patients, who previously had no intention to litigate their case, consider seriously retaining a lawyer so they can receive "real help" for their problems. The lack of a sympathetic ear, however, is only one of the sources of frustration these patients face. The use of interpreters to communicate their subjective symptoms to specialists (which may actually distort the patient's original reports [La Calle, 1987]), the lack of an adequate English vocabulary in the absence of an interpreter, and cultural expectations regarding the patient-clinician interaction are also significant contributors to the distortion of an already difficult situation. The predictable result is that patients feels unable to communicate the symptoms or make themselves understood. In either case, they perceive treatment as ineffective or totally unsatisfactory. This problem may be rooted in the cross-cultural nature of the therapeutic interaction. A clinician who is culturally different from the patient may tend to attribute pathological reasons to the behavior of a lower SES, culturally diverse patient (Malgady, Rogler, & Constantino, 1987).

How can this issue be addressed psychotherapeutically? A successful approach is what we term "symptom validation." The purpose of this strategy is to verbalize concretely the subjective experience of vague and diffuse symptoms and to make the patient feel understood. A complaint repeated constantly may be a sign that the patient needs information, reframing, or problem-solving strategies. Active listening, coupled with education, can validate the patient's experience of a common symptom while simultaneously providing impetus for progress in treatment. It also provides an opportunity for the therapist to build rapport and develop a therapeutic alliance with the patient. This approach is similar to what Cicerone (1991) has called "symptomatic treatment method."

The process involves, first, educating the patient on what symptoms are commonly present in head injury rehabilitation. Three objectives are accomplished with this technique. First, patients are given a sense of normalcy regarding their experience. They learn to see their symptoms as part of their injury. Second, the therapist can provide the patient with a realistic, yet general, time frame of what to expect at one year, 18 months, and two years post-injury in the fluctuation of their symptom severity. Through this approach, patients can be given a realistic sense of hope (Prigatano, 1986). This helps patients learn to anticipate and interpret fluctuations in symptom resolution as a natural process of their rehabilitation. Since symptom identification is a process that can be done in a structured manner throughout therapy, patients can also be reminded that they are experiencing what they were told to expect. At eight months post-injury, for instance, patient AA remarked: "I'm now going through what you told me some time ago."

Third, patients should learn explicitly that a few symptoms will remain with them for a prolonged period of time or as permanent sequelae of their injury (Ponsford et al., 1995). Head-injured patients will typically become severely depressed or report "regression" in their experience of rehabilitation when their symptom-specific recovery peaks (Prigatano & Fordyce, 1986). They should be told to expect this experience and that then they will face two choices—denial (e.g., "I won't go back to work until I'm 100% fine.") or acceptance (e.g., "I lost certain abilities, but I can go on with my life.").

Following the education of patients on what symptoms to expect as sequelae of their head injury, they are encouraged to list their symptoms exhaustively. Beginning with the most severe to the most trivial, the clinician takes detailed notes of the patient's complaints, including their nature, frequency, severity, diurnal or nocturnal variation, triggers of or related symptoms (e.g., photosensitivity and headaches, tinnitus and initial insomnia, etc.), palliatives, and history of treatment. Because history of treatment may vary with the context of therapy, when, in the rehabilitation process, the patient is seeking psychotherapy, the clinician should pay particular attention to potential abuse of pain killers or nonprescription medication as a coping mechanism. In our experience, patients will readily report the use of prescribed medications; however, only after much probing will they admit to taking pain killers on their own. Other patients will resort to "homeopathic," herbal, and nontraditional medicine as a means to cope with their symptomatology. Spiritual approaches to well-being (faith healing, *santería, limpiezas,* etc.) will also be explored by patients. For those who believe that a curse has been placed on them *("me embrujaron"),* the concern over spiritual matters will actually heighten anxiety as they attribute symptom severity or mishaps to unseen evil forces. We discuss "spiritualizing" as a reframing technique later in this chapter.

Finally, patients should be asked about their expectations of outcome in the treatment of their symptom presentation. Response to this question provides the clinician with a measure of the patient's level of awareness into their deficits. It also allows the clinician to set treatment goals for education, target behaviors, and reality testing. The symptoms identified by the patient can become the target behaviors for an effective treatment plan. Following the identification, measurement, and analysis of the behavior, behavioral interventions can be identified for specific symptoms that can later be empirically evaluated (Burke & Lewis, 1986; Burke & Wesolowski, 1988; Drudge et al., 1986; Wesolowski & Burke, 1989).

The therapist can thus develop his/her treatment planning using rich behavioral information, establishing rapport with the patient, and providing a new framework for patients to understand their symptoms. Rather than being concerned with "insight," the focus is on education of the patient about symptomatology and recovery (Mittenberg & Burton, 1994).

Perhaps headaches are the most commonly reported symptom (Jensen & Nielsen, 1990), even after two years post-injury (Ponsford et al., 1995). Martin (1993) provides a comprehensive approach to the assessment and treatment of headaches using a cognitive behavioral model. He describes eight general steps that can be useful in management of headaches but that can also be extrapolated for use with musculoskeletal pain, dizziness, tinnitus, and other difficulties resulting from the injury. Martin's program consists of (1) education, (2) relaxation training, (3) cognitive training focusing on maladaptive thoughts and beliefs, (4) imagery training, (5) attention-diversion training, (6) modification of immediate antecedents, (7) modification of life-style factors aimed at increasing hobbies and interests, and (8) training in time management and problem solving.

Limitations

There are several limitations to this approach. The first and most obvious problem with this strategy is that it can be manipulated by the patient for secondary gains. Some patients will generate an unending list of symptoms in subsequent sessions. Second, some patients may interpret the therapist's approach as validating the patient's subjective severity of the symptoms rather than empathizing with the patient's perception that his/her symptoms are severe (Chelune, Heaton, & Lehman, 1986). Third, there are anosognosic patients who never admit to any symptomatology and have little or no insight into their recovery (Deaton, 1986). Finally, there are those patients who are so severely impaired from the injury that their condition makes this technique useless.

To address some of the above limitations, clinicians should emphasize the fact that feeling overwhelmed by symptoms is common but that most patients also experience dramatic changes/decline in the experience of their symptoms over a period of time.

Change is not only to be expected, it is inevitable. For those patients who change their list of symptoms constantly for secondary gains, paradoxical interventions have proven useful (O'Hanlon, 1987). Every time their list changes, the emphasis on their control over the previous symptoms is emphasized. If malingering is suspected, patients can be asked to experience the symptom while in the office so the therapist can understand it better. They can then be asked to experience a different symptom that is less severe. The patient can be told to choose to always experience the more severe symptom first, so the other symptoms are not so distressing.

Paradoxical therapy uses the symptoms to change them. O'Hanlon (1987) suggests that the frequency, duration, time, location, intensity, quality, circumstance, or sequence of the symptoms can be changed. To deal with resistant and frivolous symptomatology, he also suggests creating a short-circuit of the symptom pattern, interrupting part of the sequence from occurring ("derailing"), adding or subtracting elements from the sequence, breaking up a symptom into smaller parts, isolating the symptom from its larger pattern, and reversing the pattern and linking the occurrence of the symptom-pattern to another pattern. The clinician's judgment, experience, and assessment skills should guide the choice and use of these interventions during therapy.

Case Study #1

XN, a 26-year-old male, suffered a nondepressed skull fracture over the left fronto-temporo-parietal area, with intraparenchymal hemorrhage and right hemiparesis. He also presented with a transcortical motor aphasia. He was hospitalized for two months in an acute rehabilitation center. He was referred for outpatient psychotherapy with the general complaint of depression five months post-discharge from the hospital. The patient complained that he had gone to multiple sessions with different doctors since the time of his discharge; however, he had not been given any details about his medical condition nor told of a treatment plan for his many symptoms. He was angry that none of the clinicians involved in his treatment seemed to be interested in him as much as in providing a service to him. During the first session, the patient was asked to describe his symptoms in detail. His symptoms included (1) word finding difficulty, (2) mild dysarthria with some stuttering, (3) poor concentration, (4) dysnomias, (5) paragrammatism, (6) mild writing difficulties, (7) poor reading comprehension, (8) memory difficulties, (9) decreased sensation in his right hand, (10) neurovegetative signs (appetite, sleep, libido, and energy disturbance), (11) depression, (12) irritability, (13) right sided weakness, (14) dragging of his right foot, and (15) headaches. His original BDI score was 36. XN was then asked to assign levels of severity to the symptoms and to rate them. He was particularly bothered by the right-sided weakness and his "inability to speak well," which resulted in depression. During the second session, the patient was educated on the process of recovery and how his symptoms fit the post-traumatic head injury syndrome. He was also given a sense of what symptoms he could have control over (depression, neurovegetative signs, irritability) and which symptoms could change with time and therapy (right-sided weakness, speech and writing problems). While the patient was told that some symptoms could remain with him as permanent sequelae of the injury, no symptoms were identified in this regard. The next five sessions focused on the management of the neurovegetative signs and the irritability. Rapport was established early on by the fact that listening to and providing education about his symptoms clarified many of the patient's concerns and worries. By the tenth session, his BDI score was 15. In subsequent sessions, the therapist had to clarify the results of findings from other disciplines. This meant close follow-up with physicians and other therapists so the patient would obtain a clear picture of his physical and cognitive progress. Emphasis shifted to management of symptoms and goal setting. During the sixteenth session (11 months post-injury), the patient began seriously considering vocational rehabilitation. However, he felt the prospects for future employment were dim, given his persistent symptoms. We made a second list of symptoms, and this time, he identified (1) short-term memory problems, (2) moderate word-finding difficulties, (3) general right-sided weakness, (4) severe pulsating headaches, and (5) constant musculoskeletal pain of his back. The patient was presented with the symptoms from the initial session. The process of his recovery was reviewed, allowing the patient to evaluate what factors made a difference in his progress. Emphasis was placed on how he managed to solve the majority of his symptoms. New goals were identified to target the remaining symptoms. The patient was reminded that he may have to live with some of his current symptoms as permanent sequelae of the injury. The patient was discharged from therapy after 20 sessions, with a decrease in severity of the symptoms noted above but no resolution. Eighteen months post-injury, the patient returned briefly for an evaluation of his disability status. At that time, his symptoms included (1) mild headaches, (2) numbness of the right side of his face, (3) musculoskeletal pain of his lower back, (4) word-finding difficulty, (5) poor reading comprehension. Progress was discussed with the patient in terms of the severity of the symptoms. For instance, his right-sided weakness had resolved to "numbness of the right side of his face." The issue of permanent sequelae of the injury was processed. The patient was now willing to accept that his life could go on despite his limitations. He eventually became a clothes salesman.

To aid in the process of symptom validation, we offer a list of symptoms in Spanish to use with the patient. Table 28.1 summarizes a list of common post-concussive symptomatology in English and Spanish.

JOURNALING

This technique is very similar to symptom validation and is particularly appropriate with patients who have had mild head injuries. Patients' educational background will be important and at least six years of education or more should be expected. The main difference between symptom validation and this approach is that it requires the patient to keep the record of symptoms and to log them with some reasonable frequency. This strategy consists of asking patients to make at least two entries a week in a notebook, diary, or journal of any sort. The therapist can provide this material (a simple notebook will suffice). In it, patients list all of their symptoms with a rating of severity (1–10, 10 being the most severe). Patients are also asked to write a thought next to the symptom (i.e., "How does the symptom make me feel?"). This can be done during the first three weeks of therapy as a structured "homework" assignment. The task may be repeated every 6–8 sessions or at the discretion of the clinician. The purpose of the task is three-fold: (1) it forces the patient to express in concrete terms what otherwise is usually a non-specific, subjective complaint; (2) it creates a "baseline" of the symptoms while providing the patient with a record of an emotional coping style toward the sequelae of his/her injury; and (3) it eventually becomes a concrete measure of progress that can empower the patient.

This strategy is particularly helpful when patients become painfully aware that they will have to live with certain symptoms for the rest of their lives. Looking back at the number, the severity, and the quality of the symptoms they have overcome can be

Table 28.1: Symptom Identification (English/Spanish)

Symptom	Spanish Equivalent (vernacular)	Selected Treatment References
PHYSICAL		
tinnitus	zumbido en el oido	
headaches	dolores de cabeza	Martin (1993)
fatigue	cansancio, fatiga, sin ganas, sin energía	
dizziness	mareos	
photosensitivity	sensibilidad a la luz, le molesta la luz	
poor balance	problemas del balance/siente que se va a caer	
loss of sensation of body parts	hormigueo, se le duerme alguna parte del cuerpo, entumecimiento	
pain (general)	dolor	Caudil (1995)
insomnia	insomnia, falta de sueño, no puede dormir	Morin (1993)
EMOTIONAL/SOCIAL		
anxiety	mal de los nervios/ansiedad/angustia/desespero	Greenber & Padesky (1993)
depression	tristeza/congoja/depresión/pena	Freeman & DeWolf (1992)
irritability/aggression	ira/enojo/rabia/coraje/agresividad	Silver & Yodofsky (1994)
	enfadado/corajudo/bravo/enojado/irritable	
obssessions	obsesiones	
rigidity	rigidez	
impulsivity	problemas de	
	... impulsividad	
	... hace las cosas sin pensar	
inappropriatenes	dice/hace cosas	Lane et al. (1989)
	... indebidas	Lewis et al. (1988)
	... soeces	
	... grocerías	
	... vulgaridades	
	... actúa mal	
COGNITIVE		
concentration	dificultades	
	... concentrándose	
	... poniendo atención	
	... siguiendo el hilo de la conversación	
memory	problemas de memorie	Parenté & Anderson-Parenté (1991)
	... se le olvidan las cosas	
	... pierde sus cosas	
	... se olvida de lo que le dicen	
	... se olvida de lo que hizo/dijo	
	... no se acuerda del pasado	
language problems	problemas	Williams & Long (1986)
	.. encontrando palabras	
	... entendiendo lo que le dicen	
	... leyendo/entendiendo lo que lee	
	... escribiendo	
	... no tiene sentido lo que dice	
	... dice una palabra por la otra	
speech problems	problems del habla	
	... tartamudea	
	... "habla arrastrado"	
	... pronuncia mal	
	... dice una letra por la otra	
	... no se entiende lo que dice	
perceptual deficits	cambio en la capacidad de	
	... ver	
	... oir	
	... oler	
	... gustar	
	... sentir (físicamente)	
disorientation	pierde sentido de	
	... el tiempo,	
	... el espacio (no sabe donde está)	
	... persona (no sabe quién es)	

reassuring to patients. One important link in the empowerment process is the distinction between the perception of symptom severity and ability to maintain normal daily functioning (Cicerone, 1991). They tend to realize how much they have changed, how emotions always accompany symptoms, and how they respond typically when faced with certain types of symptoms (see Table 28.2).

Limitations

This approach is limited by the educational experience of the patient, by the type of injury suffered, and by the degree of initiation or resistance from the patient toward therapy. Patients with a fifth grade education or less will find this task daunting and uninteresting. Patients with severe musculoskeletal injuries may be unable to use their dominant right hand to write. Other patients may be alexic or agraphic following their head injury or may have some significant language problem. Patients who are resistant to change because of secondary gains, anosognosia, or patient-therapist interaction may sabotage this technique. Thus, it should be used carefully with certain mild head-injured patients who present with multiple complaints or who are high functioning and significantly depressed about their future or the perceived loss of functioning.

Table 28.2: Journaling

Date	Symtpom	Severity (1–10)	Thought	Feeling

Fecha	Síntoma	Intensidad (1–10)	Pensamiento	Sentimiento

In summary, *symptom validation* and *journaling* are intended to create rapport between the patient and the clinician by validating their subjective experience of discomfort post-injury while managing to accomplish the following objectives:

- Create a list of target behaviors for treatment.
- Develop a baseline of problems with which to measure progress in the future.
- Give the patient a time frame to expect change.

The steps involved in these strategies include educating the patient on what general symptoms accompany post-injury recovery and exhaustive listing of the patient's symptoms.

STRUCTURING

Trauma deeply affects the daily routine of its victims. The loss of a regulated life with predictable schedules is detrimental to the patient's self-esteem, sense of purpose, and emotional well being. Depression settles in not only as a function of their feeling overwhelmed by an event that will change their lives in indiscernible yet dramatic way but also as a perception of the limitations affecting their daily lives. There is a sense of dependency on family members or therapists to get dressed, walk, eat, complete tasks, groom, or travel from one place to another according to the severity of the injury (Lezak, 1986). These limitations give the patient a sense of helplessness and may affect evaluations of self-worth in significant ways. Irritability is a common response; withdrawal is another. During the few weeks or months after the injury, patients may be the most depressed because they experience the greatest limitations.

The concept of a structured routine is paramount to recovery. The purpose of this technique is self-explanatory. The clinician works closely with the patient, his family, and whenever possible, with ancillary staff (recreational, occupational and speech therapists, social workers, etc.) to provide as much structure to the schedule of the patient as possible when he/she reintegrates back into the community.

Aside from vocational rehabilitation and follow-up visits with different physicians (if any), patients discover the unpleasant challenge of having plenty of time to spare. Many patients will not undergo a formal rehabilitation program, and months may go by before they engage in a meaningful routine. Other patients have moved back home after completing the insurance-allowed time at a rehabilitation center to find that the house is never to their liking, that there are plenty of things to complain about, and that, suddenly, everyone in the family has become an annoyance to him/her (Lezak, 1988; Gainotti, 1993). There is a third kind of patient who lives in vocational rehabilitation limbo because the severity of their orthopedic injuries significantly limits their options for placement, even though they may have no significant cognitive restrictions to return to their usual and customary occupation.

These patients learn to become keenly attuned to a wide spectrum of symptoms in their daily life primarily because they have ample idle time on their hands. Depression, irritability, sleep disturbance, boredom, and anxiety all appear to become exacerbated with unstructured time at home. For some Latino male patients, finding themselves in culturally unexpected roles of taking care of house chores is usually a reason for heightened anger/aggressiveness. Suddenly, there is reason to complain about issues they never noticed in the house before. There is little that the children or the spouse can do that seems to please the patient. The patient feels incapacitated, questions his/her self-worth, worries about perceptions from family members, has to justify his/her degree of "disability" with clear symptoms before the family, and feels like a total failure. This was the case with MT, a 37-year-old male who fell 30 feet to the ground. He perceived that the children and his spouse had lost respect for him because the family was in such financial distress. His orthopedic restrictions did not allow him to return to construction work, which he had done since he was 17. His 10-hour work days were now reduced to watching TV, arguing with his children, and worrying out loud about his future employability. Crying, yelling, withdrawal, and conflicts with family members increased significantly. His wife stated: "I need him out of the house, or we will all go crazy."

Anger is among the most common symptoms reported by patients and their family members during rehabilitation (Mittenberg & Burton, 1994; Silver & Yodofsky, 1994; Cicerone, 1989; Schwab et al., 1993). But anger, like much of the patient's emotions, can be redirected into energy. Energy can be destructive or constructive. Few things provide a smoother channeling of raw emotional energy than a focused set of practical goals. *Structuring* is a technique used in therapy to provide such goals for the patient. Returning to a predictable, purposeful set of activities allows patients to channel their energy productively. It gives them a sense of control over their immediate environment, provides them with positive feedback on their progress, and helps them achieve short-term realistic goals.

But creating a structured environment for the patient is a challenge to the clinician, as it requires more involvement in the life of the patient than one-hour weekly sessions in a formal office setting. The therapist needs to thoroughly evaluate the patient's life setting. Information on his/her living situation, family members, family obligations/roles, actual schedule (i.e., what the patient does throughout the day every day of the week), and potential resources (extended family, support system, "compadres," community resources, insurance-provided resources, etc.) will be crucial in identifying specific activities that will bring a sense of structure back into the patient's life. The therapist will find himself/herself coordinating activities, leading case conferences, and making follow up calls to family members, insurance adjusters, case managers, and others involved in order to facilitate structure for the patient.

Case Study #2

JG was a 40-year-old male who was in a motor vehicle accident and sustained a mild head injury (GCS of 12) with multiple trauma. He was unemployed and living at home when he was referred to therapy. His major complaint was significant depression at home with severely disturbed sleep. He was taking antidepressants, anxiolytics, and sleep medication to no avail. He indicated that he was sick of doctors because no one could "really" help him. He wanted desperately to have a full night's sleep but couldn't. He perceived all the treatment he received up to that point as a failure. "All they do is give me these stupid pills, talk to me for 5 minutes and that's it. They never tell me anything, they don't say whether I will get worse or better, they don't explain anything. Meanwhile, I feel I am getting worse. Nothing is helping me." His initial BDI score was 41. When asked about his daily routine, he reported that he never got up at the same time in the mornings, he ate a brunch by 10:30 A.M., cleaned around the house a bit, took a *siesta* from 12:30 to about 3:00 in the afternoon, and babysat his children when they returned from school at 3:00 P.M. until 5:30 P.M. when his wife returned home from work. He then ate dinner with the family by 6:30 P.M. and watched television until 12:30 or 1:00 A.M., although he admitted never going to bed at a regular time. He only had regular treatment appointments with a psychiatrist and a neurologist every six weeks.

After listing his symptoms and evaluating his daily routine, the treatment of this patient consisted, first, of regulating his sleep schedule, since it was the issue he was most concerned about. The patient was instructed to stop taking any naps during the day and to avoid getting out of bed when waking up at night. The wife reported that she would listen to the patient get up at 3:00 A.M. to go into the kitchen and then turn on the TV in the living room. This needed to end. Efforts were made to identify specific activities during the day which he could agree to perform on a consistent basis. First, he needed a regular waking time. The wife reported that the patient could walk their daughter to school (about 3 blocks) every morning. He readily agreed to it (his wife had not brought it up before, because she felt he was "too ill" for that sort of activity). That meant JG now had to wake up at least by 7:00 A.M. every morning to take his daughter to school by 7:30. Second, it was learned that a *"compadre"* had a business where the patient could go during the afternoons to do some light cleaning or simply to chat with his *"compadre."* That took care of the napping time. Finally, the patient was educated on how to use progressive muscle relaxation with imagery while in bed to avoid getting up in the middle of the night. JG was specifically instructed to change plans whenever he woke up during the night. His plan up to that point had been to eat, to watch TV, or to engage in some activity around the house in the middle of the night. The new plan was simple—he was to stay in bed so he could fall asleep as soon as possible. He was told that even if he did not fall asleep immediately, relaxing while in bed would provide him with enough rest for the next morning.

JG was resistant at first, stating that his problem was severe and quite unique. The tasks were broken down into manageable units. It took two weeks and multiple phone calls to implement a structured time for taking his child to school and then to start visiting his *compadre* regularly. Meanwhile the patient was educated on using progressive muscle relaxation with imagery. JG was then instructed to use it every time he woke up in the middle of the night. The instructions were kept to a minimum: "When you wake up, use the same relaxation technique *in bed* that you learned in the office. Your goal is to go back to sleep." Three weeks later, his BDI score was 18. The patient reported that he could successfully stay in bed, and after 10–15 minutes, fall asleep again using the relaxation technique. He was taking his child to school regularly. Six weeks into therapy, the patient had a structured, predictable daily schedule. This impacted his self-perception of depression and improved his overall sense of self-esteem. He was reinforced for "taking control" of an unmanageable problem through hard work. This then became a model for working on other problem areas later on and moving on to vocational rehabilitation.

The above case illustrates that these patients usually have more resources than one would expect during the initial presentation. Unless the therapist involves the family and is willing to become an active participant in learning about the patient's life and environment, these resources will remain untapped. Involving the family in treatment usually yields rich information about the patient's functioning that may otherwise remain unknown because the patient is either ignoring or discarding it as a potential asset for the rehabilitation process.

JG was unique in that he had a support system and resources that eventually were useful to him. Many Latino patients, particularly recent immigrants or those who work here to send money to their country of origin, will not have such resources. Structuring, nevertheless, can be effectively used in finding meaningful activities for the patient to restore a sense of control over his/her life. We offer several ideas for providing structure for this population in the United States:

- Taking ESL classes.
- Visiting the library, reading about previous areas of work, hobbies, literature, doing ESL homework, etc.
- Spending time in a family business (if any). Family is used here broadly to include all those in the patient's social network that he/she considers family.
- Depending on their judgment and level of functioning, participating actively in child care (preparing lunches, walking children to school, picking them up, supervising their play, etc.).
- Continuing an exercise routine from rehabilitation, going to a gym on a regular basis.
- Volunteering in church/community activities, centers, or hospitals (folding letters, announcements, helping with food/clothes distribution, etc.).

Limitations

This technique may be hampered by the patient's unwillingness to cooperate, by the lack of resources in his environment, by the patient's educational background and range of interests/abilities, and by the willingness of the therapist to become involved in the patient's treatment and set up a reasonable schedule that the patient can follow. Additionally, this process may require constant fine-tuning, as patients may develop anxiety or frustration from attempting to engage in activities that may actually be beyond their reach. When using this technique, the neuropsychological evaluation results can be used as a guideline to capitalize on the cognitive/social strengths of the patient.

REFRAMING

Reframing will serve here as an umbrella for describing paradoxical/cognitive behavioral interventions with this population. In addition to the use of *reframing* as a general skill, the specific reframing of spiritual issues (*spiritualizing*) and the use of *guided imagery* are presented in this section.

Reframing can follow the steps outlined by Haley (1991): focusing on the present and on interactions, understanding symptoms as communications, bypassing insight as the basis of change, and concentrating on the rearranging of the patient's situation as the cause and continuance of psychological change.

Focusing on the Present

Many head-injured patients review the past in a ruminating way, using "if-only" thoughts. Others are significantly depressed about the future and what will become of them and their families. CJ, a 49-year-old male who suffered a penetrating head wound in the right temporo-parietal area, said: "My family depends on me, I have to go to work. This rehabilitation is nice but not for me. I am a man of action, not of words. I need to work." The patient was told that he had already begun to take care of his family by working on his rehabilitation. "Rehabilitation is your new job." This resonated well with the patient, as he needed a concrete answer for his question that dealt with the here and now. Thus, the reframing process should focus on shifting the perspective of the process—from tragedy to challenge, from future to present, from unmanageable issues to manageable issues.

Focusing on Interactions

Rather than abstracting from the patient's interactions as indicative of subconscious mechanisms, the interactions can be measured in terms of social skills strengths or deficits (Cicerone, 1989) to be managed behaviorally (Burke & Lewis, 1986; Whitehouse, 1994).

Understanding Symptoms as Communications

This was addressed earlier in the symptom validation technique.

Bypassing Insight

Since insight-oriented therapy may be neither useful nor popular with head-injured patients (Mittenberg & Burton, 1986; Deaton, 1986), the patient will benefit most from experiences that relate to his/her immediate needs in concrete ways. Real life anecdotes or stories about recovery (gleaned from the clinician's experience) can be useful in providing the patient with models of coping. Extrapolating from Barker's (1985) suggestions, anecdotes and stories of other patients can be used to

- make or illustrate points, instead of sounding moralistic or "preachy";
- suggest solutions to problems by discussing how another patient solved a similar situation;

- help patients to recognize themselves by recognizing aspects of their behavior or reactions in their rehabilitation;
- increase motivation, telling them about successful rehabilitation cases;
- embed directives, by stating in the story which specific directive given by the therapist was successfully used by the patient in the story;
- decrease resistance, presenting ideas for change indirectly;
- model a way of communicating (e.g., how a patient learned to communicate "bottled up emotions" or difficult feelings during rehabilitation); and
- remind them of their own resources, pointing out how other patients discovered strength focusing on intact skills.

Spiritualizing

The event resulting in brain damage is a tragedy that does not have a satisfactory explanation. Many patients feel punished by God or think that it is the natural consequence of their previous mistakes in life. Others wonder why their efforts to be upright people resulted in an accident from the malice/negligence of another person or from a request to perform a task they were not properly trained for or did not have adequate protection to perform. Yet other people see their fate as part of destiny.

Since the phenomenology of the patient (especially low SES patients) will be significantly different from that of the therapist, clinicians should be careful not to dismiss it or belittle it as *irrational* thoughts but should, instead, use it as a therapeutic tool. The use of the patient's phenomenology to reevaluate his/her situation can be quite therapeutic. ST, a 27-year-old who fell four stories to the ground, honestly believed his accident was a sign of punishment from God. During the session, it was suggested to him that God may have actually saved him from dying. A week later the patient returned to therapy having pursued this issue in his mind and having attended mass over the weekend. His statement then was "God spared me for some good reason. I have to go on living." Alternatively, many a patients will tend to ponder on the meaning of life. Their sense of fragility is heightened after the injury. They have unclear ideas of what their life will be like in the future. They may turn to religion as an answer.

The patient's religious inclinations can be effectively used as a therapeutic aid. However, cultural awareness, knowledge, and respect for these issues are crucial. Jocularity, sarcasm, cynicism, and confrontation regarding the patient's spirituality will negatively affect the therapeutic relationship. This may prove particularly challenging if the therapist comes from a very diverse cultural and ethnic background. If the therapist is either totally ignorant of or antagonistic toward religion, he/she should abstain from intervening in this area.

Case Study #3

LL, a 48-year-old married man, sustained a head injury in a motor vs. pedestrian accident. He sustained a basilar skull fracture, a subdural hematoma, and multiple musculoskeletal trauma. His GCS at the scene was 13, and 11 at the E.R. There was no loss of consciousness. As a result of his injury, he developed anosmia, sinus problems, tinnitus, headaches, and difficulties with his sleep-wake cycle. He was seen in therapy three months post-injury. He reported experiencing hypervigilance, flashbacks, nightmares, and neurovegetative signs (sleep disturbance, decreased appetite, anergia, decreased libido). However, he denied feeling sad or down-hearted because, "God spared me from the jaws of death. He has a purpose for my life." Emotional wellness was framed in the context of his belief system. "God would want you to be emotionally healthy." He was educated on how people recover after head injury and what he could expect in the process. The therapist's respect for the patient's belief system facilitated rapport and allowed him to share his feelings. Problem-solving techniques using his spiritual background were used (e.g., "How would God have you react in this situation?"). As time passed and the patient became aware of his slow healing symptoms, he talked about being taught patience by God. He soon engaged in a structured schedule, serving as a volunteer in his church. He derived much pleasure from it because he believed he was serving God. He then began taking some religious education training to "be a better servant." This ended up as a complimentary addition to his cognitive rehabilitation, since he had to read, learn new information, and retrieve it on demand during exams. "My memory is not as good as before. I have to read things twice and have to take a lot of notes. But with all that, I still managed to get an A minus on the test. God is helping me." However, the first author found significant limitations trying to help this patient with his sexual adjustment. He was unable to sleep after sexual intercourse and would become very irritable the day after because he was so tired. His spouse was unwilling to consider sexual intercourse during the day because "it was unnatural," and she would not consider sex during the early mornings or on the weekends because she felt that their teenage children would be offended if they realized what was happening in their bedroom. His wife felt that she was helping him significantly by abstaining from sex. Any other form of sexual foreplay or activity aside from intercourse was emphatically rejected. The patient "learned patience" and reported that he was going to accept it until he got better.

The previous vignette illustrates that "spiritualizing" can be a powerful reframing tool if used respectfully and in addition to other structured psychotherapeutic approaches. It serves the purpose of advancing psychological recovery in post-injury by using the patient's phenomenology. There are many limitations to it including the patient's use of religion to deny problems, the disguising of psychopathology under the auspices of religion, and the sabotaging of therapy with messages from a higher source. A good source to deal with these issues is Thurman (1989). As with any of the strategies discussed in this chapter, it is ultimately up to the clinician's judgment what approach is best for the client.

Guided Imagery

Imagery can be quite effective in treating head injured patients. One common image used during the initial sessions is that of "water in the desert." It goes something like this:

> Think of your situation as a trip through the desert. To cross the desert you must have water. Without it you die. This time in your life is like a desert, your level of energy is your water. Some people use their energy to worry, to get angry at themselves, to blame others for their problems, to fantasize about things they can not change. They soon discover they have little energy to focus on treatment. It is as if they used their water to clean the sand off their shoes in the middle of the desert. They simply wasted it. Other people use their energy to change the things they can change, to work as hard as they can in (occupational, physical, cognitive) therapy, to set goals they can achieve, to learn new ways of doing things. They make it through the desert of rehabilitation just fine. You have to choose how you will use your energy. It is like water in the desert.

Imagery can be used to address a variety of issues. Patients may be resistant to this technique at first; however, they can be reminded that they already engage in active imagery work. Some have strong fantasies of what they will be doing after rehabilitation or what they will look like after orthopedic surgery is completed. Others fantasize about looking the same as before or feeling the way they did prior to their injury. Much of the content in their imagery is negative (Cicerone, 1991). The therapist then works on reframing the use of this strong skill as a tool for empowerment.

Imagery should follow the steps outlined by Edwards (1989): life event visualization, reinstatement of a dream or daytime image, and focusing feelings. The image should be explored for idiosyncratic meanings through prompted soliloquy, prompted dialogue, prompted descriptions of what is happening, and prompted transformation (therapist interventions during the imagery to guide the patient through the process). Restructuring can take place through summary and reframing, directed dialogue, and directed transformation. Since these issues have been discussed in the literature (Edwards, 1989; Edwards, 1990; Langengan, 1987), they will not be discussed here in any further detail.

The more problem-focused the technique, the greater its success. Symptom-specific interventions can be successful because the patient can generalize its benefits. The patient can be "prescribed" to use the same imagery sequence at home at the onset of a symptom or at specific times during the day as stress inoculation methods. The literature (Ridoch & Humphreys, 1994) shows that this form of imagery is effective with sleeplessness, pain management, phobias, and other sequelae of head injury.

CC, for instance, was quite fearful of driving his car alone after his motor vehicle accident. He would report significant anxiety with autonomic manifestations when getting into the car to drive. Guided imagery consisted of progressive desensitization techniques and directed transformations. The patient was made aware of his negative images before driving the car, which were systematically replaced with positive ones. When he was cleared for driving, he only used side streets but was eventually able to use the freeways and drive safely.

This technique will be of limited use with concrete, anxious, and impulsive patients. Similarly, some patients' subjective experience of pain can be so distressing and their coping style so limited that regardless of the efforts at guiding patients through positive imagery, they may simply not respond.

CONCLUSION

Psychotherapeutic treatment of head-injured Latino patients has not received attention in the literature. This chapter provides several practical suggestions on the use of psychotherapeutic skills to treat this population. However, it is expected that they would be useful with head-injured patients regardless of their ethnicity. The use of *Symptom Validation, Journaling, Structuring* and *Reframing*, which have been previously reported in the cognitive behavioral/paradoxical therapy literature, were presented. These techniques should be used at the clinician's discretion and at any time during the therapeutic relationship. While not empirically validated thus far, these techniques represent what our Latino patients have taught us about recovery from head injury. Much is yet to be learned about how support systems affect this population in their adjustment and how permanent sequelae affect low-educated, low-skilled laborers with few resources in this country. More importantly, we need to learn how cultural variables interact with long-term sequelae of head injury to impact family functioning and community reintegration among the Hispanic population. This chapter is but a small contribution to the treatment of this understudied group.

Caminante no hay camino,
se hace camino al andar.

—Machado

REFERENCES

Baker, P.A. (1985). *Using metaphors in therapy.* New York: Brunner/Mazzel.

Bohnen, N.I., Van Zutphen, W., Twijnstras, A., Wijnen, G., Bongers, J., & Jolles, J. (1994). Late outcome of mild head injury: Results from a controlled postal survey. *Brain Injury, 8,* 701–708.

Bott, J., & Klinger, E. (1986) Assessment of guided affective imagery: Methods for extracting quantitative and categorical variables from imagery sequences. *Imagination, Cognition & Personality, 5,* 279–293.

Burke, W.H., & Lewis, F.D. (1986). Management of maladaptive social behavior of a brain-injured adult. *International Journal of Rehabilitation Research, 9,* 335–342.

Burke, W.H., & Wesolowski, M.D. (1988). Applied behavioral analysis in head injury rehabilitation. *Rehabilitation Nursing, 13,* 186–188.

Caudill, M.A. (1995). *Managing pain before it manages you.* New York: Guilford Press.

Chelune, G.J., Heaton, R.K., & Lehman, R.A. (1986). Relation of neuropsychological and personality test results to patients' complaints of disability. In G. Goldstein & R. Raster (Eds.), *Advances in clinical neuropsychology* (Vol. 3). New York: Plenum Press.

Cicerone, K.D. (1989). Psychoterapeutic interventions with traumatically brain-injured patients. *Rehabilitation Psychology, 34,* 105–114.

———. (1991). Psychotherapy after mild traumatic brain injury: Relation to the nature and severity of subjective complaints. *Journal of Head Trauma Rehabilitation, 6,* 30–43.

Cole, J.R. (1992). Psychosocial rehabilitation. In P.M. Deustch & K.B. Fralish (Eds.), *Innovations in head injury rehabilitation* (pp. 1–32). New York: Matthew Bender.

Deaton, A.V. (1986). Denial in the aftermath of traumatic brain injury: Its manifestations, measurement, and treatment. *Rehabilitation Psychology, 78,* 107–126.

Drudge, O.W., Rosen, J.C., Peyser, J.M., & Peniadz, J. (1986). Behavioral and emotional problems and treatment in chronically brain-impaired adults. *Annals of Behavioral Medicine, 8,* 9–14.

Edwards, D.J. (1989). Cognitive restructuring through guided imagery: Lessons from Gestalt therapy. In A. Freeman, K. M. Simon, L. E. Beutler, & H. Arkowitz, (Eds.), *Comprehensive handbook of cognitive therapy.* New York: Plenum.

———. (1990). Cognitive therapy and the restructuring of early memories through guided imagery. *Journal of Cognitive Psychotherapy, 4,* 33–50.

Fordyce, D.J., & Roveceh, J.P. (1986). Changes in perspectives of disability among patients, staff and relatives during rehabilitation of brain injury. *Rehabilitation Psychology, 31,* 217–229.

Freeman, A., & DeWolf, R. (1992). *The 10 dumbest mistakes smart people make and how to avoid them.* New York: Harper Collins.

Gainotti, G. (1993). Emotional and psychosocial problems after brain injury. *Neuropsychological Rehabilitation, 3,* 259–277.

Greenberg, D., & Padesky, C. A. (1995). *Mind over mood: A cognitive therapy treatment manual for clients.* New York: Guilford Press.

Haley, J. (1991). *Advanced techniques of hypnosis and therapy.* San Francisco: Jossey-Bass Publishers.

Jensen, O.K. & Nielsen, F.F. (1990). The influence of sex and pre-traumatic headache on the incidence and severity of headache after head injury. *Cephalgia, 10,* 285–293.

LaCalle, J.J. (1987). Forensic psychological evaluations through an interpreter: Legal and ethical issues. *American Journal of Forensic Psychology 5,* 29–43.

Lane, I.M., Wesolowski, M.D., & Burke, W.H. (1989). Teaching socially appropriate behavior to eliminate holding in a brain-injured adult. *Journal of Behavior Therapy and Experimental Psychiatry, 20,* 79–82.

Langenbahn, D.M. (1987). The use of visual imagery and self-instruction for memory rehabilitation with closed head injury patients. *Dissertation Abstracts International, 47* (11-B), 4654.

León-Carrión, J. (1994). *Daño Cerebral: Guía para familiares y cuidadores.* Madrid: Siglo XXI de España Editores.

Lewis, F.D., Nelson, J., Nelson, C., & Reusink, P. (1988). Effects of three feedback contingencies on the socially inappropriate talk of brain-injured adults. *Behavior Therapy, 19,* 203–211.

———. (1986). Psychological implications of traumatic brain damage for the patient's family. *Rehabilitation Psychology, 31,* 241–250.

Lezak, M.D. (1988). Brain damage is a family affair. *Journal of Clinical and Experimental Neuropsychology, 10,* 111–123.

Malgady, R.G., Rogler, L.H. & Constantino, G. (1987). Ethnocultural and linguistic bias in mental health evaluation of Hispanics. *American Psychologist, 42,* 228–234.

Martin, P.R. (1993). *Psychological management of chronic headaches.* New York: Guilford.

McAllister, T.W. (1994). Mild traumatic brain injury and the post-concussive syndrome. In J.M. Silver, S.C. Yudofsky, & R.E. Hales (Eds.), *Neuropsychiatry of traumatic brain injury* (pp. 357–392). Washington, DC: American Psychiatric Press.

Mittenberg, W., & Burton, D.B. (1994). A survey of treatments for post-concussive syndrome. *Brain Injury, 8,* 429–437.

Morin, C.M. (1993). *Insomnia: Psychological assessment and management.* New York: Guilford Press.

O'Hanlon, W.H. (1987). *Taproots: Underlying principles of Milton Erickson's therapy and hypnosis.* New York: Norton.

Padesky, C.A., & Greenberg, D. (1995). *Clinician's guide to mind over mood.* New York: Guilford Press.

Parenté, R. & Anderson-Parenté, J. (1991). *Retraining memory: Techniques and applications.* Houston, TX: CSY Publishing.

Parker, R.S. (1990). *Traumatic brain injury and neuropsychological impairment.* New York: Springer Verlag.

Ponsford, J.L., Olver, J.H., & Curran, C. (1995). A profile of outcome: Two years after traumatic brain injury. *Brain Injury, 9,* 1–10.

Ponton, M.O., Satz, P., Herrera, L., Ortiz, F., Urrutia, C., Young, R., D'Elia, L., Furst, C.J., and Namerow, N. (1996). Normative data stratified by age and education for the Neuropsychological Screening Battery for Hispanics (NeSBHIS): Initial report. *Journal of the Int'l. Neuropsychological Society, 2,* 96–104.

Prigatano, G.P. & Fordyce, D.J. (1986). Cognitive dysfunction and psychosocial adjustment after brain injury. In G.P. Prigatano (Ed.), *Neuropsychological rehabilitation after brain injury* (pp. 1–17). Baltimore: John Hopkins University Press.

Ridoch, M.J., & Humphreys, G.W. (1994). *Cognitive neuropsychology and cognitive rehabilitation.* Hove, UK: Lawrence Earlbaum Associates.

Silver, J.M., & Yudofsky, S.C. (1994). Aggressive disorders. In J.M. Silver, S.C. Yudofsky, & R.E. Hales (Eds.), *Neuropsychiatry of traumatic brain injury* (pp. 313–355). Washington, DC: American Psychiatric Press

Thurman, C. (1989). *The lies we believe.* Nashville, TN: Thomas Nelson Publishers.

Wesolowski, M.D., & Burke, W.H. (1989). Behavior management techniques. In P. Deutsch & K. Fralish (Eds.), *Innovations in head injury rehabilitation.* New York: Matthew Bender.

Whitehouse, A.M. (1994). Applications of cognitive therapy with survivors of head injury. *Journal of Cognitive Psychotherapy: An International Quarterly, 8,* 141–160.

Williams, J.M., & Long, C.J. (Eds.). (1987). *The rehabilitation of cognitive disabilities.* New York: Plenum Press.

29

Economic and Legal Aspects of Neuropsychological Rehabilitation

Robert D. Voogt

Robert Voogt & Associates, Inc.
New Orleans, LA

INTRODUCTION: ECONOMIC AND LEGAL ISSUES IN BRAIN INJURY REHABILITATION

In much the same way stones thrown into a pond cause ever-widening ripples, a traumatic brain injury (TBI) makes an impact on the injured, their families and friends, their communities, and, finally, on the economy of their countries. The costs of diagnosis, treatment, rehabilitation, and long-term care will continue to mount as medical advances prolong the lives of the injured, and these costs play a direct part in the escalating cost of healthcare in general.

Background

Before considering the legal and economic implications of TBI, it is essential to understand the functions of the brain and the damage caused by TBI. The brain is responsible for an individual's consciousness, thought, memory, reason, judgement, and feelings. It also organizes and integrates many of the body's systems. Because of the brain's complexity, a brain injury is a combination of medical and social problems rather than a single diagnosis.

Despite their causes, brain injuries produce devastating long-term effects that change almost every aspect of the injured person's life. The final neurological outcome following a head injury depends on which part of the brain was injured and how severe the injury was. The individual's health and capabilities prior to the injury also play a role in his/her recovery.

Functional outcomes of persons with TBI are generally classified as mild, moderate, or severe. These classifications can help to diagnose the extent of the injury and to predict an individual's prognosis.

A mild brain injury may occur without a loss of consciousness (Voogt, 1990). It may be accompanied by contusions or lacerations that affect the brain. Because mild brain injuries can occur without concussions or obvious signs of trauma, they can be easily overlooked by witnesses who may not feel that medical intervention is warranted. If the injured person is examined by a physician, these minor brain injuries may not reveal themselves in routine examinations. A person who sustains a mild brain injury may have any or all of the following symptoms: scalp tenderness, confusion, dizziness, and generalized motor weakness. The injured person may experience headaches, insomnia, and trouble concentrating for several days after the injury. If these symptoms persist despite negative tests, the injured person may be dismissed as a malingerer.

Moderate brain injury usually includes a loss of consciousness and may include post-traumatic amnesia. Individuals with moderate brain injury may be able to function in their daily tasks, but they will have difficulty with higher level thought functions such as planning, reasoning, problem solving, and remembering. These individuals will need limited supervision and assistance to complete the tasks of daily living.

When an individual sustains a severe brain injury, he/she can no longer perform the tasks of daily living without continuous care. Such individuals cannot care for themselves safely and cannot care for others. People who sustain severe brain injury also demonstrate a myriad of motor and behavioral problems.

Because persons with TBI undergo such profound transformation, their family members often express the feeling that the person they once knew and loved has disappeared. The "new" family member may be disagreeable and difficult to care for. As family members cope with the physical and mental changes in the injured person, they will realize that the home setting may no longer provide a suitable and safe environment. The family must then begin the complicated task of determining a life care plan for the brain-injured person, a process that includes accurately estimating the cost of such care. This task becomes more difficult as healthcare becomes more expensive in general.

Rising Healthcare Costs

There can be no disputing the contention that healthcare costs have become a major problem in the economies of most countries. According to Reinstein (1993), medical costs in the United States are estimated to have risen 119% in the decade 1980–1990. In that same period, the cost of hospitalization rose 162%. To put these figures in perspective, the rate of inflation from 1980 to 1990 was 51%.

An overview of America's total budget shows that in the same period, healthcare costs increased from $275 billion (9% of the GNP) to $600 billion (12% of the GNP). It is estimated that these costs will climb to $1.5 trillion dollars (15% of the GNP) by the year 2000 (Reinstein, 1993) and that by the year 2030, healthcare costs could account for 41% of the country's GNP (Waldo, Sonnefeld, Lemieux, & McKusick, 1992).

As staggering as these numbers are, they only include costs that are funded by governmental agencies and do not take into account the indirect costs medical care places on families and communities. Because of their complexity, TBIs are one of the primary causes of rising healthcare costs.

Overview of Costs Associated with TBI

Each year in the United States, approximately 2 million people suffer mild to moderate TBIs, and an additional 100,000 people sustain severe TBIs (Voogt, 1995). These individuals will require healthcare that is expensive on both short-term and long-term levels.

Once a TBI is diagnosed, a person may require lengthy periods of rehabilitation. Estimates put the cost of TBI rehabilitation at $3 billion in 1990 (Longwell, 1991) and $10 billion in 1992 (Mullins, 1992). For those whose injuries require full-time assisted living, costs can range from $250 per diem at home with assistance to $500 per diem in a medically based facility. At an average per diem rate of more than $375, annual care can cost close to $140,000 (Table 29.1). The Brain Injury Association estimates the medical cost of TBIs in the United States to be $48.3 billion annually (Voogt, 1995).

Table 29.1: Breakdown of Daily Costs by Facility for TBI Patients

Community-Based Residential Care	$350 per day
Long-term Medical Care Facility	$500 per day
At home with 24-hour Care	$250 per day
At home with 24-hour LPN	$400 per day
Average per day	$375

Significant expense is incurred by patients who are in a persistent vegetative state. The care for such patients ranges from $2,000 to $10,000 a month, depending on the amount of medical care the patient requires and the region where the care is provided (Cranford, as cited in McCormick, 1991). That translates to an annual expenditure nationwide of $120 million to $1.2 billion to care for these patients. If a patient is ventilator-dependent, costs of care can easily triple (Ibid.).

Patients who have fully regained consciousness from their injuries but who still display significant impairments can profit from post-acute treatment programs. The cost of these programs can run from $350 to more than $1,500 per day (Voogt, 1994). These programs are designed for patients with impairments involving mobility, coordination, strength, speech and language, active exercise, cognition, memory, safety, activities of daily living, the ability to work, verbal or physical aggression, and emotional control. The cost of the future healthcare depends on the type and amount of care needed, ranging from the very minimal, where an individual is monitored from a distance, to around-the-clock care in an intensive healthcare setting with support from therapists and physicians.

Cost Grows as Care Improves

These already high costs will continue to grow as the survivorship rates for those incurring TBIs improve. Antibiotics and other medical interventions have enabled many of the injured to survive their initial traumas, and improved medical emergency treatments and new techniques in neurosurgery now enable many more to live longer lives. However, the majority of those who survive a severe brain injury each year will experience dramatic, life-long compromises of their lifestyles and will require complex medical care throughout their lives. There are also thousands of children who suffer brain injuries, often at birth, who will require life-long care.

In addition to those who experience severe brain trauma, millions more experience minor to moderate brain injuries such as blows to the head during automobile accidents or falls. Sometimes these injuries cause subtle deficits. Other times, these individuals undergo notable personality changes as a result of frontal lobe damage. Most TBIs also involve some emotional changes, either from the brain injury itself or as a reaction to the loss of function. These patients need emotional support and therapy to learn to recognize and control their behaviors (Voogt, 1994).

Overview of the Damage Caused by Brain Injury

Damage to the cortical and subcortical systems, which are associated with executive function, can cause problems that make an individual's return to independent living impossible. Skills such as planning, organizing, and setting goals are often lost (Stuss & Benson, 1986).

In much the same way as a person with a physical disability uses a wheelchair or walker, a person who has sustained a brain injury will require a personal assistant to help with those tasks the brain is unable to do. The inability to perform these executive functions often keeps a person with brain injury from resuming his/her previous vocation. The loss of executive functioning is often more devastating than the loss of ambulation. When given the choice of resuming physical activities (such as walking) or regaining the ability to perform these executive functions, many people with TBI would rather have the brain function they had before their injuries.

Because the disabilities caused by TBIs aren't as visible as physical disabilities, people with TBIs are often dismissed as having no problems at all or as malingerers or hypochondriacs. When their injuries cause them to take legal action, their lawyers often focus on their orthopedic injuries, unaware that the permanent brain damage their clients have suffered will keep them disabled for the rest of their lives (Voogt, 1994).

Persons with TBIs may appear "normal" to observers; they may have few physical signs of their dysfunction. But upon examination, a specialist can perceive that the individual with a TBI cannot process information and may be unable to remember instructions for more than a few minutes. Consequently, it is difficult for these individuals to carry out therapy, and they may require a highly structured environment for a longer period of time. Other common deficits include impaired word-finding ability, poorly organized written or verbal communication, an inability to solve problems, and difficulty in expressing thoughts and emotions.

After sustaining a TBI, individuals may express a myriad of emotions from profound depression to inappropriate elation. They may show verbal and physical aggression and such defense mechanisms as anxiety, denial, fear, and unproductive reactions. The direct costs—those for medical care and rehabilitation—are obvious; less obvious are the indirect costs of TBIs.

Indirect Costs

In addition to costs for medical treatment and long-term care, the loss to society of productive, taxpaying wage-earners must be included in the total cost of TBIs. Ninety percent of families dealing with a family member's TBI report a reduction in income, which can mean a $4 billion loss to the economy (Ashley, 1990). Unfortunately, people with TBI are discouraged from returning to work after rehabilitation because earning an income could cause them to lose the Social Security and Medicaid benefits they receive. Justin Dart, former chairman of the President's Committee on the Employment of Persons with Disabilities, has estimated that the contributions these individuals could make to the tax base would equal the annual U.S. deficit (Voogt, 1995). Calculating the amount of lost wages caused by TBIs is more complicated than simply multiplying the injured person's annual salary by the number of productive years lost.

Calculating Wage Loss

When assessing the vocational cost of a TBI, one must consider both wage loss and earning capacity. Gamboa (1994) stated that the wage loss can be calculated for older workers by simply multiplying their annual salary times the years they had left before retirement. But for younger workers, one must calculate the approximate level of education and expertise they might have achieved before computing the value of their lost wage-earning years.

It is important to note that the terms "mild," "moderate," and "severe" do not always correlate with the amount of lost wages. For example, most of us would categorize the inability to remember names as a "mild" or "moderate" disability when compared to the inability to walk. But if one's job prior to the TBI was that of a salesman, this so-called "mild" disability could result in the loss of a substantial number of sales. A writer, on the other hand, may cope better with an inability to walk than would a lumberjack or custodian, who would lose his/her job altogether.

Persons with brain injuries may also develop emotional problems such as impulsivity, moodiness, disinhibition, anger, loss of patience, and an inability to control one's emotions. These problems can make it difficult for survivors to hold down a job, get along with co-workers and family members, and deal with the public.

Indirect economic costs to society include the loss of social spending by people who have become incapacitated by brain injury. They do not purchase the homes, cars, restaurant meals, clothes, or recreational equipment they might have bought had they remained employed.

Although many European countries have subsidized medical programs that absorb the costs of rehabilitation and assisted living, these nations also incur a loss in spending by people with TBIs. Haase (1992) estimated the cost to Denmark of lost wages due to traffic accidents as 407 million Deutschmarks in 1990.

Costs to Family Members

Because the majority of those receiving TBIs require assistance of varying degrees, spouses or other family members must either leave their jobs or reduce their work hours in order to take care of their loved one who has sustained a TBI. Often these family members must also give up their social lives because of the difficulty of obtaining respite help.

When a parent sustains a brain injury, the family often must pay a caregiver to watch the children, a handyman to cut the grass and make household repairs, and a housekeeper to help keep the home running smoothly. The burden on the remaining parent becomes acute, and he/she can be vulnerable to emotional and physical illnesses resulting from the strain (Bush, 1994).

Emotional Costs to Family Members

Although families play a major role in facilitating the rehabilitation of a person with TBI, they are often neglected by healthcare professionals. Common problems in these families include isolation, depression, anxiety, and fatigue. Family members often find themselves bearing the brunt of the injured person's verbal and physical outbursts (Voogt, 1990).

Families may begin by denying that a loved one has sustained a permanent injury. They may expect the individual with a TBI to "snap out of it" and return to his/her former behavior. Once the family realizes the extent of the injury and the effect it will have on the lifestyle of their relative, they may experience profound depression and regret. A closure occurs when the family accepts the disability and makes plans for a new lifestyle for themselves and for the injured person.

When a family member suffers a TBI, the family can be devastated financially. A study by McMordie and Barker (1988) reported that 90% of the spouses of TBI survivors reported a reduction in family income. Forty-seven percent of the spouses reported they had to borrow money; 26% lost personal possessions; and 9% had to declare bankruptcy.

Hedonic Damages

Another loss that must be considered is the loss of the ability to enjoy one's life. The term "hedonic damages" (Smith, 1994) refers to the impairment individuals with brain injury experience in their ability to enjoy life. In the past, brain injury was known to cause a loss of earning potential, but little consideration was given to putting a dollar figure on the loss of enjoyment of life itself. This is understandable, given the difficulty of determining the value of enjoyment of life.

However, this loss can be calculated using a psychologist's estimate as to the percent of the loss the patient is suffering, ranging from severe to moderate to mild and then using the full value of a life (placed at approximately $2.3 million) to calculate the partial loss (Smith, 1994).

Identical injuries may cause varying degrees of hedonic damage to different people, depending upon the types of activities they enjoyed before their injuries and the way their injuries keep them from enjoying these activities in the future.

Range of Cost

Calculating the direct and indirect costs of TBI remains complicated. The exact figure most often cited regarding the cost of future care is $4–$5 million (Voogt, 1995). But because individual needs vary greatly, the actual cost of such care ranges from $3 million to almost $20 million, exclusive of hedonic losses and lost wages (Voogt, 1994). On an individual level, an accurate estimation of the costs of a TBI is necessary so that an adequate financial care plan can be drawn up.

Preparing a Life Care Plan

Preparing a life care plan for a person with TBI is a multi-step process. Before an estimate of life care needs can be made, a rehabilitation specialist must interview the person with TBI and his/her family members and review records of professionals who have treated the individual. Next, the specialist prepares a narrative detailing the individual's pre-injury status including education, vocation, relationships and achievements. A rehabilitation team must decide which forms of rehabilitation will best serve the client. A cost report is then prepared itemizing the medical, evaluative, therapeutic, and treatment costs; an estimate of the duration and frequency of these costs; and the cost per unit of service. The report should include related costs such as counseling, support care, and equipment.

The likelihood of inflation is considered when estimating the cost of future care. The cost report must then factor in the present value and discount. These calculations can be done with a variety of inflation and discount values and are available through computerized programs.

Other considerations include the community and state in which the person lives and the estimated number of years for which the person will require aid. There is a sample Life Care Plan at the end of this chapter.

LEGAL ISSUES IN TBI

TBI has created a multitude of legal issues. After an accident, blame is often sought so that a party can be found responsible for the cost of care for the injured party. In the United States and, increasingly, in many European countries, this contributes to the rise of third party lawsuits. In these cases, it is more profitable for the plaintiff if the responsible party is also a corporation or an entity that has great financial resources or superior insurance coverage. For people sustaining TBIs, there is a direct relationship between quality of life and financial resources. As such, the healthcare issues in TBI frequently become part of legal complications, and the individual's quality of life becomes compromised. One problem is the lack of lawyers who are capable of representing individuals with TBIs. Often, lawyers do not have expertise in TBI and lack the resources to obtain the services of those who do.

Many injured persons are, therefore, forced to look to their health insurance to cover their rehabilitation and daily living expenses. But the major medical policies in the United States and other countries frequently do not pay for long-term rehabilitation and almost never cover lifetime rehabilitation. The result is that individuals often receive intervention that ensures their survival but find their rehabilitation is cut short because the insurance industry is not interested in investing the sum of money required.

As managed care policies proliferate, fewer and fewer individuals will have insurance carriers willing to cover comprehensive, long-term rehabilitations. This is unfortunate, and short-term intervention accomplishes little.

Those who turn to the federal and state governments for assistance will also meet with disappointment. These agencies frequently will provide nursing home services which are not necessarily appropriate for people with TBI. More effective, but deemed too expensive, is long-term rehabilitation.

The situation is equally grim for children injured before age 18. Neither the United States nor most other countries have appropriate facilities for these children. Therefore, most children with TBI remain at home, often impacting the economic and emotional lives of their parents and siblings. In the United States, parents often look to state government agencies for help, but these agencies are not adequate to provide the wide variety of services necessary for long-term help for these children.

Some individuals with TBIs have brought suit against governmental agencies in the United States because these agencies failed to provide proper rehabilitation and, instead, housed these individuals in locked psychiatric units where they subsequently developed psychiatric problems. Ironically, the cost of providing these inappropriate services is often more than the cost of providing appropriate services in a private setting.

Worldwide, most governments provide acute care, but rarely do they provide the intervention that will make a significant difference in the individual's quality of life or the ability of these individuals to regain a portion of the life they had before their injuries.

People with TBIs are often deemed unable to make decisions regarding their treatment or the expenditure of their funds. Often, they feel imprisoned in rehabilitative facilities and press for release at the same time that their medical advisors counsel family members to keep their loved ones in such facilities. Family members, in turn, often feel guilty for forcing their loved ones to remain in rehabilitation and allow them to return home.

Reaching a Settlement

When lawsuits are filed, an individual with a brain injury may believe that he/she should settle out of court rather than press his/her case. Unscrupulous or unskilled lawyers may counsel these individuals to accept judgements that seem adequate but that, in reality, will not cover the costs of life-long rehabilitation and care. One reason an early settlement is undesirable is that, many times, the full consequences of a TBI cannot be assessed for several years (Buzard, 1994).

Choosing the most qualified attorney to litigate a case involving TBI can help the injured person obtain a suitable settlement. Lawyers involved in TBI suits can be retained on a contingency fee; that is, the attorney does not receive a fee unless the injured person receives a settlement. The attorney's fee is an agreed-upon percentage of the settlement. This practice means that a family of little means can still afford to retain an experienced attorney to litigate their loved one's case.

Simkins and Craig (1994) suggest that a law firm may need to spend as much as $50,000 in preparing a minor TBI lawsuit. People considering such litigation should be sure the firm they are retaining can afford such an expenditure. They should also inquire as to the amount of experience the lawyers in the firm have had with TBI cases and what the results were in these past lawsuits.

Adjustment for Inflation

Settlements awarded to persons with TBIs must be adjusted to reflect inflation. The present value of a settlement is the value, in today's dollars, of the amount of money that must be set aside to meet annual fiscal needs of the lifetime of a person with a catastrophic injury. Present value takes into account the increase rate and the discount rate of a given commodity or service. The real increase rate for medical services between 1947 and 1991 has been 2.26% over the general rate of inflation. The real average annual increase of medical commodities over the same period has been less than general inflation, a negative value of -0.56%. In the case study shown at the end of this chapter, the discount rate used is 1.07%, which is the real rate of interest of high grade municipal bonds.

The discount rate is offset by the increase rate to determine the present value. Therefore, for medical service, the present value would have to increase annually by the difference between the increase rate and the discount rate or 1.19% per annum. Medical commodities would be decreased by 1.63% (see pp. 545–550.)

Providing for Vocational Rehabilitation

Any settlement should include the costs required to ensure a program of vocational rehabilitation for the person with TBI. Vocational rehabilitation is not only a cost-effective treatment, it contributes greatly to increased quality of life.

The focus of rehabilitation in the past has been to spend large sums of money in initial treatment by physical and occupational therapists and speech-language pathologists. After a period of time has passed, many patients state that they can cope with their physical limitations but desperately need vocational training. There is no available research indicating that certain amounts of therapeutic interventions in the acute stage will make a significant difference long-term vs. spending these dollars for long-term care or rehabilitation (Voogt, 1995).

A study by Abrams, Barker, Haffey, and Nelson (1993) showed the value of vocational rehabilitation for 142 persons with TBI. The majority of these clients had been employed at the time of their injuries. At the time of discharge, 94 of these clients were evaluated using the Glasgow Outcome Scale; all but two were rated either severely or moderately disabled.

The clients were enrolled in an individualized return-to-work program at Sharp Memorial Rehabilitation Center in San Diego, California. A cost-benefit analysis of the program showed the return to taxpayers to be four-fold (Abrams et al., 1993). The intangible benefit of such a program is the increased self-esteem most people with disabilities feel when they are able to lead productive lives.

FINANCIAL CONTRIBUTIONS TO THE HEALTHCARE INDUSTRY

At the same time that TBI consumes billions of healthcare dollars, it also contributes to the profits of the healthcare industry. In 1970, there were no rehabilitation facilities earmarked for patients with TBI; today, there are more than 3,000 (Voogt, 1995). The gross revenue in TBI rehabilitation centers was $3 billion in 1990. By 1992, that figure had become $10 billion, and it has continued to escalate (Voogt, 1995).

The growth in rehabilitation centers has resulted in increased demand for attendants, aides, therapists, nurses, and other medical professionals. These patients also purchase wheelchairs and other specialized equipment. Scientists in almost every country take part in research and education programs designed to study TBIs, and a variety of companies seek to produce new therapeutic equipment to help persons with disabilities lead fuller lives.

Resources created through financial settlements increase the overall economic value of TBI. These "lump sum" settlements are often invested, increasing the amount of capital available for borrowing.

PREVENTION

One way to hold down the cost of TBIs is to stress prevention. For example, many countries have explored the possibility of requiring all motorcyclists to wear helmets to reduce head injuries. Motorcycle accidents are a prime cause of head injuries, and because the victims are almost always young, the cost of long-term care is prohibitive. In a study (Rivara, Dicker, Bergman, Dacey, & Herman, 1988) of 105 motorcycle victims hospitalized at a major trauma center in Seattle, Washington, it was found that total direct costs for these patients for a mean of 20 months were more than $2.7 million with an average of $25,764 per patient. Of this amount, 60% was spent on initial hospital care, and 23% went toward rehabilitation care or readmission for treatment. Most of this care was paid for by public funds such as Medicaid. It is clear that public laws mandating safety measures such as helmets can save public money spent on care and rehabilitation. Seat belts and air bags will significantly improve outcomes after auto accidents.

TBIs such as these create a group of government-dependent individuals. In the group above, none of the patients had been dependent on public assistance prior to their accidents. They became medically indigent because of their long hospital stays. Less than 1% of these charges were paid directly by the patient or his/her family (Rivara et al., 1988).

Although safety devices such as helmets, seat belts, and air bags can prevent serious injury during an accident, it is even more effective to prevent such accidents from occurring at all. Stringent drinking-and-driving laws in many European countries reduce accidents caused by drunken drivers. The Brain Injury Association estimates that more than half of those who suffer brain injury are intoxicated at the time.

Violence, especially domestic violence, also causes many incidents of TBI. Shaking and physical abuse of children and gunshot wounds in teen-teenagers are two causes of TBIs in young people.

Maintaining national speed limits also helps lessen the frequency of accidents that lead to TBIs. Other effective preventative efforts include education in schools, holding manufacturers accountable for faulty products, and discounting automobile insurance for those who consistently use safety devices such as seat belt and air bags.

WHO SPEAKS FOR THE BRAIN INJURED?

Men and women with TBIs make up a large group of citizens worldwide. This group does not have the lobbying power of the American Medical Association or the large insurance companies. Nor do they have the clout of the rehabilitation industry. But brain injury rehabilitation has become a major economic force throughout the world. It is the most costly disability that occurs on a regular basis throughout the world. Compromises will have to be made in order to provide the services these people need. Otherwise, a new class of citizens will develop a lifestyle that is less than desirable. Individuals with brain injuries will continue to be placed in psychiatric facilities where the cost of care is high and the suitability is inappropriate.

The amount of money brain-injured individuals receive in settlements can in no way overcome the significant tragedy they have incurred. Individuals with TBI have great difficulty voicing their wants, opinions, and desires, especially if they have little insight into the injuries they have sustained. It is easy, therefore, for big government systems and healthcare providers, as well as the insurance industry, to take advantage of this population and to fail to provide them with the necessary care or resources they desperately need.

The healthcare industry needs to be revolutionized throughout the world so that individuals who have sustained TBI can receive the care they desire to lead the most productive and satisfying lives they are capable of living.

A SAMPLE CASE

Following is an example of a comprehensive Life Care Plan prepared for a patient injured in an automobile accident. Estimating the present and future costs of a TBI is time-consuming and complex, but it is essential to follow each step of the procedure to ensure that an adequate amount of money is set aside to provide for the life-long needs of the patient.

Patient History

An accurate patient history is essential so that the lifestyle of the client before he/ she suffered injuries can be compared with the lifestyle of the client after the injuries. A patient history should paint a picture of the life the client led including education, hobbies, daily responsibilities, and job skills.

The patient, identified in this sample case as Jane Smith, was born in 1960 and lived in the Midwest with her husband and two young children. She had a high school diploma and some college education and worked in a real estate office, where her duties included bookkeeping, accounting, record-keeping, and typing. She enjoyed sports and was a vigorous, active spouse and parent. Her hobbies included gardening, fishing, camping, and playing cards.

Smith was injured at the age of 31 when the car she was driving was in a head-on collision with a semi-truck. When she was taken to the emergency room of a nearby hospital, she had abrasions to her face and forehead, a jagged laceration on her left wrist, pain in the wrist and elbow, and tenderness in the right hip.

By the next day, she had visible bruising on her face, breasts, thigh, arm, and abdomen, as well as a dislocated toe. Several days later, she had developed blackened eyes and a large hematoma in her right inner groin. The physician who examined her noted that she had five fractured ribs and a possible skull fracture.

This began a three-year ordeal for Smith, who was referred to neurosurgeons, neurologists, psychiatrists, physical therapists, a neuropsychologist, a psychiatrist, orthopedists, and internal medicine specialists. She was eventually diagnosed with the following:

- Closed head injury
- Chronic pain syndrome
- Post-traumatic stress disorder
- Headaches
- Myofascial pain
- Disk bulge at L5-S1
- Mild disk herniation at L4-L5
- Hyperlipidemia
- Depression
- Right jaw pain

Smith's disabilities had caused her to give up almost all of the activities she had enjoyed prior to her accident. She could no longer care for her children, prepare meals, take part in her hobbies of fishing and gardening, or work in an office. She had trouble concentrating or following simple directions (as in a recipe) and was easily fatigued. Her children noted that her personality had changed; she was quick to anger and had outbursts and irritability. Her husband was forced to shoulder the burden of keeping house and child care. She had a loss of interest in sexual relations and had pain with intercourse.

Smith had difficulty performing such basic tasks as using a can opener and baiting a fishing hook. She suffered from dizziness. Because of cognitive impairments and a slowed reaction time, she could no longer drive safely.

At the time of this evaluation, Smith's life expectancy was 46.6 more years (according to 1989 statistics from the U.S. Department of Health and Human Services).

Medical History

The Medical History should give complete details of the injury, subsequent evaluations and treatments, and a list of physical and mental impairments. Copies of the reports issued by each specialist the client consults should be included in the Medical History. In an actual Medical History, the names and addresses of hospitals, treatment centers, and physicians would be included in the narrative.

Smith was the restrained driver in a vehicle that had a head-on collision with a semi-truck. Because her driver's door was damaged extensively, she required extraction. At the scene of the injury, she complained of pain to her left elbow, face, and left foot; she denied loss of consciousness.

Smith was taken to a general hospital where her facial abrasions were treated and glass particles were removed. X-rays were negative, and she was discharged from the emergency room after three hours.

The following day, her personal physician examined her and noted abrasions between her eyes and severe abrasions on her nose and her forehead. She had bruises to both breasts, her left thigh, right arm, and right abdomen. A dislocated left foot third toe was reduced. She received Silvadene for her facial abrasions.

The remainder of the Medical History should narrate in detail each visit the client made to each physician and treatment facility. Each injury should be described in detail (e.g., "She had a large 3-cm-by-8-cm hematoma to her right groin, and it was felt that she had experienced leaking from an artery.").

Physical and Mental Limitations

This section gives a review of the patient's current condition, gathered from the medical reports and a personal interview with the client and his/her family. It is important to enumerate each impairment the client has, including those which have an intangible worth, so that an accurate estimate can be made of the total worth of her disability.

Jane Smith has been under the care of several physicians since her injury on January 1, 1991. She has been evaluated and treated by physicians who specialize in orthopedics, neurology, psychiatry, internal medicine, and rehabilitation.

She has been found to have the following physical and mental limitations:

Physical Limitations
- Neck pain radiating to the shoulder blades
- Low back pain radiating to the right lower extremity
- Awkward gait
- Decreased walking, standing, and climbing tolerance
- Dizziness and headache
- Easily fatigued
- Sleep disturbances
- Changes in sense of taste and smell
- Weight loss
- Swelling and numbness in lower extremities
- Impairments in balance
- Decreased upper extremity coordination
- Decreased ability to lift, reach, and grasp
- Limited ability to twist and bend
- Decreased ability to cook and to perform household tasks
- Unable to perform gardening, shopping
- Unable to go canoeing
- Unable to pick up children
- Unable to return to former employment
- Unable to drive

Cognitive Impairments
- Flat affect
- Memory impairments
- Repeats stories often
- Impairments in decision making and problem solving
- Poor reasoning
- Decreased attention and concentration
- Difficulty with abstract reasoning
- Limitations in judgement
- Word-finding difficulties
- Difficulty following instructions
- Becomes confused when watching a movie
- Loss of patience with children
- No longer plays with children
- Unable to anticipate or to meet children's needs

Psychological Difficulties
- Sadness
- Irritability
- Increased anxiety
- Decreased frustration tolerance
- Changes in self-image
- Lowered self-esteem
- Decreased socialization
- Changes in family relationships
- Mood swings
- Frequent crying
- Outbursts of anger

Rehabilitation Services

This section of the Life Care Plan should outline the need the person with brain injury has for rehabilitation services and describe the types of services most appropriate to the client's injuries.

Jane Smith is no longer able to manage her day-to-day affairs and participate in her children's lives. Her inability to handle the responsibilities of a wife, mother, and full-time office worker have left her frustrated, angry, and depressed. She also suffers chronic pain, weakness, and cognitive impairments. She desperately wants to regain function and continue her productive life. She has developed depression, as well as generalized cognitive limitations and motor slowing. She requires assistance with household, family, and money management. She must cope daily with many adjustments and compromises resulting from the physical, psychological, and emotional sequelae associated with a closed head injury.

Mrs. Smith will require a variety of services and support for the remainder of her life. The overall plan for these services must include medical, therapeutic, psychological, vocational, and social support. The required services/items, duration, and frequencies are outlined in the Cost Report.

Because of the complicated course of Mrs. Smith's injury, she will require ongoing medical intervention, including neurological services to assist with management of post-traumatic headaches, post-concussive syndrome, and myofascial pain. She is at increased risk for post-traumatic seizures and hydrocephalus. These conditions may not be evident and will require periodic CT Scans, MRIs, and EEGs to validate whether symptoms present. An orthopedist will be necessary to assist with the possibility of future fractures, osteoporosis, and arthritis.

Mrs. Smith has decreased range of motion secondary to pain; additional evaluations may be indicated should her mobility continue to be problematic. A physiatrist would be called upon to help with evaluating the physical, occupational, and recreational therapy Mrs. Smith requires. The physiatrist can also assist with equipment needs.

Mrs. Smith will need the services of a psychiatrist to assist her in dealing with such psychological issues as depression and anxiety. She may also require medication management, psychological testing, and counseling.

An internist would best serve Mrs. Smith by coordinating her overall medical needs. Due to her facial fractures, she will need periodic dental cleaning and check-ups. She may also require nerve conduction studies, discography, myelograms, orthopedic X-rays, and blood work.

Mrs. Smith will need the services of a physical and occupational therapist to improve her strength, endurance, stamina, and ability to assist with the activities of daily living. Cognitive remediation would be important to help her develop strategies to improve memory and executive function. A recreational therapist would help Mrs. Smith increase her social opportunities.

Counseling and social support will be necessary on an individual, couple, and family basis to improve positive couple and family interactions, role adaptation, and social involvement. Additional evaluations would include driver's, work/ gardening/functional capacity, vocational, and psychological evaluations. A case manager is necessary to coordinate these services and provide accountability.

Mrs. Smith also requires the services of a handyman, housekeeper, and lawn maintenance individual. She will require a cane, a reclining/lift chair, grab bars, toilet armrests, bath safety bench/combination bath mat, and wall-mounted personal shower. She will incur additional equipment costs should her physical state deteriorate with the aging process.

Future plans for pain management may require a neuromuscular stimulator, mentor TENS, and portable biofeedback. She will probably require medication for the rest of her life.

Because Mrs. Smith is now so dependent upon her family, plans must be made to provide services for her when this is no longer an option. She will require support on a 24-hour basis. It is also necessary to consider the complications that Mrs. Smith may develop, such as osteoporosis, degenerative disk disease, and degeneration in her affected joints.

COST REPORT

The cost report (Tables 29.2–29.11) gives a comprehensive listing and description of all services essential in meeting the client's needs and the approximate price of these services in the client's geographical area.

Table 29.2: Medical Evaluations and Treatment

Service or Item		Duration	Frequency	Cost Per Unit
Dentist		Life	1–2/year	$55–$128
Neurosurgeon				
	Initial Evaluation	Once	Once	$75
	Follow-up Visits	Life	1/year	$35
Neurologist				
	Initial Evaluation	Once	Once	$180
	Follow-up Visits	Life	1/year	$60–$75
Orthopedic Surgeon				
	Initial Evaluation	Once	Once	$36–$130
	Follow-up Visits	Life	1/year	$33–$105
Internal Medicine				
	Initial Evaluation	Once	Once	$50
	Follow-up Visits	Life	1/year	$35
Pain Management				
	Evaluation	Once	Once	$140
	Treatment Program	Once	19-day out-pt. program	$11,000

Table 29.3: Therapeutic Evaluations

Service or Item	Duration	Frequency	Cost Per Unit
Neuropsychological	Once	Once	$880
Occupational Therapy	Life	1/year	$100
Physical Therapy	Life	1/year	$100
Cognitive Remediation	For 10 years	1/year	$100
Recreational Therapy	Once	Once	$105
Driver's Evaluation	Once	Once	$385
Vocational Evaluation	Once	Once	$500–$700 (Estimated)

Table 29.4: Treatment Program

Service or Item	Duration	Frequency	Cost Per Unit
Comprehensive Post-Acute Residential Rehabilitation Program	For 6–12 Months	Daily	$350–$575/day
Counseling (self)	For 1–2 Years	1/week	$70/session
Counseling (marital)	For 1 Year	1/week	$70/session
Counseling (children)	For 1–2 Years	1/week	$70/session
Counseling (group)	For 1–2 Years	1/week	$45/session
Occupational Therapy	For 1 Year	1-3/week	$100/visit
Physical Therapy	For 1 Year	3/week	$100/visit
	After 1 Year/For Life	4/year	$100/visit
Cognitive Remediation	For 3–5 Years	3/week	$100/visit
Recreational Therapy	For 1 Year	1/week	$132/visit
Support Care	Life	24 hours/day	$11–$17/hr.
Child Care	For 10 Years	8 hours/day	$10/hour
Life Long Living Facility	Life	Daily	$350/day
Case Manager	Life	2/month	$80/visit

Table 29.5: Support Care

Service or Item	Duration	Frequency	Cost Per Unit
Handyman	Life	4 hrs./month	$25/hr.
Lawn Maintenance	Life	25/year	$35/visit
Housekeeper	Life	I/week	$40/visit

Table 29.6: Equipment

Equipment for Activities of Daily Living			
Service or Item	Duration	Frequency	Cost Per Unit
Grab Bars	Life	2/ten years	$34
Toilet Armrest	Life	I/three years	$37
Bath Safety Bench	Life	I/year	$70
Equipment for Pain Management			
Sys*Stim Neuromuscular Stimulator	Life	I/seven years	$1,994
Mentor TENS	Life	I/seven years	$325
Replacement Pads	Life	I pkg./month	$10–$21
Conductivity Gel	Life	I box/two years	$29

Table 29.7: Care Cost for Jane Smith

ONE TIME OR NON-YEARLY COST

Medical Evaluation and Treatment	388
Pain Management	11,140
Comprehensive Rehabilitation	124,875
Therapeutic Evaluation	2,970
Treatment Program	95,264
Counseling	18,070
Child Care	292,000
TOTAL ONE TIME OR NON-YEARLY COST	$544,707

YEARLY COST

	At Home With 24-hour Support Care	In Facility
Medical Evaluation and Treatment	344	344
Therapeutic Evaluation	200	-0-
Treatment Program	124,960	129,670
Support Care	4,155	-0-
Equipment	621	621
TOTAL YEARLY COST	$130,280	$130,635

Table 29.8: Economic Analysis Totals (see pp. 547–550)

Totals: at Home		
	Cumulative Value	Present Value
Medical Services (A)	9,971,227.00	7,603,776.00
Medical Commodities (B)	25,245.00	20,279.00
Non-Medical Services (C)	238,879.00	186,523.00
Totals	**$10,235,351.00**	**$7,810,578.00**
Totals: in Facility		
	Cumulative Value	Present Value
Medical Services (D)	10,329,461.00	7,876,956.00
Medical Commodities (B)	25,245.00	20,279.00
Non-Medical Services		
Totals	**$10,354,706.00**	**$7,897,235.00**

(A) (B) (C) (D) See pp. 547–550, Tables 29.9–29.12

Table 29.9: (A) Medical, Therapeutic, and Treatment Services at Home, Economic Loss Breakdown Analysis

Discount Rate: 1.07%		Increase Rate: 2.26%		Life Expectancy: 80
Age	Year	Annual Costs	Present Value	Cumulative Present Value
35	1996	125,505.00	125,505.00	125,505.00
36	1997	128,341.00	126,983.00	252,488.00
37	1998	131,242.00	128,478.00	380,966.00
38	1999	134,208.00	129,990.00	510,956.00
39	2000	137,241.00	131,521.00	642,477.00
40	2001	140,343.00	133,070.00	775,547.00
41	2002	143,515.00	134,636.00	910,183.00
42	2003	146,758.00	136,222.00	1,046,404.00
43	2004	150,075.00	137,825.00	1,184,230.00
44	2005	153,466.00	139,448.00	1,323,678.00
45	2006	156,935.00	141,090.00	1,464,768.00
46	2007	160,481.00	142,751.00	1,607,519.00
47	2008	164,108.00	144,432.00	1,751,951.00
48	2009	167,817.00	146,133.00	1,898,084.00
49	2010	171,610.00	147,853.00	2,045,937.00
50	2011	175,488.00	149,594.00	2,195,531.00
51	2012	179,454.00	151,355.00	2,346,886.00
52	2013	183,510.00	153,137.00	2,500,023.00
53	2014	187,657.00	154,940.00	2,654,964.00
54	2015	191,898.00	156,765.00	2,811,728.00
55	2016	196,235.00	158,610.00	2,970,338.00
56	2017	200,670.00	160,478.00	3,130,816.00
57	2018	205,205.00	162,367.00	3,293,183.00
58	2019	209,843.00	164,279.00	3,457,462.00
59	2020	214,585.00	166,213.00	3,623,676.00
60	2021	219,435.00	168,170.00	3,791,846.00
61	2022	224,394.00	170,150.00	3,961,996.00
62	2023	229,465.00	172,154.00	4,134,150.00
63	2024	234,651.00	174,181.00	4,308,330.00
64	2025	239,955.00	176,231.00	4,484,562.00
65	2026	245,378.00	178,306.00	4,662,868.00
66	2027	250,923.00	180,406.00	4,843,274.00
67	2028	256,594.00	182,530.00	5,025,804.00
68	2029	262,393.00	184,679.00	5,210,483.00
69	2030	268,323.00	186,853.00	5,397,336.00
70	2031	274,387.00	189,053.00	5,586,390.00
71	2032	280,588.00	191,279.00	5,777,669.00
72	2033	286,930.00	193,531.00	5,971,201.00
73	2034	293,414.00	195,810.00	6,167,011.00
74	2035	300,045.00	198,116.00	6,365,126.00
75	2036	306,826.00	200,448.00	6,565,574.00
76	2037	313,761.00	202,808.00	6,768,382.00
77	2038	320,852.00	205,196.00	6,973,578.00
78	2039	328,103.00	207,612.00	7,181,190.00
79	2040	335,518.00	210,056.00	7,391,247.00
80	2041	343,101.00	212,530.00	7,603,776.00
TOTALS		**$ 9,971,227.00**		**7,603,776.00**

Table 29.10: (B) Medical Commodities at Home or in Facility, Economic Loss Breakdown Analysis

Discount Rate: 1.07%		Increase Rate: -0.56%		Life Expectancy 80
Age	Year	Annual Costs	Present Value	Cumulative Present Value
35	1996	621	621	621
36	1997	618	611	1,232
37	1998	614	601	1,833
38	1999	611	591	2,425
39	2000	607	582	3,006
40	2001	604	573	3,579
41	2002	600	563	4,142
42	2003	597	554	4,696
43	2004	594	545	5,242
44	2005	590	536	5,778
45	2006	587	528	6,306
46	2007	584	519	6,825
47	2008	581	511	7,336
48	2009	577	503	7,839
49	2010	574	495	8,333
50	2011	571	487	8,820
51	2012	568	479	9,299
52	2013	564	471	9,770
53	2014	561	463	10,233
54	2015	558	456	10,689
55	2016	555	449	11,138
56	2017	552	441	11,579
57	2018	549	434	12,014
58	2019	546	427	12,441
59	2020	543	420	12,861
60	2021	540	414	13,275
61	2022	537	407	13,682
62	2023	534	400	14,082
63	2024	531	394	14,476
64	2025	528	388	14,863
65	2026	525	381	15,245
66	2027	522	375	15,620
67	2028	519	369	15,989
68	2029	516	363	16,352
69	2030	513	357	16,709
70	2031	510	352	17,061
71	2032	507	346	17,407
72	2033	504	340	17,747
73	2034	502	335	18,082
74	2035	499	329	18,411
75	2036	496	324	18,735
76	2037	493	319	19,054
77	2038	491	314	19,368
78	2039	488	309	19,676
79	2040	485	304	19,980
80	2041	482	299	20,279
TOTALS		**25,245**		**20,279**

Table 29.11: (C) Non-Medical Support Services at Home, Economic Loss Breakdown Analysis

Discount Rate:	1.07%	**Increase Rate:**	**0.96%**	Life Expectancy: 80
Age	Year	Annual Costs	Present Value	Cumulative Present Value
35	1996	4,155	4,155	4,155
36	1997	4,195	4,150	8,305
37	1998	4,235	4,146	12,451
38	1999	4,276	4,141	16,593
39	2000	4,317	4,137	20,730
40	2001	4,358	4,132	24,862
41	2002	4,400	4,128	28,990
42	2003	4,442	4,123	33,114
43	2004	4,485	4,119	37,233
44	2005	4,528	4,114	41,347
45	2006	4,572	4,110	45,457
46	2007	4,615	4,106	49,563
47	2008	4,660	4,101	53,664
48	2009	4,704	4,097	57,760
49	2010	4,750	4,092	61,852
50	2011	4,795	4,088	65,940
51	2012	4,841	4,083	70,023
52	2013	4,888	4,079	74,102
53	2014	4,935	4,074	78,176
54	2015	4,982	4,070	82,246
55	2016	5,030	4,065	86,312
56	2017	5,078	4,061	90,373
57	2018	5,127	4,057	94,430
58	2019	5,176	4,052	98,482
59	2020	5,226	4,048	102,530
60	2021	5,276	4,043	106,573
61	2022	5,327	4,039	110,612
62	2023	5,378	4,035	114,647
63	2024	5,429	4,030	118,677
64	2025	5,482	4,026	122,703
65	2026	5,534	4,021	126,724
66	2027	5,587	4,017	130,741
67	2028	5,641	4,013	134,754
68	2029	5,695	4,008	138,762
69	2030	5,750	4,004	142,766
70	2031	5,805	4,000	146,766
71	2032	5,861	3,995	150,761
72	2033	5,917	3,991	154,752
73	2034	5,974	3,987	158,739
74	2035	6,031	3,982	162,721
75	2036	6,089	3,978	166,699
76	2037	6,147	3,974	170,672
77	2038	6,206	3,969	174,642
78	2039	6,266	3,965	178,607
79	2040	6,326	3,961	182,567
80	2041	6,387	3,956	186,523
TOTALS		**238,879**		**186,523**

Table 29.11: (D) Medical, Therapeutic, and Treatment Services in Facility, Economic Loss Breakdown Analysis

Discount Rate: 1.07%		Increase Rate: 2.26%		Life Expectancy 80
Age	Year	Annual Costs	Present Value	Cumulative Present Value
35	1996	130,014	130,014	130,014
36	1997	132,952	131,545	261,559
37	1998	135,957	133,094	394,652
38	1999	139,030	134,661	529,313
39	2000	142,172	136,246	665,559
40	2001	145,385	137,850	803,409
41	2002	148,671	139,473	942,883
42	2003	152,030	141,116	1,083,998
43	2004	155,466	142,777	1,226,775
44	2005	158,980	144,458	1,371,233
45	2006	162,573	146,159	1,517,392
46	2007	166,247	147,880	1,665,272
47	2008	170,004	149,621	1,814,893
48	2009	173,846	151,383	1,966,275
49	2010	177,775	153,165	2,119,440
50	2011	181,793	154,968	2,274,409
51	2012	185,901	156,793	2,431,202
52	2013	190,103	158,639	2,589,841
53	2014	194,399	160,507	2,750,347
54	2015	198,793	162,397	2,912,744
55	2016	203,285	164,309	3,077,053
56	2017	207,880	166,243	3,243,296
57	2018	212,578	168,201	3,411,497
58	2019	217,382	170,181	3,581,678
59	2020	222,295	172,185	3,753,862
60	2021	227,319	174,212	3,928,074
61	2022	232,456	176,263	4,104,338
62	2023	237,709	178,339	4,282,676
63	2024	243,082	180,438	4,463,115
64	2025	248,575	182,563	4,645,678
65	2026	254,193	184,712	4,830,390
66	2027	259,938	186,887	5,017,277
67	2028	265,812	189,088	5,206,365
68	2029	271,820	191,314	5,397,679
69	2030	277,963	193,566	5,591,245
70	2031	284,245	195,845	5,787,091
71	2032	290,669	198,151	5,985,242
72	2033	297,238	200,484	6,185,727
73	2034	303,956	202,845	6,388,572
74	2035	310,825	205,233	6,593,805
75	2036	317,850	207,650	6,801,454
76	2037	325,033	210,094	7,011,549
77	2038	332,379	212,568	7,224,117
78	2039	339,891	215,071	7,439,188
79	2040	347,572	217,603	7,656,791
80	2041	355,427	220,165	7,876,956
TOTALS		**10,329,461**		**7,876,956**

REFERENCES

Abrams, D., Barker, L., Haffey, W., & Nelson, H. (1993). The economics of return to work for survivors of traumatic brain injury: Vocational services are worth the investment. *Journal of Head Trauma Rehabilitation, 8*(4), 59–76.

Ashley, M. (1990). Cost/benefit analysis for post acute rehabilitation of the TBI patient. *Journal of Insurance Medicine, 22,* 156–161.

Bush, G. (1994). Financing quality of life following severe traumatic brain injury. In C. Simkins (Ed.), *Analysis, understanding and presentation of cases involving traumatic brain injury* (pp. 239–249). Washington, DC: National Brain Injury Foundation.

Buzard, A.V. (1994). Special considerations in identifying and litigating the "mild" head injury case. In C. Simkins (Ed.), *Analysis, understanding and presentation of cases involving traumatic brain injury* (pp. 297–308). Washington, DC: National Brain Injury Foundation.

Gamboa, A.M., Jr. (1994). The vocational economic consequences of traumatic brain injury. In C. Simkins (Ed.), *Analysis, understanding and presentation of cases involving traumatic brain injury* (pp. 199–212). Washington, DC: National Brain Injury Foundation.

Haase, J. (1992). Social-economic impact of head injury. *Acta Neurochir, 55,* 75–79.

Longwell, J. (1991). Synergos stays above brain rehab downturn. *Orange County Business Journal, 14,* 4.

McCormick, B. (1991). Not enough data on lives, costs: No one knows how many people are in a persistent vegetative state. *American Medical News, 34,* 23.

McMordie, W.R., & Barker, S.L. (1988). The financial trauma of head injury. *Brain Injury, 2*(4), 357–364.

Mullins, R. (1992). Federal investigations put spotlight on brain injury treatment centers. *The Business Journal-Milwaukee, 10,* S7.

Reinstein, L. (1993). Healthcare financing in the 1990s, part I. *The Physiatrist, 9,* 1–2. (In *Journal of Head Trauma Rehabilitation,* 1993, *8*(4), 2.

Rivara, F., Dicker, B., Bergman, A., Dacey, R., & Herman, C. (1988). The public cost of motorcycle trauma. *Journal of the American Medical Association, 260,* 221–223.

Simkins, C., & Craig, A. (1994). A lay person's guide to selecting and retaining the most qualified attorney in cases involving traumatic brain injury. In C. Simkins (Ed.), *Analysis, understanding and presentation of cases involving traumatic brain injury* (pp. 285–289). Washington, DC: National Brain Injury Foundation.

Smith, S. (1994). Hedonic damages: Evaluating the loss of enjoyment of life. In C. Simkins (Ed.), *Analysis, understanding and presentation of cases involving traumatic brain injury* (pp. 429–443). Washington, DC: National Brain Injury Foundation.

Stuss, D., & Benson, D. (1986). *The frontal lobes.* New York: Raven Press.

Voogt, R. (1994). Costs of long term healthcare. In Simkins, C. (Ed.), *Analysis, understanding and presentation of cases involving traumatic brain injury* (pp. 229–238). Washington, DC: National Head Injury Foundation.

———. (1995). Costs of TBI more than economic. *ADVANCE for Physical Therapists, 6,* 6,28.

Voogt, R., & Groteguth, M. (1990). Damages: Rehabilitation and life care needs after a traumatic brain injury. *American Jurisprudence Proof of Facts,* 3rd Series, *9,* 37.

Waldo, D., Sonnefeld, S., Lemieux, J., & McKusick, D. (1992). Healthcare spending may reach 40% of GNP. *Business & Health, 10,* 22.

INDEX

553